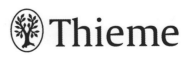

Neurosurgical Emergencies

Third Edition

Christopher M. Loftus, MD
Clinical Professor
Department of Neurosurgery
Temple University Lewis Katz School of Medicine
Philadelphia, Pennsylvania

Thieme
New York • Stuttgart • Delhi • Rio de Janeiro

Executive Editor: Timothy Y. Hiscock
Managing Editor: Sarah Landis
Director, Editorial Services: Mary Jo Casey
Assistant Managing Editor: Nikole Connors
Production Editor: Sean Woznicki
International Production Director: Andreas Schabert
International Marketing Director: Fiona Henderson
International Sales Director: Louisa Turrell
Director of Sales, North America: Mike Roseman
Senior Vice President and Chief Operating Officer: Sarah Vanderbilt
President: Brian D. Scanlan

Library of Congress Cataloging-in-Publication Data

Names: Loftus, Christopher M., editor.
Title: Neurosurgical emergencies / [edited by] Christopher M. Loftus.
Other titles: Neurosurgical emergencies (Loftus)
Description: Third edition. | New York : Thieme, [2018] | Includes
    bibliographical references.
Identifiers: LCCN 2017022406 | ISBN 9781626233331 (print)
Subjects: | MESH: Neurosurgical Procedures | Emergencies | Brain
    Diseases—therapy | Spinal Cord Diseases—therapy | Brain
    Diseases—diagnosis | Spinal Cord Diseases—diagnosis
Classification: LCC RD598 | NLM WL 368 | DDC 617.4/8—dc23 LC
record available at https://lccn.loc.gov/2017022406

Important note: Medicine is an ever-changing science undergoing continual development. Research and clinical experience are continually expanding our knowledge, in particular our knowledge of proper treatment and drug therapy. Insofar as this book mentions any dosage or application, readers may rest assured that the authors, editors, and publishers have made every effort to ensure that such references are in accordance with **the state of knowledge at the time of production of the book.**

Nevertheless, this does not involve, imply, or express any guarantee or responsibility on the part of the publishers in respect to any dosage instructions and forms of applications stated in the book. **Every user is requested to examine carefully** the manufacturers' leaflets accompanying each drug and to check, if necessary in consultation with a physician or specialist, whether the dosage schedules mentioned therein or the contraindications stated by the manufacturers differ from the statements made in the present book. Such examination is particularly important with drugs that are either rarely used or have been newly released on the market. Every dosage schedule or every form of application used is entirely at the user's own risk and responsibility. The authors and publishers request every user to report to the publishers any discrepancies or inaccuracies noticed. If errors in this work are found after publication, errata will be posted at www.thieme.com on the product description page.

Some of the product names, patents, and registered designs referred to in this book are in fact registered trademarks or proprietary names even though specific reference to this fact is not always made in the text. Therefore, the appearance of a name without designation as proprietary is not to be construed as a representation by the publisher that it is in the public domain.

© 2018 Thieme Medical Publishers, Inc.
Thieme Publishers New York
333 Seventh Avenue, New York, NY 10001 USA
+1 800 782 3488, customerservice@thieme.com

Thieme Publishers Stuttgart
Rüdigerstrasse 14, 70469 Stuttgart, Germany
+49 [0]711 8931 421, customerservice@thieme.de

Thieme Publishers Delhi
A-12, Second Floor, Sector-2, Noida-201301
Uttar Pradesh, India
+91 120 45 566 00, customerservice@thieme.in

Thieme Publishers Rio de Janeiro, Thieme Publicações Ltda.
Edifício Rodolpho de Paoli, 25ª andar
Av. Nilo Peçanha, 50 – Sala 2508,
Rio de Janeiro 20020-906 Brasil
+55 21 3172-2297 / +55 21 3172-1896

Cover design: Thieme Publishing Group
Typesetting by DiTech Processing Solutions

Printed in India by Replika Press Pvt Ltd   5 4 3 2 1

ISBN 978-1-62623-333-1

Also available as an e–book:
eISBN 978-1-62623-343-0

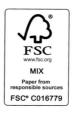

This third edition of *Neurosurgical Emergencies* is dedicated, like the second was, to the memory of the late Professor John C. VanGilder of the University of Iowa. He was my mentor for professional advancement and scholarship, and one of the most dedicated academic neurosurgeons—with a heart sincerely devoted to teaching and intellectual growth—that I have ever had the privilege to work with. I would also like to recognize the generations of residents I have trained at Iowa, Oklahoma, and at Temple, and with whom the transfer of knowledge has always been an even exchange.

Christopher Loftus

Contents

Continuing Medical Education Credit Information and Objectives

Learning Objectives

Upon completion of this activity, participants should be able to:

1. Identify and triage true neurosurgical emergencies
2. Discuss the most current diagnostic methods and system-oriented approach to neurosurgical emergencies
3. Describe the most current data on surgical management of neurosurgical emergency conditions.

Accreditation and Designation

The AANS is accredited by the Accreditation Council for Continuing Medical Education (ACCME) to provide continuing medical education for physicians.

The AANS designates this enduring material for a maximum of 15 *AMA PRA Category 1 Credits*™. Physicians should claim only the credits commensurate with the extent of their participation in the activity.

Method of physician participation in the learning process for this text book: The Home Study Examination is online on the AANS website at: http://www.aans.org/Education/Books/Neurosurgical-Emergencies

Estimated time to complete this activity varies by learner, and activity equaled up to 15 *AMA PRA Category 1 Credits*™.

Release and Termination Dates

Original Release Date: 10/17/2017
CME Termination Date: 10/17/2020

Disclosure Information

The AANS controls the content and production of this CME activity and attempts to ensure the presentation of balanced, objective information. In accordance with the Standards for Commercial Support established by the Accreditation Council for Continuing Medical Education, authors, planning committee members, staff, and any others involved in planning in education content and the significant others of those mentioned must disclose any relationship they or their co-authors have with commercial interests which may be related to their content. The ACCME defines, "relevant financial relationships" as financial relationships in any amount occurring within the past 12 months that create a conflict of interest.

Those (and the significant others of those mentioned) who have disclosed a relationship* with commercial interests are listed below.

Name	Organization	Relationship
Issam A. Awad, MD, MSc, FACS, MA (hon)	NIH/NINDS Nurami Medical, Inc.	Grants/Research Support Consultant Fees
Nicholas M. Barbaro, MD, FACS	NINDS	Grants/Research Support
Eli M. Baron, MD	Elsevier: book authorship royalty McGraw Hill: book authorship royalty	Other Financial Support Employee (any industry), Other Financial Support
Frederick A. Boop, MD, FAANS, FACS, FAAP	Medtronic	Consultant Fees
David J. Donahue, MD	Meditech, Medtronic	Consultant Fees
José M. Ferro, MD, PhD	Boehringer Ingelheim	Consultant Fee, Speaker's Bureau
Joshua E. Heller, MD	Nuvasive, SI Bone, Conva Tec, Providence Medical Technology	Consultant Fees, Grants/Research Support
Lawrence J. Hirsch, MD	Eisai, Upsher-Smith Ceribell, Monteris, Neurospace, Sun Neurosience, Engage Therapeutics Neurospace	Industry Grant Support Consultant Fees Honorarium
George I. Jallo, MD	Johnson & Johnson	Consultant Fees
Bong-Soo Kim, MD, FAANS	Medssey, USA Korean Spinal Neurosurgery Society	Grants/Research Support Honorarium
A. David Mendelow, PhD, FRCS	Stryker, Draeger R. Teeter provided the tables for the inversion group of patients.	Consultant Fees Grants/Research Support
Michael J. Schneck, MD	Baxter	Stock/Shareholder Directly Purchased
Phillip A. Tibbs, MD	Wenzel Spine	Grants/Research Support
Shelly D. Timmons, MD, PhD, FACS, FAANS	AO Neuro / AO Foundation, Centers for Disease Control Pennsylvania Neurosurgical Society, American College of Surgeons	Board/Trustee/Office/rLeadership position specifically with a neurosurgical or medical-related associated/non-profit or similar entity, Honorarium Board/Trustee/Officer/Leadership position specifically with a neurosurgical or medical-related associated/non-profit or similar entity
Vincent C. Traynelis, MD	Medtronic Globus Medical	Consultant Fees, Other Financial Support Other Financial Support
Alexander R. Vaccaro, MD, PhD, MBA	Medacorp, Guidepoint Global, Gerson Lehrman Group, Atlas Spine, Medtronics, Stryker Spine AO Spine	Consultant Fees Board/Trustee/Officer/Leadership position specifically with a neurosurgical or medical-related associated/non-profit or similar entity

* Relationship refers to receipt of royalties, consultantship, funding by research grant, receiving honoraria for educational services elsewhere, or any other relationship to a commercial interest that provides sufficient reason for disclosure.

Those (and the significant others of those mentioned) who have reported they do not have any relationship with commercial interests:

Name:

Paul D. Ackerman, MD
P. David Adelson, MD, FACS, FAAP
Douglas E. Anderson, MD
Agnieszka Ardelt, MD, PhD, FAHA
H. Alexander Arts, MD, FACS
William W. Ashley Jr., MD, PhD, MBA
Ahmed J. Awad, MD
Christopher D. Baggott, MD
Julian E. Bailes, MD
José Biller, MD, FACP, FAAN, FANA, FAHA
Alexa Bodman, MD
E. Antonio Chiocca, MD, PhD, FAANS
Diana Aguiar de Sousa, MD
Neha S. Dangayach, MD
Michael G. Fehlings, MD, PhD, FRCSC, FACS
Kenneth A. Follett, MD, PhD
Linden E. Fornoff, MD
Kimberly A. Foster, MD
Charles Francoeur, MD
Zach Fridirici, MD
Aradia X. Fu, MD
Anand V. Germanwala, MD, FAANS
James Tait Goodrich, MD, PhD, DSci (Honaris Causa)
Errol Gordon, MD
Bhuvanesh Govind, MD
Daipayan Guha, MD
Walter A. Hall, MD
Farid Hamzei-Sichani, MD
Griffith R. Harsh IV, MD, MA, MBA
Jason Heth, MD
John H. Honeycutt, MD
Omer Q. Iqbal, MD
Rajiv R. Iyer, MD
Jack Jallo, MD, PhD
Stephen J. Johans, MD

G. Alexander Jones, MD
Michael Jones, MD
Matthew Kircher, MD
Daphne D. Li, MD
Christopher M. Loftus, MD*
Allan R. Martin, BASc, MD
Michael D. Martin, MD
Stephan A. Mayer, MD, FCCM
Jamal McClendon Jr., MD
Joshua E. Medow, MD, MS, FAANS, FACS, FNCS, FAHA, FCCM
Michael P. Merchut, MD, FACP, FAAN
Vincent J. Miele, MD, FACS, FAANS
Christine C. Nelson, MD, FACS
Russell P. Nockels, MD, FAANS
Edward K. Nomoto, MD
Paolo Nucifora, MD, PhD
Margaret Pain, MD
Roy A. Patchell, MD
Courtney Pendleton, MD
Pierpaolo Peruzzi, MD, PhD
Kalmon D. Post, MD
Vikram C. Prabhu, MD, FACS, FAANS
Daniel K. Resnick, MD, MS
Margaret Riordan, MD
Richard B. Rodgers, MD, FAANS, FACS
Syed Omar Shah, MD, MBA
Kashif A. Shaikh, MD
James A. Smith, MD
Drew A. Spencer, MD
Kevin N. Swong, MD
Hieu H. Ton-That, MD, FACS
Asterios Tsimpas, MD, MSc, MRCSEd
Mazda K. Turel, MD
Michael P. Wemhoff, MD
Christopher E. Wolfla, MD, FAANS

* Educational Content Planners.

Foreword

Excluding degenerative spine surgeries, it is estimated that about one-third of neurosurgical procedures are performed as emergencies in the developed world. In developing countries with limited resources where injuries are increasingly endemic, more than half of the procedures performed are classified as an emergency.

Whereas there are many books and papers that focus on covering the topic of a single neurosurgical emergency such as traumatic brain injury (TBI) and spine cord injury (SCI), vascular malformations like ischemia, sinus thrombosis and hematomas, brain and spine tumors, infectious diseases, hydrocephalus, etc., to my knowledge this is the only reference that covers all of the above-mentioned in a single book.

What do various neurosurgical emergencies share in common that they should be included together in such a book?

1) In most neurosurgical units, the surgical on-call duties cannot be divided according to different subspecialities in neurosurgery, as only very large universities can afford to implement a subspeciality emergency system. Therefore, training of the expert neurosurgeon on call should include a number of possible surgeries. A classic exception to this rule has historically been complex spinal approaches (for example, anterior dorsal and lumbar spine routes), and surgical or endovascular management of subarachnoidal hemorrhage.

2) Many of these emergencies require pre- and post-operative access to intensive care units. The medical management of different kinds of brain and spine emergencies is similar: Avoid fatal intracranial hypertension with proper monitoring, prevent secondary brain and spinal cord damage, and evaluate the possibility of a second surgery.

3) The hospital organization to treat neurosurgical emergencies includes different pathologies; the availability of OT personnel necessarily covers different surgeries. It does not make sense to have nurses trained only in trauma surgery and not in vascular or spine emergencies.

4) Neurosurgical units in many parts of the world are limited, and the question of centralization of patients from the referral area of the unit is crucial. Different protocols must be integrated since the available resources like ICU beds are often limited, and head injury centralization policies need to be integrated with the vascular and spine cases. If we extend the indications for transfer of TBI or SCI patients to a single neurosurgical division located within such a trauma center, there will be insufficient resources to properly admit vascular patients or pediatric patients.

5) So-called "extreme" medical and surgical managements are common. The severe brain damage and consequent intracranial hypertension associated with TBI, SAH and brain ischemia requires basically the same extreme medical (barbiturates, hypothermia....) and surgical (cranial decompression) approach. Also, many prospective clinical randomized studies are similar, as are the ethical issues recently related to these types of surgeries.

Often young neurosurgical trainees ask to be trained in complicated elective surgeries such as skull base, endoscopic, vascular and complex spine surgery. But in the course of their responsibilities they will encounter neurosurgical emergencies like the ones reported in this book, and very often they face the challenge of having to quickly decide the indications for and the propriety of surgery. The ethical issues related to decisions regarding extreme emergency surgeries are complicated and cannot be consider superficially. As neurosurgeons we must balance all aspects of our demanding specialty, and this includes emergency neurosurgery.

The first edition of this book was published in 1994 by AANS, and the second edition was co-published in 2008 by AANS and Thieme. Today you hold this third edition in your hands. The success and continuation of this book demonstrates the value of the topic to the neurosurgical community and the desire for a single resource covering the spectrum of neurosurgical emergencies.

I congratulate editor Dr. Loftus and all the authors of this important contribution to the neurosurgical literature.

Franco Servadei, MD
Department of Neurosurgery
Humanitas University and Research Hospital
Milan, Italy

Preface

Twenty-two years ago, under the publications program of the American Association of Neurological Surgeons (AANS), we produced the first edition of Neurosurgical Emergencies in two volumes. The topic had not been previously addressed in monograph form, and those two little blue volumes enjoyed gratifyingly broad acceptance and (mostly) favorable reviews; they were best sellers, at least by neurosurgical standards. After the first edition was published, I had the privilege of chairing the AANS Publications Committee and steering it through some difficult financial times, during which we successfully negotiated a new publications partnership agreement with Thieme Medical Publishers. My thanks, as always, to president of Thieme Brian Scanlan for helping us through those uncertain times which are now well behind us.

One of the major products for the new Thieme partnership was a second, updated edition of Neurosurgical Emergencies. It took us some time to complete the effort, punctuated primarily by my change of venue from chairman at the University of Oklahoma to chairman at Temple University in Philadelphia. We hearkened to the critiques of the first edition, considered the previous manuscripts carefully, and ¬revised, replaced, and expanded as we thought best, to bring forth a truly modern and updated volume. It was then, as now, the editor's and the publisher's sincere hope that current and future generations of readers would find the product useful and worth the effort. Again the book, published as a single volume in large folio, was enthusiastically received, and I was pleased to see that the second edition was translated into Chinese as well.

Last year Thieme approached me to produce a third edition, which you have in front of you. The Thieme team responsible for this edition is new, Timothy Hiscock and Sarah Landis, equally as effective and professional as their predecessors, and the book is substantively new as well. I worked carefully to keep chapters that were of value, refresh those that needed updating, and weave in new material and new ideas. As is always true with an edited text, the organizational framework and overall design are my own, but the true knowledge base is the sum of the individual chapter authors' contributions, and great thanks are due them for their excellent contributions. All of them are friends and esteemed colleagues.

We stand ready, as always, to produce a fourth edition if and when the time seems right, but for now, I offer this one as the most current and comprehensive treatment of Neurosurgical Emergencies that we could assemble.

Christopher M. Loftus, MD

Contributors

Paul D. Ackerman, MD
Attending Neurosurgeon
Northwestern Neurosurgical Associates
Chicago, Illinois

P. David Adelson, MD, FACS, FAAP
Director
Barrow Neurological Institute at
    Phoenix Children's Hospital
Diane and Bruce Halle Endowed Chair for
    Pediatric Neurosciences
Chief
Department of Pediatric Neurosurgery/Children's
    Neurosciences
Professor and Chief
Department of Neurological Surgery
Department of Child Health
University of Arizona
College of Medicine
Phoenix, Arizona
Professor
Department of Neurological Surgery
Mayo Clinic
Rochester, Minnesota
Adjunct Professor
Ira A. Fulton School of Biological and Health Systems
    Engineering
Arizona State University
Pediatric Neurosurgery Fellowship Program (Director)/
    Barrow Neurological Institute
Phoenix, Arizona

Douglas E. Anderson, MD
Professor and Chair
Department of Neurological Surgery
Loyola University School of Medicine
Maywood, Illinois

Agnieszka Ardelt, MD, PhD, FAHA
Associate Professor of Neurology and Surgery
    (Neurosurgery) Director
Neurosciences Critical Care Co-director
Comprehensive Stroke Center
University of Chicago
Chicago, Illinois

H. Alexander Arts, MD, FACS
Professor of Otolaryngology and Neurosurgery
Program Director, Neurotology Fellowship Program
Medical Director, Cochlear Implant Program
Department of Otolaryngology – Head & Neck Surgery
University of Michigan
Ann Arbor, Michigan

William W. Ashley Jr., MD, PhD, MBA
Director, Cerebrovascular, Endovascular, and Skull Base
    Neurosurgery
Department of Neurosurgery
Chief, Division of Neurointerventional Radiology
Department of Radiology
Sinai Hospital of Baltimore
The Sandra and Malcolm Berman Brain & Spine Institute
Baltimore, Maryland

Ahmed J. Awad, MD
Resident
Department of Neurosurgery
Medical College of Wisconsin
Milwaukee, Wisconsin
Faculty of Medicine and Health Sciences
An-Najah National University
Nablus, Palestine

Issam A. Awad, MD, MSc, FACS, MA (hon)
The John Harper Seeley Professor
Surgery (Neurosurgery), Neurology and the Cancer Center
    Director of Neurovascular Surgery University of Chicago
    Medicine and Biological Sciences
Chicago, Illinois

Christopher D. Baggott, MD
Chief Resident
Department of Neurological Surgery
University of Wisconsin Hospitals and Clinics
Madison, Wisconsin

Julian E. Bailes, MD
Chair, Department of Neurosurgery
NorthShore University HealthSystem
Clinical Professor, University of Chicago
Pritzker School of Medicine
Evanston, Illinois

Nicholas M. Barbaro, MD, FACS
Betsey Barton Professor and Chair of Neurosurgery
Indiana University School of Medicine
Medical Director
Indiana University Health Neurosciences Center
Indianapolis, Indiana

Eli M. Baron, MD
Attending Neurosurgeon
Cedars Sinai Institute for Spinal Disorders
Los Angeles, California

José Biller, MD, FACP, FAAN, FANA, FAHA
Professor and Chairman
Department of Neurology
Loyola University Chicago
Stritch School of Medicine
Maywood, Illinois

Alexa Bodman, MD
Resident
Department of Neurosurgery
SUNY Upstate Medical University
Syracuse, New York

Frederick A. Boop, MD, FAANS, FACS, FAAP
JT Robertson Professor of Neurosurgery and
    St Jude Professor of Pediatric Neurosurgery
University of Tennessee Health Sciences Center
Semmes-Murphey Clinic
Memphis, Tennessee

E. Antonio Chiocca, MD, PhD, FAANS
Harvey W. Cushing Professor of Neurosurgery
Established by the Daniel E. Ponton Fund
Harvard Medical School
Neurosurgeon-in-Chief and Chairman,
    Department of Neurosurgery
Co-Director, Institute for the Neurosciences
Brigham and Women's/ Faulkner Hospital
Surgical Director, Center for Neuro-oncology
Dana-Farber Cancer Institute
Boston, Massachusetts

Neha S. Dangayach, MD
Assistant Professor
Departments of Neurosurgery and Neurology
The Mount Sinai School of Medicine
New York, New York

Diana Aguiar de Sousa, MD
Department of Neurosciences and Mental Health
    (Neurology)
Hospital de Santa Maria
Faculty of Medicine
University of Lisbon
Lisbon, Portugal

David J. Donahue, MD
Department of Neurosurgery
Cook Children's
Fort Worth, Texas

Michael G. Fehlings, MD, PhD, FRCSC, FACS
Professor of Neurosurgery
Vice Chairman Research
Department of Surgery
Co-Director Spine Program
Halbert Chair in Neural Repair and Regeneration
University of Toronto
Toronto, Canada

José M. Ferro, MD, PhD
Professor
Department of Neurosciences and Mental Health
Hospital de Santa Maria
University of Lisbon
Lisbon, Portugal

Kenneth A. Follett, MD, PHD
Professor and Chief
Nancy A. Keegan and Donald R. Voelte,
    Jr., Chair of Neurosurgery Division of Neurosurgery
University of Nebraska Medical Center
Omaha, Nebraska

Linden E. Fornoff, MD
Neurosurgery Resident
University of Nebraska Medical Center
Omaha, Nebraska

Kimberly A. Foster, MD
Assistant Professor
Department of Neurosurgery
University of New Mexico
Albuquerque, New Mexico

Charles Francoeur, MD
Division of Critical Care
Department of Anesthesiology and Critical Care
CHU de Québec-Université Laval
Québec, Canada

Zach Fridirici, MD
Resident
Department of Otolaryngology Head and Neck Surgery
Loyola University Medical Center
Maywood, Illinois

Aradia X. Fu, MD
Fellow
Department of Epilepsy
Yale University School of Medicine
New Haven, Connecticut

Anand V. Germanwala, MD, FAANS
Associate Professor and Residency Program Director
Department of Neurological Surgery
Loyola University Stritch School of Medicine
Maywood, Illinois

James Tait Goodrich, MD, PhD, DSci (Honaris Causa)
Director, Division of Pediatric Neurosurgery
Leo Davidoff Department of Neurological Surgery
Associate Professor
Departments of Neurological Surgery, Pediatrics,
    Plastic and Reconstructive Surgery
Albert Einstein College of Medicine
Montefiore Medical Center
Bronx, New York

Errol Gordon, MD
Assistant Professor
Departments of Neurosurgery and Neurology
The Mount Sinai School of Medicine
New York, New York

Bhuvanesh Govind, MD
Resident
Department of Neurological Surgery
Thomas Jefferson University
Philadelphia, Pennsylvania

Daipayan Guha, MD
Resident
Division of Neurosurgery
University of Toronto
Toronto, Canada

Walter A. Hall, MD
Professor
Department of Neurosurgery
SUNY Update Medical University
Syracuse, New York

Farid Hamzei-Sichani, MD, PhD
Department of Neurological Surgery
Mount Sinai Medical Center
New York, New York

Griffith R. Harsh IV, MD, MA, MBA
Professor and Vice Chairman
Department of Neurosurgery
Associate Dean (Postgraduate Medical Education)
Stanford School of Medicine
Director, Stanford Brain Tumor Center
Co-Director, Stanford Pituitary Center
Stanford, California

Joshua E. Heller, MD
Assistant Professor
Departments of Orthopedic Surgery and Neurosurgery
Thomas Jefferson University Hospital
Philadelphia, Pennsylvania

Jason Heth, MD
Associate Professor
Department of Neurosurgery
University of Michigan Medical School
Ann Arbor, Michigan

Lawrence J. Hirsch, MD
Professor of Neurology, Yale University School of Medicine
Chief, Division of Epilepsy and EEG
Co-Director, Yale Comprehensive Epilepsy Center
New Haven, Connecticut

John H. Honeycutt, MD
Medical Director, Neurosurgery
Medical Director, Neurotrauma
Co-director of the Jane and John Justin Neurosciences
    Center
Cook Children's
Fort Worth, Texas

Omer Q. Iqbal, MD
Research Professor
Department of Pathology
Loyola University Medical Center
Maywood, Illinois

Rajiv R. Iyer, MD
Resident
Department of Neurosurgery
Johns Hopkins School of Medicine
Baltimore, Maryland

George I. Jallo, MD
Clinical Practice Director of Pediatric Neurosurgery
Professor of Neurosurgery
Johns Hopkins All Children's Hospital
St. Petersburg, Florida

Jack Jallo, MD, PhD
Professor
Department of Neurological Surgery
Thomas Jefferson University
Philadelphia, Pennsylvania

Stephen J. Johans, MD
Resident
Department of Neurological Surgery
Loyola University Stritch School of Medicine
Maywood, Illinois

G. Alexander Jones, MD
Assistant Professor
Department of Neurological Surgery
Loyola University Stritch School of Medicine
Maywood, Illinois

Michael Jones, MD
Department of Neurological Surgery
Loyola University Medical Center
Maywood, Illinois

Bong-Soo Kim, MD, FAANS
Attending Neurosurgeon
Associate Professor
Department of Neurosurgery
Temple University Lewis Katz School of Medicine
Philadelphia, Pennsylvania

Matthew Kircher, MD
Assistant Professor
Department of Otolaryngology
Loyola University
Maywood, Illinois

Daphne D. Li, MD
Resident
Department of Neurological Surgery
Loyola University Stritch School of Medicine
Maywood, Illinois

Christopher M. Loftus, MD
Clinical Professor
Department of Neurosurgery
Temple University Lewis Katz School of Medicine
Philadelphia, Pennsylvania

Allan R. Martin, BASc, MD
Resident
Division of Neurosurgery
Department of Surgery
University of Toronto
Toronto, Canada

Michael D. Martin, MD
Associate Professor
Department of Neurosurgery
University of Oklahoma
Norman, Oklahoma

Stephan A. Mayer, MD, FCCM
William T. Gossett Endowed Chair
Chair, Department of Neurology
Co-Director, Neuroscience Institute
Henry Ford Health System
Detroit, Michigan

Jamal McClendon Jr., MD
Department of Neurosurgery
Mayo Clinic
Phoenix, Arizona

Joshua E. Medow, MD, MS, FAANS, FACS, FNCS, FAHA, FCCM
Endovascular Neurosurgeon and Neurointensivist
Director of Neurocritical Care
Neurocritical Care Fellowship Director
Neurosurgery Quality Improvement Chair
Associate Professor of Neurosurgery and
    Biomedical Engineering (Tenured)
University of Wisconsin School of Medicine and
    Public Health Madison, Wisconsin

A. David Mendelow, PhD, FRCS
Professor
Department of Neurosurgery
Newcastle University
Newcastle General Hospital
Newcastle Upon Tyne, England

Michael P. Merchut, MD, FACP, FAAN
Professor
Department of Neurology
Loyola University Stritch School of Medicine
Maywood, Illinois

Vincent J. Miele, MD, FACS, FAANS
Clinical Assistant Professor
Department of Neurosurgery
University of Pittsburgh
Pittsburgh, Pennsylvania

Christine C. Nelson, MD, FACS
Professor, Ophthalmology and Visual Sciences
Bartley R. Frueh, M.D. and Frueh Family Collegiate
    Professor in Eye Plastics and Orbital Surgery
Professor, Department of Surgery, Plastic Surgery Section
University of Michigan
Ann Arbor, Michigan

Russell P. Nockels, MD, FAANS
Professor/Vice Chair
Department of Neurological Surgery
Loyola University Medical Center
Maywood, Illinois

Edward K. Nomoto, MD
Cedars Sinai Institute for Spinal Disorders
Los Angeles, California

Paolo Nucifora, MD, PhD
Assistant Professor
Departments of Radiology and Neurology
Loyola University Stritch School of Medicine
Maywood, Illinois

Margaret Pain, MD
Resident
Department of Neurosurgery
Icahn School of Medicine at Mount Sinai
New York, New York

Roy A. Patchell, MD
Director
Department of Neuro-oncology
National Brain Tumor Center at the Capital Institute for
    Neurosciences
Pennington, New Jersey

Courtney Pendleton, MD
Resident
Department of Neurological Surgery
Thomas Jefferson University Hospital
Philadelphia, Pennsylvania

Pierpaolo Peruzzi, MD, PhD
Instructor
Department of Neurosurgery
Brigham and Women's Hospital
Harvard Medical School
Boston, Massachusetts

Kalmon D. Post, MD
Chairman Emeritus, Department of Neurosurgery
Professor
Departments of Neurosurgery & Medicine
Mount Sinai Health System
New York, New York

Vikram C. Prabhu, MD, FACS, FAANS
Professor
Department of Neurological Surgery and Radiation
    Oncology
Loyola University Stritch School of Medicine
Maywood, Illinois

Daniel K. Resnick, MD, MS
Professor and Vice Chairman
Department of Neurosurgery
University of Wisconsin School of Medicine and Public Health
Madison, Wisconsin

Margaret Riordan, MD
Clinical Instructor
Department of Neurosurgery
Stanford Health Care
Stanford, California

Richard B. Rodgers, MD, FAANS, FACS
Assistant Professor
Department of Neurological Surgery
Indiana University School of Medicine
Goodman Campbell Brain and Spine
Indianapolis, Indiana

Michael J. Schneck, MD
Professor
Departments of Neurology and Neurosurgery
Loyola University Medical Center
Maywood, Illinois

Syed Omar Shah, MD, MBA
Assistant Professor of Neurology and Neurological Surgery
Department of Neurological Surgery
Thomas Jefferson University
Division of Critical Care and Neurotrauma
Jefferson Hospital for Neurosciences
Philadelphia, Pennsylvania

Kashif A. Shaikh, MD
Resident
Department of Neurosurgery
Indiana University School of Medicine
Indianapolis, Indiana

James A. Smith, MD
Resident
Department of Neurosurgery
University of Kentucky
Lexington, Kentucky

Drew A. Spencer, MD
Resident
Department of Neurological Surgery
Northwestern University
Chicago, Illinois

Kevin N. Swong, MD
Resident
Department of Neurological Surgery
Loyola University Stritch School of Medicine
Maywood, Illinois

Phillip A. Tibbs, MD
Professor and Chair
Department of Neurosurgery
Director
Spine Center
University of Kentucky
Lexington, Kentucky

Hieu H. Ton-That, MD, FACS
Associate Professor
Department of Surgery
Loyola University Medical Center
Maywood, Illinois

Shelly D. Timmons, MD, PhD, FACS, FAANS
Professor of Neurosurgery
Vice Chair for Administration
Director of Neurotrauma
Penn State University College of Medicine
Milton S. Hershey Medical Center
Hershey, Pennsylvania

Vincent C. Traynelis, MD
Director, Neurosurgery Spine Fellowship Program
Professor, Department of Neurosurgery
Director, Neurosurgery Residency Program
Rush University Medical College
Chicago, Illinois

Asterios Tsimpas, MD, MSc, MRCSEd
Cerebrovascular, Endovascular & General Neurosurgeon
Assistant Professor of Neurosurgery & Radiology
Neurosurgery Clerkship Director
Loyola University Stritch School of Medicine
Maywood, Illinois

Mazda K. Turel, MD
Department of Neurosurgery
Rush University Medical Center
Chicago, Illinois

Alexander R. Vaccaro, MD, PhD, MBA
Richard H. Rothman Professor and Chair of
   Orthopedic Surgery
Professor of Neurosurgery
Co-Director, Spinal Cord Injury Center
Co-Chief, Spine Surgery
President, Rothman Institute
Thomas Jefferson University Hospital
Philadelphia, Pennsylvania

Michael P. Wemhoff, MD
Resident
Department of Neurological Surgery
Loyola University Stritch School of Medicine
Maywood, Illinois

Christopher E. Wolfla, MD, FAANS
Professor
Department of Neurosurgery
The Medical College of Wisconsin
Milwaukee, Wisconsin

1 Assessment of Acute Loss of Consciousness

Michael P. Merchut and José Biller

Abstract

Assessment of acute loss of consciousness is a clinically challenging task, as the examiner needs to quickly determine the etiology of coma and direct the most appropriate treatment towards recovery, whenever possible. After briefly reviewing the pathophysiology of coma, this chapter emphasizes the clinical approach and rational management of patients in coma from different causes.

Keywords: brain CT and MRI scans, brain herniation, coma, drug overdose, hypothermia, hypoxia, locked-in syndrome, loss of consciousness, oculocephalic and oculovestibular reflexes

1.1 Introduction

Coma is the extreme state of unconsciousness, with an apparently "sleeping" patient unresponsive to even painful stimuli. The relevant pathophysiology was perhaps most capably reviewed by Plum and Posner[1] in their landmark monograph *Stupor and Coma*. The clinical approach to patients in coma is emphasized in this chapter.

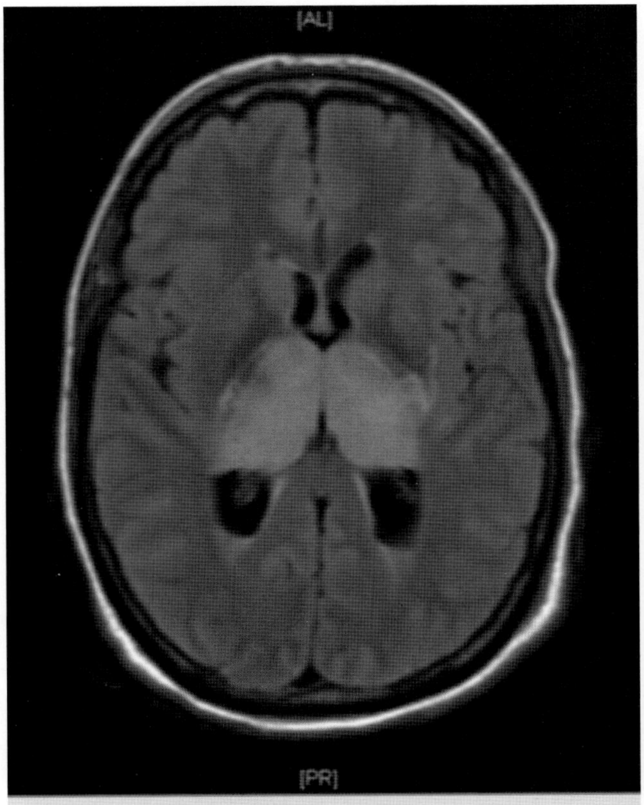

1.2 Pathophysiology of Coma

Wakefulness or alertness is critically dependent upon the "ascending reticular activating system" (ARAS), a functional component of the complex neuronal network within the reticular formation of the upper brainstem. The ARAS extends from the tegmental midpons to midbrain to thalamic intralaminar nuclei and basal forebrain, from which there are widespread cortical projections, especially to the frontal lobes and limbic system.[2] Large structural lesions directly interrupting this pathway, as in the rostral brainstem or bilateral thalamus, would cause unconsciousness (▶ Fig. 1.1), whereas a unilateral, hemispheric lesion (e.g., a frontal lobe embolic infarction) would not do so, unless it indirectly impaired the ARAS by means of pressure effect. Typically, the latter occurs in the setting of severe, perilesional edema creating a midline shift that compresses the thalamic intralaminar nuclei of the diencephalon (▶ Fig. 1.2). In the absence of midline shift or pressure on the diencephalon, coma could be produced by extensive, bilateral lesions (e.g., severe head trauma) destroying widespread cortex or disrupting most of the thalamocortical or corticocortical projections.[3] Metabolic processes producing coma generally do so by impairing bilateral or diffuse areas of cerebral cortex, which are far more sensitive to hypoxia, hypoglycemia, and drug effects than the brainstem.

Patients resuscitated from cardiopulmonary arrest may be in coma for a few days and then appear to be intermittently awake. Spontaneous breathing, roving eye movements, and other reflexive behavior occur, but cortical responsiveness or

Fig. 1.1 Magnetic resonance image (fluid-attenuated inversion recovery series) showing bilateral thalamic lesions in a comatose, immunosuppressed patient with West Nile Virus rhomboencephalitis.

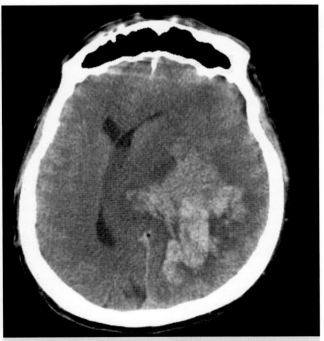

Fig. 1.2 Computer tomography image showing large cerebral hemorrhage with midline shift.

communication never returns. The functional condition of this static, anoxic encephalopathy was previously called the chronic or persistent vegetative state (PVS). More recently, PVS has been renamed the "unresponsive wakefulness syndrome."[4] Patients showing limited, occasional signs of responsiveness, such as visual tracking, were felt to be in a "minimally conscious state."[5] Some fortunate survivors may have a more complete recovery.

Other causes of coma (e.g., cerebral metastases, hemorrhage) may be progressive in nature, leading to death if not recognized and treated early. The cause of coma in a patient must thus be diagnosed rapidly and any potential treatment begun as soon as possible. Since the clinical bedside neurologic examination of the comatose patient is limited to an assessment of brainstem reflexes, the patient's history, when available, becomes a valuable piece of information. The rapidity and manner in which the patient became comatose, as well as past medical history, current medications or procedures, and recent symptoms or illness, may all provide important clues as to the cause of coma.

1.3 Clinical Evaluation of Comatose Patients

Observation of the sudden onset of coma strongly suggests intracranial hemorrhage, extensive brainstem infarction or multiple cerebral embolic infarcts, or cerebral hypoperfusion from cardiac arrhythmia or heart block. An excruciating headache just prior to loss of consciousness points towards aneurysmal rupture with subarachnoid hemorrhage. Metabolic disorders producing coma usually are preceded by a period of confusion or delirium, if that history is obtainable, although drug overdosage, whether accidental or intentional, may abruptly lead to coma. New medications or dose adjustments should be scrutinized, and any "medical alert" bracelets checked for a history of epilepsy, diabetes, or warfarin use. Serious head or cervical spine trauma is suggested by where the patient is found (e.g., the foot of the stairs) or by signs of external injury, if eyewitnesses are not present. A preceding febrile illness makes meningoencephalitis or brain abscess more likely in a comatose patient, although signs of infection may be lacking in the immunocompromised.

While any historical clues are being obtained, other medical personnel must immediately ensure the adequacy of the "ABCs" (airway, breathing, circulation) in the comatose patient. The vital signs themselves may suggest the cause of coma, as in circulatory shock, from hypovolemia, sepsis, or cardiogenic causes. Hypoventilation may signal direct involvement of vital medullary cardiorespiratory centers by an extensive brainstem hemorrhage or infarction, or indirectly by means of tonsillar herniation from cerebral or cerebellar edema. In the setting of head trauma, apnea may be due to an unsuspected, severe, high cervical spinal cord injury. Acute neuromuscular disorders leading to global paralysis (e.g., myasthenic crisis, severe Guillain–Barré syndrome) may also cause respiratory weakness, although those patients typically remain conscious despite having the "locked-in syndrome."

Increased blood pressure is a frequent reactive phenomenon in the setting of acute cerebral hemorrhage or infarction without impaired consciousness, but extremely elevated blood pressure may actually reflect the primary cause of coma: hypertensive encephalopathy, or a thalamic or basal ganglia hemorrhage from uncontrolled essential hypertension or sympathomimetic drug use (e.g., cocaine). In the setting of rising brain edema with incipient tonsillar herniation, an abrupt rise in blood pressure may be accompanied by bradycardia and decreased respirations: Cushing's reflex.

Febrile comatose patients most often have systemic or central nervous system infections. Other causes of fever, as suggested by the clinical scenario present, include malignant hyperthermia from anesthesia, neuroleptic malignant syndrome, serotonin syndrome, heatstroke, and anticholinergic overdose. Patients found outdoors in winter, however, may be comatose from hypothermia, which requires urgent rewarming. If the body core temperature drops further below 35°C, even brainstem reflexes may be lost, and the patient appears to be brain dead.

Certain features of the general physical examination may also help with the etiology of coma. Cutaneous periorbital ("raccoon eyes") and mastoid ("Battle's sign") hemorrhages reflect skull fractures, as do cerebrospinal fluid (CSF) otorrhea and rhinorrhea, incriminating head trauma as the prime cause of coma in someone "found down on the ground."[6] A jaundiced patient with gross ascites may be in hepatic coma. Diffuse petechiae and ecchymoses may point towards a systemic coagulopathy and the likelihood of an intracranial hemorrhage, whereas "palpable purpura" is a sign of meningococcemia and coexistent meningitis. Nuchal rigidity may develop from meningeal infection or subarachnoid bleeding but may be undetectable when the patient is fully comatose.[7] If there is any question of trauma, however, the neck and head should not be rotated or flexed until a cervical spine fracture or instability is radiographically excluded. A preretinal or subhyaloid hemorrhage on funduscopic examination is associated with a subarachnoid hemorrhage.[7] The discovery of papilledema confirms elevated intracranial pressure of diverse etiology, but it takes at least 2 to 4 hours to develop after an acute cerebral or subarachnoid hemorrhage.[8] Subungual (splinter), palmar, plantar, or retinal (Roth's spot) hemorrhages suggest infective endocarditis as the source of cerebral emboli or abscesses in a comatose patient with a heart murmur.

Although the neurologic examination of comatose patients is limited, it correlates with the level of dysfunction in the central nervous system and changes if there is any rostral to caudal progression of edema, hemorrhage, or ischemia down the brainstem.[3] Bedside neurologic signs of clinical deterioration, however, develop at variable rates in different patients. The main features of the bedside neurologic examination are breathing pattern, motor function or responsiveness, and assessment of the pupils and ocular reflexes.

The pattern of respiration is often impossible to evaluate, since most comatose patients are initially intubated or mechanically ventilated. Furthermore, the correlation of specific lesions with certain breathing patterns is inexact.[9] Cheyne–Stokes respiration, or crescendo/decrescendo tidal volumes alternating with apneas, may occur in patients with slowed circulation time from heart failure, or in systemically ill elderly patients, as well as those in coma from bihemispheric cerebral lesions. Unrelenting hyperventilation is found more commonly with a primary pulmonary disorder (e.g., acute respiratory distress syndrome) and only rarely from an isolated midbrain lesion. Irregular, erratic breathing is typical of ataxic breathing, the precursor of respiratory arrest from involvement of the cardiorespiratory centers in the medulla.[10]

Spontaneous or stimulus-induced movements of the patient should be observed. Movement of a limb on command, or after a painful stimulus (sternal rub, nailbed compression, or rubbing the supraorbital ridge or angle of the jaw), is prognostically better than unresponsiveness. Spontaneous or stimulus-provoked decorticate posturing (unilateral or bilateral flexion of upper limbs with extension of lower limbs) occurs with dysfunction at the level of the cerebral hemispheres or diencephalon. Decerebrate posturing (unilateral or bilateral extension of upper and lower limbs) occurs with dysfunction at the level of the red nucleus (midbrain).[10] Attempts to elicit the Babinski sign may lead to a "triple flexion" response, with flexion at the hip, knee, and ankle, indicative of a corticospinal tract lesion.[7] Asterixis may be observed bilaterally with passive extension of the hands or feet and, along with myoclonic jerks and tremulousness, suggests a metabolic cause of coma. Unilateral asterixis is seen with contralateral thalamic, midbrain, or parietal lobe lesions.[11] Myoclonus or myoclonic jerks appear as sudden, shock-like muscle contractions of a limb or entire body, often triggered by tactile stimuli, and frequently seen with anoxic encephalopathy. Any other subtle, rhythmical, repetitive movements should be noted, such as twitching of the eyelid, face, or limb or lateral gaze deviation with persistent nystagmus. These movements may be the only clinical signs of nonconvulsive or "electrical" status epilepticus, which may be the primary or major contributing cause of coma. Not all repetitive eye movements are epileptic, however. Ocular bobbing, a cyclical, fast jerk of both eyes downward, with a slower return to primary position, usually occurs with pontine lesions with poor prognosis.[12] Any intubated, motionless, unresponsive patient with spontaneously blinking, opened eyes must be assessed for the de-efferented state of the locked-in syndrome (e.g., extensive pontine infarction from basilar artery occlusion). The examiner may be surprised to find that such a patient reliably answers yes-or-no questions by blinking once or twice.

The examination of the pupils and the pupillary light reflex is a simple task, yet associated with a few pitfalls. Normal pupilloconstriction to a light stimulus involves efferent parasympathetic fibers with the third cranial nerve at the level of the midbrain. Thus, a lesion of the dorsal midbrain or third cranial nerve(s) produces larger, dilated, unreactive pupil(s). The sympathetic pupillodilator fibers leave the hypothalamus, descend the brainstem into the cervicothoracic spinal cord, exit into the sympathetic (stellate) ganglia, and ascend the carotid arteries to the orbit. Brainstem lesions caudal to the midbrain, therefore, disrupt these pupillodilator fibers, leaving tiny, pinpoint, but reactive pupils. A comatose patient with pinpoint pupils will not always harbor a pontine lesion, however, since such pupils also occur with a narcotic drug overdose or in glaucoma patients using cholinergic (pilocarpine) eyedrops. Coma-producing lesions elsewhere tend to cause somewhat small, but reactive pupils, which are the usual finding in conscious elderly patients. Metabolic causes of coma also produce small pupils of equal size, with the light reflex preserved even after loss of other cranial nerve or brainstem reflexes (corneal, oculocephalic, oculovestibular, and gag reflexes).[13]

The finding of an enlarged, dilated, nonreactive pupil in an unresponsive patient is an ominous finding, generally representing uncal herniation from an ipsilateral mass. In such unconscious patients, computed tomography (CT) and magnetic resonance imaging (MRI) studies reveal that coma is produced by severe horizontal compression and shift of the diencephalon, which precedes obscuration of the perimesencephalic cisterns and pressure on the uncus itself.[14,15] Horizontal shift and distortion of the upper brainstem, containing the ARAS, more readily creates coma than similar degrees of vertical displacement of the brainstem from tonsillar herniation. Horizontal pineal displacement of 3 to 4 mm correlates with drowsiness, 6 to 8 mm with stupor, and over 8 mm with coma.[14]

The oculocephalic and oculovestibular reflexes (▶Fig. 1.3) are both normal brainstem reflexes, most readily elicited and observed when cortical inhibition is reduced or absent. Once a cervical spine injury is ruled out, gentle, passive rotation of the patient's head toward the left normally produces conjugate lateral rolling of both eyes to the right, and vice versa. Put another way, during lateral head rotation, the patient's eyes tend to keep looking at the examiner when observing the patient "face to face." This is the oculocephalic reflex or "doll's eyes" maneuver.

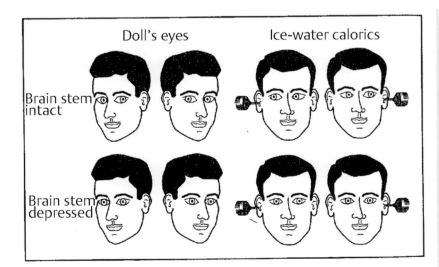

Fig. 1.3 Ocular reflexes. The eyes normally roll opposite to the turn of the head (doll's eyes or oculocephalic reflex), and the eyes slowly turn toward the ear irrigated with ice water (cold caloric or oculovestibular reflex). (Modified with permission from Collins RC. Neurology. Philadelphia, PA: WB Saunders; 1997.)

The oculovestibular, or "cold caloric," reflex may be preserved or persist after the oculocephalic reflex is absent. With the patient's head elevated about 30 degrees, ice water irrigation of the ear canal normally produces some turbulence or movement of endolymphatic fluid within the labyrinthine semicircular canals, causing a slow, tonic deviation of both eyes toward the irrigated ear. Lateral nystagmus, with rapid component to the opposite ear, requires some cortical function and is thus not usually observed in the comatose subject. Care should be taken to ensure against a false-negative response, instilling at least 50 cc of ice water for an adequate test stimulus. If cerumen or debris occludes the ear canal, a normal response may be prohibited. Water should not be instilled into an ear canal with a ruptured tympanic membrane, because of the risk of infection.

Failure to elicit ocular reflexes may occur without a brainstem lesion, however. Absent oculovestibular reflexes in particular may be secondary to preexistent labyrinthine trauma, mastoiditis, or drug toxicity. Both of these ocular reflexes are readily suppressed by benzodiazepines and barbiturates, whether previously given therapeutically, or taken in overdose by the unconscious patient. In the case of the trauma patient with facial injuries, maxillary fractures could restrict the extraocular muscles and create a false-negative ocular reflex.

These main features of the clinical neurologic examination (breathing pattern, motor function, pupils, and ocular reflexes) should be recorded periodically as the patient is treated and observed for improvement or deterioration. Paramedical personnel often use the Glasgow Coma Scale or Full Outline of UnResponsiveness (FOUR) score to quickly and serially grade comatose patients.[16] Loss of all brainstem reflexes in an apneic, comatose patient signals brain death, which is diagnosed when a known cause of coma (e.g., prolonged hypoxia) is severe enough to irreversibly destroy cerebral hemispheres and brainstem, with no improvement after a sufficient period of treatment and observation. Hypothermia (core body temperature below 32°C), circulatory shock (systolic blood pressure below 90 mm Hg), and drug intoxication must have been appropriately treated here. The recommended period of observation preceding the diagnosis of brain death in adults is 6 hours; a period of 12 hours to 2 days is suggested for children.[17] In addition to documentation of absent brainstem reflexes, the apnea test should be done to verify failure of the medullary respiratory center (no visible breaths despite reaching a partial pressure of carbon dioxide [pCO_2] of 60 mm Hg or greater, after 10 minutes of mechanical ventilation with 100% O_2). Historically, in the United States, an isoelectric, "flat-line" electroencephalogram (EEG) was sought to demonstrate absence of cortical function. Since remnants of brain wave activity were still occasionally found in patients with overwhelming loss of cortical neurons, the current ancillary test of choice is a radioisotope brain scan depicting absent intracranial blood flow.

1.4 Initial Management for Comatose Patients (▶Fig. 1.4)

As previously mentioned, the adequate functioning of the ABCs must be ensured. Poor airway protection or aspiration risk mandates intubation even if there is spontaneous respiration. Extreme hypertension, hypotension, fever, hypothermia, and cardiac arrhythmia require urgent treatment and may be primary causes of coma. Since persistent hypoglycemia leads to permanent cortical damage, it must be quickly ruled out with a fingerstick glucose reading, or by giving an intravenous (IV) bolus of 50% dextrose empirically. Thiamine 100 mg IV should be given immediately prior to any glucose infusion to prevent precipitation of Wernicke's encephalopathy in malnourished or alcoholic patients. Antidotes for narcotic (naloxone) or benzodiazepine (flumazenil) overdosage only awaken the patient temporarily; although this serves a diagnostic purpose, withdrawal convulsions may occur with flumazenil. Blood work for electrolytes, glucose, renal and hepatic function, calcium, creatine kinase, ammonia, thyroid-stimulating hormone (TSH), blood count, prothrombin time (PT), and activated partial thromboplastin time (aPTT) should be sent, in addition to an arterial blood gas (with carbon monoxide level if indicated) and a urine drug screen. Blood, urine, and CSF cultures are sent if indicated. Comatose patients resuscitated from cardiac arrest have better neurologic outcomes if treated with hypothermia within a 6-hour window, achieving a core temperature of 32 to 34°C for 24 hours, followed by slow rewarming.[18]

A CT brain scan is urgently done if there are signs of a structural central nervous system (CNS) lesion or history of head trauma, or after the failure to find a metabolic cause of coma or response to therapy (e.g., volume replacement or correction of hypoglycemia). Structural supratentorial lesions are suggested by asymmetrical neurologic deficits of movement, posturing, reflexes, or gaze; a dilated, fixed pupil; or a partial or secondarily generalized seizure. Structural infratentorial lesions are suggested by early development of quadriplegia, apnea, and loss of cranial nerve or brainstem reflexes. Patients with ischemic infarction may need an urgent brain MRI scan, or even CT angiography or MR angiography, in evaluation for acute interventions such as mechanical thrombectomy. When patients deteriorate from extensive middle cerebral artery infarction (▶Fig. 1.5) despite optimal medical support, decompressive hemicraniectomy with dural expansion within 48 hours of stroke onset improves survival in patients under age 60. Family members need to be informed, however, that at least half of these survivors will have severe disability postoperatively. Suboccipital craniectomy for progressive cerebellar infarction is also effective, with typically better functional outcomes.[19]

Metabolic causes of coma usually impair behavior or alter consciousness prior to development of symmetrical neurologic deficits. The pupillary light reflex here is typically preserved even when other brainstem reflexes are lost. Tremulousness, myoclonic jerks, bilateral asterixis, and primarily generalized seizures occur in toximetabolic coma. In patients without an obvious cause of coma and normal brain CT, an EEG should be performed to rule out nonconvulsive, "electrical" status epilepticus. Instead of obvious tonic–clonic body and limb movements, the patient may only exhibit subtle, repetitive nystagmus, or twitches of the face, as a manifestation of continuous, generalized seizures on EEG. In the absence of status, the EEG may document the diffuse brain wave slowing expected of encephalopathy, or perhaps the triphasic waves typical of renal or hepatic failure.

Management Algorithm for Comatose Patients

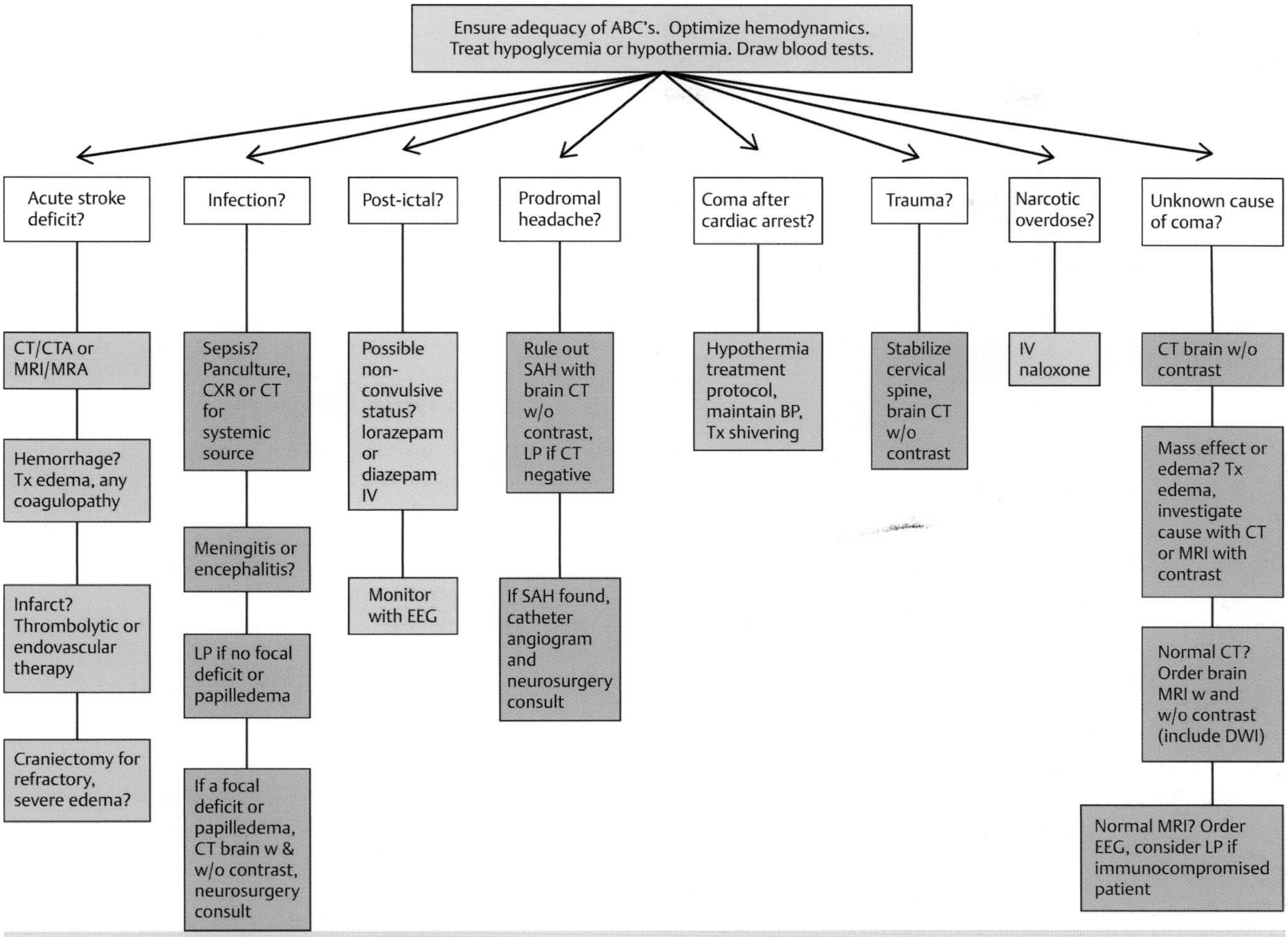

Fig. 1.4 Management algorithm for comatose patients. ABC, airway, breathing, circulation; CTA, computed tomography angiogram; MRA, magnetic resonance angiogram; Tx, treat; CXR, chest X-ray; SAH, subarachnoid hemorrhage; DWI, diffusion-weighted images; LP, lumbar puncture.

1.5 Specific Management of Comatose Patients

1.5.1 Coma from Structural Lesions with Symmetrical Neurologic Deficits

It is rare for a single lesion which causes coma to have symmetrical neurologic findings. One not-to-be-missed example is the locked-in syndrome, usually associated with an extensive, bilateral pontine infarction from basilar artery occlusion. Such a patient has preserved vertical gaze and may communicate by blinking, despite quadriplegia, facial diplegia, lateral gaze paralysis, and respiratory dysfunction. Other cases of locked-in syndrome do not involve structural CNS lesions but are due to profound neuromuscular paralysis with respiratory failure, yet consciousness is preserved. Examples include myasthenic crisis and fulminant Guillain–Barré syndrome, with global areflexia in the latter. In the absence of observers describing a history of progressive weakness, the examiner sees a paralyzed, ventilated patient with normal brain scan and EEG. A portable electromyogram (EMG) in the intensive care unit may best demonstrate the presence of an underlying severe neuromuscular transmission defect or acute demyelinating neuropathy.

A deep cerebral hypertensive hemorrhage, in the thalamus or basal ganglia, with or without rupture into the ventricles, often produces coma and quadriplegia. Subtle asymmetries of limb spasticity or gaze deviation, in conjunction with a history of headache and sudden neurologic deterioration, serve to localize the problem and its likely cause.

The paramedian thalamic syndrome may be difficult to diagnose at bedside. The patient is stuporous or hypersomnolent, requiring continuous noxious stimuli to stay awake. A vertical gaze deficit and variable degrees of quadriparesis, as well as bilateral asterixis, are due to bilateral infarction of the dorsal midbrain, extending into the intralaminar thalamic nuclei (ARAS) and thus impairing consciousness.[20]

Cerebral venous thromboses occur in patients with hypercoagulable conditions, sepsis, and the peripartum state. Superior sagittal sinus thrombosis produces headache, seizures, possibly bilateral deficits, and parasagittal hemorrhagic infarcts. It may be difficult to detect the "empty delta sign," from thrombus in

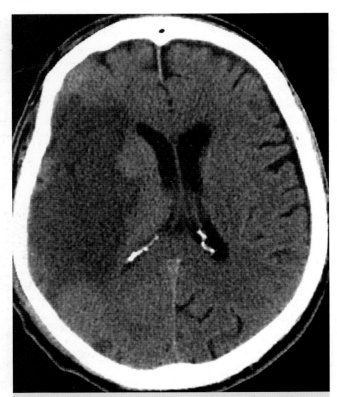

Fig. 1.5 Computer tomography image showing middle cerebral artery infarction with midline shift.

the superior sagittal sinus, as seen with infused brain CT; brain MRI is a more sensitive test. Thrombosis of deep cerebral veins may more rapidly lead to coma and a poorer prognosis, since these veins drain the dorsal thalamus, basal ganglia, choroid plexi, and periventricular white matter.[21]

Acute hydrocephalus may be heralded by headache, visual obscurations, and increasing somnolence, prior to coma. If caused by a pineal region tumor, Parinaud's syndrome may be present: impaired upgaze and light-near dissociation of the pupil (normal pupilloconstriction with viewing a nearby object, but not with a light stimulus). Other causes of acute hydrocephalus include obstruction by pus or blood at the foramina of Luschka and Magendie, or by blood from recurrent bleeding at the subarachnoid villi.

1.5.2 Coma from Toximetabolic Causes

Drug overdosage is probably the most common, nonstructural cause of coma. Again, a careful history is critical here: what are the patient's medications, or the medications of others accessible by the patient? Is there any preceding depression, other psychiatric illness, or habitual use of recreational drugs? Intoxication may predispose to concurrent head injury, which should always be suspected, and sympathomimetic drugs such as cocaine cause cerebral infarcts or hemorrhage in young adults. Ingestion of multiple drugs or medications makes for a difficult bedside diagnosis prior to results of a drug screen, but certain drugs may be suspected on the basis of the presence of sympathomimetic, sympatholytic, anticholinergic, or cholinergic signs (▶Table 1.1).[22]

Environmental toxins capable of producing coma are usually associated with a catastrophic exposure at a chemical plant, or an industrial accident. Suicide or accidental death from carbon

Table 1.1 Clinical features of coma from drug overdoses

Syndrome	Sympathomimetic	Sympatholytic	Anticholinergic	Cholinergic
Causative drugs	Cocaine, amphetamine, ephedrine	Opiates, benzodiazepines, alcohol	Antihistamines, neuroleptics, TCAs	Insecticides (organophosphates)
Heart rate	⇧ ⇧	Normal or ⇩	⇧	Either: ⇧ ⇩
BP	⇧ ⇧	⇩	⇧	Either: ⇧ ⇩
Pupils	Large	Pinpoint	Very large to fixed	Small
Diaphoresis[a]	⇧	Normal	⇩ ⇩	⇧ ⇧
GI/GU motility[a]	⇧	Normal or ⇩	⇩	⇧ ⇧
Other features			TCAs: wide QRS on EKG	Fasciculations, lacrimation, salivation

Abbreviations: BP, blood pressure; EKG, electrocardiogram; GI, gastrointestinal; GU, genitourinary; TCA, tricyclic antidepressant.

Data from Gerace RW. Drugs part A: poisoning. In: Young GB, Ropper AH, Bolton CF, eds. Coma and Impaired Consciousness. New York, NY: McGraw-Hill; 1998:457–469.

[a]Reduced diaphoresis leads to hot, dry, flushed skin. Increased GI/GU motility includes nausea and vomiting, cramps, and diarrhea. Decreased GI/GU motility includes ileus and bladder atony. Seizures and cardiac arrhythmias may occur with any syndrome.

monoxide (CO) is a household problem, often from malfunctioning heaters or unventilated garages. The clinical features of CO poisoning may unfold slowly or abruptly, including headache, confusion, dizziness, seizures, and coma. Urgent ventilation with 100% oxygen, optimally in a hyperbaric chamber, is indicated.[23]

Coma can be produced not only by hypoglycemic conditions but also by extreme hyperglycemic, hyperosmolar states, whether by the resultant dehydration or via osmolar shifts creating brain edema during corrective treatment. Focal, asymmetrical findings, such as hemiplegia or aphasia, or partial seizures, can be solely due to severe hypoglycemic,[24] hyperglycemic,[25] or acutely hyponatremic states. Rapid correction of hyponatremia, with serum sodium rising faster than 12 mmol/L daily, can lead to central pontine myelinolysis (CPM), with quadriparesis, stupor, or coma. Subcortical lesions outside the pons may also occur with CPM.[25]

Renal or liver failure can cause delirium, with tremulousness, bilateral asterixis, and myoclonic jerks, progressing to coma if untreated. In addition, hepatic necrosis preterminally produces fulminant brain edema,[26] so it should be considered when a brain CT scan demonstrates cerebral edema in a comatose patient without clear etiology. Usually, however, signs of jaundice, ascites, and cutaneous or gastrointestinal bleeding suggest liver dysfunction. The accumulation of ammonia and related toxins affects the CNS in hepatic disease and Krebs cycle disorders. Occasionally, patients with bladder obstruction and cystitis from urease-producing bacteria may become stuporous as a result of ammonia absorbed in the bladder.[27] Certain other endocrine disasters may also produce coma. Pituitary apoplexy is the hemorrhagic infarction or acute necrosis of a pituitary tumor, impairing consciousness by compressing the hypothalamus or via adrenal failure. Extraocular palsies may be noted after a sudden, severe headache. Seizures and coma may accompany thyroid storm, along with notable tachycardia and fever.[25]

1.5.3 Coma from Unknown Causes

A brain CT scan is often performed despite no clear asymmetrical findings to suggest a structural lesion, nor signs of head trauma, but because hemodynamic support and correction of metabolic factors produced no improvement in coma. If and when the patient is stable, a brain MRI scan may be the better modality to detect hyperacute ischemic infarctions (diffusion-weighted image sequences), acute herpes simplex encephalitis, and other conditions (▶Table 1.2).[17] Unless severe anoxia or ischemia has occurred, hopefully the unresponsive patient will gradually and eventually recover from a drug overdose or metabolic encephalopathy, with aggressive medical care and support.

Table 1.2 Suggestive computer tomography and magnetic resonance imaging findings in comatose patients

Findings	Clinical probabilities
Thalamic, basal ganglia hemorrhage	Uncontrolled hypertension, sympathomimetics (cocaine)
Subarachnoid hemorrhage	Trauma, ruptured aneurysm, sympathomimetics (cocaine)
Communicating hydrocephalus	Basilar meningitis or subarachnoid bleeding
Noncommunicating hydrocephalus (fourth ventricle not dilated)	Aqueductal stenosis, pineal region mass
Parasagittal hemorrhagic infarcts	Superior sagittal sinus venous thrombosis, coagulopathy
Diffuse brain edema without blood	Severe anoxia, encephalitis, acute hepatic necrosis
Bilateral basal ganglia, subcortical white matter lesions[a]	Carbon monoxide poisoning
Bilateral pontine, midbrain, thalamic, and occipital lesions (infarcts)[a]	Basilar artery occlusion
Bilateral thalamic and temporo-occipital lesions (reversible edema)[a]	Hypertensive encephalopathy, eclampsia
Bilateral frontal and mesiotemporal lesions with edema[a]	Herpes simplex encephalitis
Patchy central pontine, perhaps other subcortical lesions[a]	Central pontine myelinolysis (dysosmolar syndrome)

Adapted from Wijdicks EFM. Altered arousal and coma. In: Wijdicks EFM, ed. Catastrophic Neurologic Disorders in the Emergency Department. 2nd ed. Oxford, UK: Oxford University Press; 2004:53–93.

[a]Findings best seen on magnetic resonance images.

References

[1] Plum F, Posner JB. The Diagnosis of Stupor and Coma. 3rd ed. Philadelphia, PA: FA Davis; 1982

[2] Moruzzi G, Magoun HW. Brain stem reticular formation and activation of the EEG. Electroencephalogr Clin Neurophysiol. 1949; 1(4):455–473

[3] Plum F, Posner JB. Supratentorial lesions causing coma. In: Plum F, Posner JB. The Diagnosis of Stupor and Coma. 3rd ed. Philadelphia, PA: FA Davis; 1982:87–151

[4] Laureys S, Celesia GG, Cohadon F, et al; European Task Force on Disorders of Consciousness. Unresponsive wakefulness syndrome: a new name for the vegetative state or apallic syndrome. BMC Med. 2010; 8:68

[5] Giacino JT, Ashwal S, Childs N, et al. The minimally conscious state: definition and diagnostic criteria. Neurology. 2002; 58(3):349–353

[6] Moulton R. Head injury. In: Young GB, Ropper AH, Bolton CF, eds. Coma and Impaired Consciousness. New York, NY: McGraw-Hill; 1998:149–181

[7] Fisher CM. The neurological examination of the comatose patient. Acta Neurol Scand. 1969; 45(Suppl 36:):–1–56

[8] Pagani LF. The rapid appearance of papilledema. J Neurosurg. 1969; 30(3):247–249

[9] Lee MC, Klassen AC, Resch JA. Respiratory pattern disturbances in ischemic cerebral vascular disease. Stroke. 1974; 5(5):612–616

[10] Plum F, Posner JB. The pathologic physiology of signs and symptoms of coma. In: Plum F, Posner JB. The Diagnosis of Stupor and Coma. 3rd ed. Philadelphia, PA: FA Davis; 1982:1–86

[11] Degos JD, Verroust J, Bouchareine A, Serdaru M, Barbizet J. Asterixis in focal brain lesions. Arch Neurol. 1979; 36(11):705–707

[12] Fisher CM. Ocular bobbing. Arch Neurol. 1964; 11:543–546

[13] Plum F, Posner JB. Multifocal, diffuse and metabolic brain diseases causing stupor or coma. In: Plum F, Posner JB. The Diagnosis of Stupor and Coma. 3rd ed. Philadelphia, PA: FA Davis; 1982:177–303

[14] Ropper AH. Lateral displacement of the brain and level of consciousness in patients with an acute hemispheral mass. N Engl J Med. 1986; 314(15):953–958

[15] Ropper AH. A preliminary MRI study of the geometry of brain displacement and level of consciousness with acute intracranial masses. Neurology. 1989; 39(5):622–627

[16] Wijdicks EFM, Bamlet WR, Maramattom BV, Manno EM, McClelland RL. Validation of a new coma scale: the FOUR score. Ann Neurol. 2005; 58(4):585–593

[17] Wijdicks EFM. Altered arousal and coma. In: Wijdicks EFM, ed. Catastrophic Neurologic Disorders in the Emergency Department. 2nd ed. Oxford, UK: Oxford University Press; 2004:53–93

[18] Hypothermia after Cardiac Arrest Study Group. Mild therapeutic hypothermia to improve the neurologic outcome after cardiac arrest. N Engl J Med. 2002; 346(8):549–556

[19] Wijdicks EFM, Sheth KN, Carter BS, et al; American Heart Association Stroke Council. Recommendations for the management of cerebral and cerebellar infarction with swelling. A statement for healthcare professionals from the American Heart Association/American Stroke Association.. Stroke. 2014; 45:1222–1238

[20] Castaigne P, Lhermitte F, Buge A, Escourolle R, Hauw JJ, Lyon-Caen O. Paramedian thalamic and midbrain infarct: clinical and neuropathological study. Ann Neurol. 1981; 10(2):127–148

[21] Crawford SC, Digre KB, Palmer CA, Bell DA, Osborn AG. Thrombosis of the deep venous drainage of the brain in adults. Analysis of seven cases with review of the literature. Arch Neurol. 1995; 52(11):1101–1108

[22] Gerace RW. Drugs part A: poisoning. In: Young GB, Ropper AH, Bolton CF, eds. Coma and Impaired Consciousness. New York, NY: McGraw-Hill; 1998:457–469

[23] Ernst A, Zibrak JD. Carbon monoxide poisoning. N Engl J Med. 1998; 339(22):1603–1608

[24] Wallis WE, Donaldson I, Scott RS, Wilson J. Hypoglycemia masquerading as cerebrovascular disease (hypoglycemic hemiplegia). Ann Neurol. 1985; 18(4):510–512

[25] Young GB, DeRubeis DA. Metabolic encephalopathies. In: Young GB, Ropper AH, Bolton CF, eds. Coma and Impaired Consciousness. New York, NY: McGraw-Hill; 1998:307–392

[26] Lee WM. Acute liver failure. N Engl J Med. 1993; 329(25):1862–1872

[27] Drayna CJ, Titcomb CP, Varma RR, Soergel KH. Hyperammonemic encephalopathy caused by infection in a neurogenic bladder. N Engl J Med. 1981; 304(13):766–768

2 Intracranial Pressure Monitoring and Management of Raised Intracranial Pressure

Syed Omar Shah, Bong-Soo Kim, Bhuvanesh Govind, and Jack Jallo

Abstract

During the last few decades, our understanding of increased intracranial pressure has improved. We now have advanced neuroimaging along with multimodality monitoring techniques that allows us to effectively manage raised intracranial pressures. With the development of dedicated neuroscience intensive care units, management of these patients has continually improved. Treatment with protocol-driven therapy has increased favorable outcomes when compared with historical controls. In this chapter, we will explain the indications and contraindication for intracranial pressure monitoring. The bulk of this chapter, however, will be dedicated to the actual medical and surgical management of patients with raised intracranial pressures.

Keywords: external ventricular device, increased intracranial pressure, intracranial pressure management, multimodality monitoring

2.1 Introduction

One of the most important and common clinical problems encountered by the neurosurgeon is managing intracranial pressure (ICP). During the last several decades, we have improved our understanding of the pathophysiology of ICP as well as treating patients with intracranial hypertension. In addition, the availability of advanced neuroimaging and multimodality monitoring technologies has resulted in effective management for the patient with central nervous system diseases associated with intracranial hypertension. Refractory intracranial hypertension has been shown to be the primary cause of death in most patients who die of central nervous system diseases such as traumatic brain injury (TBI) and stroke. However, successful management of intracranial hypertension continues to remain a challenge. Virtually no new and effective treatment modality has been identified since ICP monitoring techniques have been available for clinical practice. The goal of this chapter is to discuss up-to-date clinical management of increased ICP.

2.2 Intracranial Pressure Monitoring

The relationship between ICP and its effect on intracranial hypertension stems from the Monro–Kellie doctrine, which states that the total amount of intracranial cerebrospinal fluid (CSF), brain, and blood must remain constant, and that if any one of the components increases, it must be met by a corresponding decrease in the other components.[1] Thus, the presence of large lesions made up from one of these components can cause an increase in ICP, and depending on how much intracranial hypertension is being created, this can be a life-threatening emergency. Accurate and real-time ICP monitoring is essential for successful management of increased ICP. Intracranial pressure monitoring may provide an early warning of delayed complications. Progressive increase in ICP may indicate the development of intracerebral hemorrhage, cerebral edema, or hydrocephalus. Although refractory intracranial hypertension is a strong predictor of mortality, ICP itself does not provide a useful prognostic marker of functional outcome.

2.2.1 Indications for Intracranial Pressure Monitoring

Intracranial pressure monitoring can be used in a multitude of brain injuries, including TBI, subarachnoid hemorrhage (SAH), intracerebral hematoma, and cerebral ischemia. Generally, an ICP monitor should be placed if the condition leading to ICP elevation is amenable to treatment and ICP assessment would be of consequence in decisions for treatment or intervention. Intracranial pressure monitoring can detect changes in pressure before secondary brain injury from ICP occurs. Identifying patients who would benefit from ICP monitoring is based on clinical and radiographic evaluations. There are, unfortunately, insufficient data to support a treatment standard for ICP monitoring. The Brain Trauma Foundation guidelines recommend ICP monitoring in patients with severe head injury with an abnormal admission computed tomography scan. Severe head injury is defined as a Glasgow Coma Scale score of 3 to 8 after cardiopulmonary resuscitation. An abnormal computed tomography scan of the head is one that reveals hematomas, contusions, edema, or compressed basal cisterns. In addition, ICP monitoring is appropriate in patients with severe head injury with a normal computed tomography scan if two or more of the following features are noted at admission: age over 40 years, unilateral or bilateral motor posturing, and systolic blood pressure less than 90 mm Hg. Intracranial pressure monitoring is not routinely indicated in patients with mild or moderate head injury.[2] However, a physician may choose to monitor ICP in certain conscious patients with traumatic mass lesions. Patients with moderate head injury with contusions of the temporal lobe are an example. The tendency for such injuries to evolve over the first 24 to 48 hours, coupled with their proximity to the brainstem and physical constraint in the temporal fossa, increases the possibility of delayed precipitous deterioration presenting as herniation. Therefore, some institutions tend to monitor such patients using a minimally invasive monitor such as intraparenchymal fiber-optic monitor.

The primary goal of ICP monitoring is to maintain adequate cerebral perfusion through the use of objective data, and the ICP monitor can be stopped when ICP is in normal range for 24 to 72 hours after withdrawal of ICP therapy.

2.2.2 Contraindications for Intracranial Pressure Monitoring

There is no absolute contraindication for ICP monitoring, and there are few relative contraindications. Coagulopathy can markedly increase the risk of procedure-related hemorrhage. If possible, the placement of an ICP monitor should be delayed until the international normalized ratio (INR), prothrombin time (PT), and partial thromboplastin time (PTT) are corrected. Generally, PT should be less than 13.5 seconds or the INR should be less than 1.4. For emergent situations, fresh-frozen plasma and vitamin K can be given. The platelet count should ideally exceed 100,000/mm³, but this may be unfeasible in patients with blood disorders. Patients on antiplatelet agents have historically been given a pool of platelets, but the data to support this are limited.

2.2.3 Types and Selection of Intracranial Pressure Monitors

There are several methods of classifying ICP monitors. Intracranial pressure monitoring devices are mainly classified according to the location of the monitor and the technology used for determining ICP (▶Table 2.1). Selection of the type of ICP monitoring device depends on several factors, including the clinical presentation, the need for concomitant CSF drainage, the risks associated with particular devices, system availability, a surgeon's personal familiarity with such devices, and ease of insertion.[3]

2.3 Management of Raised Intracranial Pressure

Several different ICP thresholds have been described in the literature, and there is no clear common values that are applied in clinical practice to all neurologic disorders.[4,5,6] The threshold that defines intracranial hypertension is also uncertain but generally is considered to be greater than 20 to 25 mm Hg, but both lower and higher thresholds have been described.[7] 2007

Brain Trauma Foundation guidelines recommend keeping the ICP below 20 mm Hg in TBI patients who are in level II trauma.[8] In a consensus statement by the Neurocritical Care Society and the European Society of Intensive Care Medicine, it was recommended to use ICP to guide medical and surgical interventions, but the threshold value of ICP remains uncertain based on literature.[9]

CPP represents the pressure gradient acting across the cerebrovascular bed and is a major determinant of cerebral blood flow (CBF). In the presence of intact cerebral autoregulation, CBF remains relatively constant within a wide range of perfusion pressures. This is achieved by vasoconstrictive responses to increased CPP and vasodilatory responses to decreased CPP. Cerebral pressure autoregulation normally has lower and upper CPP limits of ~ 50 and 150 mm Hg, respectively (▶Fig. 2.1 and ▶Fig. 2.2). When CPP is outside the bounds of pressure autoregulation, CBF becomes directly dependent on CPP.

Cerebral perfusion pressure is calculated as mean arterial pressure (MAP) minus ICP: CPP = MAP − ICP. In the setting of intracranial hypertension in adult patients, maintenance of CPP above 70 mm Hg has generally been recommended. But these recommendations have changed over time, given that targets for CPP rather than ICP have not improved outcomes.[10] Thus, optimal CPP values for each individual patient may need to be identified rather than a single threshold. Moreover, true CPP measurement relies on accurate placement of the blood pressure transducer. Many clinical practices place the blood pressure transducers at the level of the heart when in fact they should be referenced to the level of the tragus. Current opinion is to maintain CPP at 50 to 70 mm Hg.

2.3.1 Pathologic Waves: Lundberg Waves

Important diagnostic information is included in ICP waveforms.[11,12,13] ICP measurements produce waveforms with three classically defined peaks as shown in ▶Fig. 2.3a. The percussion wave (P1) is the first peak, reflecting arterial pulsation from the intracranial large arteries. The tidal wave (P2) is the second

Table 2.1 Selection of the type of intracranial pressure monitoring device

Type	Advantages	Disadvantages	Comments
Ventriculostomy	Able to recalibrate Accurate, reliable Less expensive Able to drain CSF	Risk of infection, hemorrhage	The gold standard place in the lateral ventricle Can be a tunneled subcutaneously or inserted as a bolted type
Parenchymal	Less invasive than ventriculostomy Accurate, reliable Easy and quick to insert	Not able to recalibrate Expensive Unable to drain CSF	Inserted into the brain parenchyma
Subarachnoid screw/bolt	Less invasive than ventriculostomy	Unable to drain CSF	Inserted into the subarachnoid space
Subdural	Less invasive than ventriculostomy	Poor accuracy and reliability over time Unable to drain CSF	Inserted into the subdural space
Epidural	Less invasive than ventriculostomy	Poor accuracy and reliability over time Unable to drain CSF	Inserted into the epidural space

Abbreviation: CSF, cerebrospinal fluid.

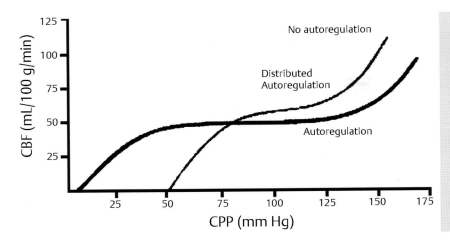

Fig. 2.1 Cerebral autoregulatory curves. CBF, cerebral blood flow. (Reproduced with permission from Marmarou A. Physiology of the cerebrospinal fluid and intracranial pressure. In: Winn RH, ed. Youman's Neurological Surgery. 5th ed. Phladelphia: Elsevier; 2004:181–183.)

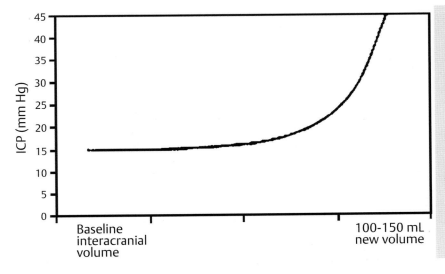

Fig. 2.2 Intracranial pressure volume curve. ICP, intracranial pressure. (Reproduced with permission from Marion DW. Pathophysiology and treatment of intracranial hypertension. In: Andrew BT, ed. Intensive Care in Neurosurgery. New York: Thieme Medical Publishers; 2003:47.)

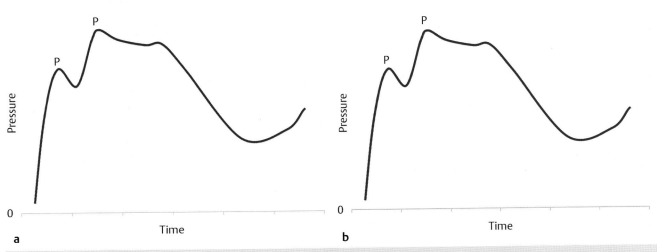

Fig. 2.3 (a) Intracranial pressure (ICP) waveform demonstrating three peaks with normal compliance state. (b) ICP waveform with compromised compliance state. P2 elevated above P1. With clinical deterioration, waveform graph does not full return to baseline state and increasingly shows elevation in the minimal ICP (ICP crisis).

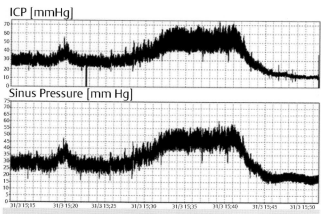

Fig. 2.4 Sample of continuous intracranial pressure recording showing gradually worsening cerebral pressure over time.

peak and reflects brain elasticity, whereas the third peak is referred to as the dicrotic wave (P3). Only the P1 and P2 waves are clinically useful.

Compromise in compliance of the brain due to intracranial hypertension manifests in pathologic "A" waves (plateau or Lundberg waves) where P2 remains elevated. The ICP increases well beyond 20 mm Hg, with peaks typically ranging from 50 to 80 mm Hg, signifying imminent brain herniation if left untreated. The plateau wave is a warning sign of deterioration of the autoregulatory curve whereby ICP is elevated to the point where CBF is compromised (▶Fig. 2.3b). Persistent increase in ICP at this point compromises CPP, engaging in a vicious cycle of further plateau waves and resultant worsening cerebral ischemia (▶Fig. 2.4). Lundberg B waves are generally of shorter duration and are increases of ICP to 20 to 50 mm Hg. B waves represent rhythmic oscillations likely related to changes in vascular tone due to vasomotor instability when CPP is at the lower limit of pressure autoregulation.

2.3.2 Medical Treatment of Raised Intracranial Pressure (▶Fig. 2.5)

Head Position

The traditional practice of elevating the head at 30 to 45 degrees above the heart to lower ICP in head-injured patients has been challenged in recent years. Some argue that patients with intracranial hypertension should be placed in a horizontal position, which maximizes CPP and reduces the severity and frequency of pressure-wave occurrence. However, ICP is generally significantly higher when the patient is in the horizontal position.[14]

Recent data indicate that head elevation to 30 degrees significantly reduces ICP without reducing CPP or CBF. The neck must be maintained in a neutral position, and compression of the jugular veins must be avoided so as not to compromise jugular venous outflow. The onset of action of head elevation is immediate.

Sedatives and Paralytics

Because agitation, anxiety, pain, and uncontrolled movement can contribute to undesirable increases in ICP and cerebral metabolic demands, the use of sedatives and pharmacologic paralytics can play an effective role in managing increased ICP, especially in severe head injury. However, such drugs can alter the neurologic examination and must be used with prudence. There is no real preference for one sedative over another; the key factor is that hypotension secondary to excessive doses of a sedative should be avoided and is more prone to occur in patients with underlying hypovolemia. Additionally, shorter-acting agents allow for intermittent clinical examination.

Propofol is being increasingly used for patients in the neurosurgical intensive care unit (ICU), particularly for head-injured patients. Propofol is potentially advantageous in this setting, given its wide dose response, short elimination half-life (24–64 minutes), and potent anticonvulsant and neuroprotective effects. In contrast with the benzodiazepines and opiates, long-term propofol use does not result in addiction or withdrawal phenomena.[15] Increasing dosage requirements, however, may occur. Whether this problem is related to tolerance or an increased rate of drug clearance remains unclear. Propofol causes hypotension, particularly in volume-depleted patients. The tendency toward hypotension with propofol can be minimized if patients have a normal intravascular volume before initiating propofol; the infusion begins at a rate of less than 20 µg/kg/min and does not increase by more than 10 µg/kg/min every 5 minutes.[16] Prolonged use (> 48 hours) of high doses of propofol (> 66 µg/kg/min) has been associated with lactic acidosis, bradycardia, and lipidemia in pediatric patients. A rare complication first reported in pediatric patients and also observed in adults is known as "propofol infusion syndrome," characterized by myocardial failure, metabolic acidosis, and rhabdomyolysis. Hyperkalemia and renal failure have also been associated with this syndrome. Hypertriglyceridemia and pancreatitis are uncommon complications.[17] This can be a fatal complication.

Morphine, fentanyl, and sufentanil are common analgesics for sedation in the ICU and do not change ICP.[18] Etomidate is used to facilitate endotracheal intubations; however, even a single bolus of etomidate can cause relative adrenal insufficiency in patients with TBI. Etomidate should be avoided.[19] Midazolam can be used alone or in combination with an opiod infusion. Care must be taken to avoid hypotension.

Although pharmacologic paralysis decreases ICP in patients with refractory intracranial hypertension, early, routine, long-term use of neuromuscular blocking agents in patients with severe head injuries to manage ICP does not improve overall outcome and may actually be detrimental because of the prolongation of their ICU stay and the increased frequency of extracranial complications, such as pneumonia and respiratory failure, associated with pharmacologic paralysis.[20]

2.3.3 Osmotic Therapy

Osmotic diuretics have been widely used in the treatment of increased ICP. Although no class I evidence has been reported for comparing the efficacy of either mannitol or hypertonic saline, class II and III evidence suggests that both agents may

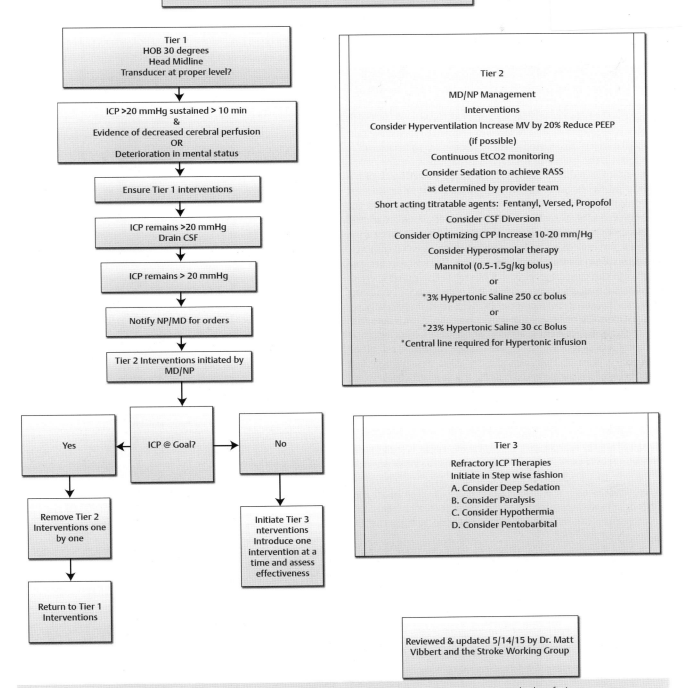

Fig. 2.5 Algorithm for elevated intracranial pressure. GCS, Glasgow Coma Scale; ICP, intracranial pressure; CPP, cerebral perfusion pressure.

Mannitol

The most commonly used diuretic is mannitol. The ICP-reducing effects of mannitol are likely to depend on several mechanisms, including an osmotic effect, a diuretic effect, and a hemodynamic effect. Traditionally, the effect of mannitol on ICP was attributed to "brain shrinkage" resulting from pulling water from the brain's interstitial space into the intravascular compartment. This effect depends on the establishment of osmotic gradients between plasma and cells. Gradients as low as 10 mOsmol/L seem to be effective in reducing ICP. It may take up to 30 minutes to develop in these patients.[22] For mannitol to be effective, the blood–brain barrier (BBB) must be preserved. Thus, an impaired BBB theoretically limits the efficacy of osmotic diuretics because an osmotic gradient cannot be formed. An osmotic gradient must be formed to drive water from the brain into the intravascular compartment. However, mannitol almost always reduces increased ICP, regardless of its cause. When 1 g mannitol/kg body weight is given over 10 minutes, a rise in serum osmolarity of 20 to 30 mOsmol/L occurs and returns to the control level in ~ 3 hours.[23] (The diuretic effect of mannitol may also contribute to ICP reduction.[21]) The direct removal of water from brain parenchyma is only partially responsible for the observed ICP reduction that follows mannitol administration. Following a bolus infusion of hyperosmolar mannitol, water is drawn from the tissues, including red blood cells, to the plasma. This immediate plasma-expanding effect reduces blood viscosity by decreasing the volume, rigidity, and cohesiveness of red blood cells.[24] Altered blood rheology results in reduced cerebrovascular resistance, increased CBF, and increased CPP. Autoregulatory vasoconstriction may then decrease cerebral blood volume (CBV) and ICP. These immediate rheologic effects of mannitol may be the primary mediators of ICP reduction.[25] Mannitol is known to open the BBB, possibly by dehydrating endothelial cells and thus causing separation of tight junctions.[26] If endothelial cells are swollen in an area of brain edema, mannitol may be of benefit in increasing CBF via increasing capillary inner diameter by decreasing the endothelial cell swelling.

Mannitol may produce immediate hypotension after rapid infusions, especially in volume-depleted patients. Renal failure is one of the most important side effects. Significant concern over renal failure often limits the use of mannitol. Although not well understood, possible mechanisms for mannitol-induced renal failure include renal afferent arteriolar vasoconstriction, renal tubular swelling, tubular vacuolation, increased intraluminal Na+ concentration at the level of macula densa, and elevation of plasma oncotic pressure.[27,28,29] Traditional treatment guidelines in clinical practice recommend that mannitol should not be administered if serum osmolarity level exceeds 320 mOsmol/L because of concern about inducing renal failure.[30,31,32] However, Gondim et al recently reported no relationship between osmolarity and renal insufficiency. Patients with preexisting conditions that are likely to impair renal function chronically appear to be at higher risk.[33]

Intermittent boluses of mannitol (0.25–1 g/kg body weight) are recommended over continuous infusion because continuous infusion is more likely to cause rebound increased ICP, particularly in cases of prolonged use of mannitol with rapid discontinuation. There are several theoretical mechanisms to explain rebound phenomenon. The most widely held explanation is penetration of osmotically active solutes into the edematous brain, their accumulation creating an unfavorable reversal of the osmotic gradient. Marshall et al have shown that reduction of ICP with a dose of 0.25 g/kg is equal to the response obtained with doses of 0.5 to 1.0 g/kg.[34]

Hypertonic Solutes

Hypertonic saline (HTS) has proven useful in the control of elevated ICP, especially when other treatments have failed. Suarez et al described eight patients (one TBI, several SAH, one glioma) administered 30-mL boluses of 23.4% HTS when refractory to mannitol.[35] All showed lowering of their ICP from a mean of 41.5 to 17 mm Hg for several hours. There was no increased serum Na+ despite multiple doses, but no change in central venous pressure (CVP) or urine output either. In another report, nine patients with cerebral vascular accident (CVA) received either 7.5% HTS or mannitol.[36] Between these patients, 30 instances of increased ICP or dilated pupils were randomly treated with either agent. An improved ICP (lowered ≥ 10%) or resolution of pupil abnormality was found in 10 of 14 patients given mannitol and all the HTS patients. A greater absolute reduction and a faster response were noted with HTS. However, the CPP improvement was better with mannitol.

Retrospective studies in children have also produced positive results. A study of 68 patients with 3% HTS therapy for refractory intracranial hypertension had good control.[37] They reported only three deaths from refractory intracranial hypertension, which was less than expected for the severity of injury. This study, however, did not include patients with "nonsurvivable injuries."[38] Gemma et al described one patient with vertebral spasm and ischemic brainstem injury after TBI.[39] The patient received 2.7% and 5.4% HTS for 48 hours each, with somatosensory evoked potentials (SSEPs) and the neurologic examination showing sustained improvement from 24 hours after initiation of therapy. Similar to mannitol and other osmotic agents, HTS's ICP-reducing effects are dependent on several mechanisms.

Hypertonic saline infusion increases the osmotic gradient between the brain and the blood and draws fluid from the interstitial space to the intravascular space.[40,41,42,43,44,45] Cerebral edema can be caused by leakage from damaged microvasculature (BBB dysfunction), vasoregulatory dysfunction, and accumulation of osmotic molecules in the interstitial and the intracellular spaces of the ischemic brain. Cell death and lysis release osmolytes into the interstitial space. Ischemic cells in the penumbra, unable to complete the metabolic cycle, collect metabolic products in the intracellular space, resulting in higher than normal parenchymal osmolarity in the entire region of the injured brain.[46,47,48] The increased serum osmolality with HTS infusion reduces the perceived osmotic gap and also reduces CSF production, which can improve intracranial compliance. Human trials showed ICP improvement for ~ 72 hours when Na+ levels increased 10 to 15 mEq/L with HTS therapy.[49,50] Hypertonic saline, as both bolus and continuous infusions, lowers ICP.[41,42,43,44,45,50] There is no evidence yet supporting one concentration of HTS above others in efficacy for controlling cerebral edema. Some studies have shown this effect to wane, and ICP increased to baseline levels when isotonic fluids were used for maintenance after an initial HTS bolus.[51,52] Even with prolonged hypernatremia, tolerance to HTS develops after several days.[50,52] The mechanism appears to be movement of cerebral osmolytes by active transport into cells in response to TBI, with increased intracellular osmolarity and loss of the osmotic gradient.[52] These osmolytes are organic molecules, including some amino acids (glutamate, glutamine, γ-aminobutyric acid, N-acetylaspartate, alanine, aspartate, and taurine), polyhydric alcohols (myoinositol), and methyl amines (creatine and glycerophosphorylcholine).[53,54] This process occurs after 3 days of a maintained hypertonic state. Sustained hyperosmolarity also increases vasopressin release and thirst, due to osmoreceptors in periventricular regions such as the lamina terminalis, which projects to the hypothalamus.[55,56]

Increases in the MAP by a hemodynamic effect of HTS infusion have been documented in human models of cardiogenic, septic, and hemorrhagic shock.[57,58,59,60,61,62,63] This has been shown to be due to multiple additive effects. HTS increases intravascular volume by causing fluid to enter the intravascular compartment.[51] It may also increase cardiac output by hormonal action.[64] The benefits of a higher MAP are accompanied by prevention of fluid overloading and hemodilution because much smaller volumes are needed. The beneficial effect on MAP is temporary (15–75 minutes) but can be extended by the addition of colloid.[39] This is likely because the intravascular volume remains higher for a longer period of time, for Na+ and Cl- can cross the capillary endothelial membranes in the rest of the body and draw intravascular fluid into the interstitial space, whereas colloids remain in the intravascular space.

Hypertonic saline therapy also has a vasoregulatory effect. Cerebral ischemia precipitated by vasomotor dysfunction is one cause of secondary brain injury.[65,66,67] Studies have also documented ischemia due to cerebral edema and vasospasm, as well as hyperperfusion in the first 2 weeks after injury.[68,69,70] Hypertonic saline therapy increases capillary vessel inner diameter and plasma volume, which counteracts vasospasm and hypoperfusion by increasing CBF. This action may come about through dehydration of endothelial cells and erythrocytes, increasing the internal diameter of vessels and improving movement of red blood cells through cerebral capillaries.[71] Hypertonic saline therapy simultaneously prevents increased ICP from hyperperfusion.[72] The net effect increases cerebral oxygen delivery and improves partial pressure of oxygen in arterial blood (PaO_2) by improved CBF and decreased pulmonary edema.[73] Primary brain injury during trauma causes extensive neuronal depolarization, increasing extracellular glutamate. Then, secondary ischemia reduces the amount of adenosine triphosphate (ATP) production, which prevents the homeostatic function of active transport transmembrane Na+/K+ exchange pumps.[74,75,76,77,78,79] The resulting lower extracellular Na+ reverses the direction of the Na+/glutamate passive cotransporter, increasing extracellular glutamate. Increased phospholipase activity and increased membrane permeability allow leakage of additional glutamate from the cell. The higher intracellular Na+ concentration opens Ca2+ channels, increasing the diffusion of water into the cell, opening stretch-sensitive channels, which allows further release of glutamate. This leads to a

positive feedback loop and can cause massive cell death.[80] Hypertonic saline can prevent pathologic glutamate release, since increased extracellular Na+ returns the Na+/glutamate pump to its normal function of glutamate reuptake. The intracellular concentrations of Na+ and Cl- and resting membrane potential are also restored. The Na+/Ca2+ pump is activated to reduce intracellular Ca2+, thereby limiting neuronal excitation.[80]

Hypertonic saline therapy has multiple immunomodulatory effects. Alterations in prostaglandin production and increases in cortisol and adrenocorticotropic hormone (ACTH) levels have been noted.[81] It has also been shown to decrease leukocyte adherence and migration.[82] Despite suppressive effects on the inflammatory system, infusion of HTS reduces the rate of infectious complications.[83] It reduces CD4+ suppression and normalizes natural killer (NK) cell activity in rat models. Hypertonic saline infusion in hemorrhagic shock models also limits the amount of bacterial translocation, reducing the risk of bacterial seeding and sepsis. Thus, HTS acts through multiple parallel complementary and interacting pathways to produce complex effects on multiple systems. The net effect is to reduce ICP and improve cardiovascular function to reduce secondary brain injury and thus, it is hoped, improve outcomes.

Hypertonic saline therapy is not without potentially adverse effects. The most serious theoretical complication of HTS therapy is the development of central pontine myelinolysis (CPM). This is the destruction of myelinated fibers after a rapid rise in serum Na+, most commonly affecting deep white matter, the pons being most susceptible. Cerebral osmolytes play a significant role in CPM, as their concentration and diffusibility affect the osmolality.[84] Literature from prospective animal studies and human case reports of correction of hyponatremia recommend increasing Na+ no more than 10 to 20 mEq/L/day.[85] However, human trials with HTS have not documented very rapid increases in Na+, with no reported cases of CPM either.[35,37,49]

The use of HTS has led to documented cases of renal insufficiency and even failure, although it is less common than with the use of other osmotic diuretics used to control cerebral edema. A quadrupled rate of renal failure in burn patients receiving HTS for resuscitation versus lactated Ringer's solution (LR) was noted, but data from this patient population, with large fluid losses, may not apply to TBI cases.[86] In 2 of 10 pediatric TBI patients with continuous HTS maintenance fluids, temporary renal insufficiency was noted, which occurred after the peak Na+ had already been passed, and was temporally associated with septic episodes. The renal failure, therefore, may not have been due to osmotic effects, but to hypotension.[50]

Hemorrhage secondary to excessive fluid resuscitation has been reported with HTS.[73,87] This is usually associated with uncontrolled primary hemorrhage. One proposed explanation for the observed coagulopathy is the dilution of plasma constituents with rapid intravascular volume expansion.[88] Decreased platelet aggregation with increased PT/PTT with 10% or more plasma replacement has also been observed.[89]

Rapid plasma volume expansion by HTS can be associated with fluid overload, particularly in patients with a preexisting heart failure. No cases of congestive heart failure or pulmonary edema were found in a retrospective study of 29 patients with SAH and hyponatremia on continuous 3% HTS infusions.[35]

Hypokalemia and hyperchloremic acidosis have both been observed when no K+ or acetate replacement was used concurrently with HTS administration.[35,45,49] These abnormalities are easily prevented by prophylactic administration of KCl and using HTS solutions with 50/50 Cl$^-$/acetate. Although HTS has been quite effective in reducing high ICPs, a rebound increase has been reported with bolus HTS doses, or after continuous HTS infusions were stopped, or even after 24 hours of continuing HTS infusion in TBI patients.[45,49,50] This may be because of the intrinsic half-life of HTS effects. However, compared with mannitol, HTS is less likely to cross the BBB and therefore less likely to cause rebound cerebral edema.[90]

2.3.4 Hyperventilation

Hyperventilation has been used in the management of intracranial hypertension for decades since Lundberg et al reported its use to lower increased ICP.[91] The reactivity of the cerebral vasculature to carbon dioxide (CO_2) is one of the primary mechanisms involved in the regulation of CBF.[92,93] Carbon dioxide reactivity involves smaller pial arteriole, and larger intracranial vessels are not significantly affected by changes in partial pressure of CO_2 in arterial blood ($PaCO_2$).[94,95] In vivo, very localized perivascular changes of $PaCO_2$ or pH can change the vascular diameter, indicating that elements of the vascular wall are responsible for effecting changes in the diameter of blood vessels. The vascular endothelium, smooth muscle cells, and extravascular cells (the perivascular nerve cells, neurons, and glia) may be involved. Changes in pH may exert their effect on smooth muscle tone through second messenger systems or by altering the Ca2+ concentration in vascular smooth muscles directly. Various agents have been identified as potential second messengers, including prostanoids, nitric oxide (NO), cyclic nucleotides, K+, and Ca2+.[96] Cerebral blood flow changes by ~ 3% for each mm Hg change in $PaCO_2$ over the range of 20 to 60 mm Hg.[97,98] The relationship between $PaCO_2$ and ICP is not linear, and the greatest effect is between $PaCO_2$ values of 30 and 50 mm Hg in humans.[99]

Carbon dioxide reactivity is preserved in most patients with severe head injury,[97,100] so hyperventilation can rapidly lower ICP through the reduction in CBV in patients with severe head injury. A recent study demonstrated that a blood volume change of only 0.5 mL was necessary to produce an ICP change of 1 mm Hg in patients with severe head injury.[101] A lower blood volume was necessary to produce a significant ICP change in patients with reduced compliance. Further, it was shown that the effects on ICP were greater during hypercapnia than during hypocapnia. In spite of the wide use of hyperventilation in the treatment of intracranial hypertension, several studies illustrate deleterious effects of hyperventilation on CBF, cerebral oxygenation, and metabolism. Using positron emission tomography imaging in the patients with severe head injury, Coles et al demonstrated that even mild hyperventilation ($PaCO_2$ < 34 mm Hg) could reduce global CBF and increase the volume of critically hypoperfused brain tissue, despite improvements in CPP and ICP.[102] Surprisingly, only a few studies have addressed the important question of whether beneficial effects on ICP remain present during prolonged hyperventilation. Only one prospective randomized clinical trial has been reported concerning the effect of hyperventilation on clinical outcome. Muizelaar et al compared the outcomes of patients who were prophylactically hyperventilated to a $PaCO_2$ of 25 mm Hg for 5 days with patients in whom the $PaCO_2$ was kept at 35 mm Hg. At both 3 and 6 months after

injury, patients with an initial Glasgow Coma Scale motor score of 4 or 5 had a significantly better outcome when they were not hyperventilated.[103,104]

Brain Trauma Foundation Guidelines recommend that prophylactic hyperventilation ($PaCO_2$ ≥ 35 mm Hg) therapy during the first 24 hours after severe TBI should not be used because it can compromise cerebral perfusion during a time when CBF is reduced. In the absence of increased ICP, chronic prolonged hyperventilation therapy ($PaCO_2$ ≥ 25 mm Hg) should be avoided after severe TBI. Jugular venous oxygen saturation (SjO_2), arterial jugular venous oxygen ($AVdO_2$) content differences, brain tissue oxygen monitoring, and CBF monitoring may help to identify cerebral ischemia if moderate hyperventilation ($PaCO_2$ < 30 mm Hg) is necessary.[2,105] Acute hyperventilation has an established role in the emergency management of acute neurologic deterioration—when there are clinical signs of herniation or acute severe elevations in ICP. Hyperventilation of brief duration may then be lifesaving until definitive management can be undertaken.[2,92,105]

2.3.5 Barbiturates

It has long been known that barbiturates can reduce ICP in a variety of clinical conditions that are associated with brain swelling.[106,107,108] The precise mechanism of ICP reduction by barbiturates is not clearly defined. One mechanism is thought to be hemodynamic alternation because of the immediate effect on ICP. Barbiturates cause a dose-dependent reversible depression of neuronal activity associated with a reduction in the cerebral metabolic rate, and it is thought that autoregulatory flow–metabolism coupling then results in reductions in CBF and CBV, thereby causing a decrease in ICP.[109,110] Barbiturates also alter cerebrovascular tone.[109,111] In addition, barbiturates act as free radical scavengers and may limit peroxidative damage to lipid membranes.[112,113,114]

Substantial side effects and complications of barbiturate therapy have been reported in the literature. They may occur despite thorough and appropriate clinical monitoring.[115,116] The most common and important complication is arterial hypotension from myocardial depression and decreased systemic vascular resistance. Hypotension caused by barbiturates is treated first with volume replacement and then with a vasopressor such as dopamine or neosynephrine, if necessary. Laboratory studies suggest that for the treatment of hypotension associated with barbiturate coma, volume resuscitation may be better than vasopressors.[117] Other complications during the treatment of intracranial hypertension with barbiturate coma include hypokalemia, respiratory complications, infectious hepatic dysfunction, renal dysfunction, and hypothermia.[115,118,119] Indications for initiating barbiturate therapy have not been clearly defined. Because of the critical hypotension associated with barbiturates, and because a neurologic examination cannot be performed during treatment, barbiturate coma is usually reserved for patients with intracranial hypertension resistant to other modalities. Thus, chances for a favorable outcome are greatest in younger patients without evidence of brainstem injury and without significant hemodynamic instability.

Pentobarbital and thiopental are relatively short-acting barbiturates. Thiopental is administered as a loading dose of 5 to 10 mg/kg, followed by a continuous infusion of 3 to 5 mg/kg per hour. Pentobarbital is also given in both loading and maintenance doses. The loading dose is 10 mg/kg, given over 30 minutes, followed by 5 mg/kg each hour for three doses. This typically provides a therapeutic level after the fourth dose. The maintenance dose is 1 to 3 mg/kg per hour, adjusted so that either the serum level is in the therapeutic range of 30 to 50 μg/mL or the electroencephalogram has a burst suppression pattern. Winer et al showed that plasma and CSF pentobarbital levels do not accurately reflect the physiologic effects of pentobarbital and recommended monitoring the electroencephalogram instead of pentobarbital levels.[120] However, if the electroencephalogram is not available immediately, initiating barbiturate therapy should not be delayed. When barbiturate therapy is undertaken, continuous monitoring of all physiologic parameters is critical. Therefore, a Swan–Ganz catheter is placed to monitor directly cardiac output, pulmonary wedge pressure, and peripheral vascular resistance in all patients.

Although high doses of barbiturate therapy have been used to treat increased ICP widely since the 1970s and several clinical trials were conducted,[106,119,121,122] none of these studies clearly proved the efficacy of barbiturates. Ward et al could not show any superiority of prophylactic barbiturate coma in a randomized trial of severely head-injured patients.[119] Schwab et al found that barbiturate coma in the therapy of increased ICP after severe hemispheric stroke can provide a short-term reduction of elevated ICP, like other conservative measures of ICP control such as osmotic therapy and hyperventilation, but that it fails to achieve sustained ICP control.[122] The most comprehensive review and meta-analysis showed that there was no evidence that barbiturate therapy in patients with acute severe head injury improved outcome. However, a randomized multicenter trial demonstrated that instituting barbiturate coma in patients with refractory ICP resulted in a 4-fold greater chance of controlling ICP.[121]

Current recommendations are that pentobarbital coma can be considered for treatment of increased ICP that is refractory to other modalities in selected patients. Patients with overwhelmingly severe injuries are not likely to benefit because their cerebral metabolic rate for oxygen ($CMRO_2$) is already markedly reduced by the injury and their outcome is already predetermined by the injury. Patients with systemic hypotension are not likely to have a good response, because hypotension limits the amount of barbiturates that can be given.

2.3.6 Hypothermia

The beneficial effects of mild to moderate hypothermia in experimental models of TBI have been demonstrated in a large number of laboratory studies.[123,124,125,126] The mechanism by which hypothermia may offer neuroprotection is not clearly defined but is thought to be multifactorial. Hypothermia can decrease the cerebral metabolic rate.[127] Autoregulatory reductions in CBF and CBV may then decrease ICP. Experimental studies in animal models have demonstrated that mild or moderate hypothermia decreases cerebral edema, reduces BBB dysfunction, and reduces extracellular levels of excitatory neurotransmitters and free radical production.[113,128,129] Adverse effects of hypothermia include a higher incidence of cardiac arrhythmias, coagulopathies, a decrease in platelet count, pulmonary infections, hypothermia-induced diuresis, pancreatitis with high serum

amylase and lipase, and electrolyte derangements. Therefore, hypothermia was applied using a strict protocol to prevent the occurrence of side effects.[124,130,131,132,133,134]

Several promising experimental trials and case series have suggested that induced hypothermia could be of benefit in reducing the risk of both the poor neurologic outcome and death in patients with severe TBI.[62,124,126,135,136,137] However, several clinical trials, including multicenter randomized trials, have reported the efficacy of induced hypothermia in decreasing the mortality and morbidity associated with severe TBI, with conflicting results.[124,125,138,139,140] McIntyre et al reviewed and analyzed 12 randomized controlled trials of therapeutic hypothermia. They found that therapeutic hypothermia was associated with a 19% reduction in the risk of death and a 22% reduction in the risk of poor neurologic outcome, compared with normothermia. Hypothermia longer than 48 hours was associated with a reduction in the risks of death and of poor neurologic outcome, compared with normothermia. Hypothermia to a target temperature between 32 and 33°C, a duration of 24 hours, and rewarming within 24 hours were all associated with reduced risks of poor neurologic outcome, compared with normothermia.[139] However, it should be noted that the meta-analysis does not indicate that mortality is lowered in groups of patients with TBI as a result of induced hypothermia as conducted in the majority of these studies. Thus, any conclusions regarding the use of hypothermia in head-injured patients are controversial and not strongly indicated by the current level of evidence.[138]

Animal studies have shown that hypothermia can alter many of the damaging effects of cerebral ischemia. Intraischemic hypothermia reduced infarct size in most occlusion models. Tissue salvage with delayed onset of hypothermia was less dramatic, but commonly observed, when hypothermia was begun within 60 minutes of stroke onset in permanent and 180 minutes of stroke onset in temporary occlusion models. Prolonged postischemic hypothermia further enhances efficacy. Studies have shown that intraischemic hypothermia is more protective than postischemic hypothermia, and more benefit is conferred in temporary than in permanent occlusion models. The efficacy of postischemic hypothermia depends on the time of initiation and the duration and depth of hypothermia.[141] Although hypothermia is remarkably neuroprotective in animal models, it may lack efficacy in human trials because it may be underdosed or overdosed. Adverse systemic effects may outweigh the benefits of brain hypothermia in a clinical trial. An open pilot study on the efficacy of induced moderate hypothermia showed hypothermia could improve clinical outcome in malignant middle cerebral artery (MCA) infarction. Some authors reported 44% mortality rate with moderate hypothermia, compared with a mortality rate of ~ 80% with standard treatment.[142,143]

2.3.7 Steroids

Glucocorticoids have been valuable adjuncts in the management of patients with intracranial tumors, both primary and metastatic. Focal neurologic deficit and decreased mental status due to peritumoral vasogenic edema may improve within hours of surgery.[144] The exact mechanism of the action of steroids remains unclear. The most common regimen is dexamethasone, but methylprednisolone can be substituted. The vasogenic edema from brain abscess may be improved with the steroid.

However, the therapeutic usefulness of steroids for abscess is controversial. Some authors believed that reducing periabscess inflammation with steroids may worsen outcome by decreasing delivery of antibiotics to the infected area.[145] Therefore, many authors recommend that steroids be reserved for cases in which mass effect is causing life-threatening herniation.[146,147] It is clear that steroids decrease the frequency of deafness and other neurologic deficits in children. Corticosteroids are now the standard of care in pediatric patients with meningitis. However, it is important to note that mortality has not been changed in studies to date.[116]

In most other situations involving increased ICP such as TBI, ischemic stroke, hemorrhage, and hypoxic encephalopathies, the routine use of steroids has not been shown to be beneficial and may be harmful.[106,148,149]

2.4 Surgical Treatment of Raised Intracranial Pressure

2.4.1 Cerebrospinal Fluid Drainage

Drainage of CSF is the most effective and rapid way of decreasing ICP. Drainage of a small amount CSF can be very effective in lowering ICP. A ventricular catheter provides for measurement of ICP and also CSF drainage for treatment of increased ICP. Because it requires penetration of the brain parenchyma in patients who often have coagulopathy, there is the risk of a ventriculostomy-related hematoma. Risk of significant hematoma requiring surgical evacuation is ~ 0.5%.[150] Infection is another important ventriculostomy-related complication. Risk factors for ventriculostomy-related infections include intracerebral hemorrhage with intraventricular hemorrhage, neurosurgical operations including operation for depressed skull fracture, ICP of 20 mm Hg or more, ventricular catheterization for more than 5 days, and irrigation of the system. Although there is no consensus regarding the use of prophylactic antibiotics with ICP monitors and ventriculostomy, most institutions use prophylactic antibiotics for ventriculostomy. Other complications of ventriculostomy include failure of optimal placement, malfunction or obstruction of drainage, and seizure.

2.4.2 Resection of Source of Mass Effect

If ICP is elevated because of a space-occupying lesion, medical intervention alone may not satisfactorily normalize ICP. Patients frequently benefit from removal of the intracranial lesion. Traumatic head injury patients with intracranial hematomas are frequently surgical candidates, depending on hematoma size, location, mass effect, or clinical condition, especially if the hematoma is epidural or subdural (▶ Table 2.2).

Surgical evacuation of spontaneous intracerebral hemorrhage remains controversial unless used as a lifesaving measure. The majority of spontaneous intracerebral hemorrhage is seated deep in the basal ganglia and thalamus and is related to hypertension. Several clinical studies have shown that no evidence of better clinical outcome was found in surgical evacuation over the best medical treatment for treatment of deep-seated intracerebral hemorrhages.[151,152] However, certain factors should be considered when evaluating surgical candidacy of patients with spontaneous intracerebral hemorrhage. Patients with significant mass effect and impending herniation may benefit from emergent surgical evacuation. However, comatose patients with evidence of lost upper brainstem reflexes and extensor posturing do poorly, regardless of surgical intervention.[153] Certainly hemorrhage in the cerebellum benefits from evacuation, especially if there are signs of obstructive hydrocephalus or compression of the brainstem, or the size of the hematoma is more than 3 cm in diameter.

For patients with a brain tumor, decision-making for surgical resection is complex unless herniation is impending. Several factors, including number, size, and location of lesions, as well as expected response of the tumor type to radiotherapy and chemotherapy, should be considered.

2.4.3 Decompressive Craniectomy

Despite the lack of prospective randomized controlled trials to define the role of decompressive craniectomy, the value of decompressive craniectomy for increased ICP associated with several neurosurgical conditions has been well reported. Disappointing experience in the past with decompressive craniectomy and lack of class I evidence, the data from recent studies on decompressive craniectomy for refractory intracranial hypertension have indicated an improved outcome compared with outcome following medical management.[154,155,156,157,158,159,160]

Most patients with an MCA stroke experience unilateral brain swelling and brain distortion that may lead to transtentorial herniation, which has up to an 80% mortality rate.[14,80,161] Recent literature reviews conclude that a significant mortality rate reduction (16–40% reduction in mortality rate), a wide therapeutic window (2–3 days), and a low incidence of intraoperative complications make decompressive craniectomy a relevant treatment in malignant MCA infarction.[162] Gupta et al reported in their review of 12 clinical series that age may be a crucial factor in predicting functional outcome after hemicraniectomy for large MCA territory infarction.[162] Good functional outcome following early emergency craniectomy for hemorrhagic infarct secondary to venous sinus thrombosis was reported, despite fixed and dilated pupils prior to operation.[163] A recent paper also describes good to excellent outcome following unilateral hemicraniectomy for poor-grade SAH patients with a large Sylvian fissure hematoma.[113] Aarabi et al found that in patients with severe head injury and brain swelling, those with an admission Glasgow Coma Scale score greater than 6 are especially good candidates for decompressive craniectomy.[154] The European Brain Injury Consortium (EBIC) and the joint Brain Trauma Foundation (BTF) and American Association of Neurological Surgeons (AANS) guidelines for severe head injuries describe decompressive craniectomy as a therapeutic option for brain edema that does not respond to conventional therapeutic measures.[105,164]

Table 2.2 Indications for surgery

Type of lesion	Indications for surgery	Timing
Acute epidural hematoma	An EDH > 30 cm³ should be surgically evacuated regardless of the patient's GCS score	It is strongly [...] with an acute [...] with anisocor [...] as soon as po:
	An EDH < 30 cm³ and with a thickness < 15 mm and with an MLS < 5 mm in patients with a GCS score > 8 without focal deficit can be managed nonoperatively with serial CT scanning and close neurologic observation in a neurosurgical center	
Acute subdural hematoma	An acute SDH with a thickness > 10 mm or an MLS > 5 mm on CT scan should be surgically evacuated, regardless of the patient's GCS score	In patients with acute SDH and indications for surgery, surgical evacuation should be performed as soon as possible
	All patients with acute SDH in coma (GCS score < 9) should undergo ICP monitoring	
	A comatose patient (GCS score < 9) with an SDH < 10 mm thick and an MLS more than 5 mm should undergo surgical evacuation of the lesion if the GCS score decreased between the time of injury and hospital admission by 2 or more points on the GCS and/or the patient presents with asymmetric or fixed and dilated pupils and/or the ICP exceeds 20 mm Hg	
Traumatic parenchymal lesions	Patients with parenchymal mass lesions and signs of progressive neurologic deterioration referable to the lesion, medically refractory intracranial hypertension, or signs of mass effect on CT scan should be treated operatively	Bifrontal decompressive craniectomy within 48 hours of injury is a treatment option for patients with diffuse, medically refractory posttraumatic cerebral edema and resultant intracranial hypertension
	Patients with GCS scores of 6–8 with frontal or temporal contusions > 20 cm³ in volume with MLS of at least 5 mm and/or cisternal compression on CT scan and patients with any lesion > 50 cm³ in volume should be treated operatively	
	Patients with parenchymal mass lesions who do not show evidence for neurologic compromise, have controlled ICP, and have no significant signs of mass effect on CT scan may be managed nonoperatively with intensive monitoring and serial imaging	
Posterior fossa mass lesions	Patients with mass effect on CT scan or with neurologic dysfunction or deterioration referable to the lesion should undergo operative intervention. Mass effect on CT scan is defined as distortion, dislocation, or obliteration of the fourth ventricle, compression or loss of visualization of the basal cisterns, or the presence of obstructive hydrocephalus	In patients with indications for surgical intervention, evacuation should be performed as soon as possible because these patients can deteriorate rapidly, thus worsening their prognosis
	Patients with lesions and no significant mass effect on CT scan and without signs of neurologic dysfunction may be managed by close observation and serial imaging	
Depressed cranial fractures	Patients with open (compound) cranial fractures depressed greater than the thickness of the cranium should undergo operative intervention to prevent infection	Early operation is recommended to reduce the incidence of infection
	Patients with open (compound) depressed cranial fractures may be treated nonoperatively if there is no clinical or radiographic evidence of dural penetration, significant intracranial hematoma, depression > 1 cm, frontal sinus involvement, gross cosmetic deformity, wound infection, pneumocephalus, and gross wound contamination	
	Nonoperative management of closed (simple) depressed cranial fractures is a treatment option	

Abbreviations: CT, computed tomography; EDH, epidural hematoma; GCS, Glasgow Coma Scale; ICP, intracranial pressure; MLS, midline shift; SDH, subdural hematoma.

2.5 Conclusion

Although successful management of intracranial hypertension remains a challenge and virtually no new and effective treatment modality has been identified, numerous clinical studies have investigated the effectiveness of management modalities of intracranial hypertension. The ineffectiveness of traditional long-standing management practices such as steroids, anticonvulsants for preventing late seizures, and chronic hyperventilation was highlighted for management of the patient with severe TBI. Although recommendations for the management of patients with intracranial hypertension are entirely based on class II and class III evidence, treatment guidelines and protocol-driven therapy for the management of patients with intracranial have increased favorable outcomes when compared with historical controls. This improvement of outcomes is a result of more rational and scientifically justified application of standard practice protocols such as the guidelines for severe TBI from the Brain Trauma Foundation.

Intracranial pressure monitoring has developed into a very useful tool for management of the patient with intracranial hypertension. It is widely accepted that a fluid-coupled system using a ventricular catheter and external transducer is considered to be the "gold standard" of ICP measurement. Ventricular ICP monitoring is the most reliable method in current use, with several advantages that include maximal accuracy, ability to recalibrate, and low cost. Intracranial pressure monitoring provides not only real-time ICP data but also prediction of outcome in patients with certain diseases, most notably severe head injury.

References

[1] Oestern HJ, Trentz O, Uranues S. Head, Thoracic, Abdominal, and Vascular Injuries: Trauma Surgery I. Berlin, Germany: Springer; 2011

[2] Brain Trauma Foundation, American Association of Neurological Surgeons, Congress of Neurological Surgeons, Joint Section on Neurotrauma and Critical Care. Guidelines for the Management of Severe Traumatic Brain Injury: Cerebral Perfusion Pressure. New York, NY: Brain Trauma Foundation; 2003 Mar 14

[3] Lang EW, Chesnut RM. Intracranial pressure: monitoring and management. Neurosurg Clin North Am 1994; 5:573–605

[4] Marshall LF, Smith RW, Shapiro HM. The outcome with aggressive treatment in severe head injuries. Part I: the significance of intracranial pressure monitoring. J Neurosurg. 1979; 50(1):20–25

[5] Marmarou A, Saad A, Aygok G, Rigsbee M. Contribution of raised ICP and hypotension to CPP reduction in severe brain injury: correlation to outcome. Acta Neurochir Suppl (Wien). 2005; 95:277–280

[6] Ratanalert S, Phuenpathom N, Saeheng S, Oearsakul T, Sripairojkul B, Hirunpat S. ICP threshold in CPP management of severe head injury patients. Surg Neurol. 2004; 61(5):429–434, discussion 434–435

[7] Resnick DK, Marion DW, Carlier P. Outcome analysis of patients with severe head injuries and prolonged intracranial hypertension. J Trauma. 1997; 42(6):1108–1111

[8] Brain Trauma Foundation. American Association of Neurological Surgeons. Congress of Neurological Surgeons. Guidelines for the management of severe traumatic brain injury. J Neurotrauma. 2007; 24:S1–S106

[9] Le Roux P, Menon DK, Citerio G, et al; Neurocritical Care Society. European Society of Intensive Care Medicine. Consensus summary statement of the International Multidisciplinary Consensus Conference on Multimodality Monitoring in Neurocritical Care: a statement for healthcare professionals from the Neurocritical Care Society and the European Society of Intensive Care Medicine. Intensive Care Med. 2014; 40(9):1189–1209

[10] Robertson CS, Valadka AB, Hannay HJ, et al. Prevention of secondary ischemic insults after severe head injury. Crit Care Med. 1999; 27(10):2086–2095

[11] Pickard JD, Czosnyka M. Management of raised intracranial pressure. J Neurol Neurosurg Psychiatry. 1993; 56(8):845–858

[12] Avezaat CJ, van Eijndhoven JH, Wyper DJ. Cerebrospinal fluid pulse pressure and intracranial volume-pressure relationships. J Neurol Neurosurg Psychiatry. 1979; 42(8):687–700

[13] Piper IR, Miller JD, Dearden NM, Leggate JRS, Robertson I. Systems analysis of cerebrovascular pressure transmission: an observational study in head-injured patients. J Neurosurg. 1990; 73(6):871–880

[14] Ropper AH. Lateral displacement of the brain and level of consciousness in patients with an acute hemispheral mass. N Engl J Med. 1986; 314(15):953–958

[15] Barr J. Propofol: a new drug for sedation in the intensive care unit. Int Anesthesiol Clin. 1995; 33(1):131–154

[16] Shafer SL. Advances in propofol pharmacokinetics and pharmacodynamics. J Clin Anesth. 1993; 5(6, Suppl 1):14S–21S

[17] De Cosmo G, Congedo E, Clemente A, Aceto P. Sedation in PACU: the role of propofol. Curr Drug Targets. 2005; 6(7):741–744

[18] Vincent JL, Berré J. Primer on medical management of severe brain injury. Crit Care Med. 2005; 33(6):1392–1399

[19] Schulz-Stübner S. Sedation in traumatic brain injury: avoid etomidate. Crit Care Med. 2005; 33(11):2723–, author reply 2723

[20] Hsiang JK, Chesnut RM, Crisp CB, Klauber MR, Blunt BA, Marshall LF. Early, routine paralysis for intracranial pressure control in severe head injury: is it necessary? Crit Care Med. 1994; 22(9):1471–1476

[21] Paczynski RP. Osmotherapy. Basic concepts and controversies. Crit Care Clin. 1997; 13(1):105–129

[22] Graham DI, Ford I, Adams JH, et al. Ischaemic brain damage is still common in fatal non-missile head injury. J Neurol Neurosurg Psychiatry. 1989; 52(3):346–350

[23] Shenkin HA, Goluboff B, Haft H. The use of mannitol for the reduction of intracranial pressure in intracranial surgery. J Neurosurg. 1962; 19:897–901

[24] Burke AM, Quest DO, Chien S, Cerri C. The effects of mannitol on blood viscosity. J Neurosurg. 1981; 55(4):550–553

[25] Schrot RJ, Muizelaar JP. Mannitol in acute traumatic brain injury. Lancet. 2002; 359(9318):1633–1634

[26] Greenwood J, Luthert PJ, Pratt OE, Lantos PL. Hyperosmolar opening of the blood-brain barrier in the energy-depleted rat brain. Part 1. Permeability studies. J Cereb Blood Flow Metab. 1988; 8(1):9–15

[27] Dziedzic T, Szczudlik A, Klimkowicz A, Rog TM, Slowik A. Is mannitol safe for patients with intracerebral hemorrhages? Renal considerations. Clin Neurol Neurosurg. 2003; 105(2):87–89

[28] Pérez-Pérez AJ, Pazos B, Sobrado J, Gonzalez L, Gándara A. Acute renal failure following massive mannitol infusion. Am J Nephrol. 2002; 22(5–6):573–575

[29] van Hengel P, Nikken JJ, de Jong GM, Hesp WL, van Bommel EF. Mannitol-induced acute renal failure. Neth J Med. 1997; 50(1):21–24

[30] Cruz J, Minoja G, Okuchi K, Facco E. Successful use of the new high-dose mannitol treatment in patients with Glasgow Coma Scale scores of 3 and bilateral abnormal pupillary widening: a randomized trial. J Neurosurg. 2004; 100(3):376–383

[31] Feig PU, McCurdy DK. The hypertonic state. N Engl J Med. 1977; 297(26):1444–1454

[32] Procaccio F, Stocchetti N, Citerio G, et al. Guidelines for the treatment of adults with severe head trauma (part II). Criteria for medical treatment. J Neurosurg Sci. 2000; 44(1):11–18

[33] Gondim FdeA, Aiyagari V, Shackleford A, Diringer MN. Osmolality not predictive of mannitol-induced acute renal insufficiency. J Neurosurg. 2005; 103(3):444–447

[34] Marshall LF, SMith RW, Rauscher LA, Shapiro HM. Mannitol dose requirements in brain-injured patients. J Neurosurg. 1978; 48(2):169–172

[35] Suarez JI, Qureshi AI, Bhardwaj A, et al. Treatment of refractory intracranial hypertension with 23.4% saline. Crit Care Med. 1998; 26(6):1118–1122

[36] Schwarz S, Schwab S, Bertram M, Aschoff A, Hacke W. Effects of hypertonic saline hydroxyethyl starch solution and mannitol in patients with increased intracranial pressure after stroke. Stroke. 1998; 29(8):1550–1555

[37] Peterson B, Khanna S, Fisher B, Marshall L. Prolonged hypernatremia controls elevated intracranial pressure in head-injured pediatric patients. Crit Care Med. 2000; 28(4):1136–1143

[38] Pfenninger J, Wagner BP. Hypertonic saline in severe pediatric head injury. Crit Care Med. 2001; 29(7):1489

[39] Gemma M, Cozzi S, Piccoli S, Magrin S, De Vitis A, Cenzato M. Hypertonic saline fluid therapy following brain stem trauma. J Neurosurg Anesthesiol. 1996; 8(2):137–141

[40] Sheikh AA, Matsuoka T, Wisner DH. Cerebral effects of resuscitation with hypertonic saline and a new low-sodium hypertonic fluid in hemorrhagic shock and head injury. Crit Care Med. 1996; 24(7):1226–1232

[41] Battistella FD, Wisner DH. Combined hemorrhagic shock and head injury: effects of hypertonic saline (7.5%) resuscitation. J Trauma. 1991; 31(2):182–188

[42] Berger S, Schürer L, Härtl R, Messmer K, Baethmann A. Reduction of post-traumatic intracranial hypertension by hypertonic/hyperoncotic saline/dextran and hypertonic mannitol. Neurosurgery. 1995; 37(1):98–107, discussion 107–108

[43] Bacher A, Wei J, Grafe MR, Quast MJ, Zornow MH. Serial determinations of cerebral water content by magnetic resonance imaging after an infusion of hypertonic saline. Crit Care Med. 1998; 26(1):108–114

[44] Freshman SP, Battistella FD, Matteucci M, Wisner DH. Hypertonic saline (7.5%) versus mannitol: a comparison for treatment of acute head injuries. J Trauma. 1993; 35(3):344–348

[45] Qureshi AI, Suarez JI, Bhardwaj A, et al. Use of hypertonic (3%) saline/acetate infusion in the treatment of cerebral edema: effect on intracranial pressure and lateral displacement of the brain. Crit Care Med. 1998; 26(3):440–446

[46] Cardin V, Peña-Segura C, Pasantes-Morales H. Activation and inactivation of taurine efflux in hyposmotic and isosmotic swelling in cortical astrocytes: role of ionic strength and cell volume decrease. J Neurosci Res. 1999; 56(6):659–667

[47] Nonaka M, Yoshimine T, Kohmura E, Wakayama A, Yamashita T, Hayakawa T. Changes in brain organic osmolytes in experimental cerebral ischemia. J Neurol Sci. 1998; 157(1):25–30

[48] Olson JE, Banks M, Dimlich RV, Evers J. Blood-brain barrier water permeability and brain osmolyte content during edema development. Acad Emerg Med. 1997; 4(7):662–673

[49] Qureshi AI, Suarez JI, Bhardwaj A. Malignant cerebral edema in patients with hypertensive intracerebral hemorrhage associated with hypertonic saline infusion: a rebound phenomenon? J Neurosurg Anesthesiol. 1998; 10(3):188–192

[50] Khanna S, Davis D, Peterson B, et al. Use of hypertonic saline in the treatment of severe refractory posttraumatic intracranial hypertension in pediatric traumatic brain injury. Crit Care Med. 2000; 28(4):1144–1151

[51] Schatzmann C, Heissler HE, König K, et al. Treatment of elevated intracranial pressure by infusions of 10% saline in severely head injured patients. Acta Neurochir Suppl (Wien). 1998; 71:31–33

[52] Trachtman H, Futterweit S, Tonidandel W, Gullans SR. The role of organic osmolytes in the cerebral cell volume regulatory response to acute and chronic renal failure. J Am Soc Nephrol. 1993; 3(12):1913–1919

[53] Lien YH, Shapiro JI, Chan L. Study of brain electrolytes and organic osmolytes during correction of chronic hyponatremia. Implications for the pathogenesis of central pontine myelinolysis. J Clin Invest. 1991; 88(1):303–309

[54] Videen JS, Michaelis T, Pinto P, Ross BD. Human cerebral osmolytes during chronic hyponatremia. A proton magnetic resonance spectroscopy study. J Clin Invest. 1995; 95(2):788–793

[55] Kobashi M, Ichikawa H, Sugimoto T, Adachi A. Response of neurons in the solitary tract nucleus, area postrema and lateral parabrachial nucleus to gastric load of hypertonic saline. Neurosci Lett. 1993; 158(1):47–50

[56] Oldfield BJ, Badoer E, Hards DK, McKinley MJ. Fos production in retrogradely labelled neurons of the lamina terminalis following intravenous infusion of either hypertonic saline or angiotensin II. Neuroscience. 1994; 60(1):255–262

[57] Walsh JC, Zhuang J, Shackford SR. A comparison of hypertonic to isotonic fluid in the resuscitation of brain injury and hemorrhagic shock. J Surg Res. 1991; 50(3):284–292

[58] Schmall LM, Muir WW, Robertson JT. Haemodynamic effects of small volume hypertonic saline in experimentally induced haemorrhagic shock. Equine Vet J. 1990; 22(4):273–277

[59] Ramires JA, Serrano Júnior CV, César LA, Velasco IT, Rocha e Silva Júnior M, Pileggi F. Acute hemodynamic effects of hypertonic (7.5%) saline infusion in patients with cardiogenic shock due to right ventricular infarction. Circ Shock. 1992; 37(3):220–225

[60] Spiers JP, Fabian TC, Kudsk KA, Proctor KG. Resuscitation of hemorrhagic shock with hypertonic saline/dextran or lactated Ringer's supplemented with AICA riboside. Circ Shock. 1993; 40(1):29–36

[61] Poli de Figueiredo LF, Peres CA, Attalah AN, et al. Hemodynamic improvement in hemorrhagic shock by aortic balloon occlusion and hypertonic saline solutions. Cardiovasc Surg. 1995; 3(6):679–686

[62] Ogata H, Luo XX. Effects of hypertonic saline solution (20%) on cardiodynamics during hemorrhagic shock. Circ Shock. 1993; 41(2):113–118

[63] Holcroft JW, Vassar MJ, Perry CA, Gannaway WL, Kramer GC. Use of a 7.5% NaCl/6% Dextran 70 solution in the resuscitation of injured patients in the emergency room. Prog Clin Biol Res. 1989; 299:331–338

[64] Tølløfsrud S, Tønnessen T, Skraastad O, Noddeland H. Hypertonic saline and dextran in normovolaemic and hypovolaemic healthy volunteers increases interstitial and intravascular fluid volumes. Acta Anaesthesiol Scand. 1998; 42(2):145–153

[65] Dickman CA, Carter LP, Baldwin HZ, Harrington T, Tallman D. Continuous regional cerebral blood flow monitoring in acute craniocerebral trauma. Neurosurgery. 1991; 28(3):467–472

[66] Hadani M, Bruk B, Ram Z, Knoller N, Bass A. Transiently increased basilar artery flow velocity following severe head injury: a time course transcranial Doppler study. J Neurotrauma. 1997; 14(9):629–636

[67] Schröder ML, Muizelaar JP, Fatouros P, Kuta AJ, Choi SC. Early cerebral blood volume after severe traumatic brain injury in patients with early cerebral ischemia. Acta Neurochir Suppl (Wien). 1998; 71:127–130

[68] Martin NA, Doberstein C, Alexander M, et al. Posttraumatic cerebral arterial spasm. J Neurotrauma. 1995; 12(5):897–901

[69] Martin NA, Patwardhan RV, Alexander MJ, et al. Characterization of cerebral hemodynamic phases following severe head trauma: hypoperfusion, hyperemia, and vasospasm. J Neurosurg. 1997; 87(1):9–19

[70] Taneda M, Kataoka K, Akai F, Asai T, Sakata I. Traumatic subarachnoid hemorrhage as a predictable indicator of delayed ischemic symptoms. J Neurosurg. 1996; 84(5):762–768

[71] Kempski O, Behmanesh S. Endothelial cell swelling and brain perfusion. J Trauma. 1997; 42(5, Suppl):S38–S40

[72] Boldt J, Zickmann B, Herold C, Ballesteros M, Dapper F, Hempelmann G. Influence of hypertonic volume replacement on the microcirculation in cardiac surgery. Br J Anaesth. 1991; 67(5):595–602

[73] Rabinovici R, Yue TL, Krausz MM, Sellers TS, Lynch KM, Feuerstein G. Hemodynamic, hematologic and eicosanoid mediated mechanisms in 7.5 percent sodium chloride treatment of uncontrolled hemorrhagic shock. Surg Gynecol Obstet. 1992; 175(4):341–354

[74] Brown JI, Baker AJ, Konasiewicz SJ, Moulton RJ. Clinical significance of CSF glutamate concentrations following severe traumatic brain injury in humans. J Neurotrauma. 1998; 15(4):253–263

[75] Bullock R, Zauner A, Woodward JJ, et al. Factors affecting excitatory amino acid release following severe human head injury. J Neurosurg. 1998; 89(4):507–518

[76] Koura SS, Doppenberg EM, Marmarou A, Choi S, Young HF, Bullock R. Relationship between excitatory amino acid release and outcome after severe human head injury. Acta Neurochir Suppl (Wien). 1998; 71:244–246

[77] Nilsson P, Laursen H, Hillered L, Hansen AJ. Calcium movements in traumatic brain injury: the role of glutamate receptor-operated ion channels. J Cereb Blood Flow Metab. 1996; 16(2):262–270

[78] Stover JF, Morganti-Kosmann MC, Lenzlinger PM, Stocker R, Kempski OS, Kossmann T. Glutamate and taurine are increased in ventricular cerebrospinal fluid of severely brain-injured patients. J Neurotrauma. 1999; 16(2):135–142

[79] Vespa P, Prins M, Ronne-Engstrom E, et al. Increase in extracellular glutamate caused by reduced cerebral perfusion pressure and seizures after human traumatic brain injury: a microdialysis study. J Neurosurg. 1998; 89(6):971–982

[80] Choi DW. Calcium: still center-stage in hypoxic-ischemic neuronal death. Trends Neurosci. 1995; 18(2):58–60

[81] Corso CO, Okamoto S, Rüttinger D, Messmer K. Hypertonic saline dextran attenuates leukocyte accumulation in the liver after hemorrhagic shock and resuscitation. J Trauma. 1999; 46(3):417–423

[82] Härtl R, Medary MB, Ruge M, Arfors KE, Ghahremani F, Ghajar J. Hypertonic/hyperoncotic saline attenuates microcirculatory disturbances after traumatic brain injury. J Trauma. 1997; 42(5, Suppl):S41–S47

[83] Coimbra R, Hoyt DB, Junger WG, et al. Hypertonic saline resuscitation decreases susceptibility to sepsis after hemorrhagic shock. J Trauma. 1997; 42(4):602–606, discussion 606–607

[84] Bourgouin PM, Chalk C, Richardson J, Duang H, Vezina JL. Subcortical white matter lesions in osmotic demyelination syndrome. AJNR Am J Neuroradiol. 1995; 16(7):1495–1497

[85] Sterns RH, Riggs JE, Schochet SS, Jr. Osmotic demyelination syndrome following correction of hyponatremia. N Engl J Med. 1986; 314(24):1535–1542

[86] Huang PP, Stucky FS, Dimick AR, Treat RC, Bessey PQ, Rue LW. Hypertonic sodium resuscitation is associated with renal failure and death. Ann Surg. 1995; 221(5):543–554, discussion 554–557

[87] Gross D, Landau EH, Assalia A, Krausz MM. Is hypertonic saline resuscitation safe in 'uncontrolled' hemorrhagic shock? J Trauma. 1988; 28(6):751–756

[88] Hess JR, Dubick MA, Summary JJ, Bangal NR, Wade CE. The effects of 7.5% NaCl/6% dextran 70 on coagulation and platelet aggregation in humans. J Trauma. 1992; 32(1):40–44

[89] Reed RL, II, Johnston TD, Chen Y, Fischer RP. Hypertonic saline alters plasma clotting times and platelet aggregation. J Trauma. 1991; 31(1):8–14

[90] Zornow MH, Scheller MS, Shackford SR. Effect of a hypertonic lactated Ringer's solution on intracranial pressure and cerebral water content in a model of traumatic brain injury. J Trauma. 1989; 29(4):484–488

[91] Lundberg N, Kjallquist A, Bien C. Reduction of increased intracranial pressure by hyperventilation. A therapeutic aid in neurological surgery. Acta Psychiatr Scand Suppl. 1959; 34(139, Suppl):1–64

[92]   Adamides AA, Winter CD, Lewis PM, Cooper DJ, Kossmann T, Rosenfeld JV. Current controversies in the management of patients with severe traumatic brain injury. ANZ J Surg. 2006; 76(3):163–174

[93]   Raichle ME, Plum F. Hyperventilation and cerebral blood flow. Stroke. 1972; 3(5):566–575

[94]   Go KG. Cerebral Pathophysiology: An Integral Approach With Some Emphasis on Clinical Implications. Amsterdam, NY: Elsevier; 1991

[95]   Giller CA, Bowman G, Dyer H, Mootz L, Krippner W. Cerebral arterial diameters during changes in blood pressure and carbon dioxide during craniotomy. Neurosurgery. 1993; 32(5):737–741, discussion 741–742

[96]   Kontos HA, Raper AJ, Patterson JL, Jr. Analysis of vasoactivity of local pH, pCO2 and bicarbonate on pial vessels. Stroke. 1977; 8(3):358–360

[97]   Cold GE. Cerebral blood flow in acute head injury. The regulation of cerebral blood flow and metabolism during the acute phase of head injury, and its significance for therapy. Acta Neurochir Suppl (Wien). 1990; 49:1–64

[98]   Obrist WD, Marion DW. Xenon techniques for CBF measurement in clinical head injury. In: Narayan RK, Wilberger J, Povlishock JT, eds. New York, NY: McGraw-Hill; 1996:471C–485C

[99]   Reivich M. Arterial pCO2 and cerebral hemodynamics. Am J Physiol. 1964; 206:25–35

[100] Stocchetti N, Mattioli C, Paparella A, et al. Bedside assessment of CO2 reactivity in head injury: changes in CBF estimated by changes in ICP and cerebral extraction of oxygen. J Neurotrauma. 1993; 10(Suppl):187

[101] Yoshihara M, Bandoh K, Marmarou A. Cerebrovascular carbon dioxide reactivity assessed by intracranial pressure dynamics in severely head injured patients. J Neurosurg. 1995; 82(3):386–393

[102] Coles JP, Minhas PS, Fryer TD, et al. Effect of hyperventilation on cerebral blood flow in traumatic head injury: clinical relevance and monitoring correlates. Crit Care Med. 2002; 30(9):1950–1959

[103] Muizelaar JP, van der Poel HG, Li ZC, Kontos HA, Levasseur JE. Pial arteriolar vessel diameter and CO2 reactivity during prolonged hyperventilation in the rabbit. J Neurosurg. 1988; 69(6):923–927

[104] Muizelaar JP, Marmarou A, Ward JD, et al. Adverse effects of prolonged hyperventilation in patients with severe head injury: a randomized clinical trial. J Neurosurg. 1991; 75(5):731–739

[105] Brain Trauma Foundation. The American Association of Neurological Surgeons. The Joint Section on Neurotrauma and Critical Care. Management and prognosis of severe traumatic brain injury, part 1: guidelines for the management of severe traumatic brain injury. J Neurotrauma. 2000; 17:451–553

[106] Dearden NM, Gibson JS, McDowall DG, Gibson RM, Cameron MM. Effect of high-dose dexamethasone on outcome from severe head injury. J Neurosurg. 1986; 64(1):81–88

[107] Piatt JH, Jr, Schiff SJ. High dose barbiturate therapy in neurosurgery and intensive care. Neurosurgery. 1984; 15(3):427–444

[108] Rea GL, Rockswold GL. Barbiturate therapy in uncontrolled intracranial hypertension. Neurosurgery. 1983; 12(4):401–404

[109] Kassell NF, Hitchon PW, Gerk MK, Sokoll MD, Hill TR. Alterations in cerebral blood flow, oxygen metabolism, and electrical activity produced by high dose sodium thiopental. Neurosurgery. 1980; 7(6):598–603

[110] Cormio M, Gopinath SP, Valadka A, Robertson CS. Cerebral hemodynamic effects of pentobarbital coma in head-injured patients. J Neurotrauma. 1999; 16(10):927–936

[111] Ochiai C, Asano T, Takakura K, Fukuda T, Horizoe H, Morimoto Y. Mechanisms of cerebral protection by pentobarbital and nizofenone correlated with the course of local cerebral blood flow changes. Stroke. 1982; 13(6):788–796

[112] Smith DS, Rehncrona S, Siesjö BK. Inhibitory effects of different barbiturates on lipid peroxidation in brain tissue in vitro: comparison with the effects of promethazine and chlorpromazine. Anesthesiology. 1980; 53(3):186–194

[113] Smith SL, Hall ED. Mild pre- and posttraumatic hypothermia attenuates blood-brain barrier damage following controlled cortical impact injury in the rat. J Neurotrauma. 1996; 13(1):1–9

[114] Demopoulos HB, Flamm ES, Pietronigro DD, Seligman ML. The free radical pathology and the microcirculation in the major central nervous system disorders. Acta Physiol Scand Suppl. 1980; 492:91–119

[115] Schalén W, Messeter K, Nordström CH. Complications and side effects during thiopentone therapy in patients with severe head injuries. Acta Anaesthesiol Scand. 1992; 36(4):369–377

[116] Wald ER, Kaplan SL, Mason EO, Jr, et al; Meningitis Study Group. Dexamethasone therapy for children with bacterial meningitis. Pediatrics. 1995; 95(1):21–28

[117] Sato M, Niiyama K, Kuroda R, Ioku M. Influence of dopamine on cerebral blood flow, and metabolism for oxygen and glucose under barbiturate administration in cats. Acta Neurochir (Wien). 1991; 110(3–4):174–180

[118] Eberhardt KE, Thimm BM, Spring A, Maskos WR. Dose-dependent rate of nosocomial pulmonary infection in mechanically ventilated patients with brain oedema receiving barbiturates: a prospective case study. Infection. 1992; 20(1):12–18

[119] Ward JD, Becker DP, Miller JD, et al. Failure of prophylactic barbiturate coma in the treatment of severe head injury. J Neurosurg. 1985; 62(3):383–388

[120] Winer JW, Rosenwasser RH, Jimenez F. Electroencephalographic activity and serum and cerebrospinal fluid pentobarbital levels in determining the therapeutic end point during barbiturate coma. Neurosurgery. 1991; 29(5):739–741, discussion 741–742

[121] Eisenberg HM, Frankowski RF, Contant CF, Marshall LF, Walker MD. High-dose barbiturate control of elevated intracranial pressure in patients with severe head injury. J Neurosurg. 1988; 69(1):15–23

[122] Schwab S, Spranger M, Schwarz S, Hacke W. Barbiturate coma in severe hemispheric stroke: useful or obsolete? Neurology. 1997; 48(6):1608–1613

[123] Biswas AK, Bruce DA, Sklar FH, Bokovoy JL, Sommerauer JF. Treatment of acute traumatic brain injury in children with moderate hypothermia improves intracranial hypertension. Crit Care Med. 2002; 30(12):2742–2751

[124] Clifton GL, Allen S, Barrodale P, et al. A phase II study of moderate hypothermia in severe brain injury. J Neurotrauma. 1993; 10(3):263–271, discussion 273

[125] Clifton GL, Miller ER, Choi SC, et al. Lack of effect of induction of hypothermia after acute brain injury. N Engl J Med. 2001; 344(8):556–563

[126] Shiozaki T, Sugimoto H, Taneda M, et al. Selection of severely head injured patients for mild hypothermia therapy. J Neurosurg. 1998; 89(2):206–211

[127] Rosomoff HL, Holaday DA. Cerebral blood flow and cerebral oxygen consumption during hypothermia. Am J Physiol. 1954; 179(1):85–88

[128] Markgraf CG, Clifton GL, Moody MR. Treatment window for hypothermia in brain injury. J Neurosurg. 2001; 95(6):979–983

[129] Globus MY, Alonso O, Dietrich WD, Busto R, Ginsberg MD. Glutamate release and free radical production following brain injury: effects of posttraumatic hypothermia. J Neurochem. 1995; 65(4):1704–1711

[130] Polderman KH, Peerdeman SM, Girbes AR. Hypophosphatemia and hypomagnesemia induced by cooling in patients with severe head injury. J Neurosurg. 2001; 94(5):697–705

[131] Reed RL, II, Johnson TD, Hudson JD, Fischer RP. The disparity between hypothermic coagulopathy and clotting studies. J Trauma. 1992; 33(3):465–470

[132] Resnick DK, Marion DW, Darby JM. The effect of hypothermia on the incidence of delayed traumatic intracerebral hemorrhage. Neurosurgery. 1994; 34(2):252–255, discussion 255–256

[133] Rohrer MJ, Natale AM. Effect of hypothermia on the coagulation cascade. Crit Care Med. 1992; 20(10):1402–1405

[134] Valeri CR, Feingold H, Cassidy G, Ragno G, Khuri S, Altschule MD. Hypothermia-induced reversible platelet dysfunction. Ann Surg. 1987; 205(2):175–181

[135] Jiang J, Yu M, Zhu C. Effect of long-term mild hypothermia therapy in patients with severe traumatic brain injury: 1-year follow-up review of 87 cases. J Neurosurg. 2000; 93(4):546–549

[136] Lyeth BGJJ, Jiang JY, Liu S. Behavioral protection by moderate hypothermia initiated after experimental traumatic brain injury. J Neurotrauma. 1993; 10(1):57–64

[137] Marion DW, Obrist WD, Carlier PM, Penrod LE, Darby JM. The use of moderate therapeutic hypothermia for patients with severe head injuries: a preliminary report. J Neurosurg. 1993; 79(3):354–362

[138] Henderson WR, Dhingra VK, Chittock DR, Fenwick JC, Ronco JJ. Hypothermia in the management of traumatic brain injury. A systematic review and meta-analysis. Intensive Care Med. 2003; 29(10):1637–1644

[139] McIntyre LA, Fergusson DA, Hébert PC, Moher D, Hutchison JS. Prolonged therapeutic hypothermia after traumatic brain injury in adults: a systematic review. JAMA. 2003; 289(22):2992–2999

[140] Shiozaki T, Hayakata T, Taneda M, et al; Mild Hypothermia Study Group in Japan. A multicenter prospective randomized controlled trial of the efficacy of mild hypothermia for severely head injured patients with low intracranial pressure. J Neurosurg. 2001; 94(1):50–54

[141] Krieger DW, Yenari MA. Therapeutic hypothermia for acute ischemic stroke: what do laboratory studies teach us? Stroke. 2004; 35(6):1482–1489

[142] Schwab S, Schwarz S, Spranger M, Keller E, Bertram M, Hacke W. Moderate hypothermia in the treatment of patients with severe middle cerebral artery infarction. Stroke. 1998; 29(12):2461–2466

[143] Schwab S, Georgiadis D, Berrouschot J, Schellinger PD, Graffagnino C, Mayer SA. Feasibility and safety of moderate hypothermia after massive hemispheric infarction. Stroke. 2001; 32(9):2033–2035

[144] French LA, Galicich JH. The use of steroids for control of cerebral edema. Clin Neurosurg. 1964; 10:212–223

[145] Davis LE, Baldwin NG. Brain abscess. Curr Treat Options Neurol. 1999; 1(2):157–166

[146] Calfee DP, Wispelwey B. Brain abscess. Semin Neurol. 2000; 20(3):353–360

[147] Mathisen GE, Johnson JP. Brain abscess. Clin Infect Dis. 1997; 25(4):763–779, quiz 780–781

[148] Bauer RB, Tellez H. Dexamethasone as treatment in cerebrovascular disease. 2. A controlled study in acute cerebral infarction. Stroke. 1973; 4(4):547–555

[149] Poungvarin N, Bhoopat W, Viriyavejakul A, et al. Effects of dexamethasone in primary supratentorial intracerebral hemorrhage. N Engl J Med. 1987; 316(20):1229–1233

[150] Narayan RK, Kishore PR, Becker DP, et al. Intracranial pressure: to monitor or not to monitor? A review of our experience with severe head injury. J Neurosurg. 1982; 56(5):650–659

[151] Batjer HH, Reisch JS, Allen BC, Plaizier LJ, Su CJ. Failure of surgery to improve outcome in hypertensive putaminal hemorrhage. A prospective randomized trial. Arch Neurol. 1990; 47(10):1103–1106

[152] Mendelow AD, Gregson BA, Fernandes HM, et al; STICH investigators. Early surgery versus initial conservative treatment in patients with spontaneous supratentorial intracerebral haematomas in the International Surgical Trial in Intracerebral Haemorrhage (STICH): a randomised trial. Lancet. 2005; 365(9457):387–397

[153] Rabinstein AA, Atkinson JL, Wijdicks EF. Emergency craniotomy in patients worsening due to expanded cerebral hematoma: to what purpose? Neurology. 2002; 58(9):1367–1372

[154] Aarabi B, Hesdorffer DC, Ahn ES, Aresco C, Scalea TM, Eisenberg HM. Outcome following decompressive craniectomy for malignant swelling due to severe head injury. J Neurosurg. 2006; 104(4):469–479

[155] Grady MS. Decompressive craniectomy. J Neurosurg. 2006; 104(4):467–468, discussion 468

[156] Jourdan C, Convert J, Mottolese C, Bachour E, Gharbi S, Artru F. [Evaluation of the clinical benefit of decompression hemicraniectomy in intracranial hypertension not controlled by medical treatment] Neurochirurgie. 1993; 39(5):304–310

[157] Polin RS, Shaffrey ME, Bogaev CA, et al. Decompressive bifrontal craniectomy in the treatment of severe refractory posttraumatic cerebral edema. Neurosurgery. 1997; 41(1):84–92, discussion 92–94

[158] Stiefel MF, Heuer GG, Smith MJ, et al. Cerebral oxygenation following decompressive hemicraniectomy for the treatment of refractory intracranial hypertension. J Neurosurg. 2004; 101(2):241–247

[159] Winter CD, Adamides A, Rosenfeld JV. The role of decompressive craniectomy in the management of traumatic brain injury: a critical review. J Clin Neurosci. 2005; 12(6):619–623

[160] Yoo DS, Kim DS, Cho KS, Huh PW, Park CK, Kang JK. Ventricular pressure monitoring during bilateral decompression with dural expansion. J Neurosurg. 1999; 91(6):953–959

[161] Hacke W, Schwab S, Horn M, Spranger M, De Georgia M, von Kummer R. 'Malignant' middle cerebral artery territory infarction: clinical course and prognostic signs. Arch Neurol. 1996; 53(4):309–315

[162] Gupta R, Connolly ES, Mayer S, Elkind MS. Hemicraniectomy for massive middle cerebral artery territory infarction: a systematic review. Stroke. 2004; 35(2):539–543

[163] Stefini R, Latronico N, Cornali C, Rasulo F, Bollati A. Emergent decompressive craniectomy in patients with fixed dilated pupils due to cerebral venous and dural sinus thrombosis: report of three cases. Neurosurgery. 1999; 45(3):626–629, discussion 629–630

[164] Maas AI, Dearden M, Teasdale GM, et al; European Brain Injury Consortium. EBIC-guidelines for management of severe head injury in adults. Acta Neurochir (Wien). 1997; 139(4):286–294

3 Invasive Multimodality Brain Monitoring

Margaret Pain, Charles Francoeur, Neha S. Dangayach, Errol Gordon, and Stephan A. Mayer

Abstract

Coma reduces the sensitivity of the neurologic examination to ongoing secondary brain injury. Multimodality monitoring (MMM) consists of an array of diagnostic tools frequently used in a critical care setting that are designed to optimize central nervous system physiology and detect secondary injury at its earliest manifestation. Intracranial pressure (ICP) and cerebral perfusion pressure (CPP) monitoring is the cornerstone of MMM. The partial pressure of oxygen in brain parenchyma ($PbtO_2$) and cerebral blood flow (CBF) sensors allow for precise determination of the adequacy of cerebral perfusion. The status of cerebral autoregulatory control can be evaluated by plotting $PbtO_2$ and CBF against CPP, and by calculating the pressure reactivity index (PRx). Tools such as intracranial electroencephalography (EEG) and continuous video EEG improve the rate of seizure detection. Microdialysis provides evidence of the metabolic consequences of central nervous system pathology and can be used to ensure adequate glucose supply, detect ischemia (which manifests as lactate/pyruvate elevation), and monitor for downstream signatures of tissue injury (glutamate and glycerol elevation). MMM sensors can be inserted via multilumen bolts and require data aggregation and display systems to allow for real-time visualization. Taken together, these devices and the physiologic relationships that they reveal can unlock powerful information about the cause and treatment of coma.

Keywords: brain tissue oxygen pressure, cerebral blood flow, cerebral perfusion pressure, coma, continuous EEG, intracranial pressure, microdialysis, multimodality monitoring

3.1 Introduction

Patients with altered mental status present formidable diagnostic and treatment challenges to physicians. Whereas mild changes in mental status can be treated symptomatically, loss of consciousness requires aggressive supportive care. Coma has a wide variety of causes and a spectrum of prognoses, each with its own treatment strategy. In the case of acute brain injury resulting from stroke, trauma, or seizures, multiple pathologic processes may be occurring simultaneously, each contributing to further secondary injury. Brain multimodality monitoring (MMM) encompasses both invasive and noninvasive technologies can provide continuous data for understanding dynamic cerebral physiology. Results from these monitors can be used to detect pathologic situations (such as increased intracranial pressure, seizures, tissue hypoxia, and metabolic crisis) in real time, allowing the clinician to act before neurologic deterioration and irreversible secondary injury occurs.

Most vital sign monitoring focuses on assessment and maintenance of cardiopulmonary stability. The designation as "vital" underscores how critical these measurements are to sustaining life in the critically ill, but not blood pressure, heart rate, or blood oxygen content can accurately describe the state of the injured brain. For decades, the most sensitive indicator of neurologic status has been the neurologic examination. The Glasgow Coma Scale (GCS) was conceived to describe the spectrum of stereotyped findings for patients with depressed level of consciousness. Lower GCS scores predict a higher likelihood of morbidity and mortality, yet they do relatively little to describe the mechanism and consequences of injury. In a comatose patient, neurologic assessment changes from a detailed description of a vast array of neurologic function to an austere approximation of the highest level of response to pain. Neurologic worsening is difficult to detect in these patients.

The primary goal of MMM is the prevention of secondary brain injury. Typically, this involves simultaneous assessment and support of brain perfusion, metabolism, and electrical activity (▶Table 3.1). This chapter addresses the fundamental concepts that underlie MMM, introduces the reader to specific techniques for addressing these concepts, and presents some suggestions for ways to develop a successful MMM system.

3.2 Intracranial Pressure and Cerebral Autoregulation

Autoregulation refers to homeostatic processes that maintain cerebral blood flow (CBF) at a constant level despite fluctuations in cerebral perfusion pressure (CPP) (▶Fig. 3.1). As the sole source of oxygen and nutrients, blood supply is the most important factor for maintaining optimal brain function. Clinical hypotension is defined, in part, by the blood pressure level at which a patient begins to develop altered mental status. Retrospective studies have also determined that hypotension significantly increases the risk of death and severe disability after brain injury.[1,2,3] Consequently, the time until blood supply is restored is one of the most important factors in determining the outcome of stroke and cardiac arrest.[4,5,6,7]

In the case of traumatic brain injury (TBI), in the absence of hypotension, it remains unclear what amount of blood flow is optimal for tissue survival and recovery. With its rich vascular supply, the brain's blood flow is directly related to CPP. An end organ in a fixed space, CPP is a function of the gradient between mean arterial blood pressure (MAP) and intracranial pressure (ICP), such that CPP = MAP − ICP. This equation is the basis for much of the science and interpretation of MMM data.

3.2.1 Physiology of Autoregulation

Investigation into cerebral autoregulation began with Nils Lassen, who demonstrated that CBF is regulated at a constant level across a wide range of CPP, from as low as 50 mm Hg to as high as 150 mm Hg in normal subjects.[8,9] When CPP is less than the lower limit of autoregulation, the cerebral arterioles are maximally dilated to permit maximal blood flow, and when CPP exceeds the upper limit, the cerebral arterioles are maximally constricted, mitigating the harmful effects of elevated perfusion pressure on the brain. Myogenic, neurogenic, metabolic, and endothelial components combine to define the upper and lower limits of autoregulatory function. Disturbances in the function or control

Table 3.1 Components of brain multimodality monitoring

Device	Physiologic parameter measured	Normal range	Pathologic condition
Continuous electroencephalography	Electrical brain activity	Alpha/delta ratio > 50% No epileptiform discharges No seizures Reactivity to stimuli	Alpha/delta ratio < 50% Epileptiform discharges Seizures No reactivity
Hemedex perfusion monitor	Cerebral blood flow (CBF)	30–50 mL/100 g/min	< 20 mL/100 g/min is indicative of ischemia assuming that metabolic demand preserved
Jugular venous oximetry	Jugular venous oxygen saturation ($SjvO_2$)	50–80%	< 50% increased oxygen extraction fraction, indicative of ischemia > 80% indicates a state of relative brain hyperemia, with reduced oxygen extraction fraction
LICOX, Raumedic	Partial pressure of oxygen in brain parenchyma ($PbtO_2$)	35–45 mm Hg	< 20 mm Hg indicative of cerebral hypoxia < 10 mm Hg severe hypoxia and likely ischemia
Cerebral microdialysis	Glucose	0.4–4.0 µmol/L	< 0.4 µmol/L is indicative of critical brain hypoglycemia
	Lactate	0.7–3.0 µmol/L	≥ 3.0 µmol/L
	Pyruvate	Unknown	Unknown
	Lactate/pyruvate ratio	< 20	> 40 indicative of ischemia and anaerobic metabolism
	Glycerol	2–10 µmol/L	> 10 µmol/L indicative of abnormal and potentially dangerous levels of glutamate release
	Glutamate	10–90 µmol/L	> 90 µmol/L indicative of cell membrane breakdown

of one or more of these factors can change the range of autoregulatory function or eliminate it completely.[10] In addition to fluctuations in pressure, cerebral vascular tone can be affected by severe hypoxia, which results in vasodilation, or extremes of partial pressure of carbon dioxide (pCO_2), which can result in vasodilation (hypercarbia) or vasoconstriction (hypocarbia).

Evidence of cerebral autoregulatory dysfunction is present in many disease states. In TBI and subarachnoid hemorrhage (SAH), patients with autoregulatory impairment have higher rates of mortality.[11] In SAH, cerebral autoregulatory dysfunction is significantly correlated with the development of delayed cerebral ischemia.[12] In ischemic stroke and carotid stenosis, cerebral autoregulatory dysfunction has been linked to infarct volume, long-term outcomes, and hemorrhagic conversion.[13,14] Finally, there is growing evidence that cerebral autoregulation and dysfunction plays a role in the development of both normal pressure and communicating hydrocephalus.[15] Improvement in hydrocephalus in these patients leads to improvement in autoregulatory control.

3.2.2 Pathologic Intracranial Pressure Elevations

Normally, ICP does not vary as a function of arterial blood pressure (ABP) or CPP. However, in states of reduced intracranial compliance, when additional volume has been added to the intracranial vault, the process of normal pressure autoregulation—resulting in vasodilation when CPP is low—can drive up ICP, a phenomenon known as "vasodilatory cascade" physiology (▶ Fig. 3.1).[16] This pathologic process is the mechanism that underlies Lundberg A and B waves: periodic elevations of ICP that occur when intracranial compliance is reduced. A waves (or

plateau waves) by definition exceed 20 mm Hg (but can exceed 100 mm Hg) and last for a minimum of 5 minutes (but can be much longer). A waves occur at irregular or random intervals, are triggered by relative hypotension, cause vasodilation, and are dangerous. The subsequent increase in ICP and reduction in CPP that results leads to more hypoperfusion and even more vasodilation, until the brain is "stuck" on a "plateau" in which ICP is elevated and CPP is reduced (▶ Fig. 3.2).[16,17] B waves also result from autoregulatory reactions to fluctuations in ABP when intracranial compliance is reduced, but they are periodic, occurring with a frequency of 0.33 to 3 cycles per minute (e.g., every 20 seconds to 3 minutes). B waves have an amplitude or less than 20 mm Hg, a duration shorter than 5 minutes, typically have a sinusoidal shape (i.e., no plateau), and are considered a marker of reduced compliance but are not directly harmful.[18]

A waves can develop suddenly, and when severe, CPP can be critically compromised. During this period, CBF and $PbtO_2$ decrease and markers of anaerobic metabolism can increase.[16] Brain MMM is designed to detect these derangements and can allow the clinician to verify that any corrective actions taken are sufficient to restore the brain to its baseline level of metabolism.

3.3 Invasive Multimodal Brain Monitoring Techniques

When developing a montage of multimodality monitors for the critically ill patient, we first ask what types of problems we are hoping to identify with the monitors. This will determine the types of monitors and timing of the setup. For example, for a patient with a large vessel occlusion and completed stroke, ICP alone may be enough to guide management, since the main

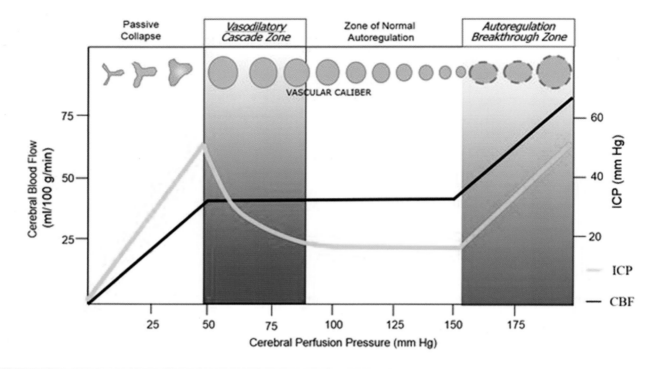

Fig. 3.1 Autoregulation allows for a constant cerebral blood flow (CBF) in the face of changing cerebral perfusion pressure (CPP) by varying vessel caliber. Over the limit of around 150 mm Hg of CPP in a healthy brain, there is endothelial injury and blood–brain barrier disruption with luxury perfusion and edema formation. Under 50 mm Hg of CPP, vasodilatation is maximal and CBF becomes directly proportional to CPP with great risks of hypoperfusion. Both hyperemia and reactive vasodilation can increase intracranial pressure (ICP) when intracranial compliance is reduced.

clinical question is if and when the patient will benefit from a surgical decompression.[19] By contrast, patients with poor grade SAH and coma are at increased risk for refractory intracranial hypertension, as well as delayed cerebral ischemia and seizures.[19,20,21] Monitors in these patients need to address all of these significant possibilities so that these complications can be recognized and reversed before causing lasting harm.

3.3.1 Intracranial Pressure and Cerebral Perfusion Pressure

Before undergoing continuous ICP monitoring, we routinely screen patients with signs and symptoms of intracranial hypertension with imaging and for signs or symptoms. Computed tomography (CT) and magnetic resonance imaging (MRI) as a rule should show evidence of increased intracranial volume (be it infarct, hematoma, tumor, cerebrospinal fluid [CSF], or vasogenic edema) and brain tissue shifting. Findings on examination such as stupor or coma, pupillary abnormalities, hyperventilation, hyperreflexia, and rigidity with motor posturing are more often a manifestation of brain shifting or herniation than a reflection of the absolute level of ICP itself. In fact, clinical signs alone are notoriously unreliable for predicting ICP. For this reason, with current technology, the only way to

truly know a patient's ICP is to directly measure it invasively. Lumbar puncture and noninvasive measurement of the optic nerve sheath diameter (> 5.5 mm indicating an 80% likelihood of increased ICP) can provide a one-time snapshot of the ICP, but even if the ICP is normal, these procedures cannot detect subsequent pathologic ICP elevations (A waves).

Physiologic Concepts

Continuous ICP and CPP monitoring is the fundamental lynchpin of brain MMM.[21] Monro, Kellie, and Burrows first studied the relationship between ICP and brain function in the 18th and 19th centuries, through studies on rabbits and human cadavers.[22,23] They correctly noted the relationship between elevated ICP and the volume of the various compartments within the skull. The Monro–Kellie doctrine states that because the adult skull has a fixed volume, an increase in the volume of any subcompartment (such as cerebral blood volume) must be met with a concomitant decrease in the volume of another subcompartment in order to maintain equal pressure. Accordingly, uncompensated increases in intracranial volume results in an increase in total ICP. In this model, blood, brain, and CSF volume all represent separate compartments. If brain volume were to increase (as in the case of cerebral edema), then other compartments (such as CSF volume) would have to decrease. Once these compensatory

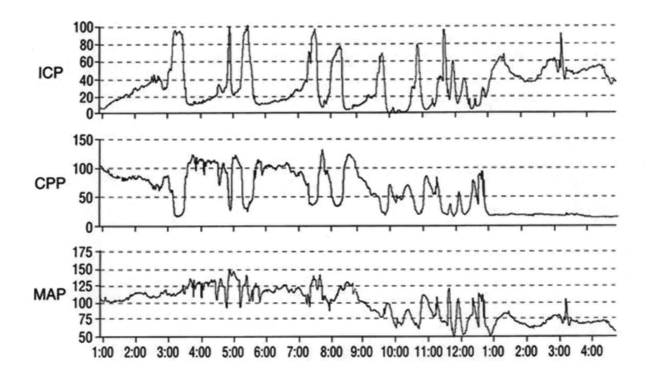

Fig. 3.2 Massive plateau intracranial pressure (ICP) elevations exceeding 80 mm Hg in a 42-year-old man with severe TBI. Note the "mirror" reduction in cerebral perfusion pressure (CPP) that occur with each ICP elevation, the progressive vasomotor instability manifesting as mean arterial pressure (MAP) fluctuations at 3:30 p.m., and the final terminal plateau wave at 1:00 a.m. In this final phase of passive collapse, the MAP and ICP tracings are identical because MAP becomes the main determinant of ICP at this point.

mechanisms are exhausted, intracranial compliance becomes progressively reduced, and even small increments in intracranial volume can lead to a drastic increase in ICP.

Intracranial Pressure and Prognosis

Intracranial pressure is clearly both an instigator and a consequence of secondary brain injury. The relationship between intracranial hypertension and mortality is well known. Retrospective case series in TBI and cardiac arrest have found an increase in the risk of morbidity and mortality when ICP consistently exceeds 22 to 25 mm Hg.[24,25,26] Current guidelines recommend that ICP be monitored in all patients with severe TBI (i.e., a GCS score of 8 or lower) in order to reduce in-hospital and 2-week postinjury mortality.[26]

Many effective treatments for intracranial hypertension exist. The most common method for treating ICP is to escalate therapy using a stepwise approach, starting with head of bed elevation and escalating to CSF drainage, sedation (and paralysis), CPP optimization, bolus osmotherapy, and hyperventilation.[27] Persistent intracranial hypertension refractory to these measures is associated with a high risk of mortality and generally should be treated with "rescue" or "salvage" hemicraniectomy. In the RESCUE ICP study, rescue craniectomy shifted nonsurvivors to survivors, but at the cost of an increased proportion of survivors with severe disability.[28] Patients who did not undergo the procedure were more likely to experience severe intracranial hypertension and had higher rates of mortality.

Intracranial Pressure Monitoring Devices

Multiple devices are currently approved for continuous ICP monitoring in the United States (▶Fig. 3.3). External ventricular drains (EVDs) have long been the gold standard for measurement and treatment of elevated ICP and hydrocephalus. At its heart, the EVD is a controlled siphon device. A fenestrated catheter is introduced through a burr hole into the lateral ventricle and threaded through the foramen of Monro. The terminus of the siphon (i.e., CSF collection receptacle) is leveled at the tragus of the ear, which is approximately the level of the third ventricle. The pressure gradient to drain the fluid is set by the level of the drain reservoir relative to the terminus of the catheter. Thus, a drain set at 15 cm will drain CSF only when the pressure at the catheter terminus is exceeds 15 cm of H_2O. This creates a simple and effective mechanism for continuous treatment of intracranial hypertension, but it has several downsides, primarily a 5 to 10% risk of ventriculostomy-related infection and lack

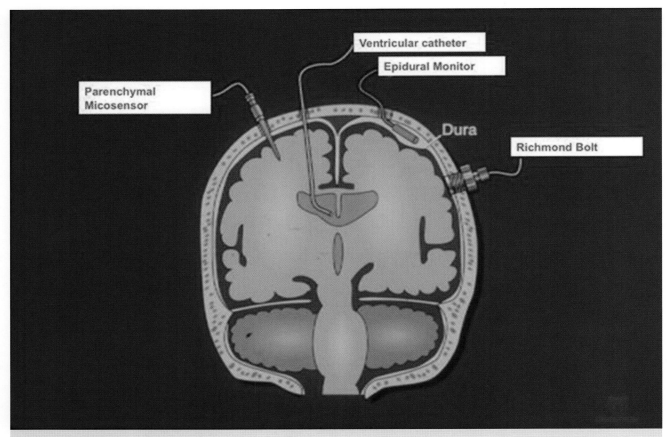

Fig. 3.3 Intracranial pressure monitoring devices.

of continuous monitoring when the system is open to drainage. For this reason, even when an EVD has been placed, it is advisable to measure ICP continuously using parenchymal probe when performing MMM.

Intraparenchymal monitors (manufactured by Camino, Codman, Spiegelberg, and Raumedic) have several advantages over EVDs as well as some disadvantages. They are easy to place, have a low risk of hemorrhage and infection, and provide continuous data. Continuous ICP is required for detecting plateau A waves as well as for calculating advanced metrics of cerebral autoregulation such as the pressure reactivity index (PRx; see below). The main disadvantage is the possibility that monitor drift can compromise data integrity, since most of these devices cannot be recalibrated to atmospheric pressure once inserted.

Less frequently utilized methods for monitoring ICP include subdural probes and epidural monitoring systems, including the hollow Richmond screw. These methods provide less reliable and robust data than current intraparenchymal options or an EVD and hence are not currently favored.

The Intracranial Pressure–Derived Pressure Reactivity Index for Assessing Autoregulation

Inherent in the process of ICP optimization is CPP optimization. If ICP reduction results in improved CBF, then improvement in CPP should accomplish the same goal. Without a mechanism for directly measuring CBF, or a surrogate for brain perfusion such as $PbtO_2$, CPP optimization has historically been directed towards maintaining a universal "one size fits all" target range. But there may be weakness to this simple approach, since all patients are obviously not the same. Early attempts at CPP-driven protocols failed to demonstrate benefit, and in some cases, they appeared to cause added harm.[29,30] This is likely to be related to the complicated and variable relationship between CBF, CPP, and cerebral autoregulation.

There are several ways to evaluate cerebral autoregulation. This adaptive characteristic of the vasculature can be quantified and analyzed as static autoregulation, whereas the rate of adaptation is referred to as dynamic autoregulation. As they both

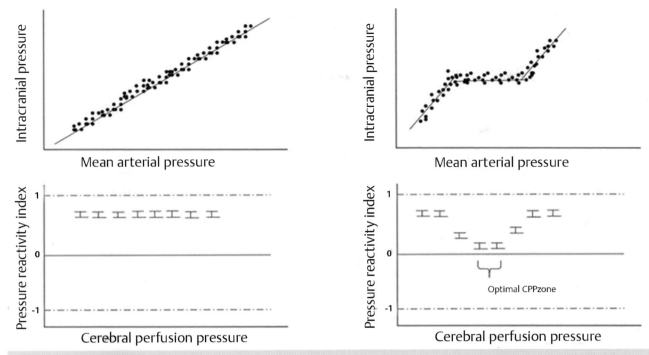

Fig. 3.4 Identifying optimal cerebral perfusion pressure. In patients with a loss of autoregulation, the relationship between intracranial pressure and mean arterial pressure appears to be linear. When the pressure reactivity index (PRx) is plotted at a specific cerebral perfusion pressure, there is no nadir in the plot, suggesting no optimal spot for autoregulation **(a)**. In patients with intact autoregulation, mean PRx values in the center of range of intact autoregulation are lower (closer to zero) than those at more extreme cerebral perfusion pressures **(b)**. CPP, cerebral perfusion pressure. (Reproduced with permission from Ko S-B. Multimodality monitoring in the neurointensive care unit: a special perspective for patients with stroke. J Stroke 2013;15:99–108.)

vary on a short-term scale, continuous monitoring, such as a running correlation coefficient, is favored over intermittent assessment such as the transient hyperemic response test.[31] The former allows derivation of a PRx, correlating 10-second clips of averaged ICP and ABP over 5 minutes.[32,33] When autoregulation is intact, slight drops in ABL result in vasodilation, which slightly increases the ICP. Thus, negative or zero values of PRx (scaled from +1 to −1) suggest appropriate cerebrovascular reactivity. Optimal CPP can be estimated by graphing PRx against CPP, with optimal CPP at the bottom of a **U**-shaped curve where PRx is most negative (▶Fig. 3.4). Steiner and colleagues showed that when observed CPP was near the derived optimal CPP, patients have improved outcomes.[34] By contrast, a positive and elevated PRx value, demonstrating autoregulatory failure, is associated with poor outcome.[31] Recent literature suggests that this information could be used to define optimal CPP for a given patient and ability to maintain optimal CPP correlates with mortality.[35] PRx has now been incorporated in recent guidelines as an adjunct to individualized decision-making process for patients with acute brain injuries.[36]

3.3.2 Brain Tissue Oxygen Monitoring

Prevention of ischemia is a central goal of neurocritical care. Brain perfusion can be studied noninvasively through CT arteriograms, CT perfusion, positron emisssion tomography (PET) imaging, and MRI, but these only provide snapshot measurements and are not practical for serial assessment. The partial

pressure of oxygen in brain parenchyma ($PbtO_2$)—normally 40 mm Hg in the cerebral cortex—can be measured directly with an intraparenchymal probe (Licox or Raumedic systems). As the product of CBF and arteriovenous oxygen content difference ($AVDO_2$; $PaO_2 - PvO_2$), values from these probes are felt to be representative of the sum of oxygen delivery, diffusion, and consumption. Hence, changes in $PbtO_2$ can be produced by increasing blood pressure and blood flow when autoregulation is impaired, improving oxygen diffusion out of the capillaries (which theoretically might occur after bolus osmotherapy), or increasing the rate of oxygen consumption (which occurs with seizures and shivering).

The optimal method for incorporating $PbtO_2$ data into clinical care remains uncertain. BOOST-2 is a clinical trial evaluating the clinical impact of $PbtO_2$ optimization in addition to conventional ICP management. Its results are expected imminently.

The oxygen reactivity index (ORx) is the Pearson correlation coefficient of $PbtO_2$ and CPP. It has been studied as a means of defining pressure passive and hyperperfusion states, with a positive correlation implying autoregulatory failure. Studies comparing PRx and ORx for predicting impaired autoregulatory failure and long-term outcomes have not shown superiority for ORx.[37]

3.3.3 Cerebral Blood Flow

Cerebral blood flow can be measured directly in the brain using thermal diffusion flowmetry (TDF; Hemedex Inc.). TDF uses the temperature differential between the probe's thermistor and temperature sensor to determine the convective and conductive heat loss to the surrounding tissue. This is mathematically correlated to regional CBF.[38] TDF technology provides real-time, continuous, and dynamic CBF data at the bedside, and TDF-derived real-time CBF (rCBF) measurements have been shown to correlate well with those obtained simultaneously using stable xenon-enhanced CT scans.[28,39] Normal rCBF values range between 40 and 70 mL/100 g/min, with rCBF less than 20 mL/100 g/min representing states of ischemia, assuming that metabolic demand is unchanged.

3.3.4 Intracortical Electroencephalography and Electrocorticography

Electrophysiology, as part of MMM, includes both surface and intracortical electroencephalography (EEG). Surface EEG, using a standard 21-electrode montage placed according to the International 10–20 system, allows detection of (mostly) nonconvulsive seizures (NCSz) and nonconvulsive status epilepticus (NCSE) in a significant proportion of brain-injured patients,[40] whether the cause is epilepsy, TBI, SAH, intracranial hypertension, or hypoxia–ischemia (▶Table 3.2). Although the evidence is sparse, most clinicians agree that both NCSz and NCSE should be treated aggressively in order to minimize secondary injury. The sooner the treatment begins, the higher the chances are of successfully terminating the seizures.[41] Whether other pathologic EEG findings in the ictal–interictal continuum deserve treatment is beyond the scope of this chapter and the object of much debate.[41]

Other information obtained with EEG, such as background reactivity and the presence of a posterior dominant rhythm or normal sleep architecture, is also useful for prognostication. In comatose patients, EEG should only be used in a continuous fashion (cEEG) for at least 48 hours in order to optimize sensitivity for the detection of seizures.[42]

Quantitaive Electroencephalography

In addition to the raw cEEG, recent technology also permits signal decomposition and analysis in an automated way using Fourier transformation, allowing quantification of amplitude, power, frequency, and rhythmicity, giving birth to quantitative EEG (qEEG). qEEG provides much faster review of long monitoring periods, and the basics of pattern recognition on qEEG can be taught to non-neurologists and nurses, enabling real-time continuous bedside monitoring. qEEG allows use of indicators such as alpha variability and the alpha/delta ratio (ADR) for detection of ischemic events.[42] For example, in one study a decrease in ADR of 40% could be used to detect delayed cerebral ischemia in SAH patients.[43]

Intracortical Electroencephalography

Subdural strip electrodes and intracortical depth electrodes are forms of intracranial invasive EEG that can detect abnormal electrophysiologic activities not visible on scalp EEG, specifically cortical spreading depolarization (CSD) and depth seizures on intracortical EEG. Intracortical EEG allows for detection of intracortical seizures that are not readily apparent on scalp EEG.[44] Using a thin wire with six discrete EEG contacts separated by 4 to 5 mm, depth EEG is usually utilized in combination with other forms of invasive brain monitoring.[45] In the first study describing this technique, approximately one third of comatose patients had no seizures detected, one third had seizures on depth and surface EEG, and one third had seizures on depth only.[44] The clinical significance of isolated seizures exclusively detected by depth EEG is not yet clear. Studies using multimodality brain monitors, however, have shown that intracortical seizures are associated with metabolic crisis after severe TBI, rising CPP and ICP, and poor outcome after aneurysmal SAH, and with CBF elevations combine with brain tissue hypoxia after cardiac arrest (▶Fig. 3.5).[46]

Electrocorticography

Electrocorticography (ECoG) involves usage of subdural strip electrodes placed on the surface of the brain. The strips have six to eight separate contacts, spaced approximately 5 mm apart. ECoG provides higher temporal and spatial resolution, less artifact, and much better signal-to-noise ratio than surface EEG. Instead of the combination of high- and low-pass filters used for traditional EEG, ECoG detects cortical spreading depolarizations (CSDs), which are slow waves of sustained direct current depolarizations in the cortex.[47] These waves are commonly observed after acute brain injury, such as severe TBI, SAH, and malignant middle cerebral artery (MCA) infarction.[47] CSD waves are associated with significant metabolic and hemodynamic changes, such as excitotoxicity, cerebral metabolic crisis, brain tissue hypoxia, and cerebral ischemia.[48] The extent to which CSD contributes to brain injury in coma states remains to be elucidated, and no treatments have been tested to date.

Table 3.2 Approximate seizure incidence in comatose patients detected by continuous electroencephalography monitoring according to underlying principal clinical diagnosis

Pathology	Electrographic seizure incidence
Ischemic stroke	5–10%
Subarachnoid hemorrhage	10–20%
Intracerebral hemorrhage	10–20%
Traumatic brain injury	20–30%
Subdural hematoma	20–30%
Hypoxic–ischemic encephalopathy	20–30%

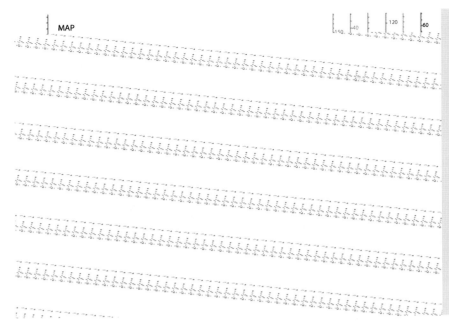

MAP

Fig. 3.5 Relationships of physiologic variables with quantitative electroencephalography (EEG) parameters (y-axes) during ictal events. The plots are 2-hour (x-axis) time recordings of (from top to bottom) mean arterial pressure (MAP), intracranial pressure (ICP), cerebral perfusion pressure (CPP), brain temperature, brain oxygen tension (PbtO$_2$), cerebral blood flow (CBF), total power EEG analysis rhymicity index, and spectrogram. During the repetitive seizure events, PbtO$_2$ consistently decreased, followed by a surge in intracranial pressure, brain temperature, and CBF. In addition, total power on the EEG is well synchronized with the rhythmicity index and the existence of high frequency waves in the spectrogram, suggesting an ictal rhythm. (Reproduced with permission from Ko SB, Ortega-Gutierrez S, Choi HA, et al. Status epilepticus-induced hyperemia and brain tissue hypoxia after cardiac arrest. Arch Neurol 2011;68:1323–1326.)

3.3.5 Brain Temperature

Fever is a common finding in patients with acute brain injury, especially in the setting of intracranial hemorrhage. Fever generates additional morbidity, since temperature elevation accelerates the metabolic rate of the damaged brain, depleting oxygen and glucose and exacerbating inflammation.[49] Therefore, prevention of fever is critical. Continuous brain tissue temperature generated by the brain tissue oxygen or CBF TDF monitor can also identify "brain thermo-pooling," a phenomenon in which brain temperature significantly exceeds core temperature.[50] A stepwise protocol for maintaining normothermia should be used in all patients.

3.3.6 Microdialysis

Although PbtO$_2$, CBF, and ICP monitoring provide a good description of systemic inputs to the brain, it is useful to assess the effect of these inputs on brain tissue. Effective delivery but ineffective utilization of blood flow, oxygen, and glucose can result in tissue damage. Microdialysis was developed in an attempt to better characterize the metabolic and biochemical environment of the brain parenchyma. It has been used for this purpose in the critical care setting for over 20 years.[51]

Equipment

Microdialysis relies on a semipermeable membrane surrounding a looped fluid-filled catheter. Dialysate fluid flowing through the inlet is fixed so that the concentration of metabolites in the outlet catheter can be measured. The semipermeable membrane excludes molecules larger than 20,000 daltons, allowing for preferential detection of the diffusion of low-molecular-weight metabolites. The system is placed into the brain parenchyma through an introducer. It can be secured to the patient by suturing to the skin or within a bolt device

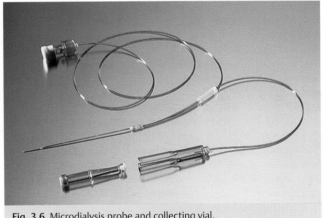

Fig. 3.6 Microdialysis probe and collecting vial.

Several physical factors affect the extrapolation and reliability of microdialysis data. The length of the catheter within the brain parenchyma and rate at which the fluid flows through the catheter determine the maximum recovery of metabolite in the dialysate. With shorter catheter length in the brain parenchyma or faster rate of fluid flow, the maximum projected recovery decreases.[52] This imposes limitations on the sampling rate, and continuous surveillance is not possible. Additionally, if the catheter is placed adjacent to structures that do not readily participate in diffusion (such as blood vessels), the rate of metabolite diffusion through the probe will be impaired.

Although several companies offer microdialysis probes and equipment, only M Dialysis (Stockholm, Sweden) offers equipment that is approved for use in humans (▶Fig. 3.6).[53] The catheter is available for either soft-tissue or bolt fixation and is intended for use with the ISCUS Flex microdialysis analyzer (Mdialysis). It is typically inserted at 10 mm into the brain parenchyma and infused at a flow rate of 0.3 µL/min, with an estimated recovery of 70% interstitial fluid composition. Sampling can be done as frequently as every 20 minutes but can be done less frequently, depending on the clinical needs of the patient.

Microdialysis Analytes

The most common target of clinical microdialysis analysis is the lactate/pyruvate ratio (LPR). In ischemic conditions, it has been demonstrated that brain tissue converts to anaerobic metabolism and pyruvate is converted to lactate rather than the citric acid cycle.[51] This alteration results in a change in the ratio of lactate and pyruvate in the brain interstitial fluid that can be detected through microdialysis. As this ratio rises, the likelihood for underlying metabolic crisis increases. Ratios greater than 25 are suggestive of crisis; ratios greater than 40 have been correlated with poor outcomes.[51]

Glucose levels in the brain interstitial liquid can reflect several different processes. In ischemic conditions, decreased delivery of glucose and a shift toward anaerobic metabolism cause a decrease in glucose concentration. In these conditions, it can be used alongside the LPR to assess the efficacy of interventions to improve ischemia. In hyperemic conditions, glucose is delivered at a rate higher than can be utilized by the tissues. During these conditions, microdialysis glucose will be elevated. Additionally, systemic hypoglycemia or hyperglycemia will be manifested in cerebral microdialysis readings.[54,55] Because of this, data concerning cerebral glucose should be interpreted in the context of systemic glucose.

As a key component of cell membrane composition, glycerol concentrations in microdialysate fluid have been hypothesized to correspond to the level of adjacent tissue injury and cell membrane breakdown. Retrospective studies of outcomes in patients with severe TBI have demonstrated survivors had lower average glycerol levels during the first 72 hours after admission.[56]

Glutamate, an excitatory neurotransmitter, has been hypothesized to be an agent of additional cell destruction during acute brain injury. It has also been observed that glutamate concentrations increase during episodes of ischemia. This is thought to be related to decreased utilization by the surrounding ischemic tissue. Patients with severe TBI who survive injury tend to have lower interstitial glutamate concentrations.[57]

3.3.7 Probe Placement, Timing, and Patient-Specific Considerations

Intraparenchymal monitors provide the advantage of measuring direct and dynamic changes in the brain. However, the data they provide reflect the conditions local to the probe and may not be reflective of anatomically distant areas.[58] Therefore, we attempt to place the probe bundles nearest to the area of injury, in areas of brain at risk, whenever possible. For example, patients with a ruptured MCA aneurysm will routinely have multimodality monitor bundles placed in the frontal lobe ipsilateral to the aneurysm. When a hemicraniectomy is performed, a small island of bone is left so that the bolt can be fixed to the ipsilateral frontal lobe at the end of the operation. For injuries without clear laterality to the insult (such as diffuse cerebral edema, meningitis, and anterior communicating artery aneurysm rupture), we prefer to place the bolt in the right frontal lobe. In the event that a right frontal EVD is also required, we

place the multimodality monitor 2 to 3 centimeters lateral and 1 to 2 centimeters anterior to Kocher's point. This arrangement usually avoids collision of the probes as well as the potential for bilateral iatrogenic injuries.

Timing of MMM placement is somewhat controversial. Although MMM can be useful in the initial neurologic resuscitation, its importance should not supersede other interventions or operations to stabilize the patient. In addition, few monitoring probes are MRI compatible, and if MRI is likely to be required within the first several days of hospitalization, it must be performed prior to monitor placement. As a result, we frequently rely on ICP readings from the EVD, MAP, and end-tidal CO_2 measurements to guide treatment until all emergent procedures and imaging studies can be acquired. As our understanding of optimal CPP improves, the timing of monitor placement is likely to become clearer.

Finally, several patient factors need to be taken into account during the planning and placement of multimodality monitors. In order to capture the most relevant pathophysiology, it is recommended that probes be placed adjacent to injured brain. In some cases, the windows of tissue available for this monitoring are quite small. For these cases, we have explored using stereotactic navigation to ensure proper probe placement. In other cases, the limits of the lesion may not be clear from a noncontrast CT scan (such as arteriovenous malformations) and additional imaging is needed prior to placement.

3.3.8 Implementation and Data Management

Even without the addition of MMM, it can be difficult for clinicians and nurses to manage all of the data produced in the intensive care unit. Although data from the monitors can be utilized for goal-directed therapy and stepwise optimization, it is far more useful when it is processed for more complex analysis, such as PRx measurements. When analyzing larger data sets for these trends, data integrity and removal of artifactual and erroneous measurements is critical in order to visualize significant trends. For the most part, maintenance of data integrity is done at the bedside. Clinicians utilizing monitors should have clear directions about escalation pathways of abnormal values, methods for assessment of dysfunctional probes, and protocols in place for timely interpretation and utilization of MMM data. Nursing staff should be trained to operate and troubleshoot the devices, continue routine nursing cares even with additional machines in the patients room, and have a basic understanding of when a device may not be connected or working properly.

On the back end, data interpretation and storage can be complicated by several factors. Many devices have their own proprietary technologies and data collection software that do not allow universal data storage. Time synchronization is another critical factor in multimodal data interpretation to allow accurate depiction of correlating data and cause-and-effect relationships. Several data acquisition and storage systems are commercially available. BedmasterEx (Excel Medical) is a hospital-based information technology program that can store high-resolution waveform data. The CNS Monitor (Moberg Research) allows for complete time synchronization of all compatible devices as well as integration with EEG, but monitors must be linked to a network in order to perform multivariate data analysis. ICM+ (Cambridge University) correlates a limited number of data types but provides time synchronization and advanced analytical tools.

3.4 Conclusion

Treatment of coma requires identification and optimization of the unique factors that contribute to brain dysfunction. As our understanding of coma has improved, several unique contributing factors have been identified to correlate to outcomes, including ICP, CBF, PbtO$_2$, and seizures. These factors can only be assessed by dedicated central nervous system monitoring. Intraparenchymal tissue monitors provide optimal assessment of the relevant variables because they are able to render continuous and direct measurement in the area of interest. Their role is likely to be clarified further as our understanding of the complex processes that underlie coma continues to evolve.

References

[1] Chesnut RM, Marshall SB, Piek J, Blunt BA, Klauber MR, Marshall LF. Early and late systemic hypotension as a frequent and fundamental source of cerebral ischemia following severe brain injury in the Traumatic Coma Data Bank. Acta Neurochir Suppl (Wien). 1993; 59:121–125

[2] Fuller G, Hasler RM, Mealing N, et al. The association between admission systolic blood pressure and mortality in significant traumatic brain injury: a multi-centre cohort study. Injury. 2014; 45(3):612–617

[3] Berry C, Ley EJ, Bukur M, et al. Redefining hypotension in traumatic brain injury. Injury. 2012; 43(11):1833–1837

[4] von Kummer R, Holle R, Rosin L, Forsting M, Hacke W. Does arterial recanalization improve outcome in carotid territory stroke? Stroke. 1995; 26(4):581–587

[5] Labiche LA, Al-Senani F, Wojner AW, Grotta JC, Malkoff M, Alexandrov AV. Is the benefit of early recanalization sustained at 3 months? A prospective cohort study. Stroke. 2003; 34(3):695–698

[6] Chen CJ, Ding D, Starke RM, et al. Endovascular vs medical management of acute ischemic stroke. Neurology. 2015; 85(22):1980–1990

[7] Hayakawa K, Tasaki O, Hamasaki T, et al. Prognostic indicators and outcome prediction model for patients with return of spontaneous circulation from cardiopulmonary arrest: the Utstein Osaka Project. Resuscitation. 2011; 82(7):874–880

[8] Lassen NA. Autoregulation of cerebral blood flow. Circ Res. 1964; 15(Suppl):201–204

[9] Lassen NA, Christensen MS. Physiology of cerebral blood flow. Br J Anaesth. 1976; 48(8):719–734

[10] Donnelly J, Budohoski KP, Smielewski P, Czosnyka M. Regulation of the cerebral circulation: bedside assessment and clinical implications. Crit Care. 2016; 20(1):129

[11] Schmidt B, Lezaic V, Weinhold M, Plontke R, Schwarze J, Klingelhöfer J. Is impaired autoregulation associated with mortality in patients with severe cerebral diseases? Acta Neurochir Suppl (Wien). 2016; 122:181–185

[12] Jaeger M, Soehle M, Schuhmann MU, Meixensberger J. Clinical significance of impaired cerebrovascular autoregulation after severe aneurysmal subarachnoid hemorrhage. Stroke. 2012; 43(8):2097–2101

[13] Jordan JD, Powers WJ. Cerebral autoregulation and acute ischemic stroke. Am J Hypertens. 2012; 25(9):946–950

[14] Budohoski KP, Czosnyka M, Smielewski P, et al. Impairment of cerebral autoregulation predicts delayed cerebral ischemia after subarachnoid hemorrhage: a prospective observational study. Stroke. 2012; 43(12):3230–3237

[15] Tanaka A, Kimura M, Nakayama Y, Yoshinaga S, Tomonaga M. Cerebral blood flow and autoregulation in normal pressure hydrocephalus. Neurosurgery. 1997; 40(6):1161–1165, discussion 1165–1167

[16] Hayashi M, Kobayashi H, Handa Y, Kawano H, Kabuto M. Brain blood volume and blood flow in patients with plateau waves. J Neurosurg. 1985; 63(4):556–561

[17] Helbok R, Olson DM, Le Roux PD, Vespa P; Participants in the International Multidisciplinary Consensus Conference on Multimodality Monitoring. Intracranial pressure and cerebral perfusion pressure monitoring in non-TBI patients: special considerations. Neurocrit Care. 2014; 21(Suppl 2):S85–S94

[18] Spiegelberg A, Preuss M, Kurtcuoglu V. B-waves revisited. Interdisciplinary neurosurgery: advanced techniques and case management. 2016; 6:13–17

[19] Komotar RJ, Schmidt JM, Starke RM, et al. Resuscitation and critical care of poor-grade subarachnoid hemorrhage. Neurosurgery. 2009; 64(3):397–410, discussion 410–411

[20] Macdonald RL. Delayed neurological deterioration after subarachnoid haemorrhage. Nat Rev Neurol. 2014; 10(1):44–58

[21] Stuart RM, Schmidt M, Kurtz P, et al. Intracranial multimodal monitoring for acute brain injury: a single institution review of current practices. Neurocrit Care. 2010; 12(2):188–198

[22] Monro A. Observations on the Structure and Functions of the Nervous System. Edinburgh, UK: Printed for, and sold by, W. Creech; 1783:176

[23] Kellie, G. On death from cold, and on congestions of the brain. In "From the Transactions of the Medico-Chirurgical Society of Edinburgh." The Royal College of Surgeons of England, 1824.

[24] Burrows G. Lumleian Lectures, On Disorders of the Cerebral Circulation: And on the Connection Between Affections of the Brain and Diseases of the Heart. Philadelphia, PA: Lea & Blanchard; 1848

[25] Gueugniaud PY, Garcia-Darennes F, Gaussorgues P, Bancalari G, Petit P, Robert D. Prognostic significance of early intracranial and cerebral perfusion pressures in post-cardiac arrest anoxic coma. Intensive Care Med. 1991; 17(7):392–398

[26] Czosnyka M, Guazzo E, Whitehouse M, et al. Significance of intracranial pressure waveform analysis after head injury. Acta Neurochir (Wien). 1996; 138(5):531–541, discussion 541–542

[27] Carney N, Totten AM, O'Reilly C, et al. Guidelines for the Management of Severe Traumatic Brain Injury. 4th ed. 2016; in press

[28] Mayer SA, Chong J. Critical care management of increased intracranial pressure. J Intensive Care Med. 2002; 17(2):55–67

[29] Hutchinson PJ, Kolias AG, Timofeev IS, et al; RESCUEicp Trial Collaborators. Trial of Decompressive Craniectomy for Traumatic Intracranial Hypertension. N Engl J Med. 2016; 375(12):1119–1130

[30] Huang SJ, Hong WC, Han YY, et al. Clinical outcome of severe head injury using three different ICP and CPP protocol-driven therapies. J Clin Neurosci. 2006; 13(8):818–822

[31] Robertson CS, Valadka AB, Hannay HJ, et al. Prevention of secondary ischemic insults after severe head injury. Crit Care Med. 1999; 27(10):2086–2095

[32] Kety SS, Schmidt CF. The effects of active and passive hyperventilation on cerebral blood flow, cerebral oxygen consumption, cardiac output, and blood pressure of normal young men. J Clin Invest. 1946; 25(1):107–119

[33] Czosnyka M, Brady K, Reinhard M, Smielewski P, Steiner LA. Monitoring of cerebrovascular autoregulation: facts, myths, and missing links. Neurocrit Care. 2009; 10(3):373–386

[34] Czosnyka M, Smielewski P, Kirkpatrick P, Laing RJ, Menon D, Pickard JD. Continuous assessment of the cerebral vasomotor reactivity in head injury. Neurosurgery. 1997; 41(1):11–17, discussion 17–19

[35] Steiner LA, Czosnyka M, Piechnik SK, et al. Continuous monitoring of cerebrovascular pressure reactivity allows determination of optimal cerebral perfusion pressure in patients with traumatic brain injury. Crit Care Med. 2002; 30(4):733–738

[36] Depreitere B, Güiza F, Van den Berghe G, et al. Pressure autoregulation monitoring and cerebral perfusion pressure target recommendation in patients with severe traumatic brain injury based on minute-by-minute monitoring data. J Neurosurg. 2014; 120(6):1451–1457

[37] Le Roux P, Menon DK, Citerio G, et al. Consensus summary statement of the International Multidisciplinary Consensus Conference on Multimodality Monitoring in Neurocritical Care: a statement for healthcare professionals from the Neurocritical Care Society and the European Society of Intensive Care Medicine. Neurocrit Care. 2014; 21(Suppl 2):S1–S26

[38] Barth M, Woitzik J, Weiss C, et al. Correlation of clinical outcome with pressure-, oxygen-, and flow-related indices of cerebrovascular reactivity in patients following aneurysmal SAH. Neurocrit Care. 2010; 12(2):234–243

[39] Jaeger M, Soehle M, Schuhmann MU, Winkler D, Meixensberger J. Correlation of continuously monitored regional cerebral blood flow and brain tissue oxygen. Acta Neurochir (Wien). 2005; 147(1):51–56, discussion 56

[40] Vajkoczy P, Roth H, Horn P, et al. Continuous monitoring of regional cerebral blood flow: experimental and clinical validation of a novel thermal diffusion microprobe. J Neurosurg. 2000; 93(2):265–274

[41] Westover MB, Shafi MM, Bianchi MT, et al. The probability of seizures during EEG monitoring in critically ill adults. Clin Neurophysiol. 2015; 126(3):463–471

[42] Claassen J, Taccone FS, Horn P, Holtkamp M, Stocchetti N, Oddo M; Neurointensive Care Section of the European Society of Intensive Care Medicine. Recommendations on the use of EEG monitoring in critically ill patients: consensus statement from the neurointensive care section of the ESICM. Intensive Care Med. 2013; 39(8):1337–1351

[43] Claassen J, Mayer SA, Kowalski RG, Emerson RG, Hirsch LJ. Detection of electrographic seizures with continuous EEG monitoring in critically ill patients. Neurology. 2004; 62(10):1743–1748

[44] Claassen J, Hirsch LJ, Kreiter KT, et al. Quantitative continuous EEG for detecting delayed cerebral ischemia in patients with poor-grade subarachnoid hemorrhage. Clin Neurophysiol. 2004; 115(12):2699–2710

[45] Waziri A, Claassen J, Stuart RM, et al. Intracortical electroencephalography in acute brain injury. Ann Neurol. 2009; 66(3):366–377

[46] Mikell CB, Dyster TG, Claassen J. Invasive seizure monitoring in the critically-ill brain injury patient: current practices and a review of the literature. Seizure. 2016; 41:201–205

[47] Vespa P, Tubi M, Claassen J, et al. Metabolic crisis occurs with seizures and periodic discharges after brain trauma. Ann Neurol. 2016; 79(4):579–590

[48] Kramer DR, Fujii T, Ohiorhenuan I, Liu CY. Cortical spreading depolarization: pathophysiology, implications, and future directions. J Clin Neurosci. 2016; 24:22–27

[49] Sakowitz OW, Santos E, Nagel A, et al. Clusters of spreading depolarizations are associated with disturbed cerebral metabolism in patients with aneurysmal subarachnoid hemorrhage. Stroke. 2013; 44(1):220–223

[50] Provencio JJ, Badjatia N; Participants in the International Multi-disciplinary Consensus . Conference on Multimodality Monitoring. Monitoring inflammation (including fever) in acute brain injury. Neurocrit Care. 2014; 21(Suppl 2):S177–S186

[51] Rossi S, Zanier ER, Mauri I, Columbo A, Stocchetti N. Brain temperature, body core temperature, and intracranial pressure in acute cerebral damage. J Neurol Neurosurg Psychiatry. 2001; 71(4):448–454

[52] de Lima Oliveira M, Kairalla AC, Fonoff ET, Martinez RC, Teixeira MJ, Bor-Seng-Shu E. Cerebral microdialysis in traumatic brain injury and subarachnoid hemorrhage: state of the art. Neurocrit Care. 2014; 21(1):152–162

[53] Galea JP, Tyrrell PJ, Patel HP, Vail A, King AT, Hopkins SJ. Pitfalls in microdialysis methodology: an in vitro analysis of temperature, pressure and catheter use. Physiol Meas. 2014; 35(3):N21–N28

[54] M Dialysis AB. www.mdialysis.com/clinical/neuro-intensive-care/products/products

[55] Magnoni S, Tedesco C, Carbonara M, Pluderi M, Colombo A, Stocchetti N. Relationship between systemic glucose and cerebral glucose is preserved in patients with severe traumatic brain injury, but glucose delivery to the brain may become limited when oxidative metabolism is impaired: implications for glycemic control. Crit Care Med. 2012; 40(6):1785–1791

[56] Kurtz P, Claassen J, Schmidt JM, et al. Reduced brain/serum glucose ratios predict cerebral metabolic distress and mortality after severe brain injury. Neurocrit Care. 2013; 19(3):311–319

[57] Clausen T, Alves OL, Reinert M, Doppenberg E, Zauner A, Bullock R. Association between elevated brain tissue glycerol levels and poor outcome following severe traumatic brain injury. J Neurosurg. 2005; 103(2):233–238

[58] Chamoun R, Suki D, Gopinath SP, Goodman JC, Robertson C. Role of extracellular glutamate measured by cerebral microdialysis in severe traumatic brain injury. J Neurosurg. 2010; 113(3):564–570

[59] Ponce LL, Pillai S, Cruz J, et al. Position of probe determines prognostic information of brain tissue PO2 in severe traumatic brain injury. Neurosurgery. 2012; 70(6):1492–1502, discussion 1502–1503

4 Management of Acute Hydrocephalus

John H. Honeycutt and David J. Donahue

Abstract

Every neurosurgeon must recognize and treat acute hydrocephalus because conditions spanning the developmental and pathologic spectrum (such as congenital and perinatal conditions, intraventricular hemorrhage and infection, subarachnoid hemorrhage, tumors and other mass lesions, and ischemic insults resulting in brain swelling with deformation or obliteration of cerebrospinal fluid [CSF] pathways) are associated with it. Even spinal disorders (i.e., tumors) can present with acute hydrocephalus. Few neurosurgical procedures produce such gratifying results as those achieved by the relief of acutely elevated intracranial pressure due to hydrocephalus. Treatment of acute hydrocephalus usually entails ventriculostomy, although lumbar puncture or endoscopic third ventriculostomy may also prove effective. Thorough understanding of the pathology underlying the patient's hydrocephalus will assure selection of the appropriate CSF diversion procedure. This chapter summarizes CSF physiology with respect to acute hydrocephalus, lists the classes of disorders associated with hydrocephalus, and details relevant operative techniques and their complications.

Keywords: acute hydrocephalus, infection, intraventricular hemorrhage, lumbar puncture, third ventriculostomy, ventriculostomy

4.1 Introduction

Acute hydrocephalus is a condition that all neurosurgeons will encounter during the course of their careers. The many etiologies of acute hydrocephalus include infection; subarachnoid hemorrhage; intracerebral or intracerebellar hemorrhage with or without intraventricular extension; sudden occlusion of cerebrospinal fluid (CSF) outflow tracts by tumor or foreign body; occlusive cerebrovascular disease; trauma; and intracranial operation. Regardless of the cause, patients can present with rapidly deteriorating neurologic conditions requiring urgent attention. "Urgent intervention," from a neurosurgical perspective, for the patient presenting in extremis with acute hydrocephalus, regardless of cause, almost always entails CSF diversion seeking to normalize intracranial pressure and allow time for further diagnostic studies or therapeutic intervention for the root cause. This chapter will discuss methods of CSF diversion in acute hydrocephalus and review some of the common causes of acute hydrocephalus. Hydrocephalus related to shunt malfunction will be covered in a different chapter.

4.2 Causes of Acute Hydrocephalus

Hydrocephalus associated with elevated intracranial pressure is the result of a derangement of normal CSF physiology in which a pressure gradient develops across the brain parenchyma from the intraventricular compartment to the extra-axial subarachnoid space.[1] This pressure gradient usually involves ventricular enlargement, ensuing parenchymal compression and obliteration of subarachnoid cisterns, forcing brain parenchyma against the inner table of the skull, which can result in neurologic compromise. Chronic or subacute processes producing a gradual derangement of CSF dynamics and progressive enlargement of the ventricles are usually better tolerated, whereas acute changes can prove fatal, either from sudden development of hydrocephalus because of an inciting event or acute deterioration in the setting of chronic hydrocephalus.

The most common cause of acquired (i.e., noncongenital) hydrocephalus is infection. Hydrocephalus in the wake of bacterial meningitis usually develops weeks after initial presentation.[2] However, there are reports in the literature of acute hydrocephalus developing within days of presentation.[2,3] Intraventricular cysts associated with parasitic infections such as neurocysticercosis can cause acute hydrocephalus by obstructing CSF outflow tracts.[4,5] Cerebellar encephalitis can produce cerebellar edema resulting in sudden obstruction of fourth ventricular CSF outflow.[6] CSF diversion in the setting of infection addresses the acute hydrocephalus until antibiotic agents take effect or the inciting inflammatory event subsides.

The second most common cause of acquired hydrocephalus is intracranial hemorrhage. Up to 27% of patients develop acute hydrocephalus following subarachnoid hemorrhage.[7,8] Many patients with intracerebral hemorrhage develop acute hydrocephalus depending on the grade and location of the hemorrhage, especially when intraventricular hemorrhage is present.[9,10,11,12] Even intracerebral hemorrhage without intraventricular extension can cause hydrocephalus when midline shift occludes the foramen of Monro, trapping the lateral ventricle. Hemorrhages deforming the cerebellum can compromise fourth ventricular outflow tracts, resulting in hydrocephalus.[13] CSF diversion addressing acute hydrocephalus improves outcomes in all these settings [11,13,14,15] save hemorrhagic dilatation of the fourth ventricle, which carries an almost 100% mortality rate.[16] ▶Fig. 4.1 shows acute hydrocephalus resulting from subarachnoid hemorrhage successfully treated by ventriculostomy.

Intraventricular mass lesions or those in the periventricular space (i.e., the foramen of Monro, the pineal region, the cerebral aqueduct, or the fourth ventricle) can all cause acute hydrocephalus or may present with an acute deterioration of a chronic condition.[17,18,19] Colloid cysts of the third ventricle are notorious for producing sudden occlusion at the foramen of Monro and sudden death (▶Fig. 4.2). Urgent CSF diversion is indicated to rescue the acutely deteriorating patient until ultimate surgical correction.[19] Clinically stable patients harboring fourth ventricular tumors, especially children, who receive steroid administration pending tumor extirpation may often avoid preoperative CSF diversion.[20]

Additional causes of acute hydrocephalus include ischemic stroke, trauma, and postoperative complications.[21,22,23,2,4,25,26] In these settings, hydrocephalus results after mass effect from hemorrhage or edema occludes CSF pathways or extends into the CSF spaces. Rarely, foreign bodies may occlude the CSF outflow tracts.[26] Diversion of CSF helps avoid further injury due to increased intracranial pressure as the primary process evolves and normal CSF absorption returns.

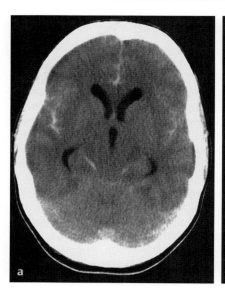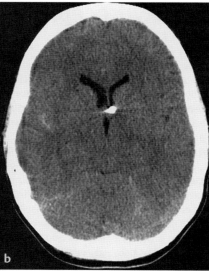

Fig. 4.1 (a) Acute hydrocephalus resulting from subarachnoid hemorrhage. Note the rounded appearance of the third ventricle and marked enlargement of the temporal horns. (b) After being treated with ventriculostomy, the ventricles are notably smaller.

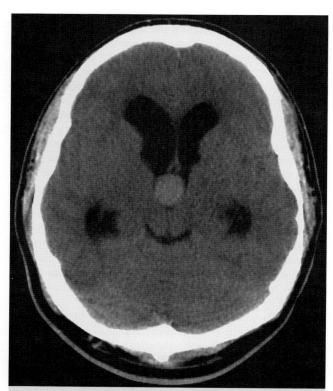

Fig. 4.2 Colloid cyst of the third ventricle and associated acute hydrocephalus. Note the colloid cyst is occluding the foramen of Monro bilaterally.

4.3 Treatment of Acute Hydrocephalus

4.3.1 Ventriculostomy

External ventricular drainage of CSF for acute hydrocephalus is the most often used CSF diversion technique. It is rapidly deployable at the bedside, has a low complication rate, and allows measurement and treatment of increased intracranial pressure. It can be lifesaving for the rapidly deteriorating patient presenting with a declining neurologic examination related to acute hydrocephalus with elevated intracranial pressure.

Ventriculostomy is not without complication. Infection, usually due to contamination by skin flora, is the most common complication and has been reported to occur with a frequency ranging from 4 to 20%.[27,28,29,30,31] Although incidence of hemorrhage associated with passing of the ventricular catheter can be up to 7%, symptomatic hemorrhage rates are less than 1%.[32] Ventricular catheter occlusion by blood products may require catheter revision, and there is a risk of suboptimal catheter positioning given the "blind" nature of the procedure.[27] Ventriculostomy associated with early aneurysm surgery has not been shown to increase the risk of rebleeding in patients suffering ventriculomegaly after subarachnoid hemorrhage,[33] but poor-grade patients still have a high risk of rebleeding after ventriculostomy.[34]

Lateral ventriculostomy may be accomplished using various techniques. Regardless of the method chosen, one must ensure that both normal coagulation and adequate platelet number and function exist. Any coagulopathy must be corrected; ideally, the platelet count surpasses 100 thousand. In this era of antiplatelet agents that may not alter the results of "standard" tests for coagulopathy, a careful medication history is essential. The risk of conservative treatment must be weighed against the potential catastrophic consequences of passing a catheter in the presence of platelet dysfunction. Neurosurgeons should keep up-to-date information on anticoagulant agents and how to counteract their effects at hand.[35] Unfortunately, hemorrhage after placement and removal is always a possibility. Using computed tomography/magnetic resonance imaging (CT/MRI) confirmation of new hemorrhage, the rates are surprisingly high (31–41%) (EVD Hemorrhage Bibliography). Fortunately, these hemorrhages rarely require evacuation but can increase external ventricular drain (EVD) malfunction rate.

CT or MRI scan confirms the diagnosis of hydrocephalus and allows the surgeon to plan the treatment. To ensure successful cannulation of the ventricle and minimize complications, careful scrutiny of the scan, especially in the face of shifted ventricular structures, and correlation of the ventricular position with other landmarks will be rewarded.

Usually the nondominant side is selected for the placement of a ventricular catheter. In the setting of intraventricular hemorrhage, we choose the lateral ventricle with the least blood to avoid rapid clogging of the catheter. In the presence of aneurysmal subarachnoid hemorrhage, a magnetic resonance angiogram (MRA), computed tomography angiogram (CTA), or even catheter angiogram can give a priori knowledge of the aneurysm location and its feeding vessels that directs the surgeons to place the ventriculostomy in a position that does not interfere with the surgical approach to the aneurysm.

Accurate catheter placement minimizes complications and preserves catheter patency. A ventricular catheter placed centrally within the ventricle, away from the choroid plexus, helps a catheter to remain functional. Frequently, insertion technique is blind and inherently inaccurate. Kitchen and colleagues' fascinating review of 183 post–EVD insertion scans showed only 40% in the ispsilateral frontal horn. Ten percent ended up within brain parenchyma. Other termini included subarachnoid space, body of lateral ventricle, third ventricle, and contralateral ventricle. Of ventricular catheters reaching an unexpected destination, 40% eventually required revision.[36] The plethora of devices seeking to address this problem attests to the frequency of suboptimal catheter positioning. Bedside computer image–guided assistance using electromagnetic technology has been shown to increase accuracy while avoiding a trip to the operating room.[37,38] Several bedside systems facilitating accurate placement without computer assistance have been shown to increase accuracy, but they are not widely used.[39]

To perform lateral ventricular puncture, we choose an entry point 1 cm anterior to the coronal suture at the midpupillary line. A small incision carried down to the skull is then fashioned at the entry point, usually utilizing a no. 15 blade. Then the periosteum is reflected, using the knife blade. Twist-drill craniostomy follows, keeping in mind the desired trajectory of the ventricular catheter through the calvarium. If necessary, the dura may be opened, using either an 18-gauge needle or a no. 11 blade. The ventricular catheter can then be advanced, stylet in place, in a trajectory orthogonal to the skull in all planes. The catheter should enter the frontal horn of the lateral ventricle at a depth of 5 to 7 cm. Sensation of an abrupt decrease in resistance to catheter passage signals ependymal transgression and ventricular entry, along with the instant appearance of CSF filling the catheter. The stylet is then removed and the catheter tunneled subcutaneously and externalized at a site distant from the entry point. The incision is closed with a nonabsorbable monofilament suture. Throughout the process, CSF egress is controlled to discourage ventricular collapse around the ventricular catheter.

An alternate method for adult lateral ventriculostomy is to localize the entry point 12 cm above the nasion in the midsagittal plane, and 3 cm from midline in the coronal plane (▶Fig. 4.3). From this point, lines are drawn toward the ipsilateral medial canthus and ipsilateral tragus. These lines provide guides for directing the ventricular catheter. The coronal plane trajectory is aligned with an imaginary plane that orthogonally intersects the skull along the medial canthus line, and the sagittal plane trajectory is lined up with an imaginary plane that orthogonally

intersects the skull along t... ter is advanced in this trajec... ed. The catheter is subseque... closed.

If lateral ventricular punctur... a trapped occipital horn withou... ent, or when a well-placed fron... ly decompress the occipital horn... prove effective. The entry point is... external occipital protuberance and... the entry point well away from the v... craniostomy is fashioned at this locat... eter is directed parallel to the long axi... cipital horn (▶Fig. 4.6).

We try to tunnel the catheter as far as possible from the skin incision. Increased distance (> 5 cm) seems to be associated with lower infection rate.[40] After tunneling, securing the ventriculostomy catheter to the skin prevents inadvertant catheter removal. At our institution, we loop the catheter and affix it to the skin at three securing suture points (▶Fig. 4.7) utilizing a special stitch, which makes it very difficult to dislodge the catheter. This stitch is illustrated in ▶Fig. 4.8. In children, we also place a simple circumferential securing stitch around the catheter at the exit site. In addition to securing stitches, we routinely place a "U" suture at the catheter exit site, with the ends left long, to close the exit site after elective catheter removal. Once secured to the scalp, the catheter is connected to a sterile drainage system.

Preventing catheter and CSF infection is always a priority. Numerous articles have documented that antibiotic- and silver-impregnated catheters can decrease infection rates (see antibiotic catheter bibliography) and now are in vogue. Antibiotic prophylaxis may be useful in preventing ventriculostomy-associated infection. In a large series, Park et al achieved an infection rate of only 8.6% in patients requiring prolonged catheterization who received prophylactic antibiotics.[30] Zingale et al showed that patients with ventriculostomies receiving only perioperative antibiotics had an 11% risk of infection versus a 3% risk for patients receiving continuous antibiotic

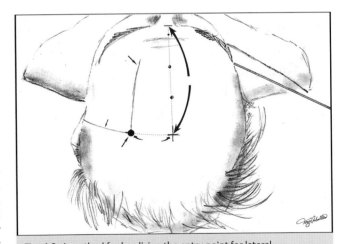

Fig. 4.3 A method for localizing the entry point for lateral ventriculostomy. Note the entry point 12 cm from the nasion in the midline and 3 cm over from the midline. Also, the tragus and medial canthus lines are shown.

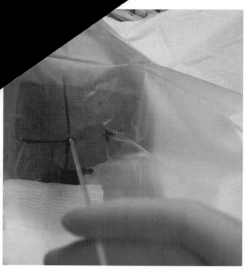

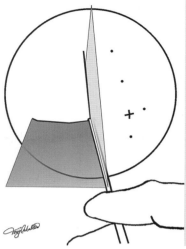

Fig. 4.4 The ventricular catheter is shown being lined up with the planes defined by the medial canthus and tragus lines. This is a line-of-sight view down the catheter. It should be noted that although it is not well represented in this figure, the catheter is medially directed toward the ipsilateral medial canthus along the medial canthus line.

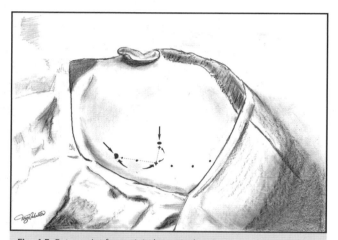

Fig. 4.5 Entry point for occipital ventriculostomy.

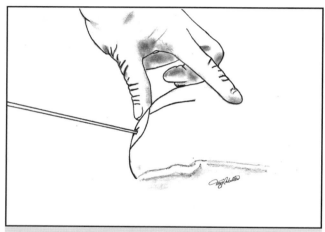

Fig. 4.6 Passing an occipital catheter. Note the catheter is passed nearly parallel with the long axis of the skull.

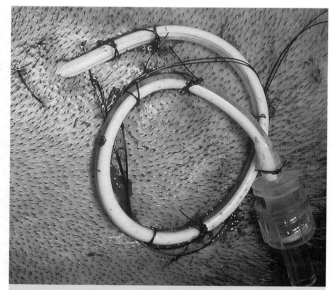

Fig. 4.7 Looping of the ventricular catheter. Note the three securing stitches. This is an important step in securing the catheter to the skin, as it greatly reduces the chances of premature removal of the catheter by the patient or by ancillary staff in performing their routine duties.

prophylaxis, although the latter tended to develop resistant bacterial or fungal infections.[31] In contrast, Murphy et al showed that postprocedure antibiotic administration has little benefit in preventing infection with use of antibiotic-coated catheters.[41] The study was conducted over 4 years, with first cohort receiving prolonged antibiotics and the second cohort receiving single dose of antibiotics at catheter insertion. This large series of 866 patients showed significantly higher rate of infection with prolonged antibiotics. Although the literature is conflicting, we routinely do not use prolonged antibiotics. Unfortunately, long-term CSF diversion is sometimes necessary. Lo et al showed in a retrospective study that duration of drainage did not correlate with infection.[42] We do not replace EVDs unless the drain malfunctions.

Using an EVD management bundle may help decrease complications. Flint et al introduced an EVD bundle to help decrease infection rates after agreement from all neurosurgeons to follow bundle protocols.[43] In 2016, the Neurocritical Care Society published their recommendations for EVD implantation and management.[44] Both of these studies used evidence-based guidelines to help implement their bundled protocols. Unfortunately, there is little class I data to help create the guidelines.

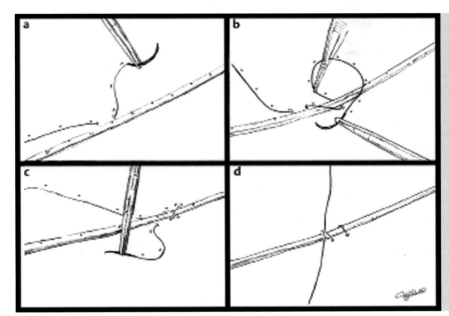

Fig. 4.8 The securing suture. **(a)** The first throw is placed parallel to the catheter. **(b)** The suture is then looped over the catheter, then passed under the catheter, and passed back over the catheter again to catch the catheter in the loop. **(c)** The second throw is then placed in the opposite direction to the first throw, parallel to and on the opposite side of the catheter. **(d)** The suture is looped around the catheter in a similar fashion to that shown in **(a)**, and the ends of the suture are tied together.

4.3.2 Lumbar Puncture/Lumbar Drainage

There are reports in the literature showing that lumbar CSF diversion in the setting of subarachnoid hemorrhage is an acceptable treatment for hydrocephalus while avoiding the potential complications of ventriculostomy.[45,46] Patients with hydrocephalus unassociated with supratentorial or infratentorial masses, obstructive mass lesion in the CSF pathways, or shift of the intracranial structures and whose basilar cisterns appear open on scans are candidates.

Hydrocephalus in this situation may be managed by repeated lumbar puncture or by placement of a lumbar drainage catheter. The latter obviates repeated lumbar punctures; however, drain output must be monitored carefully lest overdrainage and its complications occur.

Lumbar puncture's few risks include the very small likelihood of infection or injury to the lumbar nerves or cauda equina. Although technically a complication, a persistent CSF fistula can prove useful, provided that the leak remains subcutaneous as the patient decompresses the hydrocephalus, rendering repeated lumbar punctures unnecessary.

4.3.3 Endoscopic Third Ventriculostomy

Hydrocephalus secondary to obstruction of the cerebral aqueduct is usually chronic. However, acute decompensation does occur, and such patients present with acute neurologic deterioration. Endoscopic third ventriculostomy (ETV) provides a primary intervention if the patient can tolerate the delay necessary to prepare for surgery.[19,47,48] ETV addresses the hydrocephalus without the complications associated with prolonged ventricular catheterization, ventriculoperitoneal shunt, or other CSF diversion procedure involving hardware. Long-term patency of third ventriculostomy in this situation has been reported to be as high as 80%.[48] In addition to addressing the hydrocephalus, third ventriculostomy provides an opportunity to biopsy the offending lesion. Rates of successful diagnosis have been reported to be in the 90th percentile.[47] Third ventriculostomy may be performed at the time of biopsy, with discontinuation of the ventricular catheter to increase the chances of patency of the third ventriculostomy.

Risk of ETV includes hypothalamic injury, third and sixth nerve palsies, hemorrhage, cardiac arrest, basilar artery injury, and stroke. Incurred neurologic deficits tend to be transient. The overall risks of hemorrhage and neurologic deficit have been reported to range from 8 to 15%.[47,48,49]

If the patient is rapidly deteriorating and requires immediate intervention, ventriculostomy can be performed initially[50] and ETV performed later.

4.4 Conclusion

Acute hydrocephalus can be the result of many pathologic processes. In the setting of acute hydrocephalus with a deteriorating or acutely ill patient, emergency CSF diversion proves lifesaving, stabilizes the patient, provides time for definitive treatment, and allows normal CSF dynamics to return once the underlying process has run its course. Ventriculostomy, lumbar puncture, and ETV are all viable methods for managing acute hydrocephalus. The method chosen must be tailored to the individual patient, giving consideration to the underlying pathology.

4.5 Appendix

4.5.1 EVD Hemorrhage Bibliography

Gardner PA, Engh J, Atteberry D, Moossy JJ. Hemorrhage rates after external ventricular drain placement. J Neurosurg 2009;110(5):1021–1025

Miller C, Guillaume D. Incidence of hemorrhage in the pediatric population with placement and removal of external ventricular drains. J Neurosurg Pediatr 2015;16(6):662–667

Sussman ES, Kellner CP, Nelson E, et al. Hemorrhagic complications of ventriculostomy: incidence and predictors in patients with intracerebral hemorrhage. J Neurosurg 2014;120(4):931–936

4.5.2 Antibiotic Catheter Bibliography

Atkinson R, Fikrey L, Jones A, Pringle C, Patel HC. Cerebrospinal Fluid Infection Associated with Silver-Impregnated External Ventricular Drain Catheters. World Neurosurg 2016;89:505–509

Atkinson RA, Fikrey L, Vail A, Patel HC. Silver-impregnated external-ventricular-drain-related cerebrospinal fluid infections: a meta-analysis. J Hosp Infect 2016;92(3):263–272

Keong NCH, Bulters DO, Richards HK, et al. The SILVER (Silver Impregnated Line Versus EVD Randomized trial): a double-blind, prospective, randomized, controlled trial of an intervention to reduce the rate of external ventricular drain infection. Neurosurgery 2012;71(2):394–403, discussion 403–404

Root BK, Barrena BG, Mackenzie TA, Bauer DF. Antibiotic Impregnated External Ventricular Drains: Meta and Cost Analysis. World Neurosurg 2016;86:306–315

Sonabend AM, Korenfeld Y, Crisman C, Badjatia N, Mayer SA, Connolly ES Jr. Prevention of ventriculostomy-related infections with prophylactic antibiotics and antibiotic-coated external ventricular drains: a systematic review. Neurosurgery 2011;68(4):996–1005

Stevens EA, Palavecino E, Sherertz RJ, Shihabi Z, Couture DE. Effects of antibiotic-impregnated external ventricular drains on bacterial culture results: an in vitro analysis. J Neurosurg 2010;113(1):86–92

References

[1] Greitz D. Radiological assessment of hydrocephalus: new theories and implications for therapy. Neurosurg Rev. 2004; 27(3):145–165, discussion 166–167

[2] Ulloa-Gutierrez R, Avila-Agüero ML, Huertas E. Fulminant Listeria monocytogenes meningitis complicated with acute hydrocephalus in healthy children beyond the newborn period. Pediatr Emerg Care. 2004; 20(4):233–237

[3] Frat JP, Veinstein A, Wager M, Burucoa C, Robert R. Reversible acute hydrocephalus complicating Listeria monocytogenes meningitis. Eur J Clin Microbiol Infect Dis. 2001; 20(7):512–514

[4] Shanley JD, Jordan MC. Clinical aspects of CNS cysticercosis. Arch Intern Med. 1980; 140(10):1309–1313

[5] Shandera WX, White AC, Jr, Chen JC, Diaz P, Armstrong R. Neurocysticercosis in Houston, Texas. A report of 112 cases. Medicine (Baltimore). 1994; 73(1):37–52

[6] Aylett SE, O'Neill KS, De Sousa C, Britton J. Cerebellitis presenting as acute hydrocephalus. Childs Nerv Syst. 1998; 14(3):139–141

[7] Rajshekhar V, Harbaugh RE. Results of routine ventriculostomy with external ventricular drainage for acute hydrocephalus following subarachnoid haemorrhage. Acta Neurochir (Wien). 1992; 115(1–2):8–14

[8] van Gijn J, Hijdra A, Wijdicks EF, Vermeulen M, van Crevel H. Acute hydrocephalus after aneurysmal subarachnoid hemorrhage. J Neurosurg. 1985; 63(3):355–362

[9] Sumer MM, Açikgöz B, Akpinar G. External ventricular drainage for acute obstructive hydrocephalus developing following spontaneous intracerebral haemorrhage. Neurol Sci. 2002; 23(1):29–33

[10] Chung CS, Caplan LR, Han W, Pessin MS, Lee KH, Kim JM. Thalamic haemorrhage. Brain. 1996; 119(Pt 6):1873–1886

[11] Liliang PC, Liang CL, Lu CH, et al. Hypertensive caudate hemorrhage prognostic predictor, outcome, and role of external ventricular drainage. Stroke. 2001; 32(5):1195–1200

[12] Yoshimoto Y, Ochiai C, Kawamata K, Endo M, Nagai M. Aqueductal blood clot as a cause of acute hydrocephalus in subarachnoid hemorrhage. AJNR Am J Neuroradiol. 1996; 17(6):1183–1186

[13] Greenberg J, Skubick D, Shenkin H. Acute hydrocephalus in cerebellar infarct and hemorrhage. Neurology. 1979; 29(3):409–413

[14] Hochman MS. Reversal of fixed pupils after spontaneous intraventricular hemorrhage with secondary acute hydrocephalus: report of two cases treated with early ventriculostomy. Neurosurgery. 1986; 18(6):777–780

[15] Adams RE, Diringer MN. Response to external ventricular drainage in spontaneous intracerebral hemorrhage with hydrocephalus. Neurology. 1998; 50(2):519–523

[16] Shapiro SA, Campbell RL, Scully T. Hemorrhagic dilation of the fourth ventricle: an ominous predictor. J Neurosurg. 1994; 80(5):805–809

[17] Wisoff JH, Epstein F. Surgical management of symptomatic pineal cysts. J Neurosurg. 1992; 77(6):896–900

[18] Shemie S, Jay V, Rutka J, Armstrong D. Acute obstructive hydrocephalus and sudden death in children. Ann Emerg Med. 1997; 29(4):524–528

[19] Schijman E, Peter JC, Rekate HL, Sgouros S, Wong TT. Management of hydrocephalus in posterior fossa tumors: how, what, when? Childs Nerv Syst. 2004; 20(3):192–194

[20] Maher C, Friedman J, Raffel C. Posterior fossa tumors in children. In: Batjer H, Loftus C, eds. Neurological Surgery: Principles and Practice. Philadelphia, PA: Lippincott Williams and Wilkins; 2003:985–997

[21] Wolff R, Karlsson B, Dettmann E, Böttcher HD, Seifert V. Pretreatment radiation induced oedema causing acute hydrocephalus after radiosurgery for multiple cerebellar metastases. Acta Neurochir (Wien). 2003; 145(8):691–696, discussion 696

[22] Antonello RM, Pasqua M, Bosco A, Torre P. Massive cerebellar infarct complicated by hydrocephalus. Ital J Neurol Sci. 1992; 13(8):695–698

[23] Hanakita J, Kondo A. Serious complications of microvascular decompression operations for trigeminal neuralgia and hemifacial spasm. Neurosurgery. 1988; 22(2):348–352

[24] Menéndez JA, Başkaya MK, Day MA, Nanda A. Type III occipital condylar fracture presenting with hydrocephalus, vertebral artery injury and vasospasm: case report. Neuroradiology. 2001; 43(3):246–248

[25] Karasawa H, Furuya H, Naito H, Sugiyama K, Ueno J, Kin H. Acute hydrocephalus in posterior fossa injury. J Neurosurg. 1997; 86(4):629–632

[26] Lang EK. Acute hydrocephalus secondary to occlusion of the aqueduct by a bullet. J La State Med Soc. 1969; 121(5):167–168

[27] Bogdahn U, Lau W, Hassel W, Gunreben G, Mertens HG, Brawanski A. Continuous-pressure controlled, external ventricular drainage for treatment of acute hydrocephalus—evaluation of risk factors. Neurosurgery. 1992; 31(5):898–903, discussion 903–904

[28] Roitberg BZ, Khan N, Alp MS, Hersonskey T, Charbel FT, Ausman JI. Bedside external ventricular drain placement for the treatment of acute hydrocephalus. Br J Neurosurg. 2001; 15(4):324–327

[29] Stenager E, Gerner-Smidt P, Kock-Jensen C. Ventriculostomy-related infections—an epidemiological study. Acta Neurochir (Wien). 1986; 83(1–2):20–23

[30] Park P, Garton HJ, Kocan MJ, Thompson BG. Risk of infection with prolonged ventricular catheterization. Neurosurgery. 2004; 55(3):594–599, discussion 599–601

[31] Zingale A, Ippolito S, Pappalardo P, Chibbaro S, Amoroso R. Infections and re-infections in long-term external ventricular drainage. A variation upon a theme. J Neurosurg Sci. 1999; 43(2):125–132, discussion 133

[32] Wiesmann M, Mayer TE. Intracranial bleeding rates associated with two methods of external ventricular drainage. J Clin Neurosci. 2001; 8(2):126–128

[33] McIver JI, Friedman JA, Wijdicks EF, et al. Preoperative ventriculostomy and rebleeding after aneurysmal subarachnoid hemorrhage. J Neurosurg. 2002; 97(5):1042–1044

[34] Kawai K, Nagashima H, Narita K, et al. Efficacy and risk of ventricular drainage in cases of grade V subarachnoid hemorrhage. Neurol Res. 1997; 19(6):649–653

[35] Loftus CM, ed. Anticoagulation and Hemostasis in Neurosurgery. Cham, Switzerland: Springer International Publishing; 2016

[36] Toma AK, Camp S, Watkins LD, Grieve J, Kitchen ND. External ventricular drain insertion accuracy: is there a need for change in practice? Neurosurgery. 2009; 65(6):1197–1200, discussion 1200–1201

[37] Mahan M, Spetzler RF, Nakaji P. Electromagnetic stereotactic navigation for external ventricular drain placement in the intensive care unit. J Clin Neurosci. 2013; 20(12):1718–1722

[38] Patil V, Gupta R, San José Estépar R, et al. Smart stylet: the development and use of a bedside external ventricular drain image-guidance system. Stereotact Funct Neurosurg. 2015; 93(1):50–58

[39] Ghajar JB, Gae H, Oh J, Yoon S. A guide for ventricular catheter placement. Technical note. J Neurosurg. 1985; 63(6):985–986

[40] Rafiq MF, Ahmed N, Ali S. Effect of tunnel length on infection rate in patients with external ventricular drain. J Ayub Med Coll Abbottabad. 2011; 23(4):106–107

[41] Murphy RKJ, Liu B, Srinath A, et al. No additional protection against ventriculitis with prolonged systemic antibiotic prophylaxis for patients treated with antibiotic-coated external ventricular drains. J Neurosurg. 2015; 122(5):1120–1126

[42] Lo CH, Spelman D, Bailey M, Cooper DJ, Rosenfeld JV, Brecknell JE. External ventricular drain infections are independent of drain duration: an argument against elective revision. J Neurosurg. 2007; 106(3):378–383

[43] Flint AC, Rao VA, Renda NC, Faigeles BS, Lasman TE, Sheridan W. A simple protocol to prevent external ventricular drain infections. Neurosurgery. 2013; 72(6):993–999, discussion 999

[44] Fried HI, Nathan BR, Rowe AS, et al. The insertion and management of external ventricular drains: an evidence-based consensus statement. A statement for healthcare professionals from the Neurocritical Care Society. Neurocrit Care. 2016; 24(1):61–81

[45] Poon WS, Ng S, Wai S. CSF antibiotic prophylaxis for neurosurgical patients with ventriculostomy: a randomised study. Acta Neurochir Suppl (Wien). 1998; 71:146–148

[46] Hasan D, Lindsay KW, Vermeulen M. Treatment of acute hydrocephalus after subarachnoid hemorrhage with serial lumbar puncture. Stroke. 1991; 22(2):190–194

[47] Yamini B, Refai D, Rubin CM, Frim DM. Initial endoscopic management of pineal region tumors and associated hydrocephalus: clinical series and literature review. J Neurosurg. 2004; 100(5, Suppl Pediatrics):437–441

[48] Veto F, Horváth Z, Dóczi T. Biportal endoscopic management of third ventricle tumors in patients with occlusive hydrocephalus: technical note. Neurosurgery. 1997; 40(4):871–875, discussion 875–877

[49] Fukuhara T, Vorster SJ, Luciano MG. Risk factors for failure of endoscopic third ventriculostomy for obstructive hydrocephalus. Neurosurgery. 2000; 46(5):1100–1109, discussion 1109–1111

[50] Buatti JM, Friedman WA. Temporary ventricular drainage and emergency radiotherapy in the management of hydrocephalus associated with germinoma. J Neurosurg. 2002; 96(6):1020–1022

5 The Recognition and Management of Cerebral Herniation Syndromes

Daphne D. Li and Vikram C. Prabhu

Abstract

Cerebral herniation occurs as a result of abnormal displacement of brain tissue from its physiologic compartment. This may occur as a result of an imbalance in the distribution of blood, cerebrospinal fluid (CSF), and brain tissue that occupy the intracranial space, or a mass lesion. Although not all instances of anatomical cerebral herniation are associated with significant neurologic findings or morbidity, rapidly shifting pressure gradients or expanding mass lesions often result in devastating progression of neurologic deficits associated with high risk of morbidity and mortality. Various anatomical locations of cerebral herniation—transtentorial, cerebellotonsillar, and subfalcine—result in different clinical signs that when detected early on may allow rapid diagnosis of the culpable intracranial pathology and correction of the neurosurgical emergency. In this chapter, we describe the anatomy, pathophysiology, symptoms, and general principles of management and prognosis of cerebral herniation syndromes.

Keywords: cerebellotonsillar, cerebral herniation, critical care, elevated intracranial pressure, Glasgow Coma Scale, subfalcine, transtentorial

5.1 Introduction

A dreaded complication of intracranial pathology is herniation of brain tissue across the natural boundaries of dura and bone, usually due to an expanding mass lesion that has exhausted the capability of the brain and cerebrospinal fluid (CSF) to tolerate added volume, resulting in elevated intracranial pressure (ICP). It is a validation of the Monroe–Kellie hypothesis and, unless rapidly corrected, portends a grave prognosis. The Monro–Kellie doctrine states that the skull is a rigid compartment with a fixed internal volume constituting blood (10%), CSF (10%), and brain (80%). Under normal circumstances, these three components maintain a volume and pressure equilibrium in order to maintain a normal ICP. Any increase in one of the three components must be compensated for by a decrease in the others (►Fig. 5.1). Compensatory mechanisms include displacement of CSF into the thecal sac or decrease in the volume of cerebral venous blood. A slowly expanding mass lesion such as a chronic subdural hematoma or gradually enlarging tumor may lead to severe anatomical herniation, with few initial neurologic findings and little direct morbidity.[1,2] In contrast, a rapidly expanding mass lesion or shifting pressure gradient usually results in a profound and often devastating progression of neurologic deficits, with a high risk of morbidity and mortality, if not quickly recognized and effectively treated.[3,4]

Herniation may also be confined to a particular compartment of the brain, such as the anterior, middle, or posterior cranial fossa, without a major rise in overall ICP. At times, differential CSF pressures exist across anatomical barriers, such as low intraspinal fluid pressure following a lumbar puncture (LP), may also be a cause of cerebral herniation. Herniation of cerebral contents generally leads to anatomically characteristic syndromes, although the clinical manifestations depend on the acuteness or chronicity at which herniation occurs.

The most common causes of acute herniation are intracranial hemorrhage of traumatic or spontaneous origin.[1,2,3,5,6] Regional or diffuse brain edema caused by cerebral ischemia and infarction are also common.[2,6,7] In each case, the herniation syndrome may involve structures above the tentorium, in the posterior fossa, or in both spaces. Other conditions that can precipitate cerebral herniation include acute hydrocephalus,[7] hepatic encephalopathy,[8] tumor enlargement with associated vasogenic edema,[9] and therapeutic lumbar CSF drainage.[4] The most common anatomical sites of herniation are under the falx cerebri, across the tentorium cerebelli, either downward or upward,[6] and downward across the foramen magnum.[4] In all of these situations, the neurosurgeon must be adept at the recognition and management of these important complications of central nervous system pathology.

5.2 Relevant Anatomy

5.2.1 Falx Cerebri

The falx cerebri is a sickle-shaped invagination of dura that separates the two hemispheres of the cerebral cortex. Anteriorly, the falx is quite thin and is anchored to the crista galli of the ethmoid bone. Posteriorly, it is broader and attached to the superior surface of the tentorium cerebelli. The superior aspect of the falx runs along the midline of the cranium and extends posteriorly to attach to the internal occipital protuberance. Contained within the falx are important venous structures: superiorly the superior sagittal sinus and inferiorly the inferior sagittal sinus. The lower margin of the falx is in close apposition to the corpus callosum, but it is deficient anteriorly and posteriorly, providing an escape route for a swollen cingulate gyrus to egress.

5.2.2 Tentorium Cerebelli and Incisura

The tentorium cerebelli is an arched lamina of dura that separates the cerebrum from the cerebellum. Elevated in the midline and sloping downward to attach to the petrous bone laterally and the transverse grooves of the occipital bone posteriorly, the slightly concave surface of concentric, circumferential, and radial dural bands yields little to pressure. It has been described as a "mechanically perfect means of directing forces away from the vulnerable midbrain,"[10] which passes through the incisura of the tentorium. The incisura, or tentorial notch, extends from the edges of the tuberculum sella back to the confluence of the straight sinus and the great vein of Galen.

The space between the free edge of the tentorium and the lateral border of the midbrain, forming the ambient cistern, varies in size from virtually no space, with direct contact of the midbrain and dura in up to 43% of postmortem specimens, to as

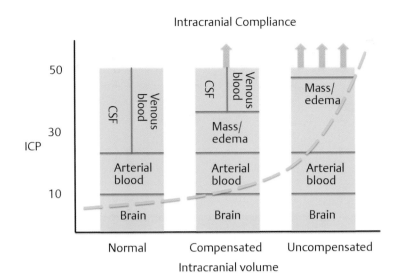

Intracranial Compliance

ICP: 50, 30, 10

Normal | Compensated | Uncompensated

Intracranial volume

(Normal column, bottom to top): Brain, Arterial blood, CSF, Venous blood

(Compensated column, bottom to top): Brain, Arterial blood, Mass/edema, CSF, Venous blood

(Uncompensated column, bottom to top): Brain, Arterial blood, Mass/edema

Fig. 5.1 Intracranial compliance as depicted in normal, compensated, and uncompensated states. The relationship between intracranial volume and ICP is not linear. As changes in intracranial volume arise, changes in CSF and venous blood volume can be made to restore some equilibrium. However, with continued mass effect, these compensatory mechanisms may be exhausted, leading to malignantly elevated ICPs. ICP, intracranial pressure; CSF, cerebrospinal fluid.

much as 7 mm of space on either side.[11] The medial margin of the uncus of the temporal lobe usually overhangs the edges of the incisura and closely approximates the more medial structures. Adler and Milhorat[12] have classified the dimensions of the tentorial notch into eight types; they noted that the amount of exposed cerebellar parenchyma within the notch and the relationship between the brainstem and the tentorial edge and brainstem position varied greatly among individuals, potentially altering susceptibility to transtentorial herniation from a supratentorial or infratentorial source.

Critical structures within the incisura include the third (oculomotor) cranial nerves, the posterior communicating and posterior cerebral (PCAs) arteries, and the midbrain. The third cranial nerves emerge from the medial aspect of the cerebral peduncles to pass through the subarachnoid space over the posterior clinoid processes anterolaterally to enter the dura at the superior margin of the cavernous sinuses. The medial margin of the uncus is immediately lateral to the third nerve in its subarachnoid course. The length, trajectory, and anatomical relationship of the third nerve to the skull base varies widely among individuals.[13] The pupilloconstrictor fibers run along the periphery of the third nerve and are exquisitely sensitive to external pressure.[12] Thus, mass effect, which compresses the uncus against the nerve, or pressure from below, which stretches or kinks it against the dural edge, results in loss of constriction, the resulting pupillary dilation being the hallmark clinical sign of transtentorial herniation.[2,6,10,11,12,13]

Superior and lateral to the third nerves are the paired posterior communicating arteries, arising anteriorly from the internal carotid arteries to run back to join the PCAs, which arise from the distal bifurcation of the basilar artery (BA). The paired PCAs course laterally over the oculomotor nerves and the free edge of the tentorium, rendering them extremely vulnerable to occlusion by downward pressure. Inferiorly, the paired superior cerebellar arteries arise from the BA to course laterally under

the tentorium; these are vulnerable to occlusion from upward herniation from the posterior fossa.

Within the incisura is located the midbrain, consisting of the cerebral peduncles anteriorly, the midportion or tegmentum, and posteriorly the tectum, composed of the superior and inferior colliculi. Through this region pass all of the fiber tracts that connect the cerebral cortex, basal ganglia, thalamus, and upper brainstem nuclei with the lower brainstem and spinal cord. Also within this region are the oculomotor and trochlear nerve nuclei, the substantia nigra, the red nuclei, the periaqueductal gray matter, and the neurons of the reticular activating system (RAS). The proximal aqueduct of Sylvius passes centrally here from the posterior third ventricle, rendering a high risk of obstructive hydrocephalus from mass effect in this area.

The blood supply to the midbrain consists of interpeduncular arteries from the distal BA and the proximal PCAs; these give rise to smaller, perforating arteries. Inferiorly, small circumferential arteries arise from the BA to irrigate the outer substance of the midbrain. These perforating arteries are all functional "end arteries" with few collateral vessels within the midbrain parenchyma. This becomes important when mechanical compression causes occlusion of these small vessels, leading to severe local ischemia.

The subarachnoid spaces of the incisura are divided into several cisterns, which may initially act as hydraulic buffers protecting the midbrain.[10,13,14] The interpeduncular cistern lies anteromedially to the cerebral peduncles, just above the prepontine cistern in the posterior fossa; others have described these together as the "basal cistern."[10] Lateral to the midbrain lies the ambient or perimesencephalic cistern. Radiographic evidence of compression or effacement of the ambient cistern gives verification of transtentorial herniation.[1,14] Compression of this cistern on the initial computed tomography (CT) of the brain has been shown to have a negative impact on prognosis in the setting of intracerebral hematoma[15] and of head injury[16]; in both cases, preservation of the cistern correlates to a far better

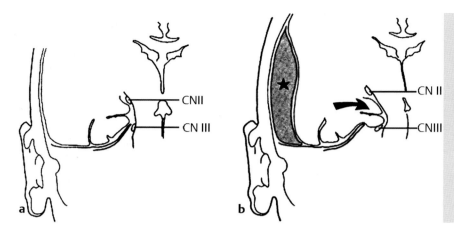

Fig. 5.2 Coronal view of the temporal lobe and adjacent midbrain. (a) The normal relationships, with preserved ambient cistern. (b) The appearance of transtentorial herniation, with downward displacement of the brain stem, medial displacement of the uncus, and compression of the oculomotor nerve and midbrain structures.

likelihood of good outcome than for those patients with compression of one or both cisterns. Posterior to the midbrain is the quadrigeminal plate cistern, also known as the "cistern of the vein of Galen."

5.3 Biomechanics and Pathology of Transtentorial Herniation

First described anatomically in 1896,[17] transtentorial herniation is the medial and caudal dislocation of brain parenchyma from the supratentorial space through the incisura (▶Fig. 5.1). Classic pathologic studies published in 1920 by Meyer[18] document medial displacement of the uncus, obliteration of the ambient cistern, compression. There may also be displacement of the oculomotor nerve, and midbrain. A deep groove is often formed along the undersurface of the ipsilateral uncus by the firm edge of the tentorium. Experimental models have since demonstrated that expansion of an intracranial mass above the tentorium results in a gradient of increased ICP, highest ipsilateral to the mass and above the tentorium, less below the tentorium, and lowest in the spinal subarachnoid space.[19] The result is medial herniation of the uncus of the temporal lobe into the ipsilateral ambient cistern, with stretching, torsion, and compression of the oculomotor nerve, compression of the midbrain itself, and occlusion of the aquaduct of Sylvius.[10,20,21,22] The stalk of the pituitary gland may be stretched across the diaphragma sellae, causing infarction of the pituitary gland itself.[21] CT shows that in severe herniation, the midbrain is rotated or twisted, and the cerebral peduncles elongated and flattened[14] (▶Fig. 5.2).

Because of contralateral displacement of the brainstem and compression of the opposite cerebral peduncle against the tentorium, Kernohan and Woltman[22] in 1929 identified a notching of the opposite side of the midbrain, later to be identified both clinically and pathologically as the "Kernohan's notch phenomenon." There may also be downward displacement of the brainstem. Using magnetic resonance imaging (MRI), Reich et al[1] showed that fully one half of patients with transtentorial herniation also had downward shift and concurrent cerebellar tonsillar herniation at the foramen magnum. Ropper[23] has shown, however, that the clinical syndrome can evolve with only horizontal displacement of the brainstem and little or no downward displacement. Reich et al[1] also showed,

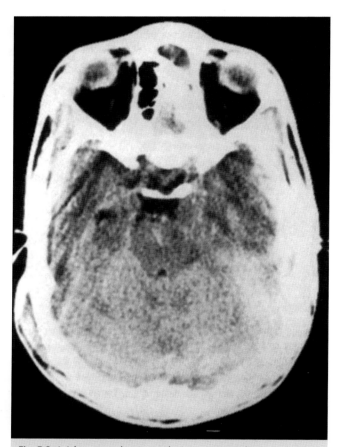

Fig. 5.3 Axial computed tomography in a patient with severe transtentorial herniation shows the midbrain to be compressed and rotated by the medial deviation of the left uncus.

using MRI, that in more chronic cases, radiographic evidence of herniation could precede clinical manifestations and identify patients with earlier, reversible clinical findings, and that resolution of clinical herniation was accompanied by reversal of radiographic findings. Transtentorial herniation causes distortion of the arteries of the posterior circulation, with stretching and occlusion of the small perforating branches that supply the upper brainstem (▶Fig. 5.3).[10,21] This may result in rupture of these small arteries, with consequent brainstem hemorrhage (Duret's hemorrhages). Hemorrhages may also occur because of initial ischemia due to vessel occlusion from downward displacement, followed by reperfusion of the infarcted areas as the displaced tissue relaxes. The PCAs are commonly occluded as they cross the incisura, resulting in characteristic infarction of one or both occipital lobes as an added complication.

Histologic changes include lipid vacuolization within the herniated uncus, with neuronal swelling and peripherally displaced nuclei. With time, surviving neurons become pyknotic and a fibrous gliosis may develop in survivors of the clinical syndrome. Edema also occurs within the brainstem, accompanied by the neuronal and white matter changes of ischemia. Thrombosed veins, venulae, and capillaries are seen, attributed to both direct compression and ischemia.[10]

5.4 Clinical Signs of Transtentorial Herniation

The classic signs of transtentorial herniation include the triad of anisocoria, with initial ipsilateral pupillary dilation, often irregular in shape,[24] loss of the light reflex, alteration in level of consciousness, and an asymmetric motor response, usually a contralateral hemiparesis. As herniation progresses, the pupillary dilation becomes bilateral and the pupils fixed and nonreactive to light.[2,6,10,11,12,18,22] Alteration in level of consciousness is usually progressive to the point of coma, from the effect of the mass lesion on ICP, global dysfunction of the cerebral hemispheres, and compression of the RAS of the midbrain. The hemiparesis is usually contralateral to the side of the mass lesion because of compression of the ipsilateral cerebral peduncle, and may be mild initially, but usually worsens to a hemiplegia as brainstem compression progresses. In ~ 25% of cases, the hemiparesis is ipsilateral to the dilated pupil, because of midbrain shift and compression of the contralateral cerebral peduncle against the opposite tentorial edge, termed the "Kernohan's notch phenomenon."[22]

5.4.1 Pupillary Function

Pupillary size and reactivity depend upon a balance between the effects of the sympathetic and parasympathetic nervous systems on the pupils. Sympathetic innervation arises from the hypothalamus and brainstem, passing through the cervical spinal cord to synapse in the intermediolateral tract of the upper thoracic spinal segments. Preganglionic fibers pass through the ventral roots of the upper thoracic spinal cord to ascend through the inferior and middle cervical sympathetic ganglia to synapse in the superior cervical ganglion. Postganglionic fibers then ascend along the internal carotid artery to enter the orbit through the superior orbital fissure with the nasociliary nerve. Fibers then enter the globe as the long ciliary nerve. Sympathetic discharges not only innervate the dilator pupillae muscles but also innervate the smooth muscle of the levators of the eyelid (Müller's muscle).

Parasympathetic innervation arises from the Edinger–Westphal nucleus, dorsal to the oculomotor nucleus in the midbrain. The preganglionic fibers travel on the periphery of the oculomotor nerve as it passes forward from the interpeduncular fossa

to enter the dural edge of the incisura and the cavernous sinus. These fibers are exquisitely sensitive to mechanical stretch or compression. After the oculomotor nerve enters the superior orbital fissure, the parasympathetic fibers pass to the ciliary ganglion and synapse. The postganglionic fibers form the short ciliary nerve, which enters the sclera to innervate smooth muscle fibers that constrict the pupil.

Transtentorial herniation of the uncus results in both direct compression and stretching or torsion of the ipsilateral oculomotor nerve itself and then compression of the oculomotor and Edinger–Westphal nuclei in the midbrain. These result in progressive loss of parasympathetic tone, with continued sympathetic innervation resulting in an enlarging and often initially irregular ipsilateral pupil.[10,15,19,24] Marshall et al[24] have shown that relatively mild increases in ICP alone may result in an irregular or dilated ipsilateral pupil. As midbrain compression and ischemia progresses, there may be loss of both parasympathetic and sympathetic innervation bilaterally, resulting in midposition (4–5 mm) pupils that are fixed to light. Marshman et al[25] have shown that rarely the dilated and fixed pupil can be contralateral to the mass lesion and thus "false localizing," possibly because of stretching of the contralateral oculomotor nerve from hemispheric mass effect and midline shift of structures well above the midbrain.

With increased pressure on the oculomotor nerve and nucleus, loss of ipsilateral extraocular movements may occur, with resulting tonic deviation of that eye laterally due to continued abducent nerve function. Other ocular findings may also be noted, such as ptosis and impaired vertical or upward gaze due to compression of the dorsal midbrain.[1,10,24]

5.4.2 Loss of Consciousness

In humans, level of consciousness reflects both level of arousal or alertness and the presence of conscious behavior or cognitive function. Normal arousal relies upon intact function of the RAS, whereas conscious behavior reflects function of the cortical hemispheres.

The RAS is a diffuse network of neurons that form a central core of the brainstem, most prominent in the midbrain. The RAS is not distinct, and its neurons are extensively interconnected, with collateral input from every major sensory pathway, particularly the spinothalamic tract and the trigeminal nerve. Numerous connections ascend into the subthalamus, thalamus, hypothalamus, and the basal forebrain structures, including the limbic system. Other connections extend diffusely and reciprocally into the neocortex.

Stimulation of the RAS produces a general activation of the cerebral cortex, in part by abolishing inhibitory input from the thalamus and the limbic system. Arousal or alertness is dependent upon the integrity of the RAS. Thus, with either direct compression or ischemia of the midbrain, there is a loss of RAS function and decrease in alertness and level of consciousness. Usually the lesion that has resulted in herniation has also affected the cortical hemispheres, either directly or through global elevation in ICP, resulting in a decrease in conscious behavior and cognitive function. Cortical lesions of increasing size usually result in a progressive decrease in level of alertness and cognitive function, associated in part with the degree of midline brain shift.[1,2,15]Alteration in the level of consciousness, a hallmark sign of transtentorial herniation, thus may result from either compression of the midbrain, affecting the function of the RAS, or dysfunction of the cerebral hemispheres in a localized or diffuse fashion.

5.4.3 Hemiparesis

Asymmetric motor findings are the third clinical manifestation of transtentorial herniation. Most often hemiparesis is due to compression of the corticospinal tracts of the ipsilateral cerebral peduncle and thus is contralateral. However, motor paresis may also result from direct compression of the ipsilateral hemisphere itself. As noted above, in ~ 25% of cases, the hemiparesis is ipsilateral to the side of herniation and the dilated pupil, because of midbrain shift to the opposite side and compression of the contralateral cerebral peduncle against the opposite tentorial edge, the Kernohan's notch phenomenon.[23]

5.5 Other Types of Cerebral Herniation

5.5.1 Upward Transtentorial Herniation

A similar clinical condition occurs when a mass lesion within the posterior fossa results in herniation of brain tissue upward through the incisura, resulting in acute impaction and compression of midbrain structures.[1,6,11,15] The usual causes are hematomas and infarctions and other mass lesions within the cerebellum such as abcess and tumors,[1,6,11,15] along with more unusual causes such as adipose graft prolapse into the posterior fossa following translabyrinthine craniotomy.[26] The usual mechanism is elevated pressure within the narrow confines of the posterior fossa, with upward displacement of the cerebellar vermis, compressing the dorsal midbrain within the incisura.[1,6,11] Upward herniation is more likely when the mass arises within the vermis itself, or when the incisura is large in size.[6] There may also be exacerbation of the pressure gradient across the tentorium by placement of a shunt or ventriculostomy above for control of secondary hydrocephalus and ICP monitoring.[1,6]

Pathologically, there is compression and distortion of the midbrain, compression of the aqueduct of Sylvius, buckling of the quadrigeminal plate, and displacement and occlusion of the vein of Galen. This venous obstruction may cause secondary hemorrhagic infarction of the diencephalons.[1,6] The distal branches of the superior cerebellar artery may become compressed against the underside of the tentorium, resulting in ischemia, edema, and infarction of the cerebellar hemispheres, aggravating the condition.[1,6]

The clinical manifestations of upward transtentorial herniation vary and in some ways are dissimilar to those of downward herniation. Level of consciousness may deteriorate to coma, often associated with small, minimally reactive pupils (so-called "pontine pupils").[6,11,15] These pupillary changes are due to direct compression of the pons, with parasympathetic papillary input from the midbrain unopposed by sympathetic tone descending through the pontomedullary region.[11,12] Cuneo et al,[6] however, have also described the initial development of anisocoria and fixed,

midposition or even large pupils due to evolving distortion and compression of the midbrain and oculomotor nerves themselves.

Also characteristic of upward herniation is the absence of vertical eye movements owing to pretectal compression. There may also be conjugate downward deviation of the eyes or skew gaze.[1,11] Flexor or extensor posturing on motor response[1,6,15] and Cheyne–Stokes respirations or hyperventilation can be noted as well.

Reich et al[1] have identified upward herniation on MRI in the sagittal plane as a cephalad deviation of the proximal opening of the aqueduct of Sylvius, above the level of the incisural line. They have also shown angulation or buckling of the quadrigeminal plate and ventral bowing and displacement of the brainstem. They noted that MRI may identify upward herniation prior to the development of extreme neurologic consequences, and that such imaging can be used to follow the course of progression or recovery of upward herniation, which correlates closely with clinical progression or recovery.

5.5.2 Cerebellotonsillar Herniation

Herniation of the cerebellar tonsils downward through the foramen magnum is the final type of brain herniation that may have immediate and devastating neurologic consequences.[1,6,10,15,18,22] Most often occurring as a result of a mass in the inferior cerebellum, the cerebellar tonsils are displaced downward through the foramen magnum, resulting in direct compression, ischemia, and infarction of the tonsils themselves, compression of the medulla oblongata, and obstruction of the foramina of Luschke and Magendie.[6] Another result of cerebellotonsillar herniation is direct compression of the pons and medulla against the clivus, with distortion or closure of the fourth ventricle. Closure of any of the ventricular outflow tracts may lead to obstructive hydrocephalus, which can further increase ICP, both above and below the tentorium.[6]

Cerebellotonsillar herniation may also occur because of a large supratentorial mass lesion, which causes elevated ICP and downward displacement of the entire brainstem.[18] After LP, with a lowered CSF pressure below the foramen magnum and an enhanced rostral–caudal pressure gradient, a supratentorial mass may result in cerebellotonsillar herniation and an abrupt clinical decline. Jennett and Stern[18] showed experimentally that a large supratentorial mass lesion was associated with mechanical distortion and downward displacement of the brainstem and tonsillar impaction into the foramen magnum. Reich et al[1] have shown, with sagittal MRI, that anatomical herniation at the foramen magnum often accompanies transtentorial herniation due to a supratentorial mass, and that such herniation may be reversed as the mass is treated and clinical herniation resolves.

The pathologic consequences of cerebellotonsillar herniation include direct mechanical compression of the medulla oblongata against the lower clivus and anterior foramen magnum, often resulting in a transverse groove along the ventral medulla.[1,6] Ischemia and infarction of the cerebellar tonsils, lower cerebellum, and the entire lower brainstem and upper spinal cord may occur because of occlusion of the vertebral arteries, their branches, and the origin of the anterior spinal artery.[1,6] Histologic changes include edema and lipid vacuolization within the herniated and compressed tissues, along with pyknotic nuclei, and poorly staining cytoplasm within the neurons of the brainstem nuclei.

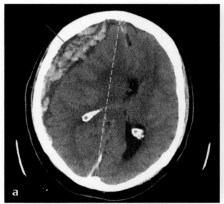 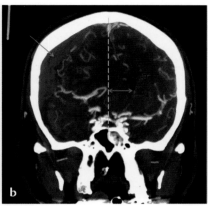

Fig. 5.4 (a) Axial computed tomography (CT) and **(b)** coronal CT angiograms demonstrating a large subdural hemotoma (blue arrows) causing significant midline shift (red double arrows) and subfalcine herniation.

Clinical Signs of Cerebellotonsillar Herniation

Clinically, rapid descent of the cerebellar tonsils and impaction of the medulla oblongata may cause sudden apnea and circulatory collapse.[1,6] Subsequent coma is more often due to respiratory and circulatory arrest than to the brainstem compression itself. Clinical signs that may precede such collapse include those of pontomedullary compression, including pontine pupils, loss of lateral eye movements, and internuclear ophthalmoplegia due to dysfunction of the abducent nerve nuclei and parapontine reticular formation. Some preservation of vertical eye movements may be retained because upper brainstem function remains intact, and "ocular bobbing" may be noted.[6]

The motor signs of pontomedullary compression may include extensor posturing, but more immediate flaccid quadriplegia occurs because of compression of the descending medullary corticospinal tracts. Respiratory changes may include immediate apnea, cluster breathing, gasping, and ataxic breathing patterns, but not the more familiar Cheyne–Stokes respirations, which are characteristic of hemispheric or midbrain–diencephalic insults.

Given the often rapid onset of abrupt and profound cardiopulmonary collapse with cerebellotonsillar herniation, it is critical that any neurologic deterioration that includes potential signs of such herniation be immediately recognized and action taken to stabilize the patient and lower ICP. This should be followed immediately by diagnostic measures to allow definitive treatment of the intracranial mass lesion causing the decline.

5.5.3 Subfalcine Herniation

This is a common form of herniation characterized by displacement of the brain, most commonly the cingulate gyrus, below the free edge of the falx cerebri. This is usually caused by a mass lesions, either hemorrhage (▶ Fig. 5.4) or tumor (▶ Fig. 5.5) in the frontal, temporal, or parietal lobe. This form of herniation may be clinically silent but is seen on imaging studies as effacement of the ipsilateral lateral and third ventricles, compression of the foramen of Monro, displacement of the septum pellucidum into the contralateral hemisphere, away from midline, and secondary dilatation of the contralateral ventricle. Clinical signs of subfalcine hernation may develop secondary to hydrocephalus or anterior cerebral artery (ACA) compression; the cingulate gyrus

herniating below the falx cerebri leads to compression of the ipsilateral ACA beneath the falx. This may lead to infarction of the territory of the distal ACA, clinically manifesting as contralateral leg weakness. Rarely, bilateral ACA compromise leading to bilateral lower extremity weakness may also be observed.

5.5.4 Cerebral Herniation as a Potential Complication of Lumbar Puncture

The possible hazards of LP in a patient with clinical papilledema were recognized soon after the introduction of this procedure into clinical practice.[27,28] The occurrence of transtentorial herniation, or more commonly, cerebellotonsillar herniation, in a patient with an intracranial mass lesion may occur within minutes of removing CSF from the lumbar region or may be delayed for hours or longer. The mechanism of herniation results from an increase in both brain volume and ICP. With a decrease in CSF pressure below the foramen magnum, there is rostral–caudal displacement of brain tissue. Herniation occurs only in the presence of some degree of obstruction of normal CSF flow between the cranial and the spinal subarachnoid spaces.[27] When there is normal free flow, the fall in lumbar CSF pressure can equilibrate within the intracranial cavity without brain displacement. LP may also exacerbate an already existing or impending herniation syndrome that is causing blockage of the subarachnoid space, either at the incisura or the foramen magnum, with clinical signs of herniation occurring only after the puncture has been performed.

Cerebral herniation after an LP is, in fact, a rare event. A large early clinical series and review of earlier reports has indicated that the incidence in patients with elevated ICP was less than 1.2%.[28] More recently, Duffy[29] reported that 7 of 52 patients with acute subarachnoid hemorrhage deteriorated clinically at the time when an LP was performed; this may have had more to do with aneurysm rebleeding in this series than with herniation occurring as a result of the puncture.

The risks of cerebral herniation make it imperative that diagnostic imaging such as CT scan be performed prior to an LP in any patient with a suspected intracranial mass or elevation of ICP.[27] In the presence of a significant mass above or below the tentorium, midline shift, or noncommunicating hydrocephalus, an LP should be avoided. If there is little mass effect and the results of CSF analysis are important to the clinical diagnosis, then an LP should be performed, understanding the possibility of what is, in fact, a very unlikely complication.

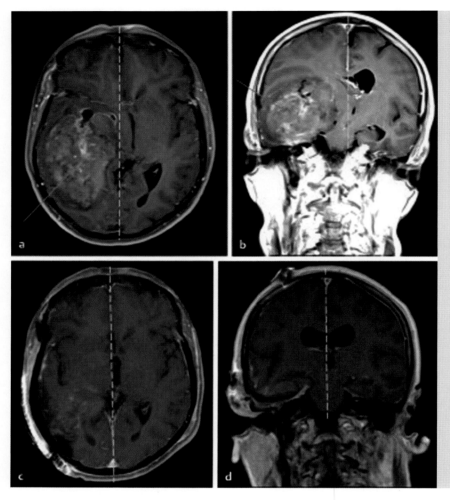

Fig. 5.5 Preoperative **(a)** axial and **(b)** coronal T1-weighted postcontrast magnetic resonance (MR) images of a patient with severe subfalcine herniation and midline shift (red double arrows) secondary to a large temporo-occipital mass lesion (blue arrows). Postoperative **(c)** axial and **(d)** coronal T1-weighted postcontrast MR images of this patient show resection of mass and significant improvement in midline shift, with no evidence of subfalcine herniation.

An acute herniation syndrome at the foramen magnum due to the use of perioperative lumbar drainage has recently been described in three patients.[4] The authors describe the development of an "acquired Chiari malformation" and the development of a negative pressure gradient between the cranial and the spinal subarachnoid spaces.

5.6 The Effect of Hypotension, Hypoxia, and Other Factors on the Neurologic Examination

Because the definition of cerebral herniation relies upon the bedside neurologic examination, it is imperative that these clinical findings accurately reflect intracranial pathology. Severe systemic hypotension, hypoxia, and hypothermia can all depress neurologic function and confound the diagnosis of cerebral herniation syndromes.

5.6.1 Cardiac Arrest and Systemic Hypotension

Systemic hypotension is a common complication of severe head injury that can markedly worsen outcome and decrease chances of survival.[30,31,32,33] Andrews et al[31] reviewed a series of 36 patients to analyze the effects of severe hypotension or preceding cardiac arrest at the time of the initial neurologic examination following head injury. Each patient had neurologic signs at the time of admission that might be consistent with a herniation syndrome. Ten patients had been successfully resuscitated from cardiac arrest, 7 had an initial systolic blood pressure (SBP) of less than 60 mm Hg, and 19 had an initial blood pressure of 60 to 90 mm Hg. The median Glasgow Coma Score (GCS) score was 3 (range: 3–8), and the neurologic findings for each group were similar. Among the 10 patients with resuscitated cardiac arrest, 4 (40%) had anisocoria and 6 (60%) had bilaterally fixed and dilated pupils; all 10 (100%) had absent corneal reflexes. Nine patients (90%) were flaccid, and one (10%) had bilaterally extensor posturing. Of the 7 patients with an initial SBP of less than 60 mm Hg, 2 (29%) had anisocoria, all had absent corneal reflexes, and all were flaccid. Of the 19 patients with an initial SBP of 60 to 90 mm Hg, 9 (47%) had anisocoria, 8 (42%) had active corneal reflexes, 4 (21%) had hemiparesis, 4 (21%) exhibited extensor posturing, and 11 (58%) were flaccid.

Each patient underwent surgical exploration and/or radiographic assessment for an underlying structural lesion causing the apparent herniation syndrome. Only 1 (10%) of the 10 patients resuscitated from cardiac arrest had a significant mass lesion; only 1 (14%) of the 7 with initially severe hypotension had a hematoma. In neither group were the findings of the initial clinical examination useful in identifying the presence or site of an intracranial mass lesion. In contrast, of the 19 patients with an initial SBP of 60 to 90 mm Hg, 13 (68%) had extra-axial hematomas ($p < 0.01$), including 78% of those with initial anisocoria. In each case, the hematoma was ipsilateral to the dilated pupil ($p < 0.05$). This study indicates that an initial SBP of at least 60 mm Hg is needed to perfuse the brain adequately and allow the neurologic examination to reflect accurately intracranial pathology. Among patients with more profound hypotension, or initial cardiac arrest, the findings of the neurologic examination reflect diffuse cerebral ischemia, not herniation.

5.6.2 Systemic Hypoxia

Systemic hypoxia is an even more common complication of severe head injury than hypotension,[30,31,33] occurring in 30% or more of patients at the time of initial evaluation. The effect of hypoxia on the neurologic examination is often complicated by systemic hypotension, which occurs because of hypoxic effects on the myocardium and peripheral vasculature. If hypotension is prevented, normal humans can tolerate an extremely low arterial oxygen tension (PaO_2) without major neurologic manifestations or sequelae. Gray and Horner[34] reported that among 22 patients with a PaO_2 of 20 mm Hg or less, 8 remained alert, 7 somnolent, and 7 comatose. Severe hypoxia usually causes clinical signs of a metabolic encephalopathy, with deterioration in level of consciousness to eventual coma, along with changes in respiratory pattern, tremor, asterixis, myoclonus, and flexor or extensor posturing.[34,35] Brainstem reflexes usually remain intact until profound anoxia has occurred, at which time there is papillary dilation and loss of the oculocephalic reflexes.[35]

It is important to recognize that any of a wide variety of metabolic insults such as hypoxia can further depress the neurologic examination, particularly in the severely injured brain. Such problems as hypothermia, severe hyper- or hypoglycemia, hyponatremia, and drug intoxications may alter level of consciousness[35] and should be considered when first evaluating any patient in coma with or without evidence of brainstem dysfunction, especially when the clinical history is unclear.

5.7 Management of Cerebral Herniation Syndromes

Treatment of acute cerebral herniation must begin upon recognition of the clinical condition and be concurrent with diagnostic studies being completed. Prolonged or persistent herniation will lead to irreversible ischemic damage to the deep midline structures of the cerebral hemispheres and the brainstem, resulting in permanent morbidity or death. The immediate goals include the reduction of elevated ICP while maintaining cerebral perfusion pressure (CPP) and oxygenation and prevention or correction of hypercarbia and acidosis.[8,36] If the cause of the herniation syndrome is unknown, then an emergent CT scan of the brain can be performed to identify if there is a directly treatable mass lesion. Lowering elevated ICP and supporting blood pressure and oxygenation are essential first steps. Blood pressure management, controlled ventilation, and intravenous infusion of mannitol are the primary means of achieving these goals. These measures allow the brain to accommodate temporarily an underlying cause of increased ICP such as a mass lesion, until definitive diagnosis and treatment can be initiated.

5.7.1 Initial Resuscitation and Management

The ABCs

The initial steps required to adequately resuscitate a patient with acute cerebral herniation are the same regardless of the cause, be it severe head injury, intracranial hemorrhage, or diffuse cerebral edema. Key to resuscitation are the ABCs: airway, breathing, and circulation. First, the patient must have an adequately protected and controlled airway. In the field, initial mask ventilation with 100% oxygen usually suffices, although often now trained prehospital staff may successfully provide orotracheal intubation before the patient arrives. Once the patient is in the emergency department, prompt endotracheal intubation should be provided if it has not already been performed. In patients with head injury, a lateral cervical radiograph should be obtained first to rule out an obvious cervical fracture or instability. Even with a negative radiograph, only gentle axial traction should be provided during intubation and extreme extension or distraction of the cervical spine should be avoided, as there is a 20% chance of significant injury despite a normal screening lateral radiograph.[37] Alternatively, nasotracheal intubation (if a major base of skull fracture is not suspected) or cricothyroidotomy may be performed. Intubation also remains a critical first step in the already hospitalized patient who develops signs of cerebral herniation, such as after mild or moderate closed head injury or after cranial surgery.

Once an airway has been established, controlled ventilation with 100% oxygen should be maintained, with the goals of improving arterial oxygenation and reversing hypercarbia and respiratory acidosis.[36] Hyperventilation can provide an immediate decrease in arterial carbon dioxide tension ($PaCO_2$), which increases the pH of blood and causes a respiratory alkalosis. This results in diffuse cerebral vasoconstriction, decreasing cerebral blood volume and lowering ICP. In patients with expanding hematomas causing transtentorial herniation, hyperventilation can temporarily result in a reversal of pupillary anisocoria as well as hemiparesis, while diagnostic studies can be performed and the hematoma identified and treated.[36,38] This is the only setting in which the Brain Trauma Foundation, American Association of Neurological Surgeons (AANS) Joint Section of Neurotrauma, and Critical Care Guidelines for the Management of Severe Head Injury support the use of hyperventilation.[4]

The risk of hyperventilation is the induction of cerebral ischemia due to excessive vasoconstriction[36] thus, as soon as diagnostic studies have been performed, if a mass lesion is identified, this should be immediately addressed and $PaCO_2$ normalized. If diagnostic studies do not identify a mass lesion, then one should bring the $PaCO_2$ to 30 to 35 mm Hg, unless further hyperventilation is guided by the use of additional monitoring to avoid ischemia, such as arteriovenous oxygen content difference ($AVDO_2$) measurement.[39] The vasoconstriction induced by hyperventilation is effective only in regions of the brain where cerebrovascular CO_2 responsiveness remains intact; therefore, ICP may respond less to hyperventilation in patients with diffuse brain injury than in those with more focal abnormalities such as hematomas, where large regions of the brain can still respond.[36] Since the latter circumstance is the case for many patients with herniation syndromes, initial hyperventilation remains an optimal initial treatment.

In patients with diffuse lesions requiring ongoing treatment of elevated ICP, the use of ongoing hyperventilation is much more controversial. Because of the risks of ischemia, and the fact that the vasoconstriction caused by hyperventilation is lost over time,[40] most practitioners now suggest normalizing the $PaCO_2$ to 30 to 35 mm Hg. Cruz,[39] however, advocate assessing global cerebral ischemia using $AVDO_2$ monitoring to guide the ongoing use of hyperventilation to the degree that it lowers ICP but does not induce ischemia.

The final step of the initial ABCs is to assess and support the circulation and blood pressure. It is critical that systemic hypotension be prevented or rapidly corrected to maintain brain perfusion. From the start, adequate intravenous access must be established. Intravascular volume resuscitation should be provided as needed to stabilize or maintain blood pressure, using a balanced salt solution such as Ringer's lactate solution. If the blood pressure is initially normal, hydration should be moderated to avoid overhydration, which may aggravate cerebral edema or lead to pulmonary edema.

In the head-injured patient, the most common cause of systemic hypotension is hemorrhagic shock. In this case, volume resuscitation should include the use of blood products.[41] Patients with multisystem injuries may have additional reasons for hypotension, such as low cardiac output due to a cardiac contusion or tamponade.[41] They may also show loss of systemic vascular resistance because of a spinal cord injury. These alternatives should be considered if the blood pressure does not respond to initial volume resuscitation, or if the clinical picture does not fit with that of hemorrhagic shock.[41]

As hemorrhagic shock is being treated with volume expansion, using crystalloids and blood products, the source of blood loss must be quickly found and controlled. Common sites of hemorrhage include the chest and abdomen, pelvis, and long bone fractures.[41] These problems must be addressed by the appropriate surgical specialist concurrent with management of the severe head injury.

There has been some enthusiasm for the use of hypertonic saline (HTS) to initially resuscitate patients with severe head injury, and to treat elevated ICP.[42] It was demonstrated that HTS solutions are effective in reducing ICP and usually improve CPP, but there was no notable superiority of such solutions to the use of conventional resuscitation and infusions of intravenous mannitol.[43] Qureshi et al[44] described the successful reversal of herniation due to supratentorial mass lesions using combinations of HTS and mannitol, barbiturates, and hyperventilation, but no clear role of hypertonic fluids in the initial resuscitation of patients with herniation has been established.

In patients with hemorrhagic shock and herniation, the use of HTS may be more appropriate, given the contraindication of use of mannitol in such patients.[42,43]

Intravenous Infusion of Mannitol

Additional steps to resuscitate a patient with acute cerebral herniation include the use of intravenous mannitol. Except in the setting of hemorrhagic shock, Andrews recommends the immediate bolus infusion of mannitol, 1.0 to 1.5 g/kg body weight.[5,36] Mannitol, a six-carbon sugar similar to glucose, is not metabolized, nor does it cross the blood–brain barrier. It remains predominantly in the intravascular space and causes a direct vasoconstriction because of its effects on blood viscosity.[45,46,47] It also has effects on red blood cell deformability and hemodilution and improved red blood cell oxygen transport.[46] All of these result in a near-immediate decrease in brain volume, improvement in intracranial compliance, and lowered ICP.[48] Mannitol improves blood flow to all parts of the brain, including the brainstem.[40] Finally, mannitol results in a somewhat more delayed osmotic dehydration of the brain. Because of the cardiovascular effects of mannitol infusion, its use is generally contraindicated in the setting of cardiovascular instability or hemorrhagic shock.[41] To avoid the risk of hypotension from rapid infusion of mannitol, it should be given at a rate no higher than 0.1 g/kg/min.[49]

The dosage of mannitol infusion in the initial management of severe head injury has historically ranged between 0.25 and 1.5 g/kg body weight.[3,36] Andrews has generally used dosages in the higher range for the initial bolus infusion. Recently, Cruz et al,[3] in a prospective randomized class I study, compared initial use of mannitol, using "conventional dosage" and "high" dosage in patients with documented subdural hematomas. Patients in the conventional-dosage group received 0.6 to 0.7 g mannitol/kg body weight, and those in the high-dosage group received a total of 1.2 to 1.4 g/kg if they did not have pupillary anisocoria, and 2.2 to 2.4 g/kg if they had anisocoria. The low-dosage group had significantly worse cerebral oxygen extraction and cerebral swelling than the high-dosage group. Preoperative improvement in anisocoria was also significantly better in the high-dosage group. After 6 months, the Glasgow Outcome Scale scores were significantly better in the high-dosage group than in those receiving the conventional dosage. The same authors have also shown that high dosage (1.4 g/kg) of mannitol was more effective than conventional dosages (0.7 g/kg) for patients with traumatic parenchymal hematomas of the temporal lobe causing abnormal pupillary response.[49] These results would seem to support strongly the use of high-dosage mannitol in patients with clinical transtentorial herniation, particularly if a hemorrhagic mass lesion has been documented to be present.

Use of Hypertonic Saline

An alternative and effective hyperosmolar agent that may be used to manage elevated ICPs is HTS.[50] As of yet, there is not a standardized protocol or concentration for the administration of HTS. HTS may be given in various concentrations (2, 3, 5, 7, or 23.5%) as a continuous infusion or as a bolus in order to achieve a goal sodium level of 150 to 155 mmol/L. By elevating the serum concentration of sodium, HTS creates an osmotic gradient, drawing fluid out of edematous cerebral tissues without crossing the blood–brain barrier. Other effects of HTS include expansion of intravascular volume, improving systemic blood pressure and CPP. HTS is also thought to induce a decrease in endothelial cell volume, which also improves circulation, decreasing hyperemia and hypoperfusion.[51] HTS is also thought to play a role in immunomodulation and reduction of CSF production.[52]

Various randomized control trials have compared HTS and mannitol as effective therapies for controlling elevated ICPs.[50] These studies have generally concluded that HTS is more effective at lowering ICPs, but without any significant difference in neurologic outcome between the two hyperosmolar therapies. Compared with mannitol, HTS is cheaper, can be given as an infusion, leads to more sustained control of ICPs, can treat concomitant hyponatremia, and lacks the hypotensive effects of mannitol. However, the use of HTS is not without its disadvantages, such as the need for central venous access in continuous infusion. The most serious risk HTS poses, although rare, is that of central pontine myelinolysis. Generally, if appropriately monitored, HTS is a safe and effective means of controlling ICPs that may be used as an alternative to, or concurrently with, mannitol.

5.7.2 Subsequent Management

After the initial management steps outlined above, it becomes imperative that the cause of herniation be identified as quickly as possible and treated directly, if possible. Upon completing endotracheal intubation, controlled ventilation with selective hyperventilation and an infusion of intravenous high-dosage mannitol are initiated, and a diagnostic CT should be performed immediately in hemodynamically stable patients.[36] CT is extremely sensitive to the presence of acute intracranial hemorrhages and other mass lesions that may cause a herniation syndrome, such as cerebral edema, tumor, or hydrocephalus. CT should also be performed prior to considering LP in any patient with a suspected mass lesion; the identification of such a mass may make LP contraindicated, unless absolutely necessary.

Of patients who are hemodynamically unstable because of traumatic injuries to the chest or abdomen, some must go directly to the operating room for treatment of these life-threatening lesions.[41] It may be impossible in such cases to obtain a preoperative CT scan. If the patient has not been resuscitated from initial cardiac arrest, or has not had profound hypotension, in which case the clinical findings of herniation are often false localizing,[31] it may be reasonable to consider performing exploratory burr holes on the side of the dilated pupil.[5] Because most traumatic lesions causing herniation are located in the epidural or subdural space, burr holes placed in the temporal, frontal, and parietal areas will be accurately identified by this rapid technique. In the case of nonlateralizing signs of herniation, the burr holes should be placed bilaterally. Intraoperative ultrasonic imaging of the brain parenchyma can further enhance the diagnostic yield of exploratory burr holes, allowing identification of parenchymal hematomas or other mass lesions.[53]

In patients with initial cardiac arrest or profound systemic hypotension, given the lower incidence of intracranial mass lesions,[31] it is not appropriate to perform exploratory burr holes, but the placement of an ICP monitor is reasonable. If the ICP is low, then no further direct treatment of intracranial physiology is appropriate except for general stabilization of the patient. If the ICP in such a case is markedly elevated, then the surgeon may decide that further surgical exploration and ultrasonic examination of the brain are appropriate to identify a treatable mass lesion.

After initial CT scanning, or upon exploratory diagnosis, the presence of a posttraumatic mass lesion should lead to immediate surgical evacuation, if feasible.[3,5,15,36,49] The presence of residual cerebral swelling after evacuating the hemorrhage should lead to consideration of an appropriately located lobectomy,[54] or a large, decompressive craniectomy,[55] or both. Decompressive craniectomy has also become a recognized treatment for herniation caused by hemispheric infarction, particularly in the nondominant hemisphere.[56] When a decompressive craniectomy is performed, it should be as large as is feasible, to fully decompress the entire hemisphere of the brain, and the bone should generally be stored in a sterile environment at minus 70°C.[55] In addition to the above-noted surgical interventions, ICP monitoring should be established at this time for subsequent patient management.[36]

Immediate surgical management of nontraumatic lesions causing herniation is also often indicated. This may include evacuation for lobar or nondominant hemispheric spontaneous hemorrhage[15] and immediate percutaneous ventricular drainage for hydrocephalus.[7] In the setting of upward tentorial herniation or tonsillar herniation at the foramen magnum, emergency management should also include evacuation of responsible mass lesions[6,9] and posterior fossa decompression as needed to decompress the cerebellum and brainstem.[4]

There may also be situations in which surgical management of a mass lesion is not indicated, such as large, deep-seated hemorrhages within the dominant hemisphere of the brain, those in the brainstem, or when a patient is elderly or has a coagulation disorder.

5.8 Prognosis in Cerebral Herniation Syndromes

Although the overall prognosis for patients with clinical herniation syndromes is poor, it is by no means hopeless. The prognosis for functional recovery may be quite good, particularly among younger patients who exhibit reversal of the clinical signs of herniation with use of mannitol and hyperventilation, and who have an intracranial mass lesion that can be surgically removed.[3,5,32,49,57]

For patients with transtentorial herniation following head trauma, the overall mortality rate is ~ 70%.[5] Among 100 such patients treated surgically, 9% had a good recovery and 9% had a moderately good outcome. Those who recovered were generally younger and had a higher initial GCS score than those who died or were severely disabled or vegetative.[5] Particularly important is the recognition of patients with an initially high GCS score who deteriorate to comatose and then herniate; the cause is often a treatable mass lesion, such as acute epidural hematoma; such patients have the best chance of functional survival with rapid resuscitation and corrective treatment.[5,29]

After traumatic herniation, age exerts a profoundly negative impact. Quigley et al[57] prospectively examined 380 patients with an initial GCS score of 3 to 5 after head injury and evaluated the effects of age, GCS score, and pupillary reactivity. They noted that when one or both pupils were nonreactive, all 96 patients older than 50 years of age, and all but one of 121 patients older than 40 years of age, were finally dead or vegetative.

Among those under 20 years of age with one or both pupils non-reactive, 11 of 72 (15%) had a functional recovery.

For patients with nontraumatic causes of herniation, the prognosis may be much better for functional recovery, as the brain itself may have intact function except for the cause of the herniation syndrome. For patients with acute hydrocephalus,[7] tumor-related cerebral edema,[9] temporal lobar hemorrhage,[15] hemispheric infarction,[55] or cerebellotonsillar herniation from lumbar drainage,[4] appropriate resuscitation and corrective reversal of mass effect can result in a satisfactory outcome.

References

[1] Reich JB, Sierra J, Camp W, Zanzonico P, Deck MD, Plum F. Magnetic resonance imaging measurements and clinical changes accompanying transtentorial and foramen magnum brain herniation. Ann Neurol. 1993; 33(2):159–170

[2] Ropper AH. Lateral displacement of the brain and level of consciousness in patients with an acute hemispheral mass. N Engl J Med. 1986; 314(15):953–958

[3] Cruz J, Minoja G, Okuchi K. Improving clinical outcomes from acute subdural hematomas with the emergency preoperative administration of high doses of mannitol: a randomized trial. Neurosurgery. 2001; 49(4):864–871

[4] Dagnew E, van Loveren HR, Tew JM, Jr. Acute foramen magnum syndrome caused by an acquired Chiari malformation after lumbar drainage of cerebrospinal fluid: report of three cases. Neurosurgery. 2002; 51(3):823–828, discussion 828–829

[5] Andrews BT, Pitts LH, Lovely MP, Bartkowski H. Is computed tomographic scanning necessary in patients with tentorial herniation? Results of immediate surgical exploration without computed tomography in 100 patients. Neurosurgery. 1986; 19(3):408–414

[6] Cuneo RA, Caronna JJ, Pitts L, Townsend J, Winestock DP. Upward transtentorial herniation: seven cases and a literature review. Arch Neurol. 1979; 36(10):618–623

[7] Muhonen MG, Zunkeler B. Management of acute hydrocephalus (landmarks and techniques). In: Loftus C, ed. Neurosurgical Emergencies. Vol. 1. Neurosurgical Topics. Chicago, IL: AANS Publications Committee; 1994:29–41

[8] Lidofsky SD, Bass NM, Prager MC, et al. Intracranial pressure monitoring and liver transplantation for fulminant hepatic failure. Hepatology. 1992; 16(1):1–7

[9] Weinberg JS, Rhines LD, Cohen ZR, Langford L, Levin VA. Posterior fossa decompression for life-threatening tonsillar herniation in patients with gliomatosis cerebri: report of three cases. Neurosurgery. 2003; 52(1):216–223, discussion 223

[10] Finney LA, Walker AE. Transtentorial Herniation. Springfield, IL: Charles C. Thomas Publishers; 1962:12–26

[11] Sunderland S. The tentorial notch and complications produced by herniations of the brain through that aperture. Br J Surg. 1958; 45(193):422–438

[12] Adler DE, Milhorat TH. The tentorial notch: anatomical variation, morphometric analysis, and classification in 100 human autopsy cases. J Neurosurg. 2002; 96(6):1103–1112

[13] Sunderland S, Hughes ESR. The pupillo-constrictor pathway and the nerves to the ocular muscles in man. Brain. 1946; 69(4):301–309

[14] Nguyen JP, Djindjian M, Brugières P, Badiane S, Melon E, Poirier J. Anatomy-computerized tomography correlations in transtentorial brain herniation. J Neuroradiol. 1989; 16(3):181–196

[15] Ross DA, Olsen WL, Ross AM, Andrews BT, Pitts LH. Brain shift, level of consciousness, and restoration of consciousness in patients with acute intracranial hematoma. J Neurosurg. 1989; 71(4):498–502

[16] Toutant SM, Klauber MR, Marshall LF, et al. Absent or compressed basal cisterns on first CT scan: ominous predictors of outcome in severe head injury. J Neurosurg. 1984; 61(4):691–694

[17] Hill L. The Physiology and Pathology of the Cerebral Circulation. London, UK: Churchill Publishers; 1896:208

[18] Meyer A. Herniation of the brain. Arch Neurol Psychiatry. 1920; 4(4):387–400

[19] Jennett WB, Stern WE. Tentorial herniation, the mid brain and the pupil. Experimental studies in brain compression. J Neurosurg. 1960; 17:598–609

[20] Jefferson G. The tentorial pressure cone. Arch Neurol Psychiatry. 1938; 40(5):857–876

[21] Howell DA. Upper brain-stem compression and foraminal impaction with intracranial space-occupying lesions and brain swelling. Brain. 1959; 82:525–550

[22] Kernohan JW, Woltman HW. Incisura of the crus due to contralateral brain tumor. Arch Neurol Psychiatry. 1929; 21(2):274–287

[23] Ropper AH. Syndrome of transtentorial herniation: is vertical displacement necessary? J Neurol Neurosurg Psychiatry. 1993; 56(8):932–935

[24] Marshall LF, Barba D, Toole BM, Bowers SA. The oval pupil: clinical significance and relationship to intracranial hypertension. J Neurosurg. 1983; 58(4):566–568

[25] Marshman LAG, Polkey CE, Penney CC. Unilateral fixed dilation of the pupil as a false-localizing sign with intracranial hemorrhage: case report and literature review. Neurosurgery. 2001; 49(5):1251–1255, discussion 1255–1256

[26] Chen TC, Maceri DR, Levy ML, Giannotta SL. Brain stem compression secondary to adipose graft prolapse after translabyrinthine craniotomy: case report. Neurosurgery. 1994; 35(3):521–523, discussion 523–524

[27] Fishman RA. Examination of the cerebrospinal fluid: techniques and complications. In: Cerebrospinal Fluid in Diseases of the Nervous System. 2nd ed. Philadelphia PA: WB Saunders; 1992:157–182

[28] Korein J, Cravioto H, Leicach M. Reevaluation of lumbar puncture; a study of 129 patients with papilledema or intracranial hypertension. Neurology. 1959; 9(4):290–297

[29] Duffy GP. Lumbar puncture in spontaneous subarachnoid haemorrhage. Br Med J (Clin Res Ed). 1982; 285(6349):1163–1164

[30] Andrews BT. Neurological monitoring. In: Intensive Care in Neurosurgery. New York, NY: Thieme Medical Publishers; 2003:21–28

[31] Andrews BT, Levy ML, Pitts LH. Implications of systemic hypotension for the neurological examination in patients with severe head injury. Surg Neurol. 1987; 28(6):419–422

[32] Andrews BT, Pitts LH. Functional recovery after traumatic transtentorial herniation. Neurosurgery. 1991; 29(2):227–231

[33] Miller JD, Sweet RC, Narayan R, Becker DP. Early insults to the injured brain. JAMA. 1978; 240(5):439–442

[34] Gray FD, Jr, Horner GJ. Survival following extreme hypoxemia. JAMA. 1970; 211(11):1815–1817

[35] Plum F, Posner JB. The Diagnosis of Stupor and Coma. 3rd ed. Philadelphia, PA: FA Davis Publishers; 1980:1–86

[36] Andrews BT. Head injury management. In: Intensive Care in Neurosurgery. New York, NY: Thieme Medical Publishers; 2003:125–136

[37] Bivins HG, Ford S, Bezmalinovic Z, Price HM, Williams JL. The effect of axial traction during orotracheal intubation of the trauma victim with an unstable cervical spine. Ann Emerg Med. 1988; 17(1):25–29

[38] Brain Trauma Foundation. American Association of Neurological Surgeons. Joint Section of Neurotrauma and Critical Care. Guidelines for the management of severe head injury. Hyperventilation. J Neurotrauma. 2000; 17:513–520

[39] Cruz J. On-line monitoring of global cerebral hypoxia in acute brain injury. Relationship to intracranial hypertension. J Neurosurg. 1993; 79(2):228–233

[40] Muizelaar JP, van der Poel HG, Li ZC, Kontos HA, Levasseur JE. Pial arteriolar vessel diameter and CO2 reactivity during prolonged hyperventilation in the rabbit. J Neurosurg. 1988; 69(6):923–927

[41] Andrews BT. Intensive Care in Neurosurgery. New York, NY: Thieme Medical Publishers; 2003

[42] Prough DS. Should I use hypertonic saline to treat high intracranial pressure? In: Valadka AB, Andrews BT, eds. Neurotrauma: Evidence-Based Answers to Common Questions. New York, NY: Thieme Medical Publishers; 2005:148–151

[43] De Vivo P, Del Gaudio A, Ciritella P, Puopolo M, Chiarotti F, Mastronardi E. Hypertonic saline solution: a safe alternative to mannitol 18% in neurosurgery. Minerva Anestesiol. 2001; 67(9):603–611

[44] Qureshi AI, Geocadin RG, Suarez JI, Ulatowski JA. Long-term outcome after medical reversal of transtentorial herniation in patients with supratentorial mass lesions. Crit Care Med. 2000; 28(5):1556–1564

[45] Muizelaar JP, Wei EP, Kontos HA, Becker DP. Mannitol causes compensatory cerebral vasoconstriction and vasodilation in response to blood viscosity changes. J Neurosurg. 1983; 59(5):822–828

[46] Burke AM, Quest DO, Chien S, Cerri C. The effects of mannitol on blood viscosity. J Neurosurg. 1981; 55(4):550–553

[47] Schrot RJ, Muizelaar JP. Is there s "best" way to give mannitol? In: Valadka AB, Andrews BT, eds. Neurotrauma: Evidence-Based Answers to Common Questions. New York, NY: Thieme Publishers; 2005:142–147

[48] Leech P, Miller JD. Intracranial volume—pressure relationships during experimental brain compression in primates. 3. Effect of mannitol and hyperventilation. J Neurol Neurosurg Psychiatry. 1974; 37(10):1105–1111

[49] Cruz J, Minoja G, Okuchi K. Major clinical and physiological benefits of early high doses of mannitol for intraparenchymal temporal lobe hemorrhages with abnormal pupillary widening: a randomized trial. Neurosurgery. 2002; 51(3):628–637, discussion 637–638

[50] Mortazavi MM, Romeo AK, Deep A, et al. Hypertonic saline for treating raised intracranial pressure: literature review with meta-analysis. J Neurosurg. 2012; 116(1):210–221

[51] Kerwin AJ, Schinco MA, Tepas JJ, III, Renfro WH, Vitarbo EA, Muehlberger M. The use of 23.4% hypertonic saline for the management of elevated intracranial pressure in patients with severe traumatic brain injury: a pilot study. J Trauma. 2009; 67(2):277–282

[52] Forsyth LL, Liu-DeRyke X, Parker D, Jr, Rhoney DH. Role of hypertonic saline for the management of intracranial hypertension after stroke and traumatic brain injury. Pharmacotherapy. 2008; 28(4):469–484

[53] Andrews BT, Mampalam TJ, Omsberg E, Pitts LH. Intraoperative ultrasound imaging of the entire brain through unilateral exploratory burr holes after severe head injury: technical note. Surg Neurol. 1990; 33(4):291–294

[54] Litofsky NS, Chin LS, Tang G, Baker S, Giannotta SL, Apuzzo ML. The use of lobectomy in the management of severe closed-head trauma. Neurosurgery. 1994; 34(4):628–632, discussion 632–633

[55] Andrews BT. Does decompressive craniectomy really improve outcome after head injury? In: Valadka AB, Andrews BT, eds. Neurotrauma: Evidence-Based Answers to Common Questions. New York, NY: Thieme Medical Publishers; 2005:163–166

[56] Carter BS, Ogilvy CS, Candia GJ, Rosas HD, Buonanno F. One-year outcome after decompressive surgery for massive nondominant hemispheric infarction. Neurosurgery. 1997; 40(6):1168–1175, discussion 1175–1176

[57] Quigley MR, Vidovich D, Cantella D, Wilberger JE, Maroon JC, Diamond D. Defining the limits of survivorship after very severe head injury. J Trauma. 1997; 42(1):7–10

6 Penetrating Cerebral Trauma

Margaret Riordan and Griffith R. Harsh IV

Abstract

Although most traumatic brain injuries in the United States are caused by blunt trauma, the percentage of penetrating cerebral injuries has been increasing in part because of gun violence. Variations in weaponry and projectile ballistic properties lead to a broad spectrum of both intracranial and extracranial damage. Current management is based on cumulative military experiences accumulated since World War I and has been modified to address the civilian population. Despite significant advancements in critical care medicine and microsurgical techniques, these injuries continue to present a formidable challenge for neurosurgeons. Treatment strategies focus on initial resuscitation, assessment of damage through imaging studies, providing appropriate supportive care, and surgical intervention when indicated.

Keywords: gunshot wound, penetrating brain injury, skull fracture, traumatic brain injury

6.1 Introduction

Each year, approximately 1.4 million people in the United States experience traumatic brain injury (TBI), and annual fatalities from TBI approach 200,000. Six thousand of these deaths involve penetrating brain injury (PBI) rather than closed head injury (CHI).[1,2,3,4,5] The percentage of TBI deaths resulting involving firearms, the most common form of PBI, is increasing, whereas that from motor vehicle accidents, the most common cause of CHI, is decreasing.[1,2,3,4,5] Early studies of PBI focused on military injuries, but changing demographics have shifted the focus to civilian injuries. Fifty percent of civilian deaths from PBI are suicide, which is most common in older white males. In urban areas, increase in gang violence has contributed to a higher incidence of PBI among civilian youth.[1,6]

Despite improved imaging, microsurgical technique, and critical care protocols (such as advanced trauma life support [ATLS]), the management of penetrating craniocerebral trauma remains challenging because of the multiplicity of mechanisms of injury and the variability of extent of intracranial damage.[6,7]

6.2 Mechanism of Injury

The extent and severity of penetrating TBI reflect characteristics of the penetrating object: shape, size, trajectory, and velocity. Although all objects damage brain traversed, the volume of the injury beyond the immediate tract is highly dependent on the object's kinetic energy. An object's kinetic energy (KE = $1/2\ mv^2$) is more influenced by its velocity (v) than its mass (m). Most low-velocity sharp projectiles, such as knives, screwdrivers, and arrows, travel 36 to 76 m/s. They cause focal injuries whose volumes depend on the object's shape and the path and depth of penetration. Little energy is transferred to surrounding tissue, which often remains unharmed. Velocities of bullets from civilian handguns are 216 to 491 m/s, from civilian rifle velocities are 820 to 960 m/s, and from military weapons are even higher.

Penetrating wounds from explosive devices, whose fragments are not aerodynamic and are thus slowed by air friction, usually resemble those from low-velocity bullets in their irregular shape and trajectory.[4,8,9]

Higher-velocity projectiles injure brain not just by direct focal disruption but also by inducing pressure waves that radiate orthogonally from the object's path. These pressure waves pass through brain, which is 75% aqueous, like ripples from a stone dropped in a puddle: proximally the waves have short wavelength and high amplitude, but as they travel through tissue, their wavelength increases and their amplitude decreases. Nearby tissue thus sustains greater disruption, but with high-velocity objects, the volume of injury can extend far beyond the initial trajectory.[10]

The injury is further augmented by cavitational forces. An object's traverse of brain displaces tissue peripherally, creating a primary tract and a cavity of greater caliber than the projectile itself. The higher the projectile's velocity and the greater its yaw (rotation along its long axis), the larger the cavity along the tract and the larger the exit site from the skull. For example, a very-high-velocity bullet may create a cavity 15 times larger than its diameter.[8] The relatively negative pressure within the cavity can draw in debris from the outside, increasing the risk of infection, and initiate cycles of cavitation and collapse that further injure the surrounding parenchyma and blood vessels.[1,8,11]

Other factors that increase brain injury include in-driven bone fragments, projectile ricochet off the inner calvarium, projectile fragmentation, and both direct and shearing disruption of intraparenchymal blood vessels, causing hematomas and subarachnoid hemorrhage.[1,8,11]

6.3 Pathology of Injury

Evidence of microscopic brain tissue damage following PBI extends beyond grossly visible damage. The projectile leaves a permanent tract of necrotic and ischemic tissues and damaged blood vessels. Peripheral to this tract lies an annulus of brain parenchyma that, although relatively less grossly disrupted, shows necrosis with axonal, neuronal, and astrocytic destruction and neutrophil infiltration. Surrounding this annulus, widespread axonal damage and injured, hyperchromatic, and vacuolated neurons are seen. This composite volume of pathologically evident injury is expanded first by cytotoxic and then by vasogenic edema. This edema is evident on imaging hours to days following trauma. Microscopic damage is not limited to that in close to the bullet tract. Perhaps reflecting the effects of shock waves, axonal injury has been found at autopsy after PBI throughout the hemispheres, brainstem, and cerebellum.[1,8,11]

At a cellular level, disruption of the neuronal and axonal structures leads to the release of free radical, glutamate, and calcium, which further injure brain parenchyma. Additionally, the damaged cells express cellular adhesion molecules and matrix metalloproteinases that trigger a localized inflammatory response and disrupt the blood–brain barrier.[12] Although this inflammatory response may contribute to tissue injury, it also facilitates tissue repair.

6.4 Physiology of Injury

Within seconds following the initial impact, a significant increase in intracranial pressure (ICP) precipitates rostrocaudal brain herniation and systemic catecholamine release, leading to hypotension. The combination of systemic hypotension and elevated ICP and the resulting decline in cerebral perfusion pressure (CPP) cause ischemic brain injury that further increases ICP. Downward cerebral herniation compresses the brainstem, leading to respiratory depression and apnea, which compounds ischemic injury.[8,12] As cerebral edema progresses, hours to days after the initial trauma, the ICP that may have subsided with autoregulation can rise again. ICP must be lowered to prevent worsening ischemic injury.

Craniocerebral missile injuries can also induce a systemic coagulopathy that worsens cerebral hemorrhage. This results from activation of the extrinsic coagulation pathway by thromboplastin from injured brain and the excessive catecholamine release after severe brain trauma.[13] Abnormalities of blood coagulation are associated with a particularly poor outcome after brain injury.

6.5 Overview of Management of Penetrating Cerebral Trauma

The current management of PBI has evolved with accumulation of experience treating military injuries. During World War I, Harvey Cushing employed early, wide débridement of necrotic tissue and debris with gentle suction and irrigation, followed by careful dural and two-layer scalp closure. He usually performed a tripod scalp incision, extensive en bloc skull débridement, and removal of all visible debris and bony fragments. Use of this technique reduced the mortality rate after PBI from 55% to 29%.[14,15,16] Throughout World War II, the mortality rates decreased further because of routine antibiotic administration, and mortality continued to decrease during the 1950 Korean War because of rapid evacuation from the battlefield via helicopter.[17,18]

During the Vietnam War, computed tomography (CT) imaging was used to identify the injured area such that surgical intervention could be more focused. Outcome studies, showing that bone and bullet fragments persist even after aggressive débridement but that these rarely cause infection, encouraged surgeons to limit débridement to removal of superficial objects and devitalized brain. Of note, analysis of PBI in the Israeli–Lebanese conflict from 1982 to 1985, found that 51% of patients had retained bone fragments after surgery, but only 0.9% of these developed a cerebral abscess.[13,15,19]

Multiple studies have also supported the importance of Cushing's prevention of cerebrospinal fluid (CSF) leakage by meticulous repair dura and scalp to avoid CSF leaks. Review of results from the 1964 Iran–Iraq war and the Israeli–Lebanon conflict also concluded that extensive débridement was not as important as prevention of CSF leakage in limiting infection, morbidity, and mortality.[13,15,19] Multivariate analysis of outcomes from the Iran–Iraq war identified CSF leakage, cranial disruption communicating brain and air sinuses, and ventricular traverse as independent predictors of infection after penetrating cerebral trauma.[13,15,19]

And the Vietnam Head Injury Study (VHIS) found a mortality of 22.8% for patients with CSF leakage versus 5.1% for those without leakage.[13,15,19] In this study, only half of the CSF leaks occurred at the wound site. Thus, current management emphasizes immediate, aggressive resuscitation, followed promptly by targeted surgical débridement and repair of CSF fistula.

6.6 Resuscitation and Initial Management

Despite improvement resulting from shorter emergency response times and advancements in paramedic care, 71% of patients with PBI still die before reaching the hospital.[1,2,6] The initial management of patients with PBI should follow the ATLS resuscitation protocols that prioritize airway protection and hemodynamic stabilization. Endotracheal intubation is indicated for patients with impaired ventilation, inability to protect their airway, and the potential for neurologic deterioration.[20,21] When inserting endotracheal and gastric tubes, extreme caution must be taken to avoid inadvertent passage into the cranial cavity, as many patients with gunshot wounds to the head have skull base and facial fractures. Extensive facial injury can complicate airway management and necessitate emergency tracheostomy.[11]

Maintenance of a systolic blood pressure of at least 90 mm Hg is recommended, as baseline hypotension is associated with a poor overall prognosis in PBI patients. Between 10 and 50% of PBI patients are hypotensive on arrival to the emergency room. Systolic blood pressure should be aggressively managed with fluid resuscitation and vasopressors if needed.[1] Intravenous access is obtained, and resuscitation is begun with isotonic normal saline (0.9%). Some patients may require transfusion with blood products such as albumin or packed red blood cells if they have an inadequate response to initial fluid resuscitation. Hypertonic saline (3% normal saline) infusions may be useful for management of elevated ICP.[11] Mannitol administration may also be necessary to lower ICP, but it should be used with caution in the setting of hypotension.

Once the patient is hemodynamically stable, a primary survey assesses the extent of the patient's injuries. A brief history, including the patient's age, events surrounding the injury, Glasgow Coma Scale (GCS) score at the scene, GCS score upon arrival in the emergency room, and postresuscitation GCS score, should be documented. A focused, rapid neurologic examination is performed to assess the level of consciousness; pupillary size, symmetry, and reaction; brainstem reflexes; motor function; and presence of spontaneous respirations. This initial information is prognostically useful, as low GCS score, unreactive pupils, and a poor neurologic examination have been associated with a poor outcome (see ▶ Box 6.1).[1,2,22,23,24]

Box 6.1 Poor Prognostic Factors

Postresuscitation Glasgow Coma Scale score < 5
Fixed and dilated pupils
Hypotension upon arrival to the emergency room
Major intracranial vascular injury
Bihemispheric injury
Obliteration of basal cisterns
Diabetes insipidus

Once the patient is hemodynamically stable, any scalp wounds can be examined in detail and débrided as necessary. The hair on the scalp should be clipped to reveal the extent of scalp damage and the presence of contaminants. Significant scalp hemorrhage can be temporarily controlled with surgical staples, Raney clips, or temporary suture until definitive operative treatment is performed. Closure of the skin also prevents CSF loss from possible dural breaches. In the case of gunshot wounds, entrance and exit wounds should be carefully examined. Lower-velocity penetrating objects such as knives and arrows should be left in place until full assessment, including radiologic studies, is performed and the object can be removed in the operating room under direct vision. The patient should be given the tetanus toxoid vaccination and prophylactic antibiotics.

6.7 Imaging

A CT scan of the head is the study of choice for evaluation of penetrating cerebral trauma and should be obtained once the patient is hemodynamically stable. Imaging allows localization of the projectile and any bullet fragments, evaluation of bony destruction, and the location of hematomas, contusions, intraventricular hemorrhage, and subarachnoid hemorrhage. In addition, CT provides prognostic value by demonstrating the extent of injury. Multilobed and bihemispheric injury, transventricular injury, thalamic and basal ganglia injury, obliteration of the basal cisterns, subarachnoid hemorrhage, and significant posterior fossa hemorrhage are each associated with a poor prognosis. Midline shift greater than 10 mm is also associated with poor prognosis; however, the entire CT scan should be taken into account, as large midline shifts in one direction can reflect the presence of a unilateral traumatic mass whose prompt evacuation may yield a favorable prognosis.[11]

Traumatic intracranial aneurysms (TICAs) occur in 3 to 42% of all cases of PBI. Blood vessel investigation is indicated if the penetrating object has traversed the frontobasal or temporal region, passed into both hemispheres, or is near the circle of Willis, or if there is extensive unexplained subarachnoid hemorrhage or intraventricular hemorrhage or a delayed hematoma. Most TICAs involve the peripheral branches of the anterior cerebral artery and middle cerebral artery. A CT angiogram can be obtained quickly, but when its interpretation is confounded by metal artifact from a bullet, digital subtraction angiography is indicated. Additionally, TICAs can develop and bleed days after the initial injury; they should be suspected if new or worsening hemorrhage is noted on follow-up imaging.[25,26,27]

Magnetic resonance imaging has no current role in penetrating cerebral trauma involving metal fragments because metal fragments create artifact and may migrate in response to the magnetic field, causing additional injury.

6.8 Surgical Management

Although retrospective studies have shown that patients with a higher postresuscitation GCS score (> 7) and focal cranial injuries that do not involve both hemispheres and that avoid the deep gray matter have a better outcome following surgical intervention, many factors must be considered when deciding how to best manage a patient.[28] For example, some patients with a lower initial GCS score but focal intracranial hematomas with significant mass effect may benefit from surgical decompression. Furthermore, when evaluating surgical candidates, complicating factors, such as administration of sedating medications for intubation or transport prior to arrival to the emergency room, must be considered. Surgical management can range from simple wound débridement in the operating room to an extensive exploration of the injury site or decompressive craniectomy, depending on the extent of the injury and the patient's clinical examination and CT findings (see ▶ Box 6.2).

Box 6.2 Relative Indications for Surgery

Glasgow Coma Scale score > 7
Mass effect on temporal lobe
Mass effect within the posterior fossa
Open depressed skull fracture
Evidence of cerebrospinal fluid leak

6.8.1 Simple Debridement

Small entrance wounds may be treated with local wound care if the scalp is not devitalized and no intracranial pathology requiring surgical evacuation is seen on CT. Superficial scalp wounds should be cleaned, débrided, and repaired to prevent infection and to prevent extensive blood loss from laceration. These wounds may be effectively treated in the emergency room by first shaving the scalp around the injured site, washing the wound with sterile saline, and closing all lacerations with staples or multilayer suturing depending on the wound's depth. Patients may be taken to the operating room if the wound is extensive.

6.8.2 Surgical Debridement

Surgery is indicated for patients with focal hematomas causing significant mass effect and urgently for those with hematomas in the temporal or posterior fossa compromising the perimesencephalic or basal cistern, respectively. Other reasons for surgical intervention include an orbitofacial wound, a need to control active hemorrhage, and evolution of an expansive intracranial lesion. The goals of surgery for penetrating cerebral trauma are evacuation of hemorrhage and wound débridement. Wounds that have devitalized scalp, bone, and dura require operative intervention to achieve a watertight reconstruction and prevent CSF leak.

After stabilization in the emergency room, the patient is taken to the operating room and positioned for optimal exposure of the injured site. The head may be placed on either a circular or a horseshoe-shaped gel headrest, or if required for positioning favorable to access, as for a suboccipital craniectomy, head pins may be applied, with care to avoid pin placement near avulsed scalp or fractured skull.

The incision is planned to avoid compromising scalp blood supply and to incorporate the scalp wound if possible. After removal of the bone flap, intact dura is exposed on all sides of the penetration. Special caution should be taken in removing depressed skull or a penetrating object from vicinity of major

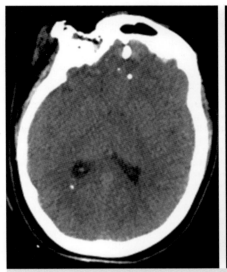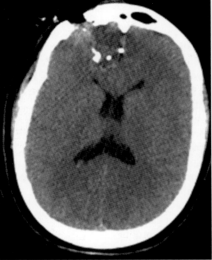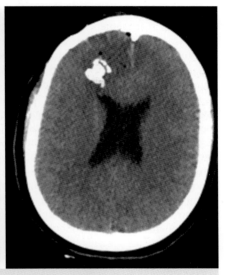

Fig. 6.1 Computed tomography images of a patient with a gunshot wound to the head showing indriven skull fragments.

venous sinuses. The subdural space is inspected, and any hematoma is evacuated. Necrotic brain tissue and foreign debris that is readily accessible are removed using a combination of gentle suction and irrigation. Meticulous hemostasis is performed. Watertight closure with pericranium, temporal or occipital fascia, or fascia lata is essential for preventing postoperative infection. Injuries that communicate intracranial space with air sinuses require repair with watertight dural closure. Proper scalp closure is important to minimize the risk of subsequent infections; if sufficient healthy tissue is lacking, tissue flaps may be required.[11]

6.8.3 Decompressive Craniectomy

The decision to replace the bone flap following débridement is multifactorial. If the skull is extensively fragmented and cannot be repaired with a good cosmetic result, the cranial defect is not filled and cranioplasty is planned for the future. Often, diffuse cerebral edema precludes the replacement of the skull flap. The preoperative CT scan may hint at extensive swelling, but severe edema may not be obvious until surgical treatment is undertaken. In such cases, decompressive craniectomy is necessary to accommodate further swelling.

6.8.4 Intracranial Pressure Monitoring

ICP monitoring can be useful in patients with cerebral edema but without a mass lesion requiring evacuation, in those for whom a reliable neurologic examination cannot be obtained, and in those needing pre- and postoperative medical management of elevated ICP. The indications for placement of an ICP monitor in PBI parallel those outlined in the guidelines for severe TBI in general: a postresuscitation GCS score less than 8, GCS score 9 to 12 in patients either requiring prolonged anesthesia or having an abnormal CT scan, and the need for constant sedation, which precludes an accurate neurologic examination.[20]

6.8.5 Illustrative Case

A patient was brought to the emergency room after being struck in the right face and head by multiple bullets during a drive-by shooting. After hemodynamic stabilization and intubation for airway protection, a neurologic examination was performed. The patient was following commands with all four extremities. The right eye was swollen shut by significant periorbital edema, and the left pupil was reactive to light. There was an obvious entry wound over the right orbit but no leakage of CSF. CT imaging showed rupture of the right globe from the bullet entry; extensive fractures of the frontal bones, anterior skull base, and air sinuses; and bifrontal hemorrhage and edema (see ▶ Fig. 6.1).

The patient was admitted to the intensive care unit (ICU) and given ceftriaxone and clindamycin. Because the significant injury to her eye and multiple facial fractures raised suspicion of CSF fistula, the patient was taken to the operating room for enucleation of her globe, exenteration of her orbit, and extensive superficial cranial debridement. The frontal dura was found to be torn in multiple places, and repair with a fascia lata graft was necessary. The deep-seated bullet and skull fragments were not removed.

In this case, the patient's presenting neurologic examination was favorable and the extensive skull base fractures and severe orbital injury warranted surgery for débridement and repair of the lacerated frontal dura.

6.9 Complications and Adjuvant Therapy

Patients with PBI require intensive care for monitoring and maintenance of CPP and monitoring for complications, including new hemorrhage, worsening edema, elevated ICP, and infection. Cardiac monitoring is also necessary, as the catecholamine release associated with severe head injury can cause myocardial ischemia. Maintenance of CPP greater than 70 mm Hg may require invasive cardiac monitoring (as large fluid shifts can occur in the early stages of injury), fluid resuscitation, and iatrogenic diuresis for management of elevated ICP. Likewise, electrolytes must also be monitored, as head injury can lead to hypothalamic–pituitary dysfunction that may manifest as diabetes insipidus or SIADH (syndrome of inappropriate antidiuretic hormone secretion), both of which are associated with worse outcome.[11]

Additionally, all patients with PBI should be observed for deep vein thromboses (DVTs) and gastrointestinal ulcerations; mechanical or chemical prophylaxis for DVTs and histamine H_2-receptor (H_2) antagonists should be used as soon as clinically permitted. As with other ICU patients who require prolonged intubation, those with PBI are at risk for respiratory complications such as pneumonia and adult respiratory distress syndrome and should be extubated in a timely manner or given a tracheostomy if extubation is not possible.

Anticonvulsant therapy following PBI is controversial. There is class I evidence showing benefit of early antiseizure prophylaxis for 7 days in TBI patients. Prophylaxis with phenytoin, phenobarbital, carbamazepine, or valproate is recommended.[29] Although long-term anticonvulsant therapy is not currently recommended, one study found that 32% of patients suffering PBI during the Iran–Iraq war developed epilepsy within the average follow-up period of 39.4 months. In particular, patients with a lower Glasgow Outcome Scale score and a focal motor neurologic deficit were particularly prone to develop epilepsy.[30] Another study that retrospectively reviewed 163 patients with posttraumatic epilepsy following either PBI or blunt head trauma found that motor deficits and encephalomalacia were common concomitants of epilepsy and thus recommended vigilance for and prompt treatment of seizures in patients with such injuries.[31]

Prophylactic use of broad-spectrum antibiotics is recommended in PBI, as infections occur in 1 to 52% of cases; the higher rates are associated with retained bone or metallic fragments, CSF fistulas, and facio-orbital entrance wounds. The most common bacteria implicated are skin flora, but gram-negative bacilli are also frequently cultured; thus, antibiotics chosen should both adequately cover these pathogens and penetrate the blood–brain barrier.[11,32,33,34,35,36,37] A prospective study of 160 patients with PHI found that a projectile trajectory through contaminated cavities, retained bone or metallic fragments, and prolonged hospital stay were risk factors for infection. Although the 59 patients given prophylactic antibiotics in this study did not have a lower infection rate than those not receiving antibiotics, since the sample size receiving prophylactic antibiotics in this study is small, surgeons may still wish to administer prophylactic antibiotic coverage to those patients at higher risk for infection.[37]

6.10 Conclusion

With the variety of weaponry available and the varying ballistic properties of projectiles, brain penetration can cause a wide range of injuries that challenge neurosurgical management. Although injury prevention should be the primary means of risk reduction, it is important to understand that PBI often requires prompt, comprehensive, and thoughtful intervention. Rapid medical resuscitation and control of bleeding are the first steps. Surgery for evacuation of space-occupying lesions that exert mass effect, for the repair of orbitofacial wounds, for débridement of extensive devitalized scalp, bone, or brain, for hemostasis, and for watertight and cosmetic closure is often needed.

References

[1]   Bizhan A, Mossop C, Aarabi JA. Surgical management of civilian gunshot wounds to the head. Handb Clin Neurol. 2015; 127:181–193

[2]   Hofbauer M, Kdolsky R, Figl M, et al. Predictive factors influencing the outcome after gunshot injuries to the head—a retrospective cohort study. J Trauma. 2010; 69(4):770–775

[3]   Levy ML, Davis SE, Mccomb JG, Apuzzo ML. Economic, ethical, and outcome-based decisions regarding aggressive surgical management in patients with penetrating craniocerebral injury. J Health Commun. 1996; 1(3):301–308

[4]   Centers for Disease Control and Prevention. Injury Fact Book 2001–2002. Atlanta, GA: Centers for Disease Control and Prevention; 2001

[5]   Ingraham C, Johnson CY. How gun deaths became as common as traffic deaths. Washington Post. December 19, 2015

[6]   Aryan HE, Jandial R, Bennett RL, Masri LS, Lavine SD, Levy ML. Gunshot wounds to the head: gang- and non-gang-related injuries and outcomes. Brain Inj. 2005; 19(7):505–510

[7]   Keong NCH, Gleave JRW, Hutchinson PJ. Neurosurgical history: comparing the management of penetrating head injury in 1969 with 2005. Br J Neurosurg. 2006; 20(4):227–232

[8]   de Lanerolle NC. Kim JH,BandakFA. Neuropathology of traumatic brain injury: comparison of penetrating, nonpenetrating direct impart and explosive blast etiologies. Semin Neurol. 2015; 35:12–19

[9]   Oehmichen M, Meissner C, König HG, Gehl HB. Gunshot injuries to the head and brain caused by low-velocity handguns and rifles. A review. Forensic Sci Int. 2004; 146(2–3):111–120

[10] Davidsson J, Risling M. Characterization of pressure distribution in penetrating traumatic brain injuries. Front Neurol. 2015; 6:51

[11] Rosenfeld JV, Bell RS, Armonda R. Current concepts in penetrating and blast injury to the central nervous system. World J Surg. 2015; 39(6):1352–1362

[12] Cunningham TL, Cartagena CM, Lu XC, et al. Correlations between blood-brain barrier disruption and neuroinflammation in an experimental model of penetrating ballistic-like brain injury. J Neurotrauma. 2014; 31(5):505–514

[13] Centers for Disease Control and Prevention, National Center for Injury Prevention and Control. Traumatic Brain Injury in the United States—A Report to Congress. Atlanta, GA: Centers for Disease Control and Prevention; 1999

[14] Amirjamshidi A, Abbassioun K, Rahmat H. Minimal débridement or simple wound closure as the only surgical treatment in war victims with low-velocity penetrating head injuries. Indications and management protocol based upon more than 8 years follow-up of 99 cases from Iran-Iraq conflict. Surg Neurol. 2003; 60(2):105–110, discussion 110–111

[15] Brandvold B, Levi L, Feinsod M, George ED. Penetrating craniocerebral injuries in the Israeli involvement in the Lebanese conflict, 1982–1985. Analysis of a less aggressive surgical approach. J Neurosurg. 1990; 72(1):15–21

[16] Rish BL, Dillon JD, Caveness WF, Mohr JP, Kistler JP, Weiss GH. Evolution of craniotomy as a debridement technique for penetrating craniocerebral injuries. J Neurosurg. 1980; 53(6):772–775

[17] Surgical management of penetrating brain injury. J Trauma. 2001; 51(2, Suppl):S16–S25

[18] West CG. A short history of the management of penetrating missile injuries of the head. Surg Neurol. 1981; 16(2):145–149

[19] Pikus HJ, Ball PA. Characteristics of cerebral gunshot injuries in the rural setting. Neurosurg Clin N Am. 1995; 6(4):611–620

[20] Brain Trauma Foundation, American Association of Neurological Surgeons, Congress of Neurological Surgeons. Guidelines for the management of severe traumatic brain injury. J Neurotrauma. 2007; 24(Suppl 1):S1–S106

[21] Kim T-W, Lee J-K, Moon K-S, et al. Penetrating gunshot injuries to the brain. J Trauma. 2007; 62(6):1446–1451

[22] Santiago LA, Oh BC, Dash PK, Holcomb JB, Wade CE. A clinical comparison of penetrating and blunt traumatic brain injuries. Brain Inj. 2012; 26(2):107–125

[23] Smith JE, Kehoe A, Harrisson SE, Russell R, Midwinter M. Outcome of penetrating intracranial injuries in a military setting. Injury. 2014; 45(5):874–878

[24] Bandt SK, Greenberg JK, Yarbrough CK, Schechtman KB, Limbrick DD, Leonard JR. Management of pediatric intracranial gunshot wounds: predictors of favorable clinical outcome and a new proposed treatment paradigm. J Neurosurg Pediatr. 2012; 10(6):511–517

[25] Bodanapally UK, Krejza J, Saksobhavivat N, et al. Predicting arterial injuries after penetrating brain trauma based on scoring signs from emergency CT studies. Neuroradiol J. 2014; 27(2):138–145

[26] Vascular complications of penetrating brain injury. J Trauma. 2001; 51(2, Suppl):S26–S28

[27] Aarabi B. Traumatic aneurysms of brain due to high velocity missile head wounds. Neurosurgery. 1988; 22(6 Pt 1):1056–1063

[28] Aarabi B, Tofighi B, Kufera JA, et al. Predictors of outcome in civilian gunshot wounds to the head. J Neurosurg. 2014; 120(5):1138–1146

[29] Antiseizure prophylaxis for penetrating brain injury. J Trauma. 2001; 51(2, Suppl):S41–S43

[30] Aarabi B, Taghipour M, Haghnegahdar A, Farokhi M, Mobley L. Prognostic factors in the occurrence of posttraumatic epilepsy after penetrating head injury suffered during military service. Neurosurg Focus. 2000; 8(1):e1

[31] Kazemi H, Hashemi-Fesharaki S, Razaghi S, et al. Intractable epilepsy and craniocerebral trauma: analysis of 163 patients with blunt and penetrating head injuries sustained in war. Injury. 2012; 43(12):2132–2135

[32] Taha JM, Haddad FS, Brown JA. Intracranial infection after missile injuries to the brain: report of 30 cases from the Lebanese conflict. Neurosurgery. 1991; 29(6):864–868

[33] Antibiotic prophylaxis for penetrating brain injury. J Trauma. 2001; 51(2, Suppl):S34–S40

[34] Aarabi B. Causes of infections in penetrating head wounds in the Iran-Iraq War. Neurosurgery. 1989; 25(6):923–926

[35] Aarabi B. Comparative study of bacteriological contamination between primary and secondary exploration of missile head wounds. Neurosurgery. 1987; 20(4):610–616

[36] Carey ME, Young H, Mathis JL, Forsythe J. A bacteriological study of craniocerebral missile wounds from Vietnam. J Neurosurg. 1971; 34(2 Pt 1):145–154

[37] Jimenez CM, Polo J, España JA. Risk factors for intracranial infection secondary to penetrating craniocere bral gunshot wounds in civilian practice. World Neurosurg. 2013; 79(5–6):749–755

7 Extra-Axial Hematomas

Shelly D. Timmons

Abstract

The term "extra-axial hematomas" is used to refer to hematomas found within the intracranial space but outside the substance of the brain itself. These lesions are among the most common emergencies encountered in neurosurgical practice and almost always occur as a result of head trauma. Brain injury is the most important contributor to mortality and morbidity from trauma, which is the leading cause of death for people under 45 years of age in the United States. Rapid evacuation of extra-axial hematomas is the mainstay of neurosurgical intervention for traumatic brain injury (TBI), and timely surgical intervention improves functional outcome and reduces mortality. For TBI patients who are initially lucid and deteriorate, four of five will have a mass lesion potentially requiring surgical evacuation, half of which are extra-axial. Most patients who present with signs of uncal or transtentorial herniation after trauma have extra-axial mass lesions, and evacuation can reverse the brainstem signs once decompression is achieved surgically.

The rapid diagnosis and transport of these injuries to allow for craniotomy and evacuation not only can save lives but prevent long-term mortality from brain compression, making recognition of the signs and symptoms and potential for rapid deterioration a hallmark of emergency care everywhere.

Keywords: craniotomy, epidural hematoma, extra-axial hematoma, hygroma, neurosurgery, neurosurgical emergency, subdural hematoma, traumatic brain injury

7.1 Introduction

The term "extra-axial hematomas" is used to refer to hematomas found within the intracranial space but outside the substance of the brain itself. These lesions are among the most common emergencies encountered in neurosurgical practice and almost always occur as a result of head trauma. Brain injury is the most important contributor to mortality and morbidity from trauma,[1] which is the leading cause of death for people under 45 years of age in the United States.[2] Rapid evacuation of extra-axial hematomas is the mainstay of neurosurgical intervention for traumatic brain injury (TBI), and timely surgical intervention improves functional outcome and reduces mortality.[3] For TBI patients who are initially lucid and deteriorate, four of five will have a mass lesion potentially requiring surgical evacuation, half of which are extra-axial.[4] Most patients who present with signs of uncal or transtentorial herniation after trauma have extra-axial mass lesions,[5,6] and evacuation can reverse the brainstem signs once decompression is achieved surgically. The entities to be discussed include acute epidural hematoma (EDH), acute subdural hematoma (aSDH), subdural hygroma, subacute subdural hematoma (sSDH), and chronic subdural hematoma (cSDH). Special considerations of posterior fossa (PF) lesions and child abuse are also presented.

7.2 Epidural Hematoma

7.2.1 Epidemiology

Epidural hematoma (►Fig. 7.1) is a relatively unusual occurrence and is most often caused by trauma, although rare instances of spontaneous occurrences in special circumstances, for example, sickle cell disease, have been reported. The overall incidence among trauma patients is estimated at between 2.7 and 4.1% of TBI patients[7,8]; however, the incidence among trauma victims in coma is higher, at 9 to 15%.[9,10] About 1% of TBI patients with normal neurologic examination and cranial fractures and 9% of patients in coma with fracture harbor an EDH.[9,11] Epidural hematoma in children is associated with fracture ~ 40% of the time, half of which are depressed, whereas fractures are uncommon with aSDHs in children.[12]

Traumatic EDH occurs most frequently in young people following high-speed accidents. In young adults, the highest incidence is between 20 and 30 years of age, and above 60 years of age EDH is unusual,[7,12,13] probably because of increasing adherence of the dura mater to the inner surface of the skull. In children, peak incidence is between 5 and 12 years, being much less common in newborns and young children.[14] Motor vehicle accidents (MVAs) account for the majority of etiologies in patients of all ages (30–73%), followed by falls (7–52%) and assault (1–19%).[15] Falls are more commonly the cause of EDH in children than are MVAs,[14,16] and children are less likely to present unconscious, to require surgery, or to have associated intracranial lesions.[16] Isolated EDHs in children are also predominantly caused by falls (68.6% in one series).[17]

Multiple (including bilateral) EDHs can occur,[8,18,19] typically in the frontal region, and are most often associated with altered sensorium without lucid interval[8] (►Fig. 7.2). These injuries have also been associated with lower Glasgow Coma Scale (GCS) score on presentation and higher mortality.[18] Epidural hematoma can extend both above and below the tentorium cerebelli. This finding may be associated with a venous sinus injury; therefore, surgical evacuation may be quite perilous. Chronic EDHs are generally smaller, more likely frontal or parietal, and present with milder, less-specific symptoms; they have excellent outcomes, whether treated operatively or observed.[19]

7.2.2 Pathogenesis

A well-described cause of EDH is a blow to the temporal region resulting in a fracture of the squamous portion of the temporal bone, with subsequent injury to the middle meningeal artery as it travels through or exits the bone. This results in arterial bleeding into the epidural space of the temporal fossa. However, recent evidence suggests that venous sources of EDH are actually more common.[20] This may be because of more frequent diagnoses being made possible by widespread rapid availability of computed tomography (CT) scanning, even in less symptomatic cases. Although expansion of EDH from arterial sources is

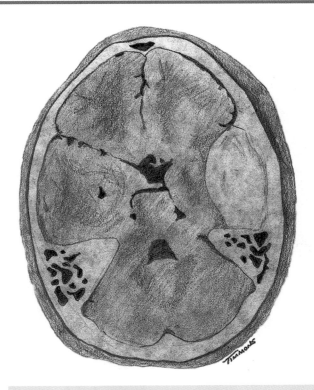

Fig. 7.1 A depiction of a large left temporal epidural hematoma with effacement of the quadrigeminal cisterns from temporal lobe displacement.

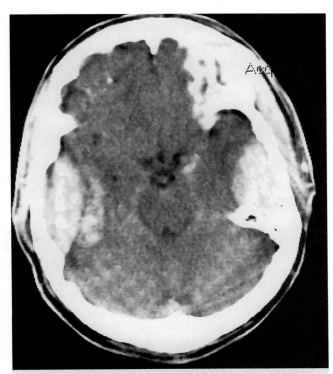

Fig. 7.2 Bilateral temporal epidural hematoma with underlying right temporal contusion/intraparenchymal hemorrhage.

treacherous and can be fatal, most EDHs are stable in size soon after trauma, as it is thought that once the dura is sheared from the inner surface of the pericranium and fills with hematoma, the cavity does not continue to expand.[13,19,21] Epidural hematomas that are potentially less rapidly expansive may be caused by a tear of a dural sinus, with or without associated overlying fracture. Tears of the bridging veins of the epidural space or diploic veins may also cause EDH. Finally, EDH is often associated with orbitofacial fractures, such as orbital roof and frontal sinus fractures, and may result from direct bleeding from bone or an associated vascular injury.

Epidural hematoma can occur intraoperatively as a result of decompression of a contralateral lesion and needs to be considered whenever intraoperative swelling or postoperative intracerebral pressure become uncontrollable. Late EDH can occur, often as a result of assault, and the outcome is generally more favorable.[19] Epidural hematomas are more likely than aSDHs to expand or to appear as new lesions on early follow-up CT but have also been shown to spontaneously reabsorb on early follow-up CT.[22,23]

7.2.3 Diagnosis

Clinical Manifestations

The classically defined "lucid interval" actually occurs in a minority of patients.[7,12,14,16,24,25,26,27] The lucid interval occurs following a blow to the head, with or without altered sensorium. There follows a period of time, up to approximately 30 minutes, in which blood is accumulating in the extradural space,

but the brain is not compressed enough to cause alteration in consciousness. When the mass effect becomes significant, brain compression and transtentorial herniation resulting in rapid loss of consciousness (and even death if untreated) can occur. The most common locations of surgically evacuated EDH are the temporal and temporoparietal regions.[7,12,14,25,28] When EDH occurs in the temporal fossa, a relatively small intracranial space, transtentorial herniation can occur rapidly via compression of the temporal lobe and compression of the brainstem.

Patients presenting in coma or deteriorating to coma preoperatively constitute 22 to 56% of EDH patients; another 12 to 42% remain conscious until surgery.[15] Other presenting findings include nausea and vomiting, hemiparesis or hemiplegia, dysphasia or aphasia, posturing, and seizure activity. Pupillary abnormalities occur in 18 to 44%, but a significant proportion of patients (3–27%) present neurologically intact.[15,29,30] Even asymptomatic patients exhibiting minor head trauma can harbor EDH diagnosed only with CT scan.[31,32] Children with isolated EDH often present with nonspecific findings of headache, vomiting, or not feeling well, leading to frequent delays in diagnosis.[14,17]

Radiographic Findings

CT scanning is the diagnostic method of choice. Since it has come into routine usage over the past four decades, its ready availability, rapid scanning capacity, and detailed resolution provide quick and accurate diagnosis of not only the size, extent, and location of the EDH but also overlying skull fractures when present. Axial imaging can, however, exclude small fractures,

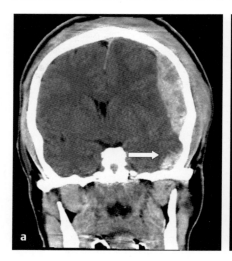
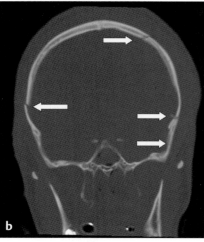

Fig. 7.3 A large left hemispheric epidural hematoma with left temporal contusion (arrow, left panel), seen on coronal CT scan. Note the overlying fractures and contralateral fracture on the bone window (arrows, right panel).

especially if they are parallel to the scanning plane, so close inspection of the scout view and/or reconstructed views in the voronal and sagittal planes is warranted. Skull X-rays do not aid in diagnosis, as ~ 35% are interpreted as normal,[29] although, especially for patients with minor head injuries, if a fracture *is* identified on plain film, CT is recommended because of the high incidence of EDH in these patients.[31]

The typical CT appearance of an EDH is a hyperdense biconvex extra-axial lesion that does not cross the bony sutures. (▸Fig. 7.1 and ▸Fig. 7.3). There may be associated relatively hypodense (either isodense or hypodense to brain) areas within the body of the hematoma suggesting a "hyperacute" or swirling blood component, thought to indicate active bleeding into the hematoma or areas of liquid blood associated with coagulopathy.[33,34] Occasionally air bubbles will be present within the hematoma (22.5–37.0%), although there is no known correlation with outcome[35] (▸Fig. 7.4). The source of air is generally from an open skull fracture or fractures through the mastoid air cells. Most EDHs are not associated with significant underlying brain injury, and postoperatively the appearance of the brain on CT quickly returns to normal.[36] Left surgically untreated, however, EDHs identified on "ultra-early" CT (< 3 hours) scans do tend to enlarge, so repeat CT within 12 hours is recommended.[22]

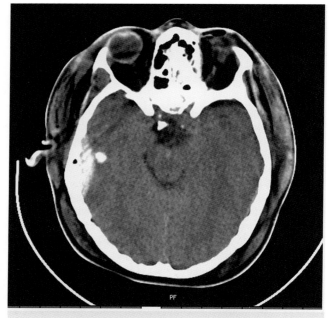

Fig. 7.4 A small bubble of air in a right temporal epidural hematoma with an underlying contusion.

7.2.4 Treatment

Operative

Craniotomy provides the most definitive form of surgical treatment of EDH. Patient selection for these lesions, which, in the CT era, have been recognized more often in asymptomatic patients, is critical. For individuals presenting in extremis, with altered level of consciousness, or neurologic deficit, the decision to operate is more straightforward. Attempts to make surgical recommendations based upon CT characteristics have been made. One group evaluated CT criteria for surgical evacuation retrospectively in a series of 33 children with EDH and found that EDH thickness > 18 mm, midline shift > 4 mm, moderate or severe mass effect, and location predicted surgery in 31 of 33 patients.[37] Evidence-based guidelines have recommended evacuation of EDH for lesions > 30 cm³ in volume and that any patient with an EDH and coma (GCS score < 9) or anisocoria

undergo evacuation as emergently as possible.[15] These authors indicated that an EDH < 30 cm³ *and* < 15 mm thick with < 5 mm midline shift in patients with GCS score > 8 and no focal deficit might be watched, with frequent serial CT and intensive observation in a neurosurgical hospital where operative therapy is immediately available, should the patient deteriorate or the radiographic appearance worsen.

Burr hole drainage as a temporizing measure has been advocated by some but has been shown to be inadequate in clinical use. Emergency burr hole exploration in one consecutive series of 100 patients prior to CT scanning resulted in a high incidence of negative exploration (44) with 6 negative explorations, despite the presence of extra-axial hematoma (4 unilateral aSDH, 1 unilateral EDH, 1 contralateral aSDH).[5] Burr hole drainage prior to transfer to an institution where definitive decompression and drainage can be done via craniotomy can result in incomplete evacuation or failure to control bleeding and may unnecessarily delay care and increase time to decompression.[38,39] Burr hole placement and irrigation of EDH in the emergency department may, however, be lifesaving if surgery is not immediately available in extremely extenuating circumstances, and results for burr hole drainage for EDH are generally better than for aSDH.[40] However, this should be a rare occurrence in organized trauma systems, as clotted blood is difficult to evacuate from a burr hole, and there is no access to the bleeding source. Thus, decompression of an inaccessible tamponaded vessel may result in additional bleeding, thereby worsening the situation.

Craniotomy for evacuation of EDH mandates identification and elimination of the source(s) of bleeding, via cauterization of vessels, waxing of bone sources, etc. Dural sinus lacerations must sometimes be repaired, plugged, or tamponaded. Epidural tack-up sutures are placed in the perimeter and the center of the craniotomy, to prevent subsequent reaccumulation of blood in the epidural space. Bone flaps are typically replaced because of the frequent absence of underlying lesions and edema, and fractures sometimes require repair. Occasionally slit durostomy to ensure the absence of aSDH is employed.

Nonoperative

In adult patients, nonoperative management can be safely employed in those EDHs with < 10 to 15 mm thickness or < 30 cm³ hematoma volume or < 5 mm midline shift, and minimal clinical symptoms, including good GCS score and normal pupillary examination.[15,23,29,41] Conservative management mandates close clinical observation and frequent radiologic follow-up, however.[42,43] Furthermore, evacuation of smaller lesions may speed recovery, shorten hospital stays, and result in fewer follow-up scans. In the face of minimal surgical risk, even small lesions are therefore sometimes evacuated. If observed, resolution of EDH typically occurs over several weeks (3–15 weeks),[21] but rarely EDH may resolve spontaneously more rapidly, most likely because of cerebral swelling associated with other injuries.[23] Factors associated with deterioration requiring surgical intervention after initial conservative therapy have included temporal location, heterogeneous density on CT, initial CT done within 6 hours of injury, and significant primary brain injury with skull fracture, causing delayed EDH not seen on ultra-early CT.[21,42,44]

7.2.5 Outcomes

Mortality in the surgical subset of EDH patients has been reported to be between 0 and 41% and is lower in the pediatric group (~ 5%).[10,11,14,28,45] Mortality has also decreased with the advent of CT scanning, development of trauma systems, and neurosurgical specialty intensive care units.[3,7,25,46,47] When examined as a contributor to mortality from TBI by lesion type in a large multicenter study, EDH had a fairly low mortality index (percent mortality × percent incidence) compared with other lesion types.[9]

Functional outcome and mortality are affected by the following clinical findings: age, neurologic status (coma or lucid interval, GCS motor score, focal neurologic deficit, pupillary status), time to evacuation/decompression (for at least a subset of patients), intracranial pressure (ICP) elevations, and medical complications.[10,11,13,27,28,48,49] Radiographic (CT) findings affecting outcome from EDH include hematoma volume, degree of midline shift, compression of cisterns, associated intracranial lesions, signs of active bleeding (heterogeneous density), presence of a skull fracture, and fracture across a meningeal artery, vein, or dural sinus.[12,13,24,27,29,50,51] Although several reports have correlated hematoma volume with outcome, at least one retrospective study found that hematoma volume did not correlate with either the preoperative neurologic condition or the 6-month outcome.[52]

Correlation of physical findings and definitive therapy is, however, important, as demonstrated in two studies showing that patients in whom the latency period between the onset of anisocoria and surgical evacuation was shorter had better outcomes and lower mortality than those for whom surgery was delayed[43,48] and in two others that correlated outcome (including mortality) to time between onset of coma and evacuation.[12,53] Others have found similar good overall outcomes after EDH without focal deficits,[12,53] but decreasing rates of good outcome with, in order, hemiparesis, hemiparesis and anisocoria, decorticate posturing, decerebrate posturing, and fixed bilateral pupils occurring preoperatively.[29] Children fare better than adults in general.[20] Mortality and outcome are improved for patients transferred directly to a neurosurgical institution over those transferred in from outlying facilities (correlating with time to evacuation).[3,26,54] This fact should be taken into account when designing trauma systems and transport protocols.

7.3 Acute Subdural Hematoma

7.3.1 Epidemiology

Although aSDH has been described in a myriad of clinical conditions (acquired coagulopathies, anticoagulation therapy, congenital bleeding disorders, arteriovenous malformations, aneurysm rupture, cancer, meningioma, cardiac surgery, spinal epidural catheter insertion, depth electrode use, cocaine use, near-drowning), the most common cause by far is trauma. Acute traumatic SDH is most often the result of vehicular-related trauma, but in older subpopulations, falls represent a higher proportion of etiologies. MVA is more often associated with a comatose state in aSDH patients, indicative of the high-velocity mechanism causing a greater degree of underlying brain trauma.[55,56]

7.3.2 Pathogenesis

Etiology of bleeding is from tearing of cortical surface arteries or veins or cerebral contusions, but often a bleeding source cannot be determined with certainty at operation.[57,58] Acute bleeding into a preexisting cSDH may also occur.[58] Arterial sources may represent a particularly treacherous entity due to rapid expansion and cerebral compression and herniation.

7.3.3 Diagnosis

Clinical Manifestations

A large proportion of aSDH patients present in coma (GCS score < 9).[7,15,59,60] Lucid intervals are sometimes seen, more frequently

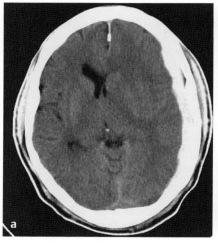
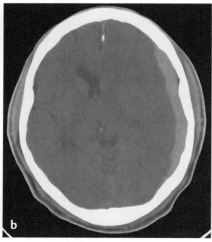

Fig. 7.5 (a) A large left hemispheric acute subdural hematoma is demonstrated on this computed tomography scan of the head, without contrast. (b) Windowing the scan differently results in better demonstration of the lesion. Mass effect on the left hemisphere, left lateral ventricle, and cisterns are noted, with midline shift proportional to the thickness of the aSDH.

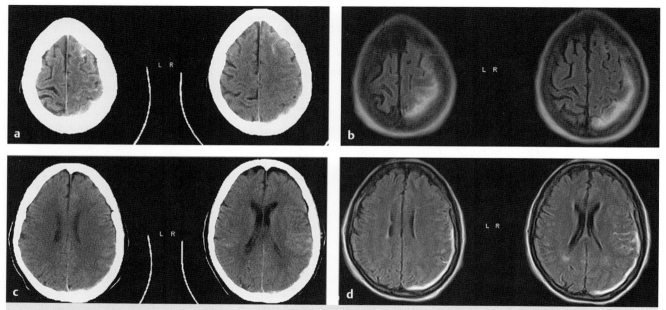

Fig. 7.6 (a–d) A small left parieto-occipital acute subdural hematoma is subtly demonstrated on the computed tomography scan of the head without contrast on the left. This lesion is actually better seen on magnetic resonance image without contrast, with the comparable T1-weighted slices shown at the right. The advanced age of this patient resulted in only slight clinical repercussions (mild right upper extremity paresis that resolved). Left frontal subarachnoid hemorrhage is also noted.

in isolated aSDH[56] and in elderly patients,[49] most likely because of the presence of cerebral atrophy that allows a collection to be harbored for longer prior to onset of mass effect from expansion of the lesion. Pupil abnormalities are noted in 30 to 50% of patients.[15] In infants with open sutures, the first signs of an aSDH may be distention of the fontanelles and/or separation of the sutures, or seizures.[61] After the sutures fuse, the presenting signs and symptoms mimic those of adults: nausea/vomiting, headache, deteriorating consciousness and neurologic status, pupillary dilation, and/or focal neurologic deficit (hemiparesis/hemiplegia or abnormal motor posturing). Isolated aSDH is seen in a minority of patients. In contrast to EDHs, most aSDHs are associated with intraparenchymal hemorrhage(s), subarachnoid hemorrhage, skull fracture, and EDH, in addition to extracranial trauma, such as facial fractures, vascular injuries, limb fractures, or thoracic or abdominal trauma.[15,36]

Radiographic Findings

CT scanning is the diagnostic modality of choice. Acute SDH appears as a hyperdense crescent-shaped extra-axial collection (▶ Fig. 7.5). Magnetic resonance imaging (MRI) can sometimes demonstrate aSDH better in cases of thin collections. Acute blood appears hyperintense on T1 and hypointense on T2 images[62] (▶ Fig. 7.6). However, MRI is usually not a feasible test to obtain in the setting of acute TBI with symptoms of aSDH, and, whereas MRI can detect some lesions not seen on CT that may aid in prognostication, surgical lesions are uniformly not

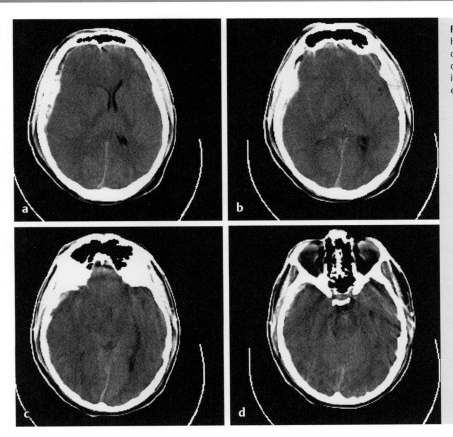

Fig. 7.7 (a-d) A thin acute subdural hematoma (aSDH) with mixed density is noted over the right hemisphere. Midline shift out of proportion to the thickness of the aSDH is indicative of right hemispheric injury and edema.

missed on CT scanning.[51,63] As described for EDH, "hyperacute" blood may also be seen in aSDH[34,64] (►Fig. 7.7).

7.3.4 Treatment

Operative

Surgical evacuation of aSDH is necessary for patients with significant mass effect, regardless of GCS score. Significant mass effect may be defined as thickness of the hematoma > 10 mm or midline shift > 5 mm.[15] Patients in whom there is less mass effect but who experience a neurologic deterioration such as a decrease in the GCS score by 2 or more points, loss of pupillary reactivity, or pupillary dilation, or who experience elevations of ICP above 20 mm Hg should also be taken to surgery for evacuation, if possible.[15] Surgical decision-making may be affected by age, as aSDH tends to be better tolerated in the elderly patient with an atrophic brain; however, elderly patients with very low GCS scores, presentation in coma, and at least one abnormal pupil uniformly do poorly, with significant contributions to mortality from preexisting conditions and multisystems failure.[65,66]

Surgical evacuation of aSDH is done via craniotomy, usually a very generous one. This may be done with or without duraplasty and bone flap removal, depending upon the degree of underlying parenchymal injury and swelling. Very thin layers of aSDH, sometimes termed "sliver" subdural hematomas, deserve special caution if accompanied by midline shift out of proportion to the size of the aSDH. The difference between the thickness of the aSDH and midline shift predicts outcome, with increasing disability and mortality when midline shift exceeds thickness by

larger and larger intervals[67] (►Fig. 7.7). This phenomenon signals significant underlying brain injury and edema, and surgical evacuation of the SDH is often helpful. Accompanying duraplasty and removal of the bone flap for delayed replacement may be necessary to accommodate significant hemispheric edema and prevent ongoing brainstem compression and elevated ICP. Intraoperative consideration must also be given to removal of underlying intraparenchymal hematomas or contusions, and much less commonly, partial lobectomy. Gentle elevation of the temporal lobe with relief of uncal herniation may be of some benefit.

Burr hole drainage is ineffective and associated with higher mortality.[49,68,69,70] In cases where CT scanning is not available, if burr hole exploration is used to detect the presence of extra-axial hematomas for subsequent evacuation via craniotomy in TBI patients with signs of transtentorial herniation or brainstem dysfunction, they should be placed first on the side corresponding to the neurologic deficit in frontal, temporal, and parietal locations, followed by contralateral burr holes if negative, to maximize the chances of identifying the lesion(s).[5]

Nonoperative

Nonoperative management is typically reserved for small subdurals without significant mass effect and minimal or no neurologic deficit.[15,71,72] Deterioration in prehospital or emergency department GCS score prompts reconsideration for surgical evacuation. For nonoperated cases, early repeat CT scan and close observation of neurologic status is mandated.[73,74] This approach should be limited to those aSDHs with thickness < 10 mm and midline shift < 5 mm, and associated with good neurologic status,[15,72,75] and requires avoidance of long-lasting sedatives and paralytic agents.[72] Most small aSDHs will resolve spontaneously, but the likelihood of progression to a surgically evacuated cSDH is increased with larger volumes and hematoma thicknesses,[76] especially in the elderly. The presence of cerebral atrophy supports nonoperative management of isolated aSDH; a history of alcohol abuse is prominent in this group,[76] in addition to advancing age.

7.3.5 Outcomes

Outcome after aSDH is worse than EDH, both with respect to mortality and functionality in survivors.[9,53,77,78,79] Mortality after aSDH ranges from 40 to 60%.[43,53,56,80] For those patients with aSDH presenting to hospital in coma requiring surgery, mortality is 57 to 68%.[15] Mortality in patients with evacuated aSDH and fixed dilated pupils was 64% in one series[43] and 97% in another.[80] In a large study correlating CT findings with outcome from the Traumatic Coma Data Bank, the volume of extracerebral mass lesions was less important than the degree of mass effect (cisternal compression, midline shift).[81] Compared with other lesion types after TBI, aSDH has the highest mortality index, accounting for 43.5% of all deaths in one large multicenter series.[9]

Clinical factors that affect functional outcome include age at presentation (with older patients faring worse), time to evacuation, admission GCS score, hypoxia or hypotension, extent of primary brain injury, duration of coma, ICP elevation duration postoperatively, mechanism of injury, presence of coagulopathy, and severity of other system injuries.[43,53,55,56,58,69,70,72,78,80,82,83] Radiographic or pathologic findings associated with outcome include other intracranial findings, diffuse axonal injury, degree of mass effect (including appearance of basal cisterns and midline shift), presence of subarachnoid hemorrhage, hematoma volume, and unilateral hemispheric edema.[43,55,56,59,60,66,70,77,78,80,84,85] Physiologic variables associated with outcome after aSDH evacuation include brain tissue oxygen tension and lactate and pyruvate concentrations in the underlying brain, indicative of the evolving primary brain injury.[86] Multimodality-evoked potentials have been used to predict outcome after surgery.[87,88]

As with EDH, increasing time from onset of coma to surgery is correlated with increasing mortality.[57,89,90,91,92,93] However, some authors have shown worse mortality with earlier surgery, probably owing to the severity of associated primary brain injuries[49,59] or the degree of mass effect.[94] Good recovery (full recovery or minimal neurologic deficit) was seen in 26% in one large series, with better outcomes in the following subgroups: isolated aSDH (81%); and isolated aSDH without coma, or those operated within 2 hours (90%).[53]

7.4 Subdural Hygroma

7.4.1 Epidemiology

Hygromas may occur as a consequence of trauma, ruptured arachnoid cysts, carcinomatosis, and a variety of other conditions. They rarely constitute a neurosurgical emergency, as they do not tend to be associated with mass effect. Hygromas are a relatively common sequela of cranial trauma (5–20% of posttraumatic lesions[74]) and may precede the development of cSDH,

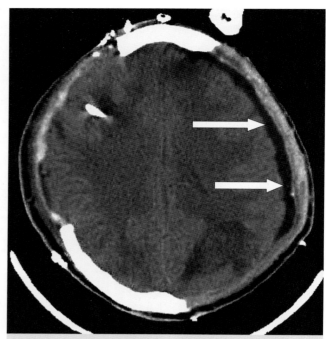

Fig. 7.8 Extra-axial fluid (hygroma) over the left convexity status post decompressive craniotomy. An early collection is also seen developing under a right-sided craniotomy defect as well.

particularly in patients without fully expanded brains (infants with less compliance, elderly patients with atrophy, and trauma survivors with encephalomalacia).[95,96]

7.4.2 Pathogenesis

Separation of the dura mater–arachnoid mater planes is required to create the potential space necessary for the formation of subdural hygromas. Once the division of the dura–arachnoid tissue plane has occurred because of trauma, cranial surgery, or other mechanism, fluid fills the potential space if the brain is not fully expanded, or the ICP is negative. (These collections are often seen after decompressive craniotomy with the bone flap left out.) See ▶ Fig. 7.8. The source of the fluid is thought to be effusion of cerebrospinal fluid (CSF) or serum from "leaky" vessels associated with neovascularization of neomembranes forming along the dura–arachnoid interface.[74] Another source of fluid is CSF egress directly from the subarachnoid space when an arachnoid breach occurs from trauma or surgery. Gravitational force on the brain does play a role in the development of hygromas, which are seen most often in the frontal regions owing to patients usually being placed supine in bed[97] and the heavier cerebrum settling to the occipital region.

7.4.3 Diagnosis

Clinical Manifestations

Most hygromas are asymptomatic but may present with neurologic deficit due to mass effect. The typical deficit is altered mental status.[98]

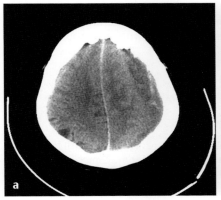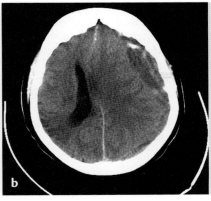

Fig. 7.9 (a, b) A large left chronic subdural hematoma (hypodense) with some subacute (isodense) and acute (hyperdense) components and midline shift.

Radiographic Findings

Subdural hygromas appear as extra-axial fluid collections isodense with CSF (hypodense to brain) on CT. Magnetic resonance imaging may also be used to make the diagnosis, and enhancement of the arachnoid may be consistent with the formation of a dural membrane[99]; this finding may be used to differentiate a true hygroma from an enlarged subarachnoid space associated with atrophy. MRI can also distinguish between hygroma and cSDH, which appear similar on CT.

7.4.4 Treatment

Treatment is usually nonoperative, but in cases in which neurologic symptoms are attributed to the hygroma, surgical evacuation with burr holes or twist-drill burr holes may be effected, with or without a drain. Most do not recur.[98]

7.5 Subacute and Chronic Subdural Hematoma

7.5.1 Epidemiology

In contrast to aSDH, cSDH is more often seen in the elderly because of the presence of cerebral atrophy.[100] Chronic SDH may occasionally be preceded by the presence of a subdural hygroma or by an sSDH.[74,89,101] Risk factors for the development of cSDH include head injury, advanced age, treatment with antiplatelet or anticoagulant drugs, bleeding disorders, hemodialysis, alcohol use or abuse, epilepsy, any condition predisposing to falls, and low ICP.[100]

7.5.2 Pathogenesis

Chronic SDH may follow significant craniocerebral trauma in younger patients, or trivial trauma or no discernible injury in the elderly. Stretching and tearing of cortical bridging veins producing hemorrhage into the subdural space is the initial mechanism. Infiltration by fibrin and fibroblasts, succeeded by formation of a membrane by the fibroblasts, then occurs. Hematoma liquefaction by phagocytes results in either resorption or enlargement, which is generally due to

recurrent small hemorrhages from the neovascularization of the membrane.[90,100] Subacute SDH is more commonly preceded by definite head trauma than cSDH.[102]

7.5.3 Diagnosis
Clinical Manifestations

Both sSDH and cSDH can present with a variety of clinical features, including hemiparesis, speech arrest, or other focal neurologic deficit; dementia; alteration in consciousness; headache; recurrent falls; seizures; transient neurologic deficits mimicking transient ischemic attacks; parkinsonism; and symptoms of raised ICP.[91,100]

Radiographic Findings

Chronic SDH is hypodense compared with brain on CT (▶ Fig. 7.9). Magnetic resonance imaging may be more useful for characterizing cSDHs at the vertex, skull base, or within the PF, and very small collections.[100] Chronic SDH may be differentiated from hygroma by the relative lack of mass effect (sulcal effacement or midline shift) seen in the latter.[74] Subacute SDH, on the other hand, is often isodense to the brain on CT. Magnetic resonance imaging can markedly enhance the detectability of sSDH, which has a hyperintense appearance on T1-weighted images.[62]

7.5.4 Treatment
Operative

Evacuation of liquefied sSDH or cSDH can generally be accomplished via burr holes and irrigation. Craniotomy may need to be employed more often in the case of sSDH, if there is a need to identify an ongoing bleeding source. In either case, multiple burr holes are desirable to ensure adequate clot removal and irrigation. Irrigation is performed until completely transparent irrigant is returned from the subdural space. Communication of irrigation between burr holes is helpful, to ensure that loculated fluid collections are not left behind. A subdural drain may be placed to facilitate drainage of residual hematoma fluid and CSF, particularly in the atrophic brain that fails to expand fully after hematoma evacuation. Closed drainage systems and gravity (without suction) are frequently employed to assist with continued postoperative drainage.[83,92] Patients at the extremes of age or who are critically ill and may not tolerate general anesthesia can sometimes be approached with bedside twist-drill burr hole drainage, particularly if the hematoma fluid is under pressure. Craniotomy with or without membrane excision is an option[103]; however, membranes have a propensity to bleed and must be adequately removed and/or coagulated if this option is employed. Membrane stripping should generally not be performed through burr holes, because hemostasis cannot be achieved, nor can adequate visualization of membrane adhesions to the brain.

Nonoperative

Small cSDHs without significant mass effect can occasionally be managed through observation. Patients must be advised that there is a risk of acute hemorrhage into a cSDH and should be admonished not to take fall risks and to take precautions against bumping their heads. The ubiquitous use of anticoagulant and antiplatelet therapy increases this risk and must be taken into consideration.

7.5.5 Outcomes

Outcome is most affected by neurologic status at the time of diagnosis and is better in those who undergo surgical treatment.[100] Mortality and morbidity are higher in elderly patients, in alcoholics, and in patients with recurrences.[90,100] Chronic SDHs can sometimes contribute to seizure; preoperative rates of seizure in the face of cSDH range from 4.3 to 6.9%.[104,105] One study demonstrated that, of 129 patients studied, no patients given prophylactic postoperative seizure medication (*n* = 73) developed seizures, but only 2 out of 56 who were not given antiepileptic drugs had early postoperative seizures, and some consideration was given to surgical technique as the cause.[106] However, the incidence of postoperative seizures has been measured as 1.8 to 18.5% in other studies.[100,102,104,107] In the series showing an 18.5% incidence, the seizures were associated with increasing morbidity and mortality, and the use of prophylactic medications significantly decreased the incidence, so they were recommended in surgically treated patients.[93] Risk factors for postoperative seizure occurrence include mixed-density lesions on preoperative CT, left-sided unilateral lesions, and chronic alcohol abuse.[105,108]

Recurrence is a frequent complication of cSDH (8–37%).[100] Greater thickness of the hematoma, existence of multiple loculations, high-density lesions (chronic mixed with acute hemorrhage) on preoperative CT, high-intensity lesions on preoperative T1-weighted MRI images, large volumes of air on postoperative CT, history of seizures, and preoperative thrombocytopenia are associated with increased recurrence, whereas diabetes mellitus and the use of both irrigation and closed drainage systems postoperatively (especially with frontal drains) may be protective.[83,90,92,109,110] Tension pneumocephalus is an unusual complication of burr hole drainage.[111,112] Development of aSDH is more common.[111] Intracerebral hematoma

formation, ischemic stroke, acute EDH, and scalp infections after cSDH evacuation have also been described.[111,113] Although rare, subdural empyema can occur with or without evacuation of cSDH.[111,114]

7.6 Special Considerations

7.6.1 Posterior Fossa

Epidural hematomas of the PF are associated with less specific clinical findings and overall better outcomes when aggressive diagnostic and follow-up imaging are used, regardless of operative or nonoperative management.[115,116] Presenting signs and symptoms include headache, nausea and vomiting, decreased level of consciousness (including sudden respiratory arrest), vertigo, diplopia, pyramidal tract signs, cerebellar signs, nuchal rigidity, papilledema, and abducens palsy.[117,118] Factors affecting outcome include effacement of perimesencephalic cisterns and/or the fourth ventricle, presence of hydrocephalus at presentation, level of consciousness prior to operation, overall GCS score (with GCS score < 9 portending poor outcome), other systemic or intracranial lesions, and timeliness of diagnosis and intervention.[101,119,120] Posterior fossa EDH is most frequently associated with direct occipital trauma, resulting in occipital or lambdoid diastatic fracture and/or linear fractures crossing the torcular or transverse sinus, with the bleeding source being the sinus or diploë.[101,121,122,123] Prompt evacuation is generally the treatment method of choice, but some PF EDHs may be managed conservatively with close clinical observation and serial radiographic follow-up. Some have advocated evacuation of PF EDH with > 10 mL volume, thickness > 15 mL, and fourth ventricular midline shift > 5 mm.[124] Magnetic resonance imaging can help to clarify volume and thickness of PF EDHs that are not well visualized on CT.[117] Posterior fossa EDHs can occur after the evacuation of a supratentorial hematoma.[125] They may also present with mixed supratentorial and infratentorial components, resulting in higher mortality rates[125,126,127] (▶ Fig. 7.10).

Posterior fossa aSDHs are less common and emergent evacuation is recommended, especially for those with thickness ≥ 10 mm, regardless of presenting status, which is most often associated with coma.[107,128] Chronic SDH of the PF is also rare.[129]

7.6.2 Child Abuse

Infants and children with extra-axial hematomas represent a special consideration. Unless the mechanism of injury is definitely known or witnessed, inflicted injury must often be considered in the differential diagnosis. Brain injuries are the most common cause of death in abused children, and aSDH is seen more often in inflicted than accidental injuries in children.[130] Mixed-density extra-axial hematomas may indicate recurrent episodes of hemorrhage associated with multiple traumas but may also represent hyperacute bleeding or admixture with CSF, so they should be interpreted with caution.[64,131,132] EDHs from inflicted injuries in children are rare,[133] and one study found no incidents of nonaccidental injury in 35 cases of *isolated* EDH.[17]

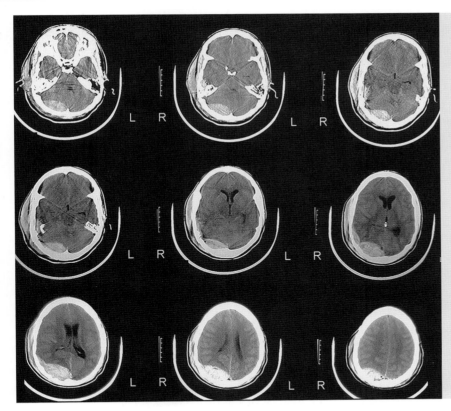

Fig. 7.10 A large right occipital (supratentorial) and posterior fossa (infratentorial) epidural hematoma (EDH). This patient presented with a lucid interval, initial Glasgow Coma Scale score = 15, followed by rapid deterioration in the emergency room. Initial computed tomography scan done at an outlying hospital had shown only a skull fracture. Emergent intubation followed by evacuation resulted in a functionally good outcome. The source of the EDH was the transverse sinus, torn by an overlying fracture.

References

[1] Gennarelli TA, Champion HR, Copes WS, Sacco WJ. Comparison of mortality, morbidity, and severity of 59,713 head injured patients with 114,447 patients with extracranial injuries. J Trauma. 1994; 37(6):962–968

[2] Miniño AM, Anderson RN, Fingerhut LA, Boudreault MA, Warner M. Deaths: injuries, 2002. Natl Vital Stat Rep. 2006; 54(10):1–124

[3] Hunt J, Hill D, Besser M, West R, Roncal S. Outcome of patients with neurotrauma: the effect of a regionalized trauma system. Aust N Z J Surg. 1995; 65(2):83–86

[4] Lobato RD, Rivas JJ, Gomez PA, et al. Head-injured patients who talk and deteriorate into coma. Analysis of 211 cases studied with computerized tomography. J Neurosurg. 1991; 75(2):256–261

[5] Andrews BT, Pitts LH, Lovely MP, Bartkowski H. Is computed tomographic scanning necessary in patients with tentorial herniation? Results of immediate surgical exploration without computed tomography in 100 patients. Neurosurgery. 1986; 19(3):408–414

[6] Uzan M, Yentür E, Hanci M, et al. Is it possible to recover from uncal herniation? Analysis of 71 head injured cases. J Neurosurg Sci. 1998; 42(2):89–94

[7] Cordobés F, Lobato RD, Rivas JJ, et al. Observations on 82 patients with extradural hematoma. Comparison of results before and after the advent of computerized tomography. J Neurosurg. 1981; 54(2):179–186

[8] Gupta SK, Tandon SC, Mohanty S, Asthana S, Sharma S. Bilateral traumatic extradural haematomas: report of 12 cases with a review of the literature. Clin Neurol Neurosurg. 1992; 94(2):127–131

[9] Gennarelli TA, Spielman GM, Langfitt TW, et al. Influence of the type of intracranial lesion on outcome from severe head injury. J Neurosurg. 1982; 56(1):26–32

[10] Seelig JM, Marshall LF, Toutant SM, et al. Traumatic acute epidural hematoma: unrecognized high lethality in comatose patients. Neurosurgery. 1984; 15(5):617–620

[11] Bricolo AP, Pasut LM. Extradural hematoma: toward zero mortality. A prospective study. Neurosurgery. 1984; 14(1):8–12

[12] Hendrick EB, Harwood-Hash DC, Hudson AR. Head injuries in children: a survey of 4465 consecutive cases at the hospital for sick children, Toronto, Canada. Clin Neurosurg. 1964; 11:46–65

[13] Bullock R, Smith RM, van Dellen JR. Nonoperative management of extradural hematoma. Neurosurgery. 1985; 16(5):602–606

[14] Maggi G, Aliberti F, Petrone G, Ruggiero C. Extradural hematomas in children. J Neurosurg Sci. 1998; 42(2):95–99

[15] Bullock MR, Chesnut R, Ghajar J, et al. Guidelines for the surgical management of traumatic brain injury. Neurosurgery. 2006; 58(3):S2–1–S2–62

[16] Jamjoom A, Cummins B, Jamjoom ZA. Clinical characteristics of traumatic extradural hematoma: a comparison between children and adults. Neurosurg Rev. 1994; 17(4):277–281

[17] Browne GJ, Lam LT. Isolated extradural hematoma in children presenting to an emergency department in Australia. Pediatr Emerg Care. 2002; 18(2):86–90

[18] Huda MF, Mohanty S, Sharma V, Tiwari Y, Choudhary A, Singh VP. Double extradural hematoma: an analysis of 46 cases. Neurol India. 2004; 52(4):450–452

[19] Bullock R, van Dellen JR. Chronic extradural hematoma. Surg Neurol. 1982; 18(4):300–302

[20] Mohanty A, Kolluri VR, Subbakrishna DK, Satish S, Mouli BA, Das BS. Prognosis of extradural haematomas in children. Pediatr Neurosurg. 1995; 23(2):57–63

[21] Hamilton M, Wallace C. Nonoperative management of acute epidural hematoma diagnosed by CT: the neuroradiologist's role. AJNR Am J Neuroradiol. 1992; 13(3):853–859, discussion 860–862

[22] Servadei F, Nanni A, Nasi MT, et al. Evolving brain lesions in the first 12 hours after head injury: analysis of 37 comatose patients. Neurosurgery. 1995; 37(5):899–906, discussion 906–907

[23] Servadei F, Staffa G, Pozzati E, Piazza G. Rapid spontaneous disappearance of an acute extradural hematoma: case report. J Trauma. 1989; 29(6):880–882

[24] Lee E-J, Hung Y-C, Wang L-C, Chung K-C, Chen H-H. Factors influencing the functional outcome of patients with acute epidural hematomas: analysis of 200 patients undergoing surgery. J Trauma. 1998; 45(5):946–952

[25] Rivas JJ, Lobato RD, Sarabia R, Cordobés F, Cabrera A, Gomez P. Extradural hematoma: analysis of factors influencing the courses of 161 patients. Neurosurgery. 1988; 23(1):44–51

[26] Jamjoom AB. The difference in the outcome of surgery for traumatic extradural hematoma between patients who are admitted directly to the neurosurgical unit and those referred from another hospital. Neurosurg Rev. 1997; 20(4):227–230

[27] Kuday C, Uzan M, Hanci M. Statistical analysis of the factors affecting the outcome of extradural haematomas: 115 cases. Acta Neurochir (Wien). 1994; 131(3–4):203–206

[28] Paterniti S, Fiore P, Macrì E, et al. Extradural haematoma. Report of 37 consecutive cases with survival. Acta Neurochir (Wien). 1994; 131(3–4):207–210

[29] Cook RJ, Dorsch NW, Fearnside MR, Chaseling R. Outcome prediction in extradural haematomas. Acta Neurochir (Wien). 1988; 95(3–4):90–94

[30] Servadei F, Faccani G, Roccella P, et al. Asymptomatic extradural haematomas. Results of a multicenter study of 158 cases in minor head injury. Acta Neurochir (Wien). 1989; 96(1–2):39–45

[31] Servadei F, Ciucci G, Morichetti A, et al. G, Taggi F. Skull fracture as a factor of increased risk in minor head injuries. Indication for a broader use of cerebral computed tomography scanning. Surg Neurol. 1988; 30(5)):364–369

[32] Servadei F, Vergoni G, Staffa G, et al. Extradural haematomas: how many deaths can be avoided? Protocol for early detection of haematoma in minor head injuries. Acta Neurochir (Wien). 1995; 133(1–2):50–55

[33] Arrese I, Lobato RD, Gomez PA, Nuñez AP. Hyperacute epidural haematoma isodense with the brain on computed tomography. Acta Neurochir (Wien). 2004; 146(2):193–194

[34] Greenberg J, Cohen WA, Cooper PR. The "hyperacute" extraaxial intracranial hematoma: computed tomographic findings and clinical significance. Neurosurgery. 1985; 17(1):48–56

[35] Cossu M, Arcuri T, Cagetti B, Brambilla Bas M, Siccardi D, Pau A. Gas bubbles within acute intracranial epidural haematomas. Acta Neurochir (Wien). 1990; 102(1–2):22–24

[36] Dolinskas CA, Zimmerman RA, Bilaniuk LT, Gennarelli TA. Computed tomography of post-traumatic extracerebral hematomas: comparison to pathophysiology and responses to therapy. J Trauma. 1979; 19(3):163–169

[37] Bejjani GK, Donahue DJ, Rusin J, Broemeling LD. Radiological and clinical criteria for the management of epidural hematomas in children. Pediatr Neurosurg. 1996; 25(6):302–308

[38] Wester K. Decompressive surgery for "pure" epidural hematomas: does neurosurgical expertise improve the outcome? Neurosurgery. 1999; 44(3):495–500, discussion 500–502

[39] Wester T, Fevang LT, Wester K. Decompressive surgery in acute head injuries: where should it be performed? J Trauma. 1999; 46(5):914–919

[40] Springer MF, Baker FJ. Cranial burr hole decompression in the emergency department. Am J Emerg Med. 1988; 6(6):640–646

[41] Chen TY, Wong CW, Chang CN, et al. The expectant treatment of "asymptomatic" supratentorial epidural hematomas. Neurosurgery. 1993; 32(2):176–179, discussion 179

[42] Bezircioğlu H, Erşahin Y, Demirçivi F, Yurt I, Dönertaş K, Tektaş S. Nonoperative treatment of acute extradural hematomas: analysis of 80 cases. J Trauma. 1996; 41(4):696–698

[43] Sakas DE, Bullock MR, Teasdale GM. One-year outcome following craniotomy for traumatic hematoma in patients with fixed dilated pupils. J Neurosurg. 1995; 82(6):961–965

[44] Poon WS, Rehman SU, Poon CY, Li AK. Traumatic extradural hematoma of delayed onset is not a rarity. Neurosurgery. 1992; 30(5):681–686

[45] Pillay R, Peter JC. Extradural haematomas in children. S Afr Med J. 1995; 85(7):672–674

[46] Lobato RD, Rivas JJ, Cordobes F, et al. Acute epidural hematoma: an analysis of factors influencing the outcome of patients undergoing surgery in coma. J Neurosurg. 1988; 68(1):48–57

[47] Jones NR, Molloy CJ, Kloeden CN, North JB, Simpson DA. Extradural haematoma: trends in outcome over 35 years. Br J Neurosurg. 1993; 7(5):465–471

[48] Cohen JE, Montero A, Israel ZH. Prognosis and clinical relevance of anisocoria-craniotomy latency for epidural hematoma in comatose patients. J Trauma. 1996; 41(1):120–122

[49] Hernesniemi J. Outcome following acute subdural haematoma. Acta Neurochir (Wien). 1979; 49(3–4):191–198

[50] Heinzelmann M, Platz A, Imhof HG. Outcome after acute extradural haematoma, influence of additional injuries and neurological complications in the ICU. Injury. 1996; 27(5):345–349

[51] Levin HS, Amparo EG, Eisenberg HM, et al. Magnetic resonance imaging after closed head injury in children. Neurosurgery. 1989; 24(2):223–227

[52] van den Brink WA, Zwienenberg M, Zandee SM, van der Meer L, Maas AI, Avezaat CJ. The prognostic importance of the volume of traumatic epidural and subdural haematomas revisited. Acta Neurochir (Wien). 1999; 141(5):509–514

[53] Haselsberger K, Pucher R, Auer LM. Prognosis after acute subdural or epidural haemorrhage. Acta Neurochir (Wien). 1988; 90(3–4):111–116

[54] Poon WS, Li AK. Comparison of management outcome of primary and secondary referred patients with traumatic extradural haematoma in a neurosurgical unit. Injury. 1991; 22(4):323–325

[55] Howard MA, III, Gross AS, Dacey RG, Jr, Winn HR. Acute subdural hematomas: an age-dependent clinical entity. J Neurosurg. 1989; 71(6):858–863

[56] Massaro F, Lanotte M, Faccani G, Triolo C. One hundred and twenty-seven cases of acute subdural haematoma operated on. Correlation between CT scan findings and outcome. Acta Neurochir (Wien). 1996; 138(2):185–191

[57] Jones NR, Blumbergs PC, North JB. Acute subdural haematomas: aetiology, pathology and outcome. Aust N Z J Surg. 1986; 56(12):907–913

[58] Shenkin HA. Acute subdural hematoma. Review of 39 consecutive cases with high incidence of cortical artery rupture. J Neurosurg. 1982; 57(2):254–257

[59] Dent DL, Croce MA, Menke PG, et al. Prognostic factors after acute subdural hematoma. J Trauma. 1995; 39(1):36–42, discussion 42–43

[60] Servadei F, Nasi MT, Giuliani G, et al. CT prognostic factors in acute subdural haematomas: the value of the 'worst' CT scan. Br J Neurosurg. 2000; 14(2):110–116

[61] Spanu G, Pezzotta S, Silvani V, Leone V. Outcome following acute supratentorial subdural hematoma in pediatric age. J Neurosurg Sci. 1985; 29(1):31–35

[62] Zimmerman RA, Bilaniuk LT, Hackney DB, Goldberg HI, Grossman RI. Head injury: early results of comparing CT and high-field MR. AJR Am J Roentgenol. 1986; 147(6):1215–1222

[63] Wilberger JE, Jr, Deeb Z, Rothfus W. Magnetic resonance imaging in cases of severe head injury. Neurosurgery. 1987; 20(4):571–576

[64] Sargent S, Kennedy JG, Kaplan JA. "Hyperacute" subdural hematoma: CT mimic of recurrent episodes of bleeding in the setting of child abuse. J Forensic Sci. 1996; 41(2):314–316

[65] Cagetti B, Cossu M, Pau A, Rivano C, Viale G. The outcome from acute subdural and epidural intracranial haematomas in very elderly patients. Br J Neurosurg. 1992; 6(3):227–231

[66] Shigemori M, Syojima K, Nakayama K, et al. The outcome from acute subdural haematoma following decompressive hemicraniectomy. Acta Neurochir (Wien). 1980; 54(1–2):61–69

[67] Zumkeller M, Behrmann R, Heissler HE, Dietz H. Computed tomographic criteria and survival rate for patients with acute subdural hematoma. Neurosurgery. 1996; 39(4):708–712, discussion 712–713

[68] Servadei F. Prognostic factors in severely head injured adult patients with epidural haematoma's. Acta Neurochir (Wien). 1997; 139(4):273–278

[69] Hatashita S, Koga N, Hosaka Y, Takagi S. Acute subdural hematoma: severity of injury, surgical intervention, and mortality. Neurol Med Chir (Tokyo). 1993; 33(1):13–18

[70] Servadei F. Prognostic factors in severely head injured adult patients with acute subdural haematoma's. Acta Neurochir (Wien). 1997; 139(4):279–285

[71] Croce MA, Dent DL, Menke PG, et al. Acute subdural hematoma: nonsurgical management of selected patients. J Trauma. 1994; 36(6):820–826, discussion 826–827

[72] Servadei F, Nasi MT, Cremonini AM, Giuliani G, Cenni P, Nanni A. Importance of a reliable admission Glasgow Coma Scale score for determining the need for evacuation of posttraumatic subdural hematomas: a prospective study of 65 patients. J Trauma. 1998; 44(5):868–873

[73] Lee KS, Bae HG, Yun IG. Small-sized acute subdural hematoma: operate or not. J Korean Med Sci. 1992; 7(1):52–57

[74] Lee KS. The pathogenesis and clinical significance of traumatic subdural hygroma. Brain Inj. 1998; 12(7):595–603

[75] Wong CW. Criteria for conservative treatment of supratentorial acute subdural haematomas. Acta Neurochir (Wien). 1995; 135(1–2):38–43

[76] Mathew P, Oluoch-Olunya DL, Condon BR, Bullock R. Acute subdural haematoma in the conscious patient: outcome with initial non-operative management. Acta Neurochir (Wien). 1993; 121(3–4):100–108

[77] Lobato RD, Cordobes F, Rivas JJ, et al. Outcome from severe head injury related to the type of intracranial lesion. A computerized tomography study. J Neurosurg. 1983; 59(5):762–774

[78] Selladurai BM, Jayakumar R, Tan YY, Low HC. Outcome prediction in early management of severe head injury: an experience in Malaysia. Br J Neurosurg. 1992; 6(6):549–557

[79] Wu JJ, Hsu CC, Liao SY, Wong Y-K. Surgical outcome of traumatic intracranial hematoma at a regional hospital in Taiwan. J Trauma. 1999; 47(1):39–43

[80] Koç RK, Akdemir H, Oktem IS, Meral M, Menkü A. Acute subdural hematoma: outcome and outcome prediction. Neurosurg Rev. 1997; 20(4):239–244

[81] Eisenberg HM, Gary HE, Jr, Aldrich EF, et al. Initial CT findings in 753 patients with severe head injury. A report from the NIH Traumatic Coma Data Bank. J Neurosurg. 1990; 73(5):688–698

[82] Klun B, Fettich M. Factors influencing the outcome in acute subdural haematoma. A review of 330 cases. Acta Neurochir (Wien). 1984; 71(3–4):171–178

[83] Wakai S, Hashimoto K, Watanabe N, Inoh S, Ochiai C, Nagai M. Efficacy of closed-system drainage in treating chronic subdural hematoma: a prospective comparative study. Neurosurgery. 1990; 26(5):771–773

[84] Ono J, Yamaura A, Kubota M, Okimura Y, Isobe K. Outcome prediction in severe head injury: analyses of clinical prognostic factors. J Clin Neurosci. 2001; 8(2):120–123

[85] Yanaka K, Kamezaki T, Yamada T, Takano S, Meguro K, Nose T. Acute subdural hematoma—prediction of outcome with a linear discriminant function. Neurol Med Chir (Tokyo). 1993; 33(8):552–558

[86] Hlatky R, Valadka AB, Goodman JC, Robertson CS. Evolution of brain tissue injury after evacuation of acute traumatic subdural hematomas. Neurosurgery. 2004; 55(6):1318–1323, discussion 1324

[87] Seelig JM, Becker DP, Miller JD, Greenberg RP, Ward JD, Choi SC. Traumatic acute subdural hematoma: major mortality reduction in comatose patients treated within four hours. N Engl J Med. 1981; 304(25):1511–1518

[88] Seelig JM, Greenberg RP, Becker DP, Miller JD, Choi SC. Reversible brainstem dysfunction following acute traumatic subdural hematoma: a clinical and electrophysiological study. J Neurosurg. 1981; 55(4):516–523

[89] Lee KS, Bae WK, Doh JW, Bae HG, Yun IG. Origin of chronic subdural haematoma and relation to traumatic subdural lesions. Brain Inj. 1998; 12(11):901–910

[90] König SA, Schick U, Döhnert J, Goldammer A, Vitzthum H-E. Coagulopathy and outcome in patients with chronic subdural haematoma. Acta Neurol Scand. 2003; 107(2):110–116

[91] Kotwica Z, Brzeziński J. Clinical pattern of chronic subdural haematoma. Neurochirurgia (Stuttg). 1991; 34(5):148–150

[92] Markwalder T-M. The course of chronic subdural hematomas after burr-hole craniostomy with and without closed-system drainage. Neurosurg Clin N Am. 2000; 11(3):541–546

[93] Sabo RA, Hanigan WC, Aldag JC. Chronic subdural hematomas and seizures: the role of prophylactic anticonvulsive medication. Surg Neurol. 1995; 43(6):579–582

[94] Kotwica Z, Brzeziński J. Acute subdural haematoma in adults: an analysis of outcome in comatose patients. Acta Neurochir (Wien). 1993; 121(3–4):95–99

[95] Ohno K, Suzuki R, Masaoka H, Matsushima Y, Inaba Y, Monma S. Chronic subdural haematoma preceded by persistent traumatic subdural fluid collection. J Neurol Neurosurg Psychiatry. 1987; 50(12):1694–1697

[96] Murata K. Chronic subdural hematoma may be preceded by persistent traumatic subdural effusion. Neurol Med Chir (Tokyo). 1993; 33(10):691–696

[97] Lee KS, Bae WK, Yoon SM, Doh JW, Bae HG, Yun IG. Location of the traumatic subdural hygroma: role of gravity and cranial morphology. Brain Inj. 2000; 14(4):355–361

[98] Stone JL, Lang RG, Sugar O, Moody RA. Traumatic subdural hygroma. Neurosurgery. 1981; 8(5):542–550

[99] Hasegawa M, Yamashima T, Yamashita J, Suzuki M, Shimada S. Traumatic subdural hygroma: pathology and meningeal enhancement on magnetic resonance imaging. Neurosurgery. 1992; 31(3):580–585

[100] Adhiyaman V, Asghar M, Ganeshram KN, Bhowmick BK. Chronic subdural haematoma in the elderly. Postgrad Med J. 2002; 78(916):71–75

[101] Mahajan RK, Sharma BS, Khosla VK, et al. Posterior fossa extradural haematoma—experience of nineteen cases. Ann Acad Med Singapore. 1993; 22(3, Suppl):410–413

[102] De Jesús O, Pacheco H, Negron B. Chronic and subacute subdural hematoma in the adult population. The Puerto Rico experience. P R Health Sci J. 1998; 17(3):227–233

[103] Hamilton MG, Frizzell JB, Tranmer BI. Chronic subdural hematoma: the role for craniotomy reevaluated. Neurosurgery. 1993; 33(1):67–72

[104] Kotwica Z, Brzeiński J. Epilepsy in chronic subdural haematoma. Acta Neurochir (Wien). 1991; 113(3–4):118–120

[105] Rubin G, Rappaport ZH. Epilepsy in chronic subdural haematoma. Acta Neurochir (Wien). 1993; 123(1–2):39–42

[106] Ohno K, Maehara T, Ichimura K, Suzuki R, Hirakawa K, Monma S. Low incidence of seizures in patients with chronic subdural haematoma. J Neurol Neurosurg Psychiatry. 1993; 56(11):1231–1233

[107] Borzone M, Rivano C, Altomonte M, Baldini M. Acute traumatic posterior fossa subdural haematomas. Acta Neurochir (Wien). 1995; 135(1–2):32–37

[108] Chen C-W, Kuo J-R, Lin H-J, et al. Early post-operative seizures after burr-hole drainage for chronic subdural hematoma: correlation with brain CT findings. J Clin Neurosci. 2004; 11(7):706–709

[109] Kuroki T, Katsume M, Harada N, Yamazaki T, Aoki K, Takasu N. Strict closed-system drainage for treating chronic subdural haematoma. Acta Neurochir (Wien). 2001; 143(10):1041–1044

[110] Jonker C, Oosterhuis HJ. Epidural haematoma. A retrospective study of 100 patients. Clin Neurol Neurosurg. 1975; 78(4):233–245

[111] Mori K, Maeda M. Surgical treatment of chronic subdural hematoma in 500 consecutive cases: clinical characteristics, surgical outcome, complications, and recurrence rate. Neurol Med Chir (Tokyo). 2001; 41(8):371–381

[112] Sharma BS, Tewari MK, Khosla VK, Pathak A, Kak VK. Tension pneumocephalus following evacuation of chronic subdural haematoma. Br J Neurosurg. 1989; 3(3):381–387

[113] Modesti LM, Hodge CJ, Barnwell ML. Intracerebral hematoma after evacuation of chronic extracerebral fluid collections. Neurosurgery. 1982; 10(6 Pt 1):689–693

[114] Dill SR, Cobbs CG, McDonald CK. Subdural empyema: analysis of 32 cases and review. Clin Infect Dis. 1995; 20(2):372–386

[115] Bor-Seng-Shu E, Aguiar PH, de Almeida Leme RJ, Mandel M, Andrade AF, Marino R, Jr. Epidural hematomas of the posterior cranial fossa. Neurosurg Focus. 2004; 16(2):ECP1

[116] Rivano C, Altomonte M, Capuzzo T, Borzone M. Traumatic posterior fossa extradural hematomas. A report of 22 new cases surgically treated and a review of the literature. Zentralbl Neurochir. 1991; 52(2):77–82

[117] d'Avella D, Cristofori L, Bricolo A, Tomasello F. Importance of magnetic resonance imaging in the conservative management of posterior fossa epidural haematomas: case illustration. Acta Neurochir (Wien). 2000; 142(6):717–718

[118] Wilberger JE, Jr, Harris M, Diamond DL. Acute subdural hematoma: morbidity and mortality related to timing of operative intervention. J Trauma. 1990; 30(6):733–736

[119] Bozbuğa M, Izgi N, Polat G, Gürel I. Posterior fossa epidural hematomas: observations on a series of 73 cases. Neurosurg Rev. 1999; 22(1):34–40

[120] Sahuquillo-Barris J, Lamarca-Ciuro J, Vilalta-Castan J, Rubio-Garcia E, Rodriguez-Pazos M. Acute subdural hematoma and diffuse axonal injury after severe head trauma. J Neurosurg. 1988; 68(6):894–900

[121] Garza-Mercado R. Extradural hematoma of the posterior cranial fossa. Report of seven cases with survival. J Neurosurg. 1983; 59(4):664–672

[122] Otsuka S, Nakatsu S, Matsumoto S, et al. Study on cases with posterior fossa epidural hematoma—clinical features and indications for operation. Neurol Med Chir (Tokyo). 1990; 30(1):24–28

[123] Koç RK, Paşaoğlu A, Menkü A, Oktem S, Meral M. Extradural hematoma of the posterior cranial fossa. Neurosurg Rev. 1998; 21(1):52–57

[124] Wong CW. The CT criteria for conservative treatment—but under close clinical observation—of posterior fossa epidural haematomas. Acta Neurochir (Wien). 1994; 126(2–4):124–127

[125] Lui TN, Lee ST, Chang CN, Cheng W-C. Epidural hematomas in the posterior cranial fossa. J Trauma. 1993; 34(2):211–215

[126] Sripairojkul B, Saeheng S, Ratanalert S, Pheunpathom N, Sriplung H. Traumatic hematomas of the posterior cranial fossa. J Med Assoc Thai. 1998; 81(3):153–159

[127] Pozzati E, Tognetti F, Cavallo M, Acciarri N. Extradural hematomas of the posterior cranial fossa. Observations on a series of 32 consecutive cases treated after the introduction of computed tomography scanning. Surg Neurol. 1989; 32(4):300–303

[128] Ersahin Y, Mutluer S. Posterior fossa extradural hematomas in children. Pediatr Neurosurg. 1993; 19(1):31–33

[129] Stendel R, Schulte T, Pietilä TA, Suess O, Brock M. Spontaneous bilateral chronic subdural haematoma of the posterior fossa. Case report and review of the literature. Acta Neurochir (Wien). 2002; 144(5):497–500

[130] Reece RM, Sege R. Childhood head injuries: accidental or inflicted? Arch Pediatr Adolesc Med. 2000; 154(1):11–15

[131] Lonergan GJ, Baker AM, Morey MK, Boos SC. From the archives of the AFIP. Child abuse: radiologic-pathologic correlation. Radiographics. 2003; 23(4):811–845

[132] Zouros A, Bhargava R, Hoskinson M, Aronyk KE. Further characterization of traumatic subdural collections of infancy. Report of five cases. J Neurosurg. 2004; 100(5, Suppl Pediatrics):512–518

[133] Shugerman RP, Paez A, Grossman DC, Feldman KW, Grady MS. Epidural hemorrhage: is it abuse? Pediatrics. 1996; 97(5):664–668

8 Spontaneous Intracerebral Hemorrhage

A. David Mendelow and Christopher M. Loftus

Abstract

Spontaneous ICH is classified both by location and by etiology. ICH with underlying structural lesions should be addressed both for the management of ICH mass and also for attention to the primary lesion. removal of idiopathic ICH, while appealing, is difficult to prove as beneficial in many cases. Cerebellar bleeds are an exception. Medical management with factor VII reduces volume and arrests bleeding but does not improve outcome. Future trends include MIS approaches and continued study of coagulation issues. New AHA guidelines for ICH are available and provided here.

Keywords: arteriovenous malformation, cerebral aneurysm, intracerebral hemorrhage, STICH, stroke

8.1 Introduction

It has long been known from postmortem studies that some strokes are caused by intracerebral hemorrhage (ICH), but a reliable premortem diagnosis was rarely made in the days before the introduction of computed tomography (CT) scanning in 1975.[1] Since the early 1980s, CT and magnetic resonance (MR) scanning have become widely available so that now essentially all patients presenting with a stroke have one of these investigations, making it possible to study the natural history of ICH and to try specific medical and surgical treatments. The treatment that has received most attention is surgical evacuation of the hematoma, but despite 30 years of research and 12 completed randomized trials, it remains uncertain whether surgical clot evacuation brings any benefits. The Surgical Trial in Intracerebral Hemorrhage (STICH), the result of which was published in 2005,[2] spanned a period from 1993 to 2004 and recruited 1,033 patients who were randomized to receive "initial conservative management" or "early surgery." Its neutral result has been instrumental in dimming enthusiasm for surgical evacuation of hematomas. When this result is meta-analyzed with those of the other completed randomized trials, the overall conclusion remains neutral. These results notwithstanding, it would be an oversimplification to dismiss surgery as a treatment for ICH. Several hypotheses of benefit from surgery have survived the results of these trials. Specifically, in some cases, the mechanistic argument for removing a clot is strong, and such cases were not well represented in trials because of a lack of equipoise in the minds of the treating surgeons. Superficial lobar hematomas, not complicated by extension into more central areas or the ventricles, were one such group. For this reason, a follow-up trial, STICH II, was performed. STICH II tested the hypothesis that early surgery compared with initial conservative treatment could improve outcome in these patients with superficial lobar ICH of 10 to 100 mL and no intraventricular hemorrhage admitted within 48 hours of ictus. This international trial undertaken in 78 centers in 27 countries, compared early surgical hematoma evacuation within 12 hours of randomization plus medical treatment with initial medical treatment alone (later evacuation was allowed if judged necessary). In the early surgery group, 174 (59%) of 297 patients had an unfavorable outcome, compared with 178 (62%) of 286 patients in the initial conservative treatment group (absolute difference: 3.7% [95% confidence interval: −4.3 to 11.6%], odds ratio: 0.86 [0.62 to 1.20]; $p = 0.367$). The STICH II results are, like STICH I, relatively neutral. STICH II confirmed that early surgery does not increase the rate of death or disability at 6 months and might have a small but clinically relevant survival advantage for patients with spontaneous superficial ICH without intraventricular hemorrhage.

8.2 Classification of Intracerebral Hemorrhage

The most useful classification scheme for ICH is based on etiology, as this is directly related to treatment options. Intracranial hemorrhages fall into two broad groups: those that arise from "ictohemorrhagic" vascular lesions and those that do not. The lesions concerned are those that can be diagnosed with currently available imaging techniques. There are a wide range of ictohemorrhagic lesions that can cause ICH: they all have in common the risk that they may bleed again in the future. This means that treating an ICH that has arisen from an ictohemorrhagic source involves the two aims of dealing with the acute hemorrhage and dealing with the cause to prevent any further hemorrhages in the future. The lesions involved are arteriovenous malformations (AVMs), cavernous malformations (CVMs), aneurysms, dural fistulae, and tumors.

Most spontaneous ICHs that present do not arise from an underlying macroscopic ictohemorrhagic lesion. They arise either from microaneurysms in the brain parenchyma, known as Charcot–Bouchard aneurysms, that are associated with hypertension or from amyloid angiopathy, which is a common component of a range of neurodegenerative disorders.

In parallel with this etiologic classification, an anatomical classification is also useful. The deficit inflicted by a hemorrhage is closely dependent on the eloquence of the brain area in which it arises. The most serious disabilities arise from hemorrhages in the left hemisphere, particularly those that are deep-seated. An important anatomical distinction is made between hemorrhages in the supratentorial compartment and those in the posterior fossa. The posterior fossa is much smaller than the supratentorial compartment and contains tightly packed eloquent vital centers. Most posterior fossa clots occur in the relatively noneloquent cerebellum and exert their clinical effects by compression rather than direct destruction of the brainstem. They also have a marked tendency to produce hydrocephalus. These factors lead to strong mechanistic arguments for surgical evacuation of posterior fossa clots in patients who deteriorate, and they have generally not been included in trials of ICH.

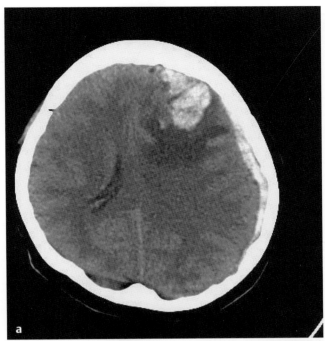

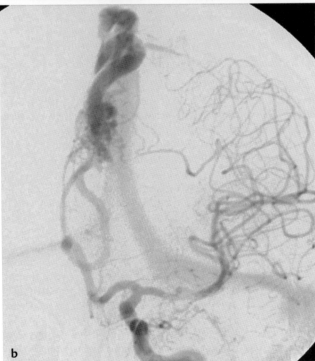

Fig. 8.1 Left frontal spontaneous intracerebral hemorrhage with associated subdural hemorrhage seen on a computed tomography scan (a). This arose from an arteriovenous malformation (AVM) that was shown on a catheter angiogram (b). The hemorrhage was managed conservatively. Elective microsurgical resection of the AVM was done after 3 weeks when the hematoma had liquefied.

8.3 Arteriovenous Malformations

Arteriovenous malformations are congenital vascular abnormalities that involve shunting of blood between arteries and

veins within the brain. They are present from birth and can give rise to hemorrhages at any age. Overall, most intracranial hemorrhages occur later in life, so those presenting in younger people are generally more likely to arise from AVMs. Other clinical features can give clues that a presenting ICH is of AVM origin. Intracranial hemorrhages are prone to provoke epilepsy and steal phenomenon, which may be associated with a history of neurologic deficit or focal epileptic activity in a similar distribution to the presenting deficit. Because AVMs are low-pressure lesions located in brain tissue that is already abnormal, when they hemorrhage, they tend to give less deficit than one would expect from the size of the clot (▶ Fig. 8.1).

There are certain systemic conditions associated with cerebral AVMs that carry both cutaneous and ocular features such as Sturge–Weber and von Hippel–Lindau syndromes. Even in the absence of a specific syndrome, evidence of cutaneous vascular malformations on the head is a suggestive clue to an underlying AVM.

Many AVMs are associated with calcification that can be seen on CT scans, and this is a strong clue to an underlying AVM, if seen with an ICH. Equally, sometimes serpiginous enhancing areas are seen that correspond to large draining veins. Definitive diagnosis is made with catheter angiography or an alternative angiographic modality such as MR or CT.

Untreated AVMs carry an annual risk of hemorrhage that ranges from 2 to 4%.[3,4] These hemorrhages are associated with a morbidity of between 38 and 53% and a mortality of 10 to 18%,[5,6,7,8] significantly lower than the rates for other ICHs. When treatment of an AVM is undertaken, these risks are not eliminated or even significantly reduced unless the AVM is completely removed or obliterated and cannot be seen on catheter angiography.[9,10,11,12] It has been reported that the hemorrhage rate may actually increase following treatment if complete elimination is not achieved.[12] Three modalities are available to treat AVMs: surgical excision, stereotactic radiosurgery, and endovascular embolization. There are some large or complex AVMs that cannot be completely obliterated even with a combination of all three of these treatments, and in such cases it is better not to embark on treatment at all. This means that it is necessary to consider whether a particular AVM has a reasonable chance of being cured before starting treatment, and the need for this judgment as well as the number of modalities involved means that large or complex AVMs are best treated in a multidisciplinary setting.

8.3.1 Surgical Excision

Surgical excision has the potential to eliminate the hemorrhage risk immediately. It has the problem of a significant operative morbidity and mortality, especially for larger and more complex lesions or those located in eloquent areas.[5,13] A particular problem with surgery is the so-called normal perfusion pressure breakthrough phenomenon.[6,7] The arteriovenous shunting effect of AVMs lowers the cerebral perfusion pressure in their immediate vicinity. This long-standing lowering of perfusion pressure leads to dilated and fragile vasculature around the AVM. If the AVM is surgically removed, local perfusion pressure is restored to normal and the fragility of this vasculature leads to a significant rate of postoperative swelling and hemorrhage formation.

8.3.2 Embolization

Like surgery, endovascular embolization has the potential to completely obliterate an AVM and afford immediate protection from hemorrhage. It is also considerably safer than surgery, with lower associated morbidity and mortality. Its main problem is that as a single treatment, it has a low obliteration rate of 0 to 22%.[14,15,16] This low obliteration rate makes it a poor stand-alone treatment, but in a multidisciplinary setting it is frequently used as a primary treatment, because it is quite often possible to tailor embolization to enhance the success rate of other treatments rather than to achieve a cure. Cases where cure is achieved can be seen as a bonus. For example, it is often possible specifically to embolize deep arterial feeders, which are particularly difficult to control surgically.[15] Or, alternatively, it may be possibly to embolize more diffuse peripheral areas of an AVM, leaving a compact nidus as a suitable target for stereotactic radiosurgery.[17] We are still at a relatively early stage in the evolution of embolization technology, with new products and techniques becoming readily available. This holds the promise of improvements in the efficacy of the technique in the future.

8.3.3 Focused Radiosurgery

Focused radiosurgery involves administering a single dose of radiotherapy that is accurately focused on the AVM. There are two groups of technology available for doing this. Linear accelerators use a single narrow X-ray beam that passes through the target but is moved through an arc so outside of the target that the radiation exposure is spread over wider areas of brain. The Gamma Knife is a single product produced by Elekta. It focuses 201 beams of gamma rays from cobalt sources onto a small target. With either type of unit, the treatment involves attaching a stereotactic frame to the patient's head, usually under local anesthetic. The patient is then imaged with the frame in place and the imaging data used to relate the geometry of the AVM to the frame. The frame is then used accurately to target the radiation dose to the lesion.

Stereotactic radiosurgery obliterates between 65 and 85% of AVMs that are less than 3 cm in diameter.[11,18,19] With larger AVMs, the total radiation dose to the surrounding brain per gray delivered to the target is increased and it is necessary to reduce the target dose accordingly. This leads to a reduced obliteration rate in larger lesions.[20,21,22] The technique is best suited to AVMs with small, compact nidi rather than more diffuse ones. A significant limitation of stereotactic radiosurgery is that it takes between 1 and 4 years following the treatment for the AVM to be obliterated, so a hemorrhage risk persists for this "latency" period.

8.4 Aneurysms

Most cerebral aneurysms lie outside the brain parenchyma in the subarachnoid space. When they rupture, they usually give rise to a subarachnoid hemorrhage, which is a clinical entity that is distinct from ICH. Frequently, a subarachnoid hemorrhage will be complicated by extension of blood into the

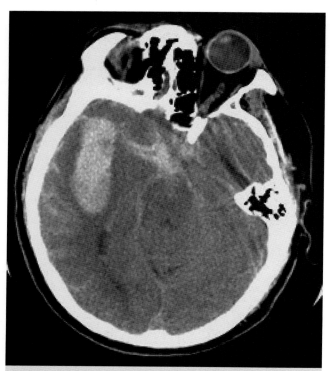

Fig. 8.2 Aneurysmal hematoma associated with subarachnoid hemorrhage, arising owing to rupture of a right middle cerebral artery aneurysm.

parenchyma, but in such cases management is usually dictated by the subarachnoid hemorrhage overall rather than the intraparenchymal component. Less frequently, an aneurysm will give rise to an ICH with little or no subarachnoid hemorrhage. Such ICHs are often devastating because aneurysms are high-pressure, high-flow lesions that are located proximally. A history of sudden severe headache, followed by collapse, and imaging findings of a hemorrhage that is adjacent to one of the proximal cerebral vessels are clues that there may be an underlying aneurysm (▶ Fig. 8.2).

Aneurysmal ICHs are unusual in that there is good evidence for clinical benefit for prompt surgical evacuation.[13,23] If an operation to remove the hematoma is being undertaken, the aneurysm can be isolated from the circulation to prevent future hemorrhage by applying a spring-loaded clip across its neck. This method of securing aneurysms is the classic surgical approach, but since the early 1990s an alternative treatment of endovascular embolization with fine, coiled platinum wire has been developed. In the context of subarachnoid hemorrhage, coiling is the better tolerated of the two treatments, but it is not quite so effective at preventing rehemorrhage.[24] For this reason, it is now favored in the treatment of aneurysms that have caused a subarachnoid hemorrhage, but in the context of ICH, when an operation is being done anyway, the argument is much weaker. Nevertheless, in the United Kingdom, there is a trend toward coiling aneurysms at the time when they are demonstrated on angiography so that there is no need for dissection around the cerebral arteries, with associated morbidity (▶ Fig. 8.3).[25]

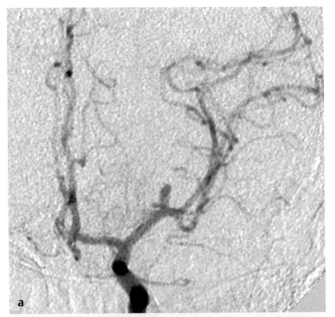

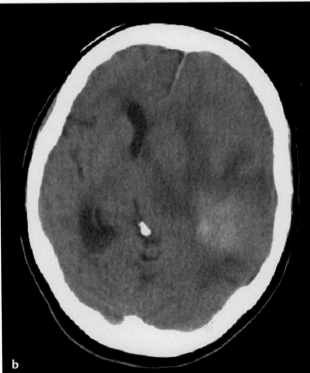

Fig. 8.3 This ruptured left middle cerebral artery aneurysm was treated by coiling (**a**). Remarkably the hematoma was well tolerated by the patient. However, there was an acute deterioration 11 days later, comprising right-sided hemiplegia and aphasia, with impairment of conscious level. The hematoma (**b**) was evacuated without need for the aneurysm to be dissected out. The patient responded well to this treatment.

8.5 Cavernous Malformations

Cavernous malformations are small nodular vascular lesions with a relatively low blood flow that cannot be seen on intra-arterial

angiography. They are indistinct at best on CT but are easily seen on MRI because they contain paramagnetic hemoglobin breakdown products of various ages (▶Fig. 8.4). They occur throughout the central nervous system and carry a variable risk of hemorrhage, ranging from some that cause repeated clinically significant hemorrhages to some that remain asymptomatic indefinitely. The hematomas they cause tend to be small, and morbidity is dependent on the eloquence of the area in which the CVM is located.[26,27] Devastating hemorrhages are rare and tend to occur with CVMs in the optic chiasm, midbrain, brainstem, or spinal cord. Because the hemorrhages are small, surgical evacuation in the acute phase is rarely justified, but once a lesion has bled, it tends to denote a high risk of recurrent hemorrhage in the future and surgical evacuation to prevent such recurrences should be considered, especially if the lesion has bled more than once.[26,28,29] The true nature of unruptured asymptomatic CVMs is unknown. Because they cannot be seen on angiography, embolization is not a treatment option, but stereotactic radiosurgery has been used. It seems to reduce the hemorrhage rate by about three quarters rather than give total protection from rebleeds, and, as with AVMs, there is a time lag of more than 1 year before the fall in rebleed rate is seen. There have been some reported cases of multiple CVMs[30] and of their sometimes being associated with previous radiotherapy.[31] There may also be an association with venous malformations, which themselves do not bleed at all.

8.6 Dural Fistulae

Dural fistulae are shunts between arteries and veins like AVMs, but unlike AVMs they are located in the dura and associated with the dural venous sinuses rather than in the brain. Their origin is unclear, but in some cases they appear to arise secondary to trauma. They may be provoked by venous sinus thrombosis and are probably not congenital. They are associated with localized raised venous pressure and a tendency to intracerebral and subdural hemorrhage. Treatment modalities available are as for AVMs: endovascular embolization, surgery, and stereotactic radiosurgery,[32] although in the case of stereotactic radiosurgery their peripheral location may make them inaccessible to this modality if they occur in someone with a large head at the frontal or occipital pole.

8.7 Brain Tumors

Some types of brain tumors are prone to hemorrhaging and may present as an apparently spontaneous ICH. The wide range of appearances of an ICH on CT or MR imaging can make it quite difficult to tell if there is an underlying tumor. One of the most reliable guides is the appearance of more mass effect than would be expected from the amount of blood alone (▶Fig. 8.5). In uncertain cases, it is helpful to repeat the imaging after a period of 6 to 12 weeks, when the changes due to the hematoma have substantially resolved. As with other ICHs, the benefits of removing the clot per se are largely unknown in most cases. Moreover, the tumors that tend to behave in this way are metastases from renal cell carcinomas or malignant melanoma, and high-grade gliomas. As such, long-term prevention of rehemorrhage is rarely the primary objective of treatment because

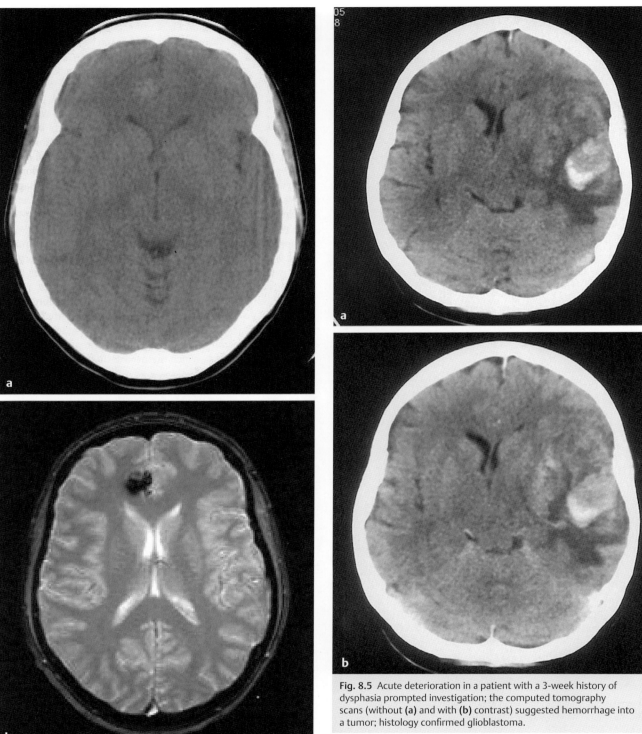

Fig. 8.4 Demonstration of intralesional hemorrhage of a right frontal cavernous venous malformation on computed tomography scan **(a)** and T2*-weighted magnetic resonance image **(b)**.

Fig. 8.5 Acute deterioration in a patient with a 3-week history of dysphasia prompted investigation; the computed tomography scans (without **(a)** and with **(b)** contrast) suggested hemorrhage into a tumor; histology confirmed glioblastoma.

of the relatively poor prognosis that these conditions carry. Surgery may be justified to remove the tumor itself.[33]

Benign tumors may occasionally give rise to hemorrhages, but this behavior is rare. Hemangioblastomas are worth noting because they are benign tumors with a reputation for hemorrhage, although the risk has been reported as only 0.24% per year.[34] Most of them arise as part of the von Hippel–Lindau syndrome. Rarely do cases arise without it.[35] Genetic testing for von Hippel–Lindau is recommended when one is diagnosed. Symptomatic hemangioblastomas usually form cystic lesions with a small, enhancing nodule in the wall. They have a predilection for the posterior fossa.[36] Their benign nature and tendency to symptomatic cyst formation or hemorrhage generally justify surgical removal.

8.8 No Ictohemorrhagic Lesion

Hemorrhages arising from microaneurysms are known as hypertensive hemorrhages. They are usually large in size and occur in the midbrain and basal ganglia. As a consequence, they often have a devastating impact. By contrast, hemorrhages arising from amyloid angiopathy tend to be located in the peripheral neocortex, particularly the occipital lobes, and to be smaller in size. Consequently, they tend to have a smaller clinical impact. Often there is evidence of previous clinically silent hemorrhages on the presenting CT scan. The two types of hemorrhage overlap in appearance and it is not always possible to discriminate between them on imaging grounds, for which reason they are normally regarded as a single group.[37] This group forms a large majority of presenting brain hemorrhages and has been the substrate for most research into the behavior of brain hemorrhages and specific treatments for them. Several surgical treatments aimed at removing ICHs are available. Conventional surgery involves an open craniotomy and clot removal under direct vision. This is increasingly being supplemented by various minimally invasive options.

8.8.1 Craniotomy and Hematoma Evacuation

Open craniotomy and removal of the clot is the surgical treatment that has the longest history; consequently, it has been the most studied. Results from animal models of ICH suggested substantial potential benefits for surgical clot removal.[38] These hopes have so far not been substantiated by randomized data collected in a clinical setting. Eight trials have been completed to date in which open surgical clot removal was the main treatment used.[2,39,40] The conclusion from this work has been that there is no evidence of any benefit from clot removal, although to dismiss the treatment wholly would be an oversimplification. There are several hypotheses of potential benefit from surgery that survive the randomized results. In some cases, there is a strong mechanistic argument for clot removal. Lobar hematomas, which are not complicated by extension into central areas or the ventricular system and are remote from eloquent areas, especially if they are associated with mass effect or recent clinical deterioration, form one such group. The decision to operate on such cases is rarely in equipoise, and so they are infrequently

recruited to randomized trials. In the STICH trial, the broader group of lobar hematomas with or without these complications formed 40% of those randomized to surgery or conservative treatment. This group of patients formed 49% of cases operated on outside of the trial in the participating centers. A retrospective subgroup analysis of this population does show beneficial trends. Most other trial data that are in the public domain do not carry enough detail to allow this subgroup to be identified retrospectively, but in those cases that do, a modest benefit is again found.

As we have noted above, the STICH II trial, like its forerunner trial STICH I, gave a neutral result regarding the superiority of conservative or surgical hematoma management. The Minimally Invasive Surgery Plus Recombinant Tissue-Type Plasminogen Activator for ICH Evacuation Trial II (MISTIE II) aimed to determine the safety of minimally invasive surgery plus recombinant tissue plasminogen activator in the setting of ICH.[41] This study compared 79 surgical patients with 39 medical patients. The study demonstrated a significant reduction in perihematomal edema in the hematoma evacuation group, with a trend toward improved outcomes. A randomized

Phase 3 clinical trial of minimally invasive hematoma evacuation (MISTIE III) is currently in progress.

The recently published American Heart Association/American Stroke Association (AHA/ASA) guidelines for the management of spontaneous ICH confirm that randomized trials have not yet demonstrated a clear benefit for surgical clot evacuation.[42]

Timing of Surgery

The logistics of clinical presentation, assessment, and transfer mean that it is very rare for an ICH to present to a neurosurgical unit in time for evacuation within 3 hours of the onset of the symptoms. The circumstances in which it is possible to perform very early surgery are found in the management of postoperative hematomas that occur on neurosurgical wards and in patients presenting with ICH who deteriorate acutely while in a neurologic unit. In the former case, almost all surgeons are confident that prompt removal of the hematoma improves outcome. Similarly, in the latter case, the decision to operate is rarely in equipoise, and in the STICH trial a substantial proportion of cases recruited to the initial conservative arm that continued to deteriorate crossed over to having surgery. For this reason, no conclusions can be drawn from the STICH trial about the effects of surgery within 3 hours of onset or deterioration.

Some cases of deterioration in hospital appear to be due to repeated hemorrhage.[43] This has led to trials of medical treatment. One treatment in particular, recombinant factor VII, showed promise in phase II trials[44,45]—but this was not confirmed in a phase III trial, which found no improvement in outcome.[46]

If the logistics of stroke management improve, it may become possible to address the question of very early surgery.

Stereotactic and Endoscopic Surgery

It is possible that minimally invasive surgical techniques may achieve benefits where open craniotomy and clot removal do not. This is most likely to be in those deep-seated hematomas where craniotomy may do more harm than good by disrupting brain overlying the clot. Several techniques have been developed. These include stereotactic clot aspiration with or without irrigating with thrombolytic agents such as urokinase, endoscopically assisted clot removal, and thrombolytic irrigation of the ventricular system for hemorrhages that involve the ventricles. Several trials of minimally invasive clot removal have so far been completed.[47,48] In the STICH trial, minimally invasive techniques were intended in 25% of patients who were randomized to surgery. A post hoc analysis shows that patients who had minimally invasive operations were more likely to have deep-seated clots; subgroup analysis accounting for the difference in the location of hematomas found that open surgery performed best, followed by conservative treatment, with minimally invasive surgery performing worst. These differences were not statistically significant. As we have said, we await the results of the MISTIE III trial for guidance on the propriety and efficacy of novel minimally invasive surgical supratentorial clot removal techniques.

8.9 Hematomas of the Cerebellum

Cerebellar hematomas are generally treated as a distinct clinical entity and are more likely to be considered an acute surgical emergency (▶ Fig. 8.6). Most trials have excluded them, and

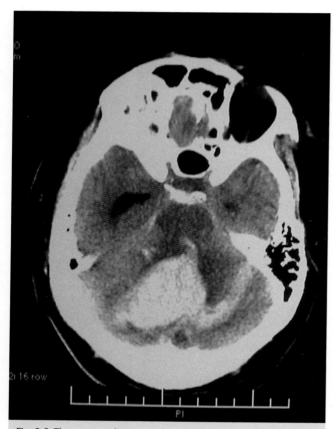

Fig. 8.6 The computed tomography scan shows appearance of a spontaneous cerebellar hemisphere hematoma, causing brainstem compression; the dilated temporal horns indicate obstructive hydrocephalus.

there is little evidence about the benefits of surgery beyond expert opinion and case series.[51,52] Hemorrhages that involve the brainstem carry a very poor prognosis, and there is little reason to believe that surgical intervention can influence this. When a hemorrhage is confined to the cerebellum, especially the lateral cerebellum, the local brain tissue damage can be tolerated with minimal deficit. When such hemorrhages cause cognitive impairment or coma, it is via either hydrocephalus or external compression of the brainstem. Both of these mechanisms are potentially amenable to surgical reversal by drainage of hydrocephalus or posterior fossa craniectomy and evacuation of the clot. Because of this potentially decisive surgical intervention, the policy adopted by most surgeons is early clot removal or observation on a neurologic ward on initial presentation and intervention with cerebrospinal fluid drainage or clot removal should the clinical picture deteriorate.

8.10 Conclusion

Experimentation on animal models of ICH has led to the theory that, in addition to causing mechanical tissue disruption and increased local tissue pressure, the clot induces destructive chemical changes that are of an ischemic or inflammatory origin in the surrounding tissue. It is suggested that such changes are mediated by diffusible agents originating within the clot.[53,54,55,56,57,58] The leading contenders are thrombin and its breakdown products.[56,57,59] These ideas suggest the possibility of developing drugs that influence the process and reduce the degree of permanent tissue damage. Animal experimentation has yielded promising results in this area,[60,61] but so far no useful treatments for humans. Necessary prerequisites, if such an approach to neuroprotection is to be possible, are first that a significant chemically mediated contribution to the neurologic damage caused by ICH in mankind does indeed exist, second that this component is permanent, and third that drugs can be found that influence it. All these features have been reported though not proven in animal models, but as yet clinical effectiveness is unproven.

All available treatments of ICH are at best limited in their effect; the condition still carries a grievous clinical impact. A successful prevention program would be worthwhile but is not immediately practical. The principal preventative measure available is control of hypertension, and Western populations have been screened and treated for it for several decades. During this time, patients have continued to present with uncontrolled hypertension and ICH. It is unknown whether more vigorous therapy targeted at people at particular risk of ICH may impact on the incidence; this merits further research. The relative rarity of ICH and the lack of known specific risk factors hamper progress at the present time. Even the role of family history is not well defined, because it is only since CT has been widely available that it has been possible to make the diagnosis accurately. This is still too recent to characterize familial patterns in conditions that principally affect an older age group. Were it possible to identify a particularly high-risk population, then it might also be feasible to gather Class I evidence on the efficacy of more focused blood pressure control with the long-term aim of finding an effective prevention strategy.

Medical therapy with recombinant factor VIIa may prove to be the best initial treatment of ICH. Unfortunately, the FAST trial showed that hemostatic therapy with rFVIIa reduced growth of the hematoma but did not improve survival or functional outcome after intracerebral hemorrhage.[46] Surgical treatment is as yet of no proven benefit. The result of 12 randomized trials is that no evidence of benefit from surgical removal of ICH has been found. The neutral trial data notwithstanding, craniotomy and clot removal are likely to be practiced in most neurosurgical units in selected groups of patients, specifically those who present at a young age or who deteriorate from an initially good conscious state with superficial lobar hematomas. Also, surgical removal will retain a role in the treatment of postoperative hematomas and those of aneurysmal origin. For the large majority of patients with ICH, surgery has not been shown to be effective at improving outcome. There are outstanding hypotheses of benefit that are currently under trial, including the subgroups mentioned above and the role of more minimally invasive techniques rather than open craniotomy for deep and intraventricular hematomas.

There is less evidence available to inform management of ICHs arising from structural ictohemorrhagic lesions. The standard approach is to treat the ICH as one would a spontaneous ICH and also to treat the underlying lesions with a view to preventing recurrent hemorrhage. Three modalities are available for such preventative treatment: surgery, stereotactic radiosurgery, and endovascular embolization.

8.11 AHA/ASA 2015 Guidelines[42]

8.11.1 Surgical Treatment of ICH: Recommendations

1. Patients with cerebellar hemorrhage who are deteriorating neurologically or who have brainstem compression and/or hydrocephalus from ventricular obstruction should undergo surgical removal of the hemorrhage as soon as possible (*Class I; Level of Evidence B*). Initial treatment of these patients with ventricular drainage rather than surgical evacuation is not recommended (*Class III; Level of Evidence C*). (Unchanged from the previous guideline)
2. For most patients with supratentorial ICH, the usefulness of surgery is not well established (*Class IIb; Level of Evidence A*). (Revised from the previous guideline)
3. Specific exceptions and potential subgroup considerations are outlined below in recommendations 3 through 6.
4. A policy of early hematoma evacuation is not clearly beneficial compared with hematoma evacuation when patients deteriorate (*Class IIb; Level of Evidence A*). (New recommendation)
5. Supratentorial hematoma evacuation in deteriorating patients might be considered as a life-saving measure (*Class IIb; Level of Evidence C*). (New recommendation)
6. Decompressive craniectomy with or without hematoma evacuation might reduce mortality for patients with supratentorial ICH who are in a coma, have large hematomas with significant midline shift, or have elevated ICP refractory to medical management (*Class IIb; Level of Evidence C*). (New recommendation)
7. The effectiveness of minimally invasive clot evacuation with stereotactic or endoscopic aspiration with or without thrombolytic usage is uncertain (*Class IIb; Level of Evidence B*). (Revised from the previous guideline)

References

[1] Hounsfield GN. Nobel Award address. Computed medical imaging. Med Phys. 1980; 7(4):283–290

[2] Mendelow AD, Gregson BA, Fernandes HM, et al; STICH investigators. Early surgery versus initial conservative treatment in patients with spontaneous supratentorial intracerebral haematomas in the International Surgical Trial in Intracerebral Haemorrhage (STICH): a randomised trial. Lancet. 2005; 365(9457):387–397

[3] Ondra SL, Troupp H, George ED, Schwab K. The natural history of symptomatic arteriovenous malformations of the brain: a 24-year follow-up assessment. J Neurosurg. 1990; 73(3):387–391

[4] Mast H, Young WL, Koennecke HC, et al. Risk of spontaneous haemorrhage after diagnosis of cerebral arteriovenous malformation. Lancet. 1997; 350(9084):1065–1068

[5] Brown RD, Jr, Wiebers DO, Torner JC, O'Fallon WM. Frequency of intracranial hemorrhage as a presenting symptom and subtype analysis: a population-based study of intracranial vascular malformations in Olmsted Country, Minnesota. J Neurosurg. 1996; 85(1):29–32

[6] Kader A, Young WL, Pile-Spellman J, et al. The influence of hemodynamic and anatomic factors on hemorrhage from cerebral arteriovenous malformations. Neurosurgery. 1994; 34(5):801–807, discussion 807–808

[7] Graf CJ, Perret GE, Torner JC. Bleeding from cerebral arteriovenous malformations as part of their natural history. J Neurosurg. 1983; 58(3):331–337

[8] Porter PJ, Willinsky RA, Harper W, Wallace MC. Cerebral cavernous malformations: natural history and prognosis after clinical deterioration with or without hemorrhage. J Neurosurg. 1997; 87(2):190–197

[9] Karlsson B, Lax I, Söderman M. Risk for hemorrhage during the 2-year latency period following gamma knife radiosurgery for arteriovenous malformations. Int J Radiat Oncol Biol Phys. 2001; 49(4):1045–1051

[10] Fournier D, TerBrugge KG, Willinsky R, Lasjaunias P, Montanera W. Endovascular treatment of intracerebral arteriovenous malformations: experience in 49 cases. J Neurosurg. 1991; 75(2):228–233

[11] Lunsford LD, Kondziolka D, Flickinger JC, et al. Stereotactic radiosurgery for arteriovenous malformations of the brain. J Neurosurg. 1991; 75(4):512–524

[12] Miyamoto S, Hashimoto N, Nagata I, et al. Posttreatment sequelae of palliatively treated cerebral arteriovenous malformations. Neurosurgery. 2000; 46(3):589–594, discussion 594–595

[13] Schaller C, Schramm J, Haun D. Significance of factors contributing to surgical complications and to late outcome after elective surgery of cerebral arteriovenous malformations. J Neurol Neurosurg Psychiatry. 1998; 65(4):547–554

[14] Yu SC, Chan MS, Lam JM, Tam PH, Poon WS. Complete obliteration of intracranial arteriovenous malformation with endovascular cyanoacrylate embolization: initial success and rate of permanent cure. AJNR Am J Neuroradiol. 2004; 25(7):1139–1143

[15] Taylor CL, Dutton K, Rappard G, et al. Complications of preoperative embolization of cerebral arteriovenous malformations. J Neurosurg. 2004; 100(5):810–812

[16] Liu HM, Wang YH, Chen YF, Tu YK, Huang KM. Endovascular treatment of brain-stem arteriovenous malformations: safety and efficacy. Neuroradiology. 2003; 45(9):644–649

[17] Henkes H, Nahser HC, Berg-Dammer E, Weber W, Lange S, Kühne D. Endovascular therapy of brain AVMs prior to radiosurgery. Neurol Res. 1998; 20(6):479–492

[18] Friedman WA, Bova FJ, Mendenhall WM. Linear accelerator radiosurgery for arteriovenous malformations: the relationship of size to outcome. J Neurosurg. 1995; 82(2):180–189

[19] Steiner L, Lindquist C, Adler JR, Torner JC, Alves W, Steiner M. Clinical outcome of radiosurgery for cerebral arteriovenous malformations. J Neurosurg. 1992; 77(1):1–8

[20] Miyawaki L, Dowd C, Wara W, et al. Five year results of LINAC radio-surgery for arteriovenous malformations: outcome for large AVMS. Int J Radiat Oncol Biol Phys. 1999; 44(5):1089–1106

[21] Kwon Y, Jeon SR, Kim JH, et al. Analysis of the causes of treatment failure in gamma knife radiosurgery for intracranial arteriovenous malformations. J Neurosurg. 2000; 93(Suppl 3):104–106

[22] Ellis TL, Friedman WA, Bova FJ, Kubilis PS, Buatti JM. Analysis of treatment failure after radiosurgery for arteriovenous malformations. J Neurosurg. 1998; 89(1):104–110

[23] Sisti MB, Kader A, Stein BM. Microsurgery for 67 intracranial arteriovenous malformations less than 3 cm in diameter. J Neurosurg. 1993; 79(5):653–660

[24] Spetzler RF, Wilson CB, Weinstein P, Mehdorn M, Townsend J, Telles D. Normal perfusion pressure breakthrough theory. Clin Neurosurg. 1978; 25:651–672

[25] Niemann DB, Wills AD, Maartens NF, Kerr RS, Byrne JV, Molyneux AJ. Treatment of intracerebral hematomas caused by aneurysm rupture: coil placement followed by clot evacuation. J Neurosurg. 2003; 99(5):843–847

[26] Porter RW, Detwiler PW, Han PP, Spetzler RF. Stereotactic radiosurgery for cavernous malformations: Kjellberg's experience with proton beam therapy in 98 cases at the Harvard Cyclotron. Neurosurgery. 1999; 44(2):424–425

[27] Porter RW, Detwiler PW, Spetzler RF, et al. Cavernous malformations of the brainstem: experience with 100 patients. J Neurosurg. 1999; 90(1):50–58

[28] Mitchell P, Hodgson TJ, Seaman S, Kemeny AA, Forster DM. Stereotactic radiosurgery and the risk of haemorrhage from cavernous malformations. Br J Neurosurg. 2000; 14(2):96–100

[29] Kondziolka D, Lunsford LD, Flickinger JC, Kestle JR. Reduction of hemorrhage risk after stereotactic radiosurgery for cavernous malformations. J Neurosurg. 1995; 83(5):825–831

[30] Maraire JN, Awad IA. Intracranial cavernous malformations: lesion behavior and management strategies. Neurosurgery. 1995; 37(4):591–605

[31] Detwiler PW, Porter RW, Zabramski JM, Spetzler RF. Radiation-induced cavernous malformation. J Neurosurg. 1998; 89(1):167–169

[32] Steiger HJ, Hänggi D, Schmid-Elsaesser R. Cranial and spinal dural arteriovenous malformations and fistulas: an update. Acta Neurochir Suppl (Wien). 2005; 94:115–122

[33] Mitchell P, Ellison DW, Mendelow AD. Surgery for malignant gliomas: mechanistic reasoning and slippery statistics. Lancet Neurol. 2005; 4(7):413–422

[34] Gläsker S, Van Velthoven V. Risk of hemorrhage in hemangioblastomas of the central nervous system. Neurosurgery. 2005; 57(1):71–76, discussion 71–76

[35] Kato M, Ohe N, Okumura A, et al. Hemangioblastomatosis of the central nervous system without von Hippel-Lindau disease: a case report. J Neurooncol. 2005; 72(3):267–270

[36] Wanebo JE, Lonser RR, Glenn GM, Oldfield EH. The natural history of hemangioblastomas of the central nervous system in patients with von Hippel-Lindau disease. J Neurosurg. 2003; 98(1):82–94

[37] Molyneux AJ, Kerr RS, Yu LM, et al; International Subarachnoid Aneurysm Trial (ISAT) Collaborative Group. International Subarachnoid Aneurysm Trial (ISAT) of neurosurgical clipping versus endovascular coiling in 2143 patients with ruptured intracranial aneurysms: a randomised comparison of effects on survival, dependency, seizures, rebleeding, subgroups, and aneurysm occlusion. Lancet. 2005; 366(9488):809–817

[38] Nehls DG, Mendelow DA, Graham DI, Teasdale GM. Experimental intracerebral hemorrhage: early removal of a spontaneous mass lesion improves late outcome. Neurosurgery. 1990; 27(5):674–682, discussion 682

[39] Batjer HH, Reisch JS, Allen BC, Plaizier LJ, Su CJ. Failure of surgery to improve outcome in hypertensive putaminal hemorrhage. A prospective randomized trial. Arch Neurol. 1990; 47(10):1103–1106

[40] McKissock W, Richardson A, Taylor J. Primary Intracerebral haematoma: a controlled trial of surgical and conservative treatment in 180 unselected cases. Lancet. 1961; 2:221–226

[41] Mould WA, Carhuapoma JR, Muschelli J, et al; MISTIE Investigators. Minimally invasive surgery plus recombinant tissue-type plasminogen activator for intracerebral hemorrhage evacuation decreases perihematomal edema. Stroke. 2013; 44(3):627–634

[42] Hemphill JC, Greenberg SM, Anderson CS, et al; American Heart Association Stroke Council. Council on Cardiovascular and Stroke Nursing. Council on Clinical Cardiology. Guidelines for the Management of Spontaneous Intracerebral Hemorrhage: a guideline for healthcare professionals from the American Heart Association/American Stroke Association. Stroke. 2015; 46(7):2032–2060

[43] Brott T, Broderick J, Kothari R, et al. Early hemorrhage growth in patients with intracerebral hemorrhage. Stroke. 1997; 28(1):1–5

[44] Mayer SA, Brun NC, Begtrup K, et al; Recombinant Activated Factor VII Intracerebral Hemorrhage Trial Investigators. Recombinant activated factor VII for acute intracerebral hemorrhage. N Engl J Med. 2005; 352(8):777–785

[45] Mayer SA, Brun NC, Broderick J, et al; Europe/AustralAsia NovoSeven ICH Trial Investigators. Safety and feasibility of recombinant factor VIIa for acute intracerebral hemorrhage. Stroke. 2005; 36(1):74–79

[46] Mayer SA, Brun NC, Begrup K, Broderick J, Davis S, Diringer MN, Skolnick BE, Steiner T; for the FAST Trial Investigators. Efficacy and safety of recombinant activated factor VII for acute intracerebral hemorrhage. N Engl J Med. 2008; 358:2127–2137

[47] Teernstra OP, Evers SM, Lodder J, Leffers P, Franke CL, Blaauw G; Multicenter randomized controlled trial (SICHPA). Stereotactic treatment of intracerebral hematoma by means of a plasminogen activator: a multicenter randomized controlled trial (SICHPA). Stroke. 2003; 34(4):968–974

[48] Hattori N, Katayama Y, Maya Y, Gatherer A. Impact of stereotactic hematoma evacuation on activities of daily living during the chronic period following spontaneous putaminal hemorrhage: a randomized study. J Neurosurg. 2004; 101(3):417–420

[49] Hosseini H, Leguerinel C, Hariz M, et al. Stereotactic aspiration of deep intracerebral haematomas under computed tomographic control, a multicentric prospective randomised trial. Cerebrovasc Dis. 2003; 16(57):S4

[50] Auer LM, Deinsberger W, Niederkorn K, et al. Endoscopic surgery versus medical treatment for spontaneous intracerebral hematoma: a randomized study. J Neurosurg. 1989; 70(4):530–535

[51] Kirollos RW, Tyagi AK, Ross SA, van Hille PT, Marks PV. Management of spontaneous cerebellar hematomas: a prospective treatment protocol. Neurosurgery. 2001; 49(6):1378–1386, discussion 1386–1387

[52] Mathew P, Teasdale G, Bannan A, Oluoch-Olunya D. Neurosurgical management of cerebellar haematoma and infarct. J Neurol Neurosurg Psychiatry. 1995; 59(3):287–292

[53] Andaluz N, Zuccarello M, Wagner KR. Experimental animal models of intracerebral hemorrhage. Neurosurg Clin N Am. 2002; 13(3):385–393

[54] Bullock R, Mendelow AD, Teasdale GM, Graham DI. Intracranial haemorrhage induced at arterial pressure in the rat. Part 1: description of technique, ICP changes and neuropathological findings. Neurol Res. 1984; 6(4):184–188

[55] Bullock R, Brock-Utne J, van Dellen J, Blake G. Intracerebral hemorrhage in a primate model: effect on regional cerebral blood flow. Surg Neurol. 1988; 29(2):101–107

[56] Yang GY, Betz AL, Chenevert TL, Brunberg JA, Hoff JT. Experimental intracerebral hemorrhage: relationship between brain edema, blood flow, and blood-brain barrier permeability in rats. J Neurosurg. 1994; 81(1):93–102

[57] Yang GY, Betz AL, Hoff JT. The effects of blood or plasma clot on brain edema in the rat with intracerebral hemorrhage. Acta Neurochir Suppl (Wien). 1994; 60:555–557

[58] Mendelow AD, Bullock R, Teasdale GM, Graham DI, McCulloch J. Intracranial haemorrhage induced at arterial pressure in the rat. Part 2: short term changes in local cerebral blood flow measured by autoradiography. Neurol Res. 1984; 6(4):189–193

[59] Figueroa BE, Keep RF, Betz AL, Hoff JT. Plasminogen activators potentiate thrombin-induced brain injury. Stroke. 1998; 29(6):1202–1207, discussion 1208

[60] Nakamura T, Keep RF, Hua Y, Schallert T, Hoff JT, Xi G. Deferoxamine-induced attenuation of brain edema and neurological deficits in a rat model of intracerebral hemorrhage. J Neurosurg. 2004; 100(4):672–678

[61] Chu K, Jeong SW, Jung KH, et al. Celecoxib induces functional recovery after intracerebral hemorrhage with reduction of brain edema and perihematomal cell death. J Cereb Blood Flow Metab. 2004; 24(8):926–933

9 Pituitary Apoplexy

Farid Hamzei-Sichani and Kalmon D. Post

Abstract

Pituitary apoplexy is a neurosurgical entity in which rapid diagnosis and prompt surgical treatment enhance the probability of good endocrinologic and neurologic outcomes. The difficulty lies in the fact that patients present with myriad signs and symptoms. Meningeal signs, visual and oculomotor disturbances, as well as endocrine deficits are all possible. Computed tomography (CT) and magnetic resonance imaging (MRI) are important in defining the pituitary tumor, the hemorrhage, and their relationship to other nearby anatomical structures. Angiography or magnetic resonance angiography (MRA) may be necessary to exclude an aneurysm. Transsphenoidal resection of the pituitary tumor and hemorrhage is the procedure of choice. It offers definitive treatment for the pituitary apoplexy as well as its underlying neoplastic pathology. It also carries with it a low morbidity and mortality, even in seriously ill patients. Intensive hormonal support is a necessary adjunct in the perioperative period, and endocrine evaluation is necessary postoperatively to establish need for long-term replacement therapy.

Keywords: addisonian crisis, emergency, macroadenoma, pituitary

9.1 Introduction

Pituitary apoplexy is a neurosurgical emergency in which prompt intervention may halt and even reverse the neurologic deficits and possible mortality. The condition results most commonly from hemorrhage or necrosis of a pituitary macroadenoma, but it can also occur in pregnancy. Pituitary apoplexy occurs in 0.6 to 10.5% of all pituitary adenomas.[1]

Bailey is commonly credited with reporting the first case of hemorrhagic necrosis of pituitary gland in 1898, followed by a formal description of the clinical syndrome of "pituitary apoplexy" by Brougham et al in a case series in 1950.[2,3] These patients presented with changes in mental status, headache, meningismus, and ocular disturbances. Since then, there has been extensive interest in this clinical condition as well as considerable debate on what the term pituitary apoplexy may encompass. In fact, there have been reports of silent pituitary apoplexy.[4] Mohr and Hardy estimated the incidence of asymptomatic hemorrhages in pituitary adenomas to be 9.9%, in contrast to 0.6% that presented with clinical findings.[5] Furthermore, Onesti et al described five patients with subclinical pituitary apoplexy yet extensive hemorrhage into a pituitary adenoma.[6]

With such a broad interpretation in the literature, it is increasingly helpful to define pituitary apoplexy by clinical findings such as sudden onset of headache, meningismus, visual impairment (field defect or decreased visual acuity), ocular abnormalities (partial or complete ophthalmoplegia), and endocrine dysfunction in varying combinations along with radiologic evidence of hemorrhage or sudden expansion of sellar contents. A review of pituitary apoplexy including major precipitating factors is provided in an excellent publication.[7]

9.2 Etiology

Basic anatomy lends insight into the genesis of pituitary apoplexy. The pituitary gland is seated in the sella turcica of the sphenoid bone, attached to the hypothalamus by the infundibulum. The cavernous sinuses are laterally located; through these pass the internal carotid arteries (ICAs), the oculomotor (III), trochlear (IV), and abducens (VI) cranial nerves, as well as the ophthalmic divisions of the trigeminal (V) cranial nerve. Superiorly, the intercavernous and circular sinuses are enclosed in the diaphragma sellae. In the suprasellar region lie the optic nerves, chiasm, and tracts.

The pituitary gland receives its vascular supply from the ICAs. The inferior hypophyseal arteries originate from the cavernous carotid and supply the posterior lobe of the pituitary gland. The superior hypophyseal arteries arise just distal to the cavernous sinus and supply the stalk and adjacent parts of the anterior lobe. The majority of the anterior lobe of the pituitary derives its blood supply from the portal system.

Brougham and colleagues proposed that rapidly growing tumors outgrow their own blood supply, resulting in ischemic infarction.[2] Rovit and Fein hypothesized that an expanding pituitary neoplasm would necessarily compress the superior hypophyseal arteries against the diaphragmatic notch, rendering the pars distalis and the tumor ischemic, necrotic, and hemorrhagic.[8] Mohanty and colleagues stated that the tumor size was directly related to vascularity and therefore larger tumors are more prone to acute vascular events.[9] Critics, however, have pointed out that even small adenomas will show evidence of hemorrhage.[6,10] Furthermore, anatomical studies have shown that the predominant blood supply of pituitary tumors is derived from the meningohypophyseal trunks.[11] Others suggest that "intrinsic" tumoral factors may cause the apoplectic event.[12] A multifactorial explanation for pituitary apoplexy is probably more appropriate.[13]

Other predictive factors have been suggested. Although the majority of cases have no precipitating event, case reports of apoplexy related to estrogen therapy, diabetic ketoacidosis, pregnancy, radiotherapy, bromocriptine, cabergoline, chlorpromazine stimulation, anticoagulation, angiography, and even cardiac surgery exist.[5,14,15,16,17,18,19,20,21,22,23,24,25,26,27,28,29,30,31] Incidences of pituitary apoplexy following closed head trauma have also been reported.[32] These observations have been attributed to vascular compromise, direct tumor necrosis, and systemic hypotension. However, whether there is a direct relationship between these conditions and pituitary apoplexy remains unproven and anecdotal. An overall review of the literature has shown that no particular type of tumor displays an increased incidence of hemorrhage, and the data in fact reflect the relative frequency of each type of tumor.[5,11,17,25,33]

In 20 consecutive patients diagnosed with pituitary apoplexy, from a series of more than 1,000 patients treated surgically for pituitary tumors by the senior author (KDP), no contradictory trends are evident. Five patients had a history of a precipitating factor. The precipitating factors were bromocriptine (two patients), radiotherapy, pregnancy, and head trauma. Hemorrhage was noted in all patients at the time of surgery and confirmed on histologic examination. In 3 cases, there was evidence of prior hemorrhage with the deposition of hemosiderin within the adenoma, and in 17 of 20 cases, necrosis was present. In four cases, the entire sample was necrotic, preventing identification of the cell type after immunohistochemical staining. Eleven adenomas were undifferentiated. There were two corticotroph cell adenomas. A Rathke's cleft cyst with hemorrhage and inflammatory response to the ruptured cyst and a reported case of metastatic adenocarcinoma were identified.[6]

9.3 Presentation

As previously mentioned, not all patients who bleed into a pituitary adenoma necessarily develop the apoplectic syndrome. The authors are in agreement with several others who consider pituitary apoplexy a clinical entity supported with pathologic evidence of hemorrhage.[2,6,8,11,17] Using this definition, the incidence of pituitary apoplexy ranges from 0.6 to 12.3%.[11,12,34,35] The 2% incidence of pituitary apoplexy found in our series is consistent with these studies. Semple and colleagues found an apoplexy incidence of about 4% (62 patients) in a series of 1,605 patients.[36]

The distribution of sexes in pituitary apoplexy is roughly equal. The largest case series was published in 1981 by Wakai and colleagues.[35] In this series of 560 consecutive pituitary adenomas, pituitary apoplexy was diagnosed in 51 patients (~ 9%), with roughly equal division between (28) males and females (23). Cardoso and Peterson noted 241 patients with pituitary apoplexy reported in the literature, 141 (58%) of whom were men.[17] Males represented 60% of the authors' personal series as well as in the Semple series.[36]

Cardoso and Peterson found that the average age of onset in 176 patients was 46.7 years (range: 6–88 years).[17] The clinical progression of pituitary apoplexy can evolve rapidly in a few hours to days.[2,6,17,37] Because of this variable presentation, it is prudent to include apoplexy in the differential diagnosis in any patient who presents with meningeal signs. In the authors' series, only 4 of 20 patients were known to have pituitary adenomas. The others had their tumors diagnosed after the apoplectic event. In the Semple series, the average time of presentation was 14.2 days after the ictus.[36] This delay was thought to be secondary to 81% not having a previous diagnosis of adenoma as well as the frequent misdiagnosis of subarachnoid hemorrhage.[38]

The presenting symptoms of pituitary apoplexy are consistent across a large number of studies.[2,5,6,8,11,12,17,25,33,34,35,39] An excruciating headache (almost ubiquitous) is characteristically retro-orbital or frontotemporal and usually precedes other symptoms or signs. The mechanism underlying the headaches is postulated to be irritation or stretching of the basal meninges or the diaphragma sellae.[17,25] Extravasation of blood into the subarachnoid space may mimic meningitis, characterized by neck stiffness, fever, and spinal pleocytosis.[40,41] Mental status changes may be evident. In addition, the cerebrospinal fluid (CSF) may become bloody or xanthochromic.[33,42]

Acute upward extension of the pituitary adenoma from a space-occupying hemorrhage, plus associated edema and necrosis, will cause compression of the optic pathways and diencephalon. Involvement of the optic pathways manifests commonly by deteriorating vision, ranging from mild to severe decrease in acuity and visual field defects. Optic discs usually appear normal, but optic atrophy and papilledema may be present. Often one eye is affected more than the other.[42,43] Associated impaired consciousness may be related to compression of the diencephalon.[17] Hemorrhage extending into the third ventricle has been reported in a large pituitary tumor with suprasellar extension.[18]

Lateral expansion of the tumor into the cavernous sinuses results in extraocular ophthalmoplegia, trigeminal dysfunction, and vascular compromise. Oculomotor (III) nerve palsy was evident in more than 50% of a series of 39 patients with pituitary apoplexy and 45% of another series of patients presenting with ophthalmoplegia, diplopia, ptosis, and mydriasis.[38,44] A sellar mass with extraocular ophthalmoplegia is highly suggestive of pituitary apoplexy. Abducens (VI) nerve involvement is rare and, if it occurs, usually follows the third nerve palsy.[17,42] Impingement of the first division of the trigeminal (V) nerve may cause facial pain and impaired corneal reflex. Damage to the sympathetic fibers that accompany the first division may give rise to a central form of Horner's syndrome.[25] There have been reports of carotid artery occlusion resulting in mental status changes and hemiparesis or hemiplegia.[44,45]

Pituitary apoplexy has been considered an endocrine emergency.[46] Hypopituitarism, either partial or complete, is a major manifestation.[36,46,47] Low basal or stimulated levels of growth hormone, corticotrophin, thyrotropin, and gonadotropins have all been documented. Worsening of preexisting endocrine abnormalities is not unusual.[25,46,47] Major morbidity and mortality can occur because of failure to treat an evolving addisonian crisis.

Conversely, spontaneous reversal of endocrine abnormalities, mostly in acromegalic patients, but also in prolactinomas and Cushing's disease, following pituitary apoplexy has been reported.[48] Clinically significant derangement of the neurohypophysis is rare.[47] Veldhuis and Hammond calculated a 4% incidence of transient and a 2% incidence of permanent diabetes insipidus.[47]

9.4 Differential and Diagnosis

Bacterial and viral meningitis, intracerebral hematoma, optic neuritis, brainstem infarction, temporal arteritis, encephalitis, transtentorial herniation, and migraine may all in one form or another mimic an acute pituitary vascular accident.[17,33,41,43,49] However, the most important entity that must be considered and excluded is an aneurysmal subarachnoid hemorrhage, also a neurosurgical emergency. Both apoplexy and subarachnoid hemorrhage may present with an altered level of consciousness, sudden headache, ocular signs, and subarachnoid hemorrhage.[17,33] The mass effect of a large anterior communicating aneurysm may likewise mimic the ocular findings of a pituitary apoplectic event.[50] It must also be kept in mind that intracranial aneurysms may be found in 7% of all pituitary tumors.[51,52] Epidermoid cysts with extension into the sella may present like apoplexy.[53]

The diagnosis of pituitary apoplexy requires radiographic evidence of hemorrhage coupled with clinical correlation.

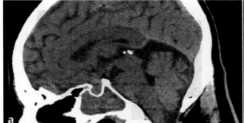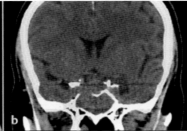

Fig. 9.1 Computed tomography scans, **(a)** axial and **(b)** coronal, showing expansion of the sphenoidal sinus by soft tissue mass and thinning of the lateral walls of the spheonid sinus.

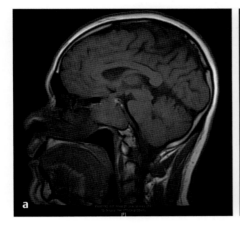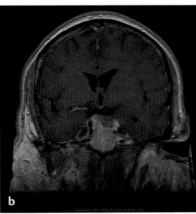

Fig. 9.2 T1-weighted **(a)** sagittal and **(b)** coronal magnetic resonance images demonstrating a sellar mass of heterogenous signal intensity, with suprasellar extension of increased signal intensity consistent with hemorrhagic pituitary macroadenoma.

Literature has demonstrated that computed tomography (CT) without contrast is most valuable the first 2 days after the hemorrhage.[54,55] It will show a hyperdense lesion consistent with new blood within a pituitary tumor, which is usually hyperdense relative to the brain[55] (▶ Fig. 9.1). After 48 hours, magnetic resonance imaging (MRI) is more sensitive, as it can better differentiate older blood from tumor and areas of necrosis from cystic changes[16,39,55,56,57] (▶ Fig. 9.2). MRI is also helpful in estimating the age and time course of the hemorrhage. Hemorrhages of less than 7 days old will appear hypointense or isointense on both T1- and T2-weighted images. A hyperintense signal will develop around the periphery of the hematoma during the second week, and signal intensity will increase throughout the hematoma on T1- and T2-weighted images after 14 days.[54] If clinically warranted, an angiogram or magnetic resonance angiogram (MRA) should be obtained if neither CT nor MRI is able to rule out a concomitant aneurysm. MRI will also best demonstrate the extension of the tumor or hemorrhage into the suprasellar space, as well as chiasmal compression and cavernous sinus extension. Earlier detection has also been reported with diffusion-weighted MRI.[58]

9.5 Treatment

The necessity for rapid action and surgical treatment of pituitary apoplexy has been well documented. There was a high rate of mortality in untreated pituitary apoplexy. In Brougham's initial 1950 review, 10 of the 12 patients died.[2] Seven years later, Uihlein and colleagues found that of the 35 cases reported in the literature, 21 patients died.[37,41] With surgical intervention, prognosis has improved immensely. Cardoso and Peterson's review of the literature from 1970 to 1984 revealed an operative mortality of only 6.7% in 105 patients.[17] In part, the improved mortality may be due to better supportive care and hormonal therapy. Medical stabilization in carefully selected pregnant patients may allow delivery and subsequent definitive surgical therapy. However, although medical management alone may stabilize a patient in acute pituitary apoplexy, it does not address the underlying pituitary adenoma. In other words, medical treatment does not eliminate the possibility of rehemorrhage, nor does it offer the greatest likelihood of full endocrine or neurologic recovery.

In the late 1950s, Uihlein was one of the first to advocate surgical intervention. His protocol consisted of hormonal support and early operation (right transfrontal craniotomy).[41] Modern literature supports this two-tier approach. Intensive steroid replacement is integral in the perioperative management.[17,39,49,59,60,61,62] It is the authors' practice to give dexamethasone 16 mg/day prior to surgery and to taper to a slightly supraphysiologic level postoperatively. Multiple authors now propose early transsphenoidal surgery to decompress the tumor and hemorrhage with less morbidity, less mortality, and better visual improvement.[18,63]

Conservative/expectant treatment of apoplexy is rarely associated with reversal of hypopituitarism and may in fact worsen the condition.[46] In the endocrine literature, follow-up of eight patients with partial or complete hypopituitarism who had undergone surgical decompression revealed normal pituitary adrenal function in seven of the eight. Good improvement was found in preoperative thyroid and gonadal dysfunction.

Untreated cases of pituitary apoplexy may show spontaneous recovery from ophthalmoplegia.[6,17,60,63,62,63,65] One prospective study, in which all patients were treated with high-dose steroids and surgery was performed only if there was no improvement in the first week, concluded that patients with visual impairment or diminished levels of consciousness would benefit from surgery. If the presentation was ophthalmoplegia, conservative treatment was just as effective.[37] Blindness, whether monocular or binocular, is a poor prognostic sign; however, early surgical treatment probably offers the greatest chance of recovery.[6,42,63,66,67] Early visual loss due to demyelination can be reversed by operative decompression, whereas prolonged pressure will cause irreversible ischemic damage.[67] Regardless, a late presentation should not preclude rapid preparation for surgery. It has been suggested that decompression may be valuable even late in the course of pituitary apoplexy. There are reports of partial visual recovery as late as 7 days after the hemorrhage.[6,67] Visual improvement in acuity seen in 76% and visual field improvement in 79% of patients, reported by Semple and colleagues, is similar to other series.[36,42,63,68] Visual improvement has been reported in completely blind eyes.[69]

Open transsphenoidal decompression of the hemorrhagic pituitary adenoma is the preferred treatment for pituitary apoplexy.[36,63,70,71] Unlike the transfrontal approach, no brain retraction is needed, and it is better tolerated by severely ill patients. Craniotomy is reserved for patients with a nonaerated sphenoid sinus, a small sella with a large suprasellar mass, a tight diaphragma with a dumbbell-shaped mass, or an associated intracerebral hematoma.[6,17]

9.6 Indications

- Diagnosis of pituitary apoplexy requires evidence of hemorrhage or rapid expansion of a pituitary mass on CT or MRI as well as clinical correlation.
- Patients often present with sudden onset of headache, meningismus, disturbances of mental status, and ocular findings such as ophthalmoplegia, visual field defects, and monocular or binocular blindness.
- Bacterial and viral meningitis, intracerebral hematoma, acute hydrocephalus, optic neuritis, brainstem infarction, temporal arteritis, encephalitis, transtentorial herniation, cavernous sinus thrombosis, and migraine may mimic an acute pituitary vascular accident.[1,72]
- Aneurysmal subarachnoid hemorrhage is the most important clinical entity to exclude before considering treatment options.[73,74]
- A ruptured Rathke's cleft cyst, though rare, may also mimic pituitary apoplexy.[75,76]
- Initial medical stabilization is mandatory in all cases and includes intravenous fluid and steroids in order to address concomitant severe hypoadrenalism. Involvement of the posterior pituitary gland is rather uncommon, with diabetes insipidus reported in only about 3% of cases.[77]
- Transsphenoidal resection is considered for those with continued neurologic deficit after initial conservative therapy.[72]
- Although visual acuity has been shown to correct as frequently with conservative management as well as with surgical intervention,[63,64,65] surgical resection offers the best chance of improving visual field defects and ophthalmoplegia.[63,78,79] Many studies have suggested that decompression

within 1 week after pituitary apoplexy may offer the best chance of visual recovery.[63,80] Others have shown improvement with decompression months after initial visual loss.[67] Jho and colleagues have proposed a classification scheme for pituitary apoplexy based on clinical and radiologic findings. This classification is a useful guide in stratifying the severity of this condition and thus may prove useful in choosing surgical versus conservative treatments.[81] However, we would like to emphasize the unique nature of each clinical scenario demanding clinical judgment on a case-by-case basis.

9.7 Preprocedure Considerations

9.7.1 Imaging

- CT without contrast is the most valuable study during the first 2 days of hemorrhage (▶ Fig. 9.1), which may show a hemorrhagic cavity with fluid/fluid level within an enhancing sellar mass.
- After 48 hours, MRI is more sensitive than CT in delineating blood from tumor and areas of necrosis from cystic changes. MRI is also helpful in estimating the age and time course of the hemorrhage. Hemorrhages less than 7 days old will appear hypo- to isointense on T1- and T2-weighted images. During the second week, a hyperintense signal can be found bordering the hematoma. By the second week, increasing hyperintensity will be seen throughout the hematoma on both T1- and T2-weighted images (▶ Fig. 9.2).
- If clinically warranted, an angiogram or MRA should be obtained in order to rule out a concomitant aneurysm.
- MRI is the best technique to evaluate extension of the tumor or hemorrhage into the suprasellar space, chiasmatic compression, and cavernous sinus extension and for proper surgical planning (endoscopic vs. microscopic transsphenoidal surgery, craniotomy).

9.7.2 Medications

- The first line of treatment for patients presenting with pituitary apoplexy is to ensure fluid and electrolyte balance and to address any pituitary dysfunction, especially an incumbent addisonian crisis. It is our common practice to give hydrocortisone 100 to 200 mg or dexamethasone 4 mg every 6 hours prior to surgery and taper to a slightly supraphysiologic level postoperatively, as major morbidity and mortality can occur because of failure to treat an evolving addisonian crisis.
- We also obtain a full endocrine panel to serve as a basis for hormonal replacement (e.g., thyroid hormone replacement) in case of hypopituitarism.
- Perioperative antibiotic treatment includes 1.5 g of cefuroxime given 30 minutes prior to initial incision (in case of allergy to penicillin, we administer vancomycin/gentamicin). We commonly continue antibiotic therapy in the postoperative periods as long as nasal packings are in place.

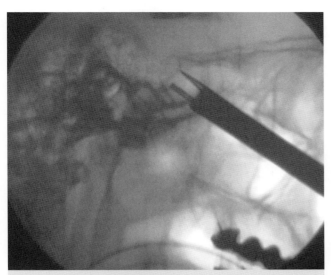

Fig. 9.3 Lateral X-ray of the skull showing the sellar floor marked by instruments passing through the nasal cavity after placement of a self-retaining speculum.

9.8 Operative Field Preparation

- After intubation, the patient's eyelids are gently taped shut and povidone–iodine is applied over the nares, cheeks, and upper lip.
- Povidone–iodine dipped swabs are used to clean the inside of both nostrils as well as under the upper lip (for possible sublabial approach).
- The right lower abdominal quadrant is prepped sterilely with a separate tray of povidone–iodine for possible harvest of fat graft.
- Fluoroscopy- or frameless image-guided navigation is employed in order to determine appropriate trajectory in a midline plane (▶ Fig. 9.3, ▶ Fig. 9.4).

9.9 Operative Procedure

- Patient is placed to far right edge of the operative table in supine position. Right arm is bent 90 degrees at elbow and secured across the chest with padding and tape.
- Head is placed in a neutral position on a soft "donut" or "horseshoe" head holder. For most accurate image-guided navigation, a Mayfield head holder may be used.
- Fluoroscopy arm is positioned at the head of the bed to obtain lateral view X-ray of the skull and clear demarcation of the sella. Alternatively, frameless image guidance is set up to allow for online intraoperative navigation.
- Surgical fields of the nasal passages and the left or right lower abdominal quadrant are prepped and draped in a sterile fashion. Abdominal fat graft may be required if CSF is encountered during the operation.
- Surgical microscope is draped and positioned for optimal visualization of the endonasal route to sella. Endoscope is set up to provide wide view of the endonasal route to sella.

- Using a handheld speculum as well as fluoroscopy/image guidance to direct the dissection toward the sella, the nasal mucosa is identified in the midline and 1 to 2 mL of lidocaine with epinephrine 1:100,000 is injected between the mucosa and nasal septum.
- A no. 15 blade is then used to make a linear incision in the mucosa, and the mucosa is dissected off the septum using a freer instrument.
- A self-retaining speculum is then placed with one blade on either side of the vomer.
- A combination of Kerrison rongeurs and pituitary instruments are used to remove the vomer, enlarging the bilateral ostia into the sphenoid sinus. The sphenoid sinus mucosa is removed.
- A small osteotome and mallet are used to fracture the sellar floor. Kerrison rongeurs are used to remove it.
- It is important to note that sphenoid sinus septations usually do not mark the midline. In contrast, vomer always marks the midline.
- The dura is exposed and incised using a no. 15 blade in a cruciate fashion.
- Ring curettes of various sizes are used to remove the infarcted hemorrhagic tumor in a stepwise fashion inferiorly and then laterally to the limits of the cavernous sinus and finally superiorly.
- After irrigation with normal saline, the previously removed bone fragments are used to reconstruct the sellar floor.
- Hemostasis is achieved and the retractor is gently removed. Using a handheld speculum, a nasal tampon is placed in the nares to ensure tight approximation of the mucosal flap to the nasal septum
- If CSF is seen during the operation, a piece of subcutaneous fat harvested from the abdomen is packed in the sinus.
- If necessary, fat tissue is harvested by making a small linear incision in the right or left lower quadrants.
- A right-sided nasal packing is almost always placed; however, the left nasal packing is placed only if CSF was seen or to achieve better hemostasis.

9.10 Postoperative Management

- Hydrocortisone or dexamethasone is continued in the immediate postoperative period.
- Left-sided nasal packing is commonly removed after 24 hours.
- The patient is monitored for any signs of addisonian crisis as well as diabetes inspidus. To this end, we strictly measure fluid intake and output and obtain daily serum sodium and osmolality. Should the patient have more than 200 mL/h of urine output over three consecutive hours, repeat serum sodium level is obtained. Desmopressin (DDAVP) is administered if serum sodium is elevated.
- On postoperative day 2, the right nasal packing is removed and the patient is discharged home if stable.
- Endocrine laboratory findings are monitored in an outpatient setting to assess the level of hypopituitarism.
- Neurosurgical, endocrine, and ophthalmology follow-up appointments are provided for all apoplexy patients.

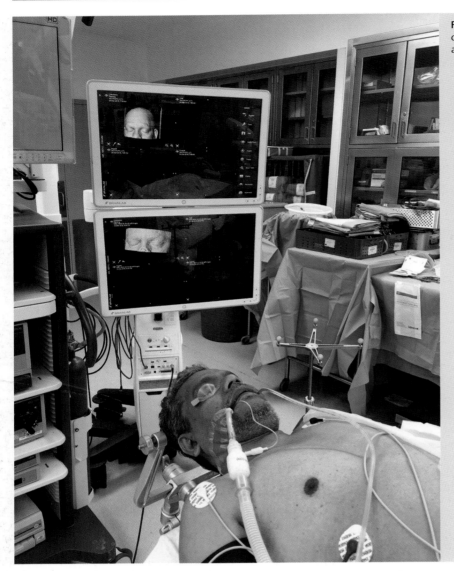

Fig. 9.4 Frameless navigation used in conjunction with an endoscopic approach is an alternative to microscopic endonasal approach.

9.11 Special Considerations

- It is our preference to use the operating microscope for the transsphenoidal approach; however, endoscopic technique may provide wider exposure. Surgeon comfort level should dictate which surgical technique is used.
- Craniotomy is reserved for patients with a nonaerated sphenoid sinus, small sella with an associated large suprasellar mass, tight diaphragma with a dumbbell-shaped mass, or an associated intracerebral hematoma.[6,17]

References

[1] Nawar RN, AbdelMannan D, Selman WR, Arafah BM. Pituitary tumor apoplexy: a review. J Intensive Care Med. 2008; 23(2):75–90

[2] Brougham M, Heusner AP, Adams RD. Acute degenerative changes in adenomas of the pituitary body—with special reference to pituitary apoplexy. J Neurosurg. 1950; 7(5):421–439

[3] Bailey P. Pathological report of a case of acromegaly with special reference to the lesions in hypophysis cerebri and in the thyroid gland and of a case of hemorrhage into the pituitary. Philadelphia Med J. 1898; 1:789–792

[4] Findling JW, Tyrrell JB, Aron DC, Fitzgerald PA, Wilson CB, Forsham PH. Silent pituitary apoplexy: subclinical infarction of an adrenocorticotropin-producing pituitary adenoma. J Clin Endocrinol Metab. 1981; 52(1):95–97

[5] Mohr G, Hardy J. Hemorrhage, necrosis, and apoplexy in pituitary adenomas. Surg Neurol. 1982; 18(3):181–189

[6] Onesti ST, Wisniewski T, Post KD. Clinical versus subclinical pituitary apoplexy: presentation, surgical management, and outcome in 21 patients. Neurosurgery. 1990; 26(6):980–986

[7] Johnston PC, Hamrahian AH, Weil RJ, Kennedy L. Pituitary tumor apoplexy. J Clin Neurosci. 2015; 22(6):939–944

[8] Rovit RL, Fein JM. Pituitary apoplexy: a review and reappraisal. J Neurosurg. 1972; 37(3):280–288

[9] Mohanty S, Tandon PN, Banerji AK, Prakash B. Haemorrhage into pituitary adenomas. J Neurol Neurosurg Psychiatry. 1977; 40(10):987–991

[10] Jeffcoate WJ, Birch CR. Apoplexy in small pituitary tumours. J Neurol Neurosurg Psychiatry. 1986; 49(9):1077–1078

[11] Kaplan B, Day AL, Quisling R, Ballinger W. Hemorrhage into pituitary adenomas. Surg Neurol. 1983; 20(4):280–287

[12] Fraioli B, Esposito V, Palma L, Cantore G. Hemorrhagic pituitary adenomas: clinicopathological features and surgical treatment. Neurosurgery. 1990; 27(5):741–747, discussion 747–748

[13] De Villiers J, Marcus G. Non-haemorrhagic infarction of pituitary tumours presenting as pituitary apoplexy. Adv Biosci. 1988; 69:461–464

[14] Alhajje A, Lambert M, Crabbé J. Pituitary apoplexy in an acromegalic patient during bromocriptine therapy. Case report. J Neurosurg. 1985; 63(2):288–292

[15] Bernstein M, Hegele RA, Gentili F, et al. Pituitary apoplexy associated with a triple bolus test. Case report. J Neurosurg. 1984; 61(3):586–590

[16] Biousse V, Newman NJ, Oyesiku NM. Precipitating factors in pituitary apoplexy. J Neurol Neurosurg Psychiatry. 2001; 71(4):542–545

[17] Cardoso ER, Peterson EW. Pituitary apoplexy: a review. Neurosurgery. 1984; 14(3):363–373

[18] Challa VR, Richards F, II, Davis CH, Jr. Intraventricular hemorrhage from pituitary apoplexy. Surg Neurol. 1981; 16(5):360–361

[19] Cooper DM, Bazaral MG, Furlan AJ, et al. Pituitary apoplexy: a complication of cardiac surgery. Ann Thorac Surg. 1986; 41(5):547–550

[20] Goel A, Deogaonkar M, Desai K. Fatal postoperative 'pituitary apoplexy': its cause and management. Br J Neurosurg. 1995; 9(1):37–40

[21] Knoepfelmacher M, Gomes MC, Melo ME, Mendonca BB. Pituitary apoplexy during therapy with cabergoline in an adolescent male with prolactin-secreting macroadenoma. Pituitary. 2004; 7(2):83–87

[22] Matsuura I, Saeki N, Kubota M, Murai H, Yamaura A. Infarction followed by hemorrhage in pituitary adenoma due to endocrine stimulation test. Endocr J. 2001; 48(4):493–498

[23] Nourizadeh AR, Pitts FW. Hemorrhage into pituitary adenoma during anticoagulant therapy. JAMA. 1965; 193:623–625

[24] Reichenthal E, Manor RS, Shalit MN. Pituitary apoplexy during carotid angiography. Acta Neurochir (Wien). 1980; 54(3–4):251–255

[25] Reid RL, Quigley ME, Yen SS. Pituitary apoplexy. A review. Arch Neurol. 1985; 42(7):712–719

[26] Shapiro LM. Pituitary apoplexy following coronary artery bypass surgery. J Surg Oncol. 1990; 44(1):66–68

[27] Shirataki K, Chihara K, Shibata Y, Tamaki N, Matsumoto S, Fujita T. Pituitary apoplexy manifested during a bromocriptine test in a patient with a growth hormone- and prolactin-producing pituitary adenoma. Neurosurgery. 1988; 23(3):395–398

[28] Silverman VE, Boyd AE, III, McCrary JA, III, Kohler PO. Pituitary apoplexy following chlorpromazine stimulation. Arch Intern Med. 1978; 138(11):1738–1739

[29] Slavin ML, Budabin M. Pituitary apoplexy associated with cardiac surgery. Am J Ophthalmol. 1984; 98(3):291–296

[30] Weisberg LA. Pituitary apoplexy. Association of degenerative change in pituitary ademona with radiotherapy and detection by cerebral computed tomography. Am J Med. 1977; 63(1):109–115

[31] Yamaji T, Ishibashi M, Kosaka K, et al. Pituitary apoplexy in acromegaly during bromocriptine therapy. Acta Endocrinol (Copenh). 1981; 98(2):171–177

[32] Holness RO, Ogundimu FA, Langille RA. Pituitary apoplexy following closed head trauma. Case report. J Neurosurg. 1983; 59(4):677–679

[33] Markowitz S, Sherman L, Kolodny HD, Baruh S. Acute pituitary vascular accident (pituitary apoplexy). Med Clin North Am. 1981; 65(1):105–116

[34] Müller-Jensen A, Lüdecke D. Clinical aspects of spontaneous necrosis of pituitary tumors (pituitary apoplexy). J Neurol. 1981; 224(4):267–271

[35] Wakai S, Fukushima T, Teramoto A, Sano K. Pituitary apoplexy: its incidence and clinical significance. J Neurosurg. 1981; 55(2):187–193

[36] Semple PL, Webb MK, de Villiers JC, Laws ER, Jr. Pituitary apoplexy. Neurosurgery. 2005; 56(1):65–72, discussion 72–73

[37] McFadzean RM, Doyle D, Rampling R, Teasdale E, Teasdale G. Pituitary apoplexy and its effect on vision. Neurosurgery. 1991; 29(5):669–675

[38] Seyer H, Kompf D, Fahlbusch R. Optomotor palsies in pituitary apoplexy. Neuroophthalmology. 1992; 12(4):217–224

[39] Castañeda Adriano H, al-Mondhiry HAB. Hemorrhagic necrosis in pituitary tumors. (Pituitary apoplexy). N Y State J Med. 1967; 67(11):1448–1452

[40] Bjerre P, Lindholm J. Pituitary apoplexy with sterile meningitis. Acta Neurol Scand. 1986; 74(4):304–307

[41] Uihlein A, Balfour WM, Donovan PF. Acute hemorrhage into pituitary adenomas. J Neurosurg. 1957; 14(2):140–151

[42] Reutens DC, Edis RH. Pituitary apoplexy presenting as aseptic meningitis without visual loss or ophthalmoplegia. Aust N Z J Med. 1990; 20(4):590–591

[43] Petersen P, Christiansen KH, Lindholm J. Acute monocular disturbances mimicking optic neuritis in pituitary apoplexy. Acta Neurol Scand. 1988; 78(2):101–103

[44] Rosenbaum TJ, Houser OW, Laws ER. Pituitary apoplexy producing internal carotid artery occlusion. Case report. J Neurosurg. 1977; 47(4):599–604

[45] Clark JD, Freer CE, Wheatley T. Pituitary apoplexy: an unusual cause of stroke. Clin Radiol. 1987; 38(1):75–77

[46] Arafah BM, Harrington JF, Madhoun ZT, Selman WR. Improvement of pituitary function after surgical decompression for pituitary tumor apoplexy. J Clin Endocrinol Metab. 1990; 71(2):323–328

[47] Veldhuis JD, Hammond JM. Endocrine function after spontaneous infarction of the human pituitary: report, review, and reappraisal. Endocr Rev. 1980; 1(1):100–107

[48] Armstrong MR, Douek M, Schellinger D, Patronas NJ. Regression of pituitary macroadenoma after pituitary apoplexy: CT and MR studies. J Comput Assist Tomogr. 1991; 15(5):832–834

[49] Haviv YS, Goldschmidt N, Safadi R. Pituitary apoplexy manifested by sterile meningitis. Eur J Med Res. 1998; 3(5):263–264

[50] Aoki N. Partially thrombosed aneurysm presenting as the sudden onset of bitemporal hemianopsia. Neurosurgery. 1988; 22(3):564–566

[51] Jakubowski J, Kendall B. Coincidental aneurysms with tumours of pituitary origin. J Neurol Neurosurg Psychiatry. 1978; 41(11):972–979

[52] Pia HW, Obrador S, Martin JG. Association of brain tumours and arterial intracranial aneurysms. Acta Neurochir (Wien). 1972; 27(3):189–204

[53] Sani S, Smith A, Leppla DC, Ilangovan S, Glick R. Epidermoid cyst of the sphenoid sinus with extension into the sella turcica presenting as pituitary apoplexy: case report. Surg Neurol. 2005; 63(4):394–397, discussion 397

[54] Glick RP, Tiesi JA. Subacute pituitary apoplexy: clinical and magnetic resonance imaging characteristics. Neurosurgery. 1990; 27(2):214–218, discussion 218–219

[55] Kyle CA, Laster RA, Burton EM, Sanford RA. Subacute pituitary apoplexy: MR and CT appearance. J Comput Assist Tomogr. 1990; 14(1):40–44

[56] Ostrov SG, Quencer RM, Hoffman JC, Davis PC, Hasso AN, David NJ. Hemorrhage within pituitary adenomas: how often associated with pituitary apoplexy syndrome? AJR Am J Roentgenol. 1989; 153(1):153–160

[57] Piotin M, Tampieri D, Rüfenacht DA, et al. The various MRI patterns of pituitary apoplexy. Eur Radiol. 1999; 9(5):918–923

[58] Rogg JM, Tung GA, Anderson G, Cortez S. Pituitary apoplexy: early detection with diffusion-weighted MR imaging. AJNR Am J Neuroradiol. 2002; 23(7):1240–1245

[59] Ayuk J, McGregor EJ, Mitchell RD, Gittoes NJ. Acute management of pituitary apoplexy—surgery or conservative management? Clin Endocrinol (Oxf). 2004; 61(6):747–752

[60] Bills DC, Meyer FB, Laws ER, Jr, et al. A retrospective analysis of pituitary apoplexy. Neurosurgery. 1993; 33(4):602–608, discussion 608–609

[61] Brisman MH, Katz G, Post KD. Symptoms of pituitary apoplexy rapidly reversed with bromocriptine. Case report. J Neurosurg. 1996; 85(6):1153–1155

[62] Lubina A, Olchovsky D, Berezin M, Ram Z, Hadani M, Shimon I. Management of pituitary apoplexy: clinical experience with 40 patients. Acta Neurochir (Wien). 2005; 147(2):151–157, discussion 157

[63] Randeva HS, Schoebel J, Byrne J, Esiri M, Adams CB, Wass JA. Classical pituitary apoplexy: clinical features, management and outcome. Clin Endocrinol (Oxf). 1999; 51(2):181–188

[64] Maccagnan P, Macedo CL, Kayath MJ, Nogueira RG, Abucham J. Conservative management of pituitary apoplexy: a prospective study. J Clin Endocrinol Metab. 1995; 80(7):2190–2197

[65] Nishioka H, Haraoka J, Miki T. Spontaneous remission of functioning pituitary adenomas without hypopituitarism following infarctive apoplexy: two case reports. Endocr J. 2005; 52(1):117–123

[66] da Motta LA, de Mello PA, de Lacerda CM, Neto AP, da Motta LD, Filho MF. Pituitary apoplexy. Clinical course, endocrine evaluations and treatment analysis. J Neurosurg Sci. 1999; 43(1):25–36

[67] Parent AD. Visual recovery after blindness from pituitary apoplexy. Can J Neurol Sci. 1990; 17(1):88–91

[68] Peter M, De Tribolet N. Visual outcome after transsphenoidal surgery for pituitary adenomas. Br J Neurosurg. 1995; 9(2):151–157

[69] Agrawal D, Mahapatra AK. Visual outcome of blind eyes in pituitary apoplexy after transsphenoidal surgery: a series of 14 eyes. Surg Neurol. 2005; 63(1):42–46, discussion 46

[70] Ebersold MJ, Laws ER, Jr, Scheithauer BW, Randall RV. Pituitary apoplexy treated by transsphenoidal surgery. A clinicopathological and immunocytochemical study. J Neurosurg. 1983; 58(3):315–320

[71] Kosary IZ, Braham J, Tadmor R, Goldhammer Y. Trans-sphenoidal surgical approach in pituitary apoplexy. Neurochirurgia (Stuttg). 1976; 19(2):55–58

[72] Murad-Kejbou S, Eggenberger E. Pituitary apoplexy: evaluation, management, and prognosis. Curr Opin Ophthalmol. 2009; 20(6):456–461

[73] Suzuki H, Muramatsu M, Murao K, Kawaguchi K, Shimizu T. Pituitary apoplexy caused by ruptured internal carotid artery aneurysm. Stroke. 2001; 32(2):567–569

[74] Okawara M, Yamaguchi H, Hayashi S, Matsumoto Y, Inoue Y, Okawara S. [A case of ruptured internal carotid artery aneurysm mimicking pituitary apoplexy] No Shinkei Geka. 2007; 35(12):1169–1174

[75] Onesti ST, Wisniewski T, Post KD. Pituitary hemorrhage into a Rathke's cleft cyst. Neurosurgery. 1990; 27(4):644–646

[76] Chaiban JT, Abdelmannan D, Cohen M, Selman WR, Arafah BM. Rathke cleft cyst apoplexy: a newly characterized distinct clinical entity. J Neurosurg. 2011; 114(2):318–324

[77] Sweeney AT, Blake MA, Adelman LS, et al. Pituitary apoplexy precipitating diabetes insipidus. Endocr Pract. 2004; 10(2):135–138

[78] Bujawansa S, Thondam SK, Steele C, et al. Presentation, management and outcomes in acute pituitary apoplexy: a large single-centre experience from the United Kingdom. Clin Endocrinol (Oxf). 2014; 80(3):419–424

[79] Rajasekaran S, Vanderpump M, Baldeweg S, et al. UK guidelines for the management of pituitary apoplexy. Clin Endocrinol (Oxf). 2011; 74(1):9–20

[80] Muthukumar N, Rossette D, Soundaram M, Senthilbabu S, Badrinarayanan T. Blindness following pituitary apoplexy: timing of surgery and neuro-ophthalmic outcome. J Clin Neurosci. 2008; 15(8):873–879

[81] Jho DH, Biller BM, Agarwalla PK, Swearingen B. Pituitary apoplexy: large surgical series with grading system. World Neurosurg. 2014; 82(5):781–790

10 Acute Management of Subarachnoid Hemorrhage

Agnieszka Ardelt and Issam A. Awad

Abstract

The annual incidence of nontraumatic subarachnoid hemorrhage (SAH) is estimated to be 2 to 22.5 cases per 100,000 people depending on the region, and despite vast improvement over the years, mortality in SAH is still approximately 30 to 40%. Clinical presentation of aneurysmal SAH is typically characterized by the "worst headache of life," but a significant proportion of patients present with a mild headache due to a sentinel hemorrhage. The Fisher score and the Hunt and Hess score are frequently used to grade SAH: they reflect the severity of disease and aid in informing the prognosis. The most devastating primary cerebral complications are aneurysmal rerupture, acute hydrocephalus, intracranial hypertension, and delayed cerebral ischemia due to vasospasm, but patients are at risk for seizures, neurogenic pulmonary edema, stress cardiomyopathy, cerebral salt wasting, infections, typical complications associated with catastrophic illness, as well as decompensation of underlying chronic illness. The mainstays of therapy are prompt recognition and diagnosis; resuscitation; transfer to a center with experience in managing the disease; blood pressure control; reversal of anticoagulation or correction of thrombocytopenia; management of acute hydrocephalus; rapid treatment (coiling or clipping) of the aneurysm; monitoring, prophylaxis, and treatment of vasospasm; prevention and treatment of complications; management of preexisting chronic illnesses; and rehabilitation.

Keywords: aneurysm clipping, aneurysm coiling, cerebral aneurysm, cerebral vasospasm, hydrocephalus, intracranial hypertension, subarachnoid hemorrhage

10.1 Introduction

The annual incidence rate of spontaneous (nontraumatic) subarachnoid hemorrhage (SAH) is estimated to be 2 to 22.5 cases per 100,000 people depending on region.[1] Patients who survive to hospital admission and receive adequate medical attention have a higher chance of survival and good outcome, but some may still succumb to rebleeding, sequelae of the initial hemorrhage, vasospasm, or medical complications. Despite vast improvement over the years, mortality in SAH is still approximately 30 to 40%.[1]

Many of the catastrophic sequelae of SAH occur in the first hours or days following the event. Prompt diagnosis and careful management in this early stage can greatly impact the overall outcome of these patients. Conversely, delayed diagnosis or negligence of one or more management principles may result in devastating and irreversible consequences.

Despite the widespread availability of modern diagnostic and treatment modalities, many patients do not reach specialized centers until hours or days following hemorrhage.[2] Even in large metropolitan areas, delayed diagnosis and delayed transfer to a center capable of definitive treatment of the problem are still prevalent, denying many patients the advantages of optimized treatment in the acute phase. There continues to be a lack of general awareness among primary and community physicians about the optimal diagnostic and therapeutic maneuvers in patients with suspected SAH. Neurosurgeons must be involved in the education of community and emergency room physicians, and in campaigns of public awareness about this entity. Few conditions in neurosurgery merit as intense and careful a diagnostic and therapeutic approach in the acute stage as SAH.

Concurrent steps are taken in each patient so as to arrive at optimal diagnosis, systemic stabilization, and management of neurologic sequelae.[3] These measures are taken while planning as early as possible the definitive treatment of the cause of SAH in each individual patient, so as to prevent the devastating consequences of rebleeding.

10.2 Clinical Presentation of Subarachnoid Hemorrhage

Recognition of the common signs and symptoms of SAH is essential for rousing clinical suspicion and eventual diagnosis.[4] Patients most commonly report a sudden onset of severe excruciating "thunderclap" headache,[5] typically "the worst of one's life." This may occur at any time, during activity or rest, but is frequently reported during intense physical activity, heavy straining, or sexual intercourse. The headache is frequently described as retro-orbital and often radiates to the nuchal area. In patients who are frequent headache sufferers, the headache induced by SAH is often different from one's more regular headaches and clearly more intense. Patients frequently report a clustering of more minor headache complaints, termed sentinel headaches, in the days or weeks preceding SAH.[6] Such warning headaches may be caused by minor hemorrhage, changes in the size of the aneurysm, and/or mass effect on nearby structures, before catastrophic rupture.

Within seconds or minutes of the intense headache, the patient may lose consciousness, suffer a seizure-like episode, or die. These phenomena are likely related to cerebral circulatory arrest, either transient or persistent, related to the elevation of intracranial pressure (ICP) at ictus. Patients who die at this stage likely do so from intracranial hypertension–related asystole or other cardiac dysrhythmia, or respiratory arrest leading to cardiac arrest. Other patients may have persistent severe debilitating headache in subsequent hours, or a less bothersome dull and nagging discomfort. Retro-orbital pain, photophobia, nuchal discomfort, and meningeal signs persist for hours and days following SAH. In cases where these initial symptoms are misinterpreted, a variety of delayed sequelae may set in prior to definitive diagnosis. New ischemic neurologic deficits, persistent unexplained meningeal symptoms, noninfectious meningitis, or hydrocephalus should raise the possibility of SAH in the preceding days or weeks. In some cases, subhyaloid retinal hemorrhages may increase suspicion of SAH in situations where the clinical scenario is not otherwise clear. Similarly, a wide variety of focal neurologic deficits may accompany the rupture of aneurysms in various brain locations and may enhance clinical suspicion.

Cranial neuropathies, e.g., abducens or oculomotor palsy, may represent elevated ICP or aneurysmal compression of the

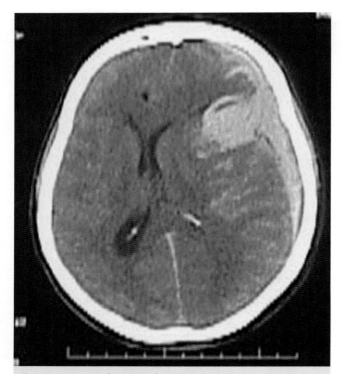

Table 10.1 Hunt and Hess grade

Grade	Neurologic status
I	Asymptomatic; or minimal headache and slight nuchal rigidity
II	Moderate to severe headache; nuchal rigidity; no neurologic deficit except cranial nerve palsy
III	Drowsy; minimal neurologic deficit
IV	Stuporous; moderate to severe hemiparesis; possibly early decerebrate rigidity and vegetative disturbances
V	Deep coma; decerebrate rigidity; moribund appearance

Table 10.2 World Federation of Neurological Surgeons subarachnoid hemorrhage grade

WFNS grade	Glasgow Coma Scale score	Major focal deficit
0 (intact aneurysm)	–	–
1	15	Absent
2	13–14	Absent
3	13–14	Present
4	7–12	Present or absent
5	3–6	Present or absent

Abbreviation: WFNS, World Federation of Neurological Surgeons.

Fig. 10.1 Computed tomography (CT) scan in comatose patient with massive subarachnoid hemorrhage and intracerebral hemorrhage (plus subdural hemorrhage). Such a patient is taken emergently for surgical evacuation of hematoma, with or without contrast-enhanced CT scan, but without taking additional time for conventional angiography.

cranial nerve, e.g., posterior communicating artery or superior cerebellar artery aneurysm compression the oculomotor nerve, depending on the clinical condition of the patient. Other focal neurologic deficits likely imply an intracerebral hemorrhage (ICH) in addition to the SAH, as is common with middle cerebral artery aneurysms (► Fig. 10.1). Vascular malformations and dural fistulae are more likely to cause ICH than SAH but could result in both. Aneurysmal hemorrhage from the anterior communicating artery, basilar summit, or posterior inferior cerebellar artery may cause intraventricular hemorrhage, and this, in turn, may cause ventricular obstruction and account for decreased level of consciousness.

10.2.1 Grading of Subarachnoid Hemorrhage

The patient's initial level of consciousness is a cardinal determinant of outcome after SAH, and it can affect treatment decisions as well as prognostication. The clinical grade can be assigned using the Hunt and Hess scale (► Table 10.1)[7] or the World Federation of Neurological Surgeons scale (► Table 10.2).[8] The former is quite simple and widely used, whereas the latter has been shown to have better positive and negative predictive values in relation to outcome, especially among high-grade patients.[9,10]

10.3 Establishing the Diagnosis of Subarachnoid Hemorrhage

The diagnosis of SAH must be made rapidly because of the dire consequences of rebleeding from an unsecured aneurysm if the diagnosis is missed.[11] SAH diagnosis is most often established with a simple nonenhanced brain computed tomography (CT) scan, which can detect the SAH in as many as 95% of cases,[12] although the sensitivity of the head CT declines with time (► Fig. 10.2). The amount of SAH is evaluated by the Fisher grading system, which has a prognostic value in predicting the risk of vasospasm and overall patient outcome (► Table 10.3).[13,14]

The nonenhanced CT scan may also provide useful localizing information about the possible source of hemorrhage. In instances where the CT scan is negative or questionable in the setting of any clinical suspicion of SAH, a lumbar puncture should be performed unless contraindicated. If performed properly, the presence of red cells in the cerebrospinal fluid (CSF) confirms clinical suspicion of SAH, but the differential diagnosis of sanguineous CSF includes the possibility of a traumatic puncture. Although a traumatic CSF should clear of blood between the first and the last tube, this cannot always be determined with certainty. In SAH, serially collected tubes will likely have a stable red cell count, without evidence of clearing. A repeat lumbar puncture at a higher level (if safe), or even several hours later, may assist in clarifying the situation. Lumbar puncture may be withheld in specific circumstances, i.e., if the head CT performed less than 6 hours after headache is negative.[15]

Xanthochromia (yellowish staining) of CSF occurs due to lysis and degradation of red blood cells and hemoglobin, appears 12 to 24 hours following SAH, and may persist for several days. The presence of xanthochromia in centrifuged CSF is consistent

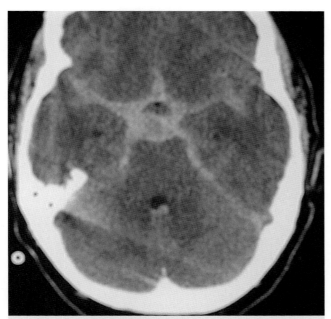

Fig. 10.2 Computed tomography (CT) scan showing polycisternal subarachnoid hemorrhage. The etiology is most likely aneurysmal.

Table 10.3 Fisher grading system of severity of subarachnoid hemorrhage

Fisher group	Blood on CT
1	No subarachnoid blood detected
2	Diffuse or vertical layers ≤ 1 mm thick
3	Localized clot and/or vertical layer > 1 mm
4	Intracerebral or intraventricular clot with diffuse or no SAH

Abbreviations: CT, computed tomography; SAH, subarachnoid hemorrhage.

with SAH, whereas a traumatic puncture will usually result in a clear supernatant. A cellular polymorphonuclear meningeal reaction may occur in the first hours after SAH and may become gradually more monocytic in subsequent days. This response and an accompanying elevated protein level may persist in CSF for 2 to 3 weeks following SAH and may be present even after the disappearance of xanthochromia and red cells. In the setting of negative or uncertain interpretation of the CT scan, a crystal clear CSF on lumbar puncture will safely and reliably exclude the possibility of significant SAH.

10.4 Establishing the Etiology of Subarachnoid Hemorrhage

The prevalence of cerebral aneurysms in the population is estimated to be between 0.2 and 7.9%, with greater prevalence in older patients.[16] This etiology is considered to be responsible for 70 to 80% of spontaneous SAH presentations. Circle of Willis, or "berry," aneurysms are known to develop at vessel bifurcations, i.e., at points of maximum hemodynamic stress. Aneurysms associated with infection or trauma tend to occur more distally in

the circulation. Eighty percent to 90% of aneurysms affect the anterior (or carotid) circulation, at the anterior communicating artery, posterior communicating artery, middle cerebral artery, or other locations. Ten percent to 20% of aneurysms affect the posterior (or vertebrobasilar) circulation, most likely at the basilar summit, the posterior inferior cerebellar arteries, or other locations. Aneurysms can be classified by shape, with the great majority of aneurysms being saccular or berry-shaped and involving an eccentric pathology of the arterial wall, usually at a branching point. A small fraction of aneurysms is fusiform, with or without saccular protrusions, reflecting more diffuse vessel wall pathology, including arteriopathy, dissection, and infection. Saccular aneurysms are classified by size: small, if less than 10 mm in diameter (78%); large, from 10 to 24 mm in diameter (20%); and giant, if more than 24 mm in diameter (2%).

The pathogenesis of saccular aneurysms is not fully understood, although their risk factors appear to be both congenital and acquired. Some systemic conditions are associated with the presence of cerebral aneurysms. These include connective tissue disorders (including Ehlers–Danlos syndrome and Marfan syndrome), autosomal dominant polycystic kidney disease, fibromuscular dysplasia, and atherosclerosis, but these account for only a small fraction of all aneurysms. Twenty percent of patients harbor multiple aneurysms. Approximately 20% of patients with aneurysms have a family history of aneurysms affecting a first-degree blood relative.[17] Hypertension and smoking appear to contribute to the risk of aneurysm formation and also to the risk of hemorrhage.[1] Risk of rupture and hemorrhage increases with larger aneurysm size.[1] The annual risk of hemorrhage for unruptured aneurysms varies between 0.1 and 5–10% per year, with highest risk in giant aneurysms. Higher rupture risk also occurs in patients who have previously hemorrhaged from another aneurysm, and in aneurysms at certain locations (basilar summit and anterior communicating arteries).[18,19]

Once diagnosis of SAH is established, a four-vessel (conventional) cerebral angiogram is the most sensitive and specific modality for diagnosis of an aneurysm, and this typically reveals the etiology of SAH (►Fig. 10.3). Modern angiographic protocols include digital subtraction techniques and rotational three-dimensional assessment of the aneurysm (►Fig. 10.4). These new protocols vastly enhance image quality and provide enhanced information for therapeutic planning.

In cases where the angiogram fails to demonstrate the etiology, magnetic resonance imaging (MRI) should be done to rule out any angiographically occult lesion as a source of hemorrhage. Repeat angiography should be performed 1 to 2 weeks after the first negative study. A contrast-enhanced CT scan, computed tomography angiogram (CTA), or magnetic resonance angiogram (MRA) may establish diagnosis of aneurysm (►Fig. 10.5, ►Fig. 10.6, ►Fig. 10.7) with less invasiveness, but also with less sensitivity than conventional angiography. These tests are used in cases where diagnosis of SAH is questionable or where risks, the patient's medical condition, or immediate availability of an angiographic facility or personnel may preclude emergent conventional angiography.

Subarachnoid hemorrhage restricted to the perimesencephalic cisterns, i.e., perimesencephalic SAH, is more likely to be associated with negative angiography (►Fig. 10.8). However, this condition must remain a diagnosis of exclusion,[20] and repeat angiography may be warranted because basilar or other posterior

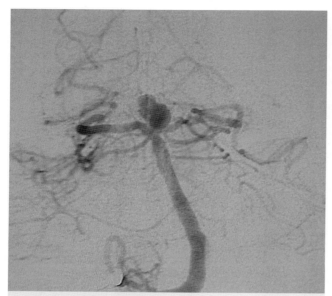

Fig. 10.3 Conventional angiogram revealing basilar summit region aneurysm.

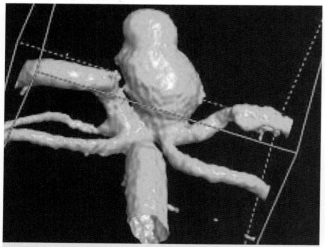

Fig. 10.4 Three-dimensional (3D) rotational angiogram in same case depicted in ▶ Fig. 10.3, revealing much more spatial resolution than in the conventional angiogram images. The information in 3D angiography can help guide therapeutic decisions regarding endovascular versus surgical intervention.

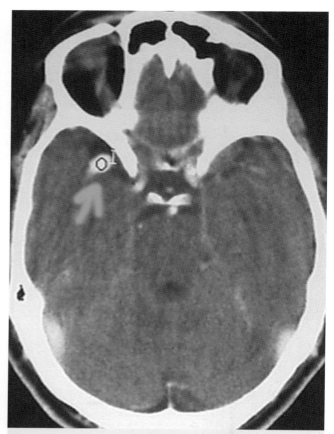

Fig. 10.5 Computed tomography (CT) scan with contrast, showing middle cerebral artery aneurysm.

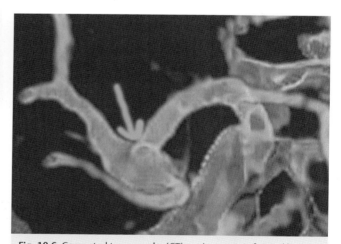

Fig. 10.6 Computed tomography (CT) angiogram, performed by computer reconstruction of thin-cut high-resolution CT scan with contrast, reveals an aneurysmal dilatation at the middle cerebral artery.

circulation aneurysms may also result in hemorrhage restricted to the perimesencephalic region.

In arterial dissection, the cerebral angiogram may reveal one of the following findings: lumenal stenosis, lumenal occlusion, double lumen sign, fusiform vessel dilatation, frank extravasation of dye, or pseudoaneurysm (▶ Fig. 10.9). An arterial dissection may be associated with normal lumenal filling on angiography; therefore, dissection is not excluded by a negative angiogram. In many cases, MRI with axial T1 sequences and MRA source images is more sensitive than catheter angiography (and the reconstructed MRA) for the diagnosis of an arterial dissection. These sequences may reveal a crescent sign, which corresponds to the hematoma in the vessel wall:

this is a bright signal surrounding the signal void of the carotid or vertebrobasilar arteries on axial T1-weighted or source images. MRI also provides an assessment of thrombosed portions of aneurysms, as in giant lesions, that may not fill on the angiogram (▶ Fig. 10.10).

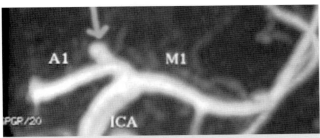

Fig. 10.7 Magnetic resonance angiogram (MRA) revealing a carotid summit berry aneurysm. This is an excellent modality for screening patients for aneurysms. A negative MRA is not sufficient to exclude aneurysm in a patient with subarachnoid hemorrhage. A1, the A1 segment of the anterior cerebral artery ICA, internal carotid artery; M1, the M1 segment of the middle cerebral artery.

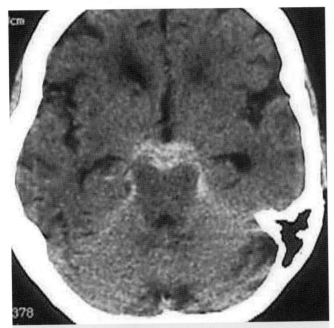

Fig. 10.8 Perimesencephalic subarachnoid hemorrhage (SAH). Cerebral angiogram did not reveal an aneurysm. A perimesencephalic SAH may also be caused by basilar aneurysm or other etiologies.

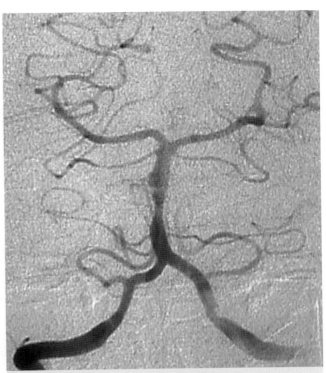

Fig. 10.9 Conventional angiogram of patient with severe subarachnoid hemorrhage, revealing dissection of the basilar artery, with double lumen and small aneurysmal dilatation.

In summary, if angiography does not reveal the source of SAH, a systematic search of other causes is undertaken, including MRI of the brain and spine, performed with and without contrast and with dissection detection protocol. These sequences have the potential to reveal occult vascular malformations, dissections, or tumors. If none is found, a repeat cerebral angiogram is performed, a week or more later, this time with external carotid selective injections in addition to traditional four-vessel views, to exclude dural fistulae. A second angiogram is not required if another etiology of SAH is found or in selected cases in which the hematoma was solely limited to perimesencephalic cisterns and the first angiogram was of excellent quality.

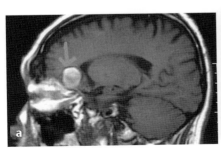

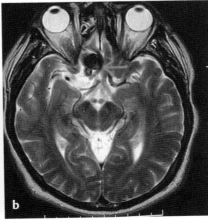

Fig. 10.10 Magnetic resonance imaging of partially thrombosed giant aneurysm. (a) T1-weighted and (b) T2-weighted imaging.

10.5 Management of Patients with Subarachnoid Hemorrhage

Current guidelines suggest that hospital centers with low volume of aneurysmal SAH patients (less than 10 patients annually) should, after initial stabilization, transfer such patients to high-volume centers with neurosciences critical care services and surgeons and endovascular specialists experienced in the management of SAH.[1]

10.5.1 Initial Medical Stabilization

Airway

The acute resuscitation of SAH patients follows the ABCs, i.e., the airway, breathing, and circulation are stabilized first.[3] In any patient with a Glasgow Coma Scale (GCS) score of 8 or less, or in those the airway cannot be protected for other reasons, endotracheal intubation is advocated. During intubation, careful attention should be paid to the blood pressure: if intracranial hypertension is suspected, the blood pressure should not be allowed to decrease to levels that could result in cerebral hypoperfusion. Hypertension should also be avoided.

Blood Pressure

Once the ABCs are addressed, blood pressure should be controlled because of the presumed presence of an unsecured vascular lesion, which may be at high risk of rebleeding. Although the specific blood pressure target is unknown, recent guidelines suggest that a systolic blood pressure less than 160 mm Hg is reasonable.[1] However, as discussed above, relative hypotension should be avoided because it could compromise cerebral perfusion, especially in the setting of elevated ICP,[21] discussed in more detail below. In selected patients, a central venous line and an arterial line may be required to assist with acute management of blood pressure. Cerebral vasodilating agents such as nitrates should not be used for blood pressure control because of the potential to exacerbate intracranial hypertension; instead, medications such as labetalol and/or nicardipine are typically used in SAH patients.

Coagulopathy

Coagulation parameters should be examined and abnormalities corrected promptly. Vitamin K inhibition should be reversed with 10 mg intravenous vitamin K and prothrombin complex concentrate, unless contraindicated. Thawed plasma can be used as well, but it takes longer to achieve international normalized ratio (INR) normalization than prothrombin complex concentrate, and its use is associated with increased frequency of pulmonary side effects such as congestion, as well as transfusion-related lung injury (TRALI). Specific antidotes and reversal agents for the novel target-specific oral anticoagulants (TSOACs) are becoming available, and these should be utilized in patients who suffer an SAH while treated with TSOACs. The first of these,

idarucizumab (Praxbind, Boehringer Ingelheim), was approved by the Food and Drug Administration (FDA) in Spring 2016 to specifically reverse the direct thrombin inhibitor (DTI) anticoagulant dabigatran (Pradaxa, Boehringer Ingelheim).[22] We anticipate that reversal agents for factor Xa inhibitors (specifically andexanet alfa)[23] may be approved by the time of publication.

Pain

Pain management in SAH patients should be optimized, preferably with short-acting narcotics such as fentanyl, but care should be taken not to oversedate patients, which could confound the neurologic examination. In some patients, a short course of steroids may be helpful for nuchal and lower back pain related to inflammation.

Transfer to a High-Volume Center

After initial stabilization, the patient should be transferred as soon as possible to a critical care environment where these specific measures are maintained along with multisystem homeostasis as further diagnostic and therapeutic interventions are planned and the patient is examined serially.

Acute Neurologic Complications

Seizures

It has been reported that up to 25% of patients with aneurysmal SAH have generalized tonic–clonic activity related to the presentation, but the etiology (i.e., whether the activity represents epileptic seizures or ischemia due to intracranial hypertension) and implications for prophylaxis and treatment with antiepileptic medications remain controversial.[24,25] In one single-center study spanning 16 years, generalized tonic–clonic activity was observed in 11% of patients within 6 hours of presentation, and although it was associated with a higher incidence of in-hospital seizures and medical and neurologic complications, it did not have an effect on outcome at 3 months.[26] In another recent study, 13.8% of patients exhibited seizures after SAH, the occurrence of which was associated with poor clinical grade on presentation and greater hematoma burden.[27] Higher electrographic seizure burden on continuous electroencephalography (EEG) is independently associated with worse outcome in SAH,[26] and patients who have persistently altered mental status should be monitored with continuous EEG so that seizures can be detected and treated.

The controversy around seizures in the acute setting of SAH exists because of a desire to prevent this type of activity if it is a cause of rebleeding, which portends a poor outcome, on the one hand, and the desire to avoid the proven adverse effects associated with long-term prophylaxis with some antiepileptic medications, on the other hand. Recent studies and guidelines suggest that 3-day prophylaxis with phenytoin (or other antiepileptics) may be a reasonable approach, and antiepileptic medications should be stopped after the aneurysm is treated.[1,28] Epilepsy after SAH is discussed below.

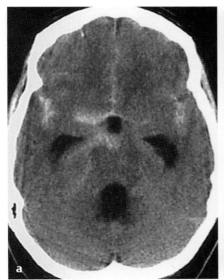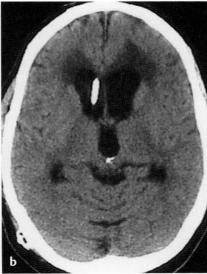

Fig. 10.11 Patient with subarachnoid hemorrhage (SAH) and severe hydrocephalus. **(a)** Diffuse SAH and ventriculomegaly; **(b)** ventriculostomy catheter in the right frontal horn.

Hydrocephalus

Hydrocephalus is reported in 15 to 20% of patients with SAH[29] and results from extravasated blood interfering with CSF circulation in the ventricles, sylvian aqueduct, or the basal cisterns. In the acute setting, hydrocephalus should be managed with emergent CSF diversion via ventriculostomy (or lumbar drainage in selected patients) whenever there is ventriculomegaly on the brain CT scan of a patient with altered mental status (▶Fig. 10.11). Ventriculostomy is a bedside procedure utilizing sterile technique and compact cranial access kits for twist drill or burr hole. Clinical improvement in 80% of the patients in whom ventriculostomy was performed has been reported.[30,31,32] External ventricular drainage allows diversion of CSF whenever ICP exceeds a certain level and may be performed continuously (by titrating the level of the drip chamber) or intermittently depending on ICP. In either case, overdrainage should be avoided because it may provoke aneurysmal rebleeding by rapid decompression of the aneurysmal transmural pressure.[11] Overdrainage may also precipitate slit ventricles and prevent further CSF drainage. Optimal ventricular drainage aims to keep ICP below 15 to 20 mm Hg. Chronic hydrocephalus after SAH is discussed below.

Intracranial Hypertension

Intracranial hypertension can be caused by several mechanisms in the acute post-SAH period, including hydrocephalus, global cerebral edema as a result of hypoxic–ischemic brain injury during transient cerebral circulatory arrest at ictus, as well as mass effect and edema associated with concomitant contusions or ICH or subdural hemorrhage. Hydrocephalus should be treated with CSF diversion as described above, whereas mass lesions such as subdural hemorrhage should be evaluated for operative treatment. Medical management of intracranial hypertension should be used emergently to stabilize patients before surgical

management, or chronically if no surgical options exist.[33] Emergent medical management involves facilitation of venous drainage through head positioning (30 degrees and midline), hyperventilation (10 rapid bagged breaths followed by adjustment of ventilator rate to achieve a partial pressure of carbon dioxide [pCO_2] of 25 to 35 mm Hg), and intravenous infusion of mannitol, 1 g/kg, or 23.4% saline if the patient has a central line (▶Fig. 10.12). Care should be taken not to hyperventilate to pCO_2 less than 25 mm Hg, as that may result in detrimental vasoconstriction and cerebral hypoperfusion. Further management of intracranial hypertension is described below.

Acute Cardiac Complications

Aneurysmal SAH has been associated with a variety of cardiac effects, including electrocardiographic changes (the so-called "cerebral T waves"), elevation of myocardial enzymes, ventricular wall motion abnormalities, and life-threatening arrhythmias.[34] A type of stress cardiomyopathy, so-called takotsubo cardiomyopathy because the shape of the heart as observed on echocardiography is similar to the shape of a Japanese pot of that name, has been described in association with SAH. Subendocardial ischemia, proportional to the severity of neurologic insult, and thus proportional to the amount of catecholamine release, may occur in some patients. Fortunately, these conditions do not alter the course of the illness in many patients, but they do require careful management during the acute phase and during the vasospasm period if they have not resolved by then. In contrast, in patients with preexisting cardiomyopathy or other systemic illnesses, these complications may become life-threatening. Echocardiography is useful in the diagnosis and follow-up of cardiac complications, but some patients may require invasive hemodynamic monitoring and interventions to augment cardiac function to prevent cerebral ischemia, especially in the vasospasm period.

Open the airway		
Position HOP at 30° and midline		
If EVD present drain 5 cc CSF		
Hyperventilate	10 rapid bagged breaths	
	Once intubated, set ventilator rate to pCO_2 goal 25-35mm Hg	
Hypertonic infusion	Mannitol, 1 g/kg IV, over 30 minutes (or 23.4% saline via central venous catheter)	
STAT head CT	If indicated, surgical treatment	
	Continued medical treatment	

Fig. 10.12 Emergent management of intracranial hypertension. CSF = cerebrospinal fluid; EVD = external ventricular drain; HOB = head of bed; pCO_2, partial pressure of carbon dioxide.

Acute Pulmonary Complications

Patients with SAH may develop pulmonary complications. Patients with poor neurologic grade are at increased risk of aspiration, atelectasis, pneumonia, or pulmonary edema.[35] Neurogenic pulmonary edema is a complication that may occur after a significant neurologic insult and consists of leakage of protein-rich fluid into the pulmonary alveoli. Neurogenic pulmonary edema is believed to be due to disruption of the endothelial barrier in response to massive sympathetic discharge. Cardiogenic pulmonary edema may be superimposed on neurogenic pulmonary edema in patients with stress cardiomyopathy.

Preexisting Medical Conditions

Patients with a myriad of associated medical conditions may sustain SAH. In general, management of SAH takes priority, and highly individualized management decisions are necessary in these complicated patients, weighing the advantages and disadvantages of every intervention with respect to the brain injury and medical condition. When possible, stabilization should be achieved for all non–life-threatening conditions while treatment of SAH is undertaken. Typically, the presence of other medical conditions increases the urgency of definitive treatment of SAH. In cases in which associated life-threatening medical problems preclude definitive treatment of SAH, supportive medical and neurologic measures are undertaken until such time as definitive therapy becomes advisable.

The management of a pregnant patient with SAH should take into consideration potential harm to the mother and fetus.[36] Often, the mother is treated urgently as if she were not pregnant, with the added specific precautions taken so as to protect the fetus and the pregnancy. In cases of SAH in the third trimester of pregnancy (and with a viable fetus), delivery managed by a high-risk obstetrics team as well as definitive management of the aneurysm should be undertaken.[37] Again, decisions are highly individualized according to the particular clinical scenario, including considerations of the condition of the mother, the fetus, the status of the pregnancy, and the difficulty of proposed

treatment of the cerebral aneurysm. Rebleeding and other sequelae of SAH account for a large number of maternal and fetal deaths, many of which would be preventable by careful and well-coordinated neurosurgical and obstetric care. Again, missed or delayed diagnosis can result in devastating consequences in many such cases.

Several legal and illegal drugs, usually stimulants, have been associated with SAH. Cocaine abuse in various forms is increasingly encountered in this setting.[38] Careful history taking in patients with SAH should screen for drug use, although denial is prevalent. Urgent drug screening on a urine sample should be obtained upon admission. Patients who hemorrhage following or during drug use are likely to harbor cerebral aneurysms, and this should be considered the most likely source of hemorrhage. Such patients are managed in an identical fashion to patients without drug use, but with added attention to potential drug overdose, withdrawal, associated medical complications from chronic drug use, and appropriate selection of antihypertensive medications for blood pressure control.

10.5.2 Management after Initial Stabilization

Rebleeding

Because the major cause of death in patients who survive an initial aneurysmal SAH is rebleeding, which may occur as early as 2 to 12 hours after presentation, SAH must be treated as a neurosurgical emergency.[11] It is standard practice to attempt to prevent rebleeding by controlling the blood pressure and treating the aneurysm rapidly. Prevention of even brief periods of hypertension is thought to be of importance in preventing rebleeding, and a systolic blood pressure goal of less than 160 mm Hg is generally accepted as reasonable.[1] The definitive treatment of vascular lesions in patients with SAH is discussed in a separate section below (see Definitive Treatment of Vascular Lesions Underlying Subarachnoid Hemorrhage). With respect to the timing of the intervention to treat the aneurysm, the literature supports early intervention to eliminate the aneurysm from the circulation, i.e., within the first 24[11] to 72[39] hours. Arterial dissection that has caused an SAH also mandates early therapeutic intervention, aimed typically at excluding the dissected segment from the circulation. If there is an inadvertent delay in the treatment of the vascular lesion, guidelines suggest the short-term use of antifibrinolytic agents (aminocaproic acid or tranexamic acid, neither of which is approved by the FDA for this indication) based on common practice at some of the centers.[1] These agents are associated with decreased rebleeding risk but may be associated with a higher incidence of delayed ischemia if used for more than 3 days.

Intracranial Hypertension

The cerebral perfusion pressure (CPP) is the pressure gradient responsible for cerebral blood flow, and its compromise results in cerebral ischemia. The CPP is defined as the difference between the mean arterial pressure (MAP) and the ICP. ICP monitoring, therefore, is used to guide CPP management whenever intracranial hypertension is suspected.[40] Elevated ICP is defined as exceeding 20 mm Hg for more than 5 minutes, and the typical ICP goal is less than 20 mm Hg, whereas the typical CPP goal is greater than 60 mm Hg. An ICP monitor should be considered in patients with GCS score of 8 or less or in those who cannot be followed with serial neurologic examinations. Intraparenchymal fiberoptic ICP monitors and intraventricular monitors are commonly used; the former is more accurate and less vulnerable to obstruction; the latter allows simultaneous drainage of CSF to treat elevated ICP.

Generally, intracranial hypertension can be treated by diverting CSF, facilitating venous outflow (thus decreasing blood volume), decreasing brain tissue volume, decreasing brain metabolic demand, improving blood rheology, or using hyperventilation (i.e., arterial vasoconstriction), thereby resulting in decreased cerebral blood flow and, consequently, arterial blood volume.[33] Head positioning, hyperventilation, intravenous mannitol or 23.4% infusion, and ventriculostomy were described above as part of emergent therapy for intracranial hypertension. If the patient requires continued management of intracranial hypertension after initial stabilization, the following approach is reasonable, although it is not informed by clinical trials, as there is a paucity of trial data on this topic.[41] First, temperature, seizures, and agitation should be controlled (to attenuate metabolic demand and, therefore, blood volume). If normothermia (36.5–37.5°C) and sedation/pain control using typical agents such as benzodiazepines and/or narcotics are insufficient, then hypothermia (temperature target 33.0–36.0°C) and induced coma (e.g., with pentobarbital drip) to attenuate metabolic demand are options. Induced coma should be monitored with continuous EEG, as no additional benefit will occur with increasing the drip rate once the EEG shows burst suppression, and virtually all such patients require central venous access for vasopressor therapy to maintain CPP. Hyperventilation is not a long-term option, as its use is complicated by tachyphylaxis, and care should be taken when restoring normocapnea, as the patient may be vulnerable to rebound intracranial hypertension.

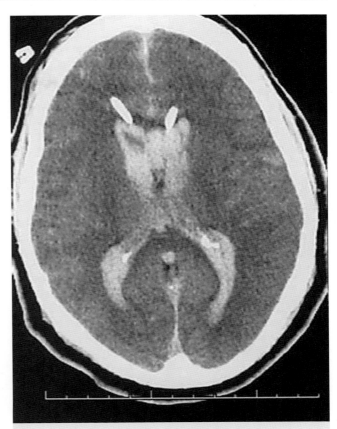

Fig. 10.13 Severe intraventricular hemorrhage from rupture of anterior communicating artery aneurysm. Note bilateral intraventricular catheters used to drain the ventricles pending endovascular treatment of the aneurysm. Subsequent clotting of the catheters required revision.

Hydrocephalus

Management of acute hydrocephalus during initial resuscitation was discussed above. Ventriculostomy may also be performed at surgery to enhance brain relaxation for access to the aneurysm and may be utilized in cases of unexplained decreased level of consciousness, regardless of ventricular size, to monitor and assist in ICP management.

Infection (ventriculitis) occurs in 5 to 20% of cases undergoing ventriculostomy and CSF drainage.[42] Risk factors for infection include duration of drainage for greater than 5 days, presence of intraventricular blood, open skull fracture, systemic infection, leak around ventriculostomy catheter, flushing of catheter, and prophylactic antibiotics. The risk of infection is minimized by optimizing sterile technique at catheter insertion, tunneling and carefully caring for the catheter exit site, and avoiding nonsterile breaches of the draining system. The use of prophylactic intravenous antibiotics is controversial, and practice varies among institutions, from intravenous use of antibiotic at ventricular drain insertion only; use of antibiotic-impregnated catheters; prophylactic administration of intravenous antibiotics for the duration of ventricular drainage; to a combination thereof. In some studies, the use of antibiotic-impregnated catheters decreases colonization and infection rates,[43] whereas long-term prophylactic systemic antibiotics may result in the growth of resistant organisms. Inflammation in the CSF can be monitored longitudinally by sampling CSF every few days, provided that the CSF sample is drawn in a sterile manner and system breaches are not too frequent, e.g., every 48 to 72 hours. CSF should be evaluated with the Gram stain, cell count, glucose level, protein level, and cultures. Ventriculostomy infections are treated by optimizing intravenous antibiotics based on culture results; changing the infected catheter if possible; or administering antibiotics through the catheter directly into the ventricles.[42]

Ventriculostomy catheters may clot and be ineffective in the setting of severe intraventricular hemorrhage. Even multiple catheters may clot rapidly and fail to prevent serious neurologic deterioration from casting of the ventricular system and associated elevated ICP (▶Fig. 10.13). Intraventricular thrombolysis is being investigated as a potential adjunct to clear the ventricular system of blood and enhance ventricular catheter patency and ICP control in selected patients. Intraventricular thrombolysis should not be used in the setting of untreated cerebral aneurysms or other vascular lesions for fear of precipitating aneurysmal rebleeding.

More than half of the patients who undergo ventriculostomy in the acute phase of SAH can be weaned from CSF drainage in the first 2 weeks after ictus. Weaning typically involves the gradual raising of the drainage threshold or intermittent clamping of the ventriculostomy catheter. Intermittent lumbar punctures can be used to aid the weaning process in selected patients who no longer exhibit ventricular system obstruction. Ventriculoperitoneal shunting, or the permanent implantation of a ventricular diversion system, is performed in patients who cannot be weaned from external ventricular drainage.[1]

Abnormalities of Sodium Homeostasis

Hyponatremia is common in patients with SAH.[35] It may result from two mechanisms: the syndrome of inappropriate antidiuretic hormone (SIADH) with free water retention and inappropriate natriuresis (also known as cerebral salt wasting) mediated by atrial natriuretic factor (ANF) and brain natriuretic peptide (BNP).[44,45] Determining the likely cause is important because the two syndromes are managed differently. Hyponatremia due to SIADH is more common after ICH than SAH and is treated with fluid restriction. Hyponatremia due to cerebral salt wasting is more common after SAH and is treated with volume and salt replacement. The distinction between the two syndromes is critical in aneurysmal SAH patients during the period of vulnerability to vasospasm, as patients can develop delayed cerebral ischemia in the setting fluid restriction. For this reason, daily fluid balance (intake vs. output), serum and urine sodium concentrations and osmolality, as well as serum uric acid should be monitored and the correct diagnosis made.

Spontaneous hypernatremia is rare after SAH: diabetes insipidus (DI) has been reported in patients with rupture of anterior communicating artery (ACOM) aneurysms.[46,47,48] DI should be treated with free water replacement and vasopressin.

Cerebral Vasospasm

Depending on the exact definition, cerebral vasospasm has been reported to affect 60 to 70% of patients after SAH. The vasospasm time window begins 3 to 5 days after the SAH and lasts for 2 to 3 weeks; the brain is vulnerable to ischemic insults during this time, and such insults negatively affect the neurologic outcome.[1] Vasospasm causes death in approximately one third of all SAH-associated deaths and serious disability from cerebral infarctions, termed delayed cerebral ischemia (DCI) or delayed ischemic neurologic deterioration (DIND), in another third of patients. Risk factors for vasospasm include the severity of SAH as assessed by clinical and radiographic grades. The breakdown products of subarachnoid blood are probably partly responsible for vasospasm in cerebral arteries following SAH.

Cerebral vasospasm is not the sole cause of poor outcome,[3] and several additional mechanisms of DCI have been postulated in recent years after studies showed that medical attenuation of vasospasm does not necessarily improve outcome.[49] To decrease the chance of poor outcome, nimodipine at 60 mg orally every 4 hours for 21 days should be started on the day of admission. Although nimodipine is a calcium channel blocker, it does not demonstrably relieve vasospasm when administered systemically; thus, its positive effects in SAH patients are likely to be due to other mechanisms, e.g., neuroprotection. Patients in the vasospasm period should be closely monitored for the development of symptoms, preferably in a neuroscience intensive care unit (ICU), and prompt treatment should be instituted, as described below. Any neurologic deterioration in the vulnerable period after SAH is presumed due to ischemic sequelae of vasospasm unless proven otherwise and attributed to other causes.

Vasospasm Monitoring

The diagnosis of symptomatic vasospasm is supported by clinical suspicion and specific evidence. Clinical suspicion that the cause of neurologic deterioration in the vasospasm period is symptomatic vasospasm should be high, and patients should be cared for by specialized ICU teams with experience in the management of this condition. Neurologic examinations should be followed frequently, e.g., hourly, during the vulnerable period. Symptomatic vasospasm can manifest as a global decrease in mentation or focal deficits. Focal deficits may result from spasm of proximal arteries most invested with extravasated blood; thus, possible clinical syndromes are highly predictable and facilitate prompt diagnosis in many cases. In addition to the neurologic examination, many centers use noninvasive means of monitoring for the development of sonographic vasospasm, i.e., daily transcranial Doppler sonography (TCD) (▶Fig. 10.14). This noninvasive bedside procedure has good sensitivity and specificity for vasospasm but requires technical expertise and experience and good acoustic windows.[49] The course of sonographic vasospasm correlates closely with the course and clinical sequelae of vasospasm detected on angiography, and its severity closely reflects clinical sequelae of brain ischemia. Emergent noninvasive vascular imaging with CT or MR angiography along with perfusion sequences may be used in selected patients in whom the clinical syndrome is ambiguous or TCD findings are nonconcordant with the clinical status of the patient. The gold standard, conventional angiography, has been largely replaced by noninvasive

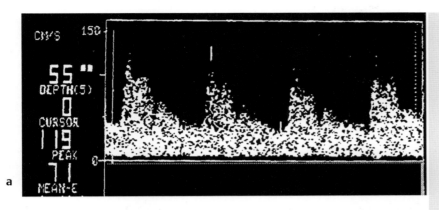
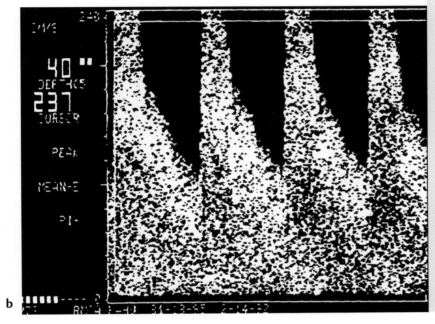

Fig. 10.14 Transcranial Doppler (TCD) insonation of intracranial artery. (a) Normal tracing with mean velocity below 100 cm/s and peak systolic velocity below 140 cm/s. (b) Severe vasospasm tracing with mean velocity exceeding 150 cm/s and peak systolic velocity exceeding 240 cm/s.

tests for the diagnosis of vasospasm, as it is associated with risk of stroke and groin complications, but it is the study of choice if endovascular therapy for vasospasm is being contemplated, as discussed below.

Vasospasm Prophylaxis

Management of patients during the time period of vulnerability to symptomatic vasospasm includes pharmacologic therapy, maintenance of euvolemia, and permissive hypertension.[50] Nimodipine, 60 mg orally or by nasogastric tube, administered every 4 hours for 21 days after SAH, has been shown to significantly decrease the prevalence and clinical sequelae of symptomatic vasospasm, although it does not prevent vasospasm per se, as discussed above.

Intravascular volume and blood pressure need to be judiciously maintained during the period of vulnerability to vasospasm, commencing as early as 2 to 3 days after SAH, as dehydration and hypotension can precipitate cerebral infarction. By then, the risk of aneurysm rebleeding ought to have been eliminated by surgery or endovascular treatment, and blood pressure is usually allowed to be elevated (permissive hypertension) as

antihypertensive medications are held. If nimodipine is found to lower the blood pressure, dosing can be changed to 30 mg every 2 hours or the drug can be held.

As with any patient with brain injury, SAH patients in the "vasospasm watch" period should be managed according to neuroprotective and critical care principles: the blood glucose and body temperature should be monitored and maintained in the normal range; enteral nutrition should be provided; and complications including deep venous thrombosis, infections, and decubitus ulcers should be treated with preventative maneuvers and diagnosed and treated rapidly if they occur.[3]

Medical Management of Symptomatic Vasospasm

Frequently, patients initially manifesting symptomatic vasospasm will develop mental status changes, hyponatremia (from cerebral salt wasting), and fever. Symptomatic vasospasm is managed with so-called Triple H therapy (hypertension, hypervolemia, hemodilution), although the details of the TripleHs vary among institutions.[51] In selected cases, endovascular therapy is utilized, as discussed below.

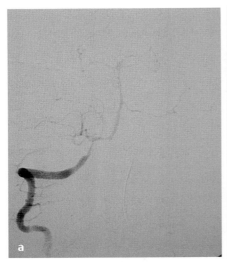
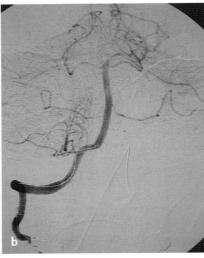

Fig. 10.15 Angiograms of severe basilar artery vasospasm. **(a)** Before and **(b)** after balloon angioplasty.

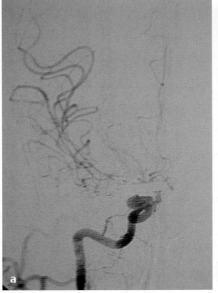
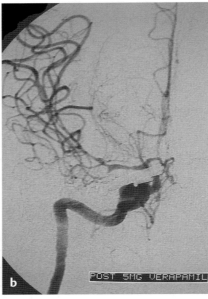

Fig. 10.16 Angiograms of severe middle cerebral artery vasospasm. **(a)** Before and **(b)** after intra-arterial verapamil infusion.

Cerebral salt wasting associated with vasospasm is treated with salt and volume administration, frequently in the form of hypertonic saline. If saline concentrations of 3% or greater are used, the patient requires central venous access. Fever is treated with antipyretic medications and cooling; and even if the etiology of fever is most likely vasospasm, potential sources of infections are diligently sought.

Although the traditional medical management approach includes hemodilution, this component is no longer actively targeted during therapy, as the appropriate degree of hemodilution was unknown and, furthermore, hemodilution could also be harmful by reducing the oxygen carrying capacity of blood.[52] Current practice maintains hemoglobin concentrations between 8 and 10 g/dL.

The hypertension component may be either permissive or induced with vasopressors (typically phenylephrine or norepinephrine), and the blood pressure should be titrated to neurologic symptoms.[53,54] Obviously, central venous access is required for this therapy. In some patients in whom endovascular therapy is not an option, very high blood pressures (in excess of 180 mm Hg) may be necessary to prevent infarction. This aggressive approach is appropriate even in the setting of other unruptured aneurysms or cardiomyopathy, as cerebral infarctions have a vastly greater negative effect on the ultimate functional outcome than complications of hypertensive therapy. The approach needs to be stopped, however, if the patient demonstrates systemic adverse effects such as myocardial infarction, pulmonary congestion, or acute kidney injury.

The hypervolemia component of Triple H usually requires the placement of a central venous line for central venous pressure (CVP) monitoring (targeting CVP > 8 mm Hg), but medically complicated patients may require other monitoring devices, including cardiac output monitors, which include several noninvasive instruments as well as all pulmonary artery catheters. Transthoracic echocardiography is also a useful adjunctive test in this setting. Some studies have recently suggested caution when employing hypervolemia, as the benefit–risk calculation

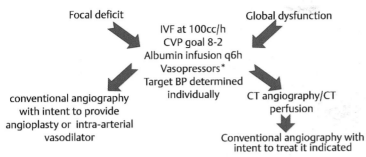

Focal deficit

Global dysfunction

IVF at 100cc/h
CVP goal 8-2
Albumin infusion q6h
Vasopressors*
Target BP determined
individually

conventional angiography
with intent to provide
angioplasty or intra-arterial
vasodilator

CT angiography/CT
perfusion

Conventional angiography with
intent to treat it indicated

*Sequential escalation after approximately 1 hour of observation
(repeated neurological evaluation) at each step, but may elect to do
endovascular treatment early

Endpoints clinical improvment or development of systemic complications
from therapy

Fig. 10.17 An algorithm for the management of symptomatic cerebral vasospasm. CT = computed tomography; CVP = central venous pressure; IVF = intravenous fluids ; BP, blood pressure.

may be less favorable than previously thought.[55] Medical augmentation of intravascular volume with fludrocortisone[56] and/or intermittent albumin infusions, e.g., 12.5 to 25 g of 25% human albumin every 6 hours, in addition to hypertonic saline are also sometimes utilized.[57]

Endovascular Management of Symptomatic Vasospasm

Selected patients with symptomatic vasospasm may be candidates for endovascular treatment.[58] Endovascular treatment of spasm consists of balloon angioplasty (▶Fig. 10.15), best used for very proximal spasm, or intra-arterial vasodilator infusions (▶Fig. 10.16), best used for distal branch vasospasm. Angioplasty is associated with greater risk of arterial rupture or dissection, especially if applied to more distal vessels, but its effect is more durable than intra-arterial pharmacologic infusions. The latter may need to be repeated several times, guided by the examination and imaging.

Selection of candidates for endovascular treatment is of great importance, but the precise threshold for endovascular intervention remains controversial, with some centers advocating early and frequent endovascular treatment of vasospasm, while other centers reserving endovascular intervention for cases where symptomatic vasospasm does not respond to medical therapy. An example of an algorithm for the management of symptomatic vasospasm is illustrated in ▶Fig. 10.17.

In summary, with aggressive monitoring, prophylaxis, and medical and endovascular therapy, morbidity from vasospasm can be minimized.

Epilepsy

Epilepsy following SAH has been variably reported as occurring in 1 to 25% of patients. A recent large population-based study in Finland that included long-term follow-up showed that the rate was 12% at 5 years.[59] Intracerebral hemorrhage was associated with higher risk of post-SAH epilepsy. Patient-specific factors should be taken into account when selecting anti-epileptic

medications, and follow-up with an epileptologist is recommended after hospital discharge.

10.6 Definitive Treatment of Vascular Lesions Underlying Subarachnoid Hemorrhage

Guidelines suggest that the decision on the type of definitive treatment should be made based on a multidisciplinary discussion among surgeons, endovascular specialists, and critical care providers, taking into account aneurysm-specific characteristics, including the location and morphology, and the clinical condition of the patient.[1] To date, there have been three prospective randomized trials comparing endovascular coiling and surgical clipping (the Kuopio study; the International Subarachnoid Aneurysm Trial [ISAT]; and the Barrow Ruptured Aneurysm Trial [BRAT]).[60]

10.6.1 Endovascular Treatment

The ISAT is the only multicenter prospective randomized trial that compares endovascular coiling to surgical treatment in 2,143 ruptured aneurysms that were deemed equally suitable for surgical clipping and endovascular coiling. This study concluded that coiling, compared with surgical treatment, was significantly more likely to result in survival free of disability 1 year after SAH.[61] The durability of the mortality effect (lower mortality with coiling), but not dependency, was sustained at 10 years of follow-up.[62] Of note, epilepsy was less common and cognitive outcomes were better in patients treated with endovascular coiling than patients treated with surgical clipping.[63,64] Recent guidelines suggest endovascular treatment for aneurysms that are thought to be treatable with either modality.[1]

One of the critiques of the ISAT was that its results may not be generalizable because less than 25% of eligible patients (1–40% at the various centers) were randomized. In part to address this criticism, the BRAT was designed as a single-center prospective randomized trial in which all patients with nontraumatic SAH were enrolled and treated either with clipping or coiling if an aneurysm was found. The group recently published their 6-year follow-up results in 408 patients that suggested that clipping and coiling resulted in similar outcomes for patients with anterior circulation aneurysms, whereas coiling produced more favorable outcomes for patients with posterior circulation aneurysms.[65] Of note, the trial is underpowered to detect small differences.

Aneurysms are more likely to rebleed after coiling than surgery and may require re-treatment. In the ISAT long-term follow-up, rebleeding was more frequent in the coiled group, but the risk was low and did not negate the mortality effect.[62] In summary, although coiling may be favored in certain cohorts (e.g., those represented in the ISAT; in aneurysms at certain locations, such as the basilar summit; and in older or sicker patients), some argue that there is no evidence that the introduction of coiling has improved overall outcome of aneurysm treatment at large neurovascular centers,[66] especially when taking into account long-term follow-up.[67]

Other endovascular interventions have an important role in the management of SAH. Parent vessel occlusion, performed with endovascular coils or glue, can be used for occlusion of distal vessels harboring aneurysm, as in mycotic and traumatic aneurysms, and aneurysms on feeding vessels of arteriovenous malformations (AVMs). Proximal parent vessel occlusion, using endovascular balloons or coils, is performed in cases of ruptured fusiform aneurysms or dissection.[68] This is preceded by balloon test occlusion under full anticoagulation and clinical monitoring and is often deferred until a patient is stabilized and awakened to tolerate test occlusion, and also until vasospasm has subsided, as occlusion of a major artery poses a significant ischemic risk during vasospasm.

Additional endovascular treatment options include stent and balloon–assisted coiling of aneurysms with broad necks.[69] Flow-diverting stents are being utilized for anatomically complex aneurysms (including ones with wide necks, fusiform shape, or associated branch arteries) that are not amenable to other treatments, and additional indications for the use of the technique are being proposed.[70]

Endovascular adjuncts, including proximal control, suction decompression, and intraoperative angiography, have greatly enhanced surgical treatment of certain aneurysms such as giant lesions and those at paraclinoid locations.[71] Endovascular coiling may be used in cases where surgery has failed completely to clip an aneurysm and the residual neck is narrow.

10.6.2 Surgical Treatment

In many cases, the definitive method for exclusion of an aneurysm and prevention of rebleeding remains surgical clipping.[72] Surgery is not favored if the patient is unstable or has a poor medical condition that puts him or her at great risk for general anesthesia and open surgery, or in a setting of intractable elevated ICP; also, as discussed above, endovascular coiling should be used instead in patients resembling those enrolled in the ISAT.

Surgery is indicated emergently for cerebral aneurysm whenever there is an associated intracerebral hematoma causing or threatening herniation syndrome, as is common with middle cerebral artery aneurysms associated with temporal clots and

anterior communicating or carotid aneurysms with deep frontal clots. If surgery for hematoma evacuation and aneurysm clipping is performed emergently, conventional angiography is not necessary, as CT angiography is usually sufficient to demonstrate the aneurysm or vascular malformation and will often preclude unexpected findings on surgery, such as a more complex lesion than anticipated. An aneurysm should always be sought and clipped at the time of hematoma evacuation, but an AVM does not always require excision in the same setting unless the patient is stable and the lesion is simple and well defined. Intraoperative or immediate postoperative angiography may be considered if there is any question about adequacy of treatment of an aneurysm, especially if a conventional angiogram was not performed preoperatively.

10.6.3 Complications of Therapy

A range of potential complications is associated with endovascular or surgical therapy. Aneurysm rupture may occur during attempted coiling or surgical clipping. Intraprocedural rupture is typically handled with emergent technical maneuvers, but it may result in untoward sequelae. Coils or clips may compromise parent vessels, parent vessel branches, or perforating vessels, and thromboembolism may occur during endovascular or surgical manipulation of blood vessels—all causing a spectrum of ischemic complications. These complications may be prevented by judicious anticoagulation during endovascular interventions, and by verification of vessel patency by micro-Doppler insonation or intraoperative angiography. Complications are treated according to the specific clinical scenario, as with interventions for brain ischemia discussed elsewhere in this text.

10.7 Conclusion

Subarachnoid hemorrhage continues to be associated with significant morbidity and mortality despite great improvements in management over the years. Despite affecting patients in the middle years of their lives, often without other preexisting or associated diseases, it is estimated that 30 to 40% of all SAH patients will die as a result of SAH. A common cause of death is neurologic injury from the initial hemorrhage, with 10 to 15% of patients estimated to die before reaching a medical facility. Many survivors are left with persistent physical, cognitive, behavioral, and emotional changes that affect their day-to-day lives.

The most common predictor of death or major disability after SAH is the patient's clinical condition at presentation.[1] Age, medical morbidities, severity of hemorrhage on CT, and aneurysm type (giant or posterior circulation) are also correlated with poor outcome. Other patients initially in good condition may deteriorate in the setting of misdiagnosis, from rebleeding, as a result of therapeutic complications, or from vasospasm or other medical or neurologic sequelae of the disease.

Much of what is discussed in this chapter and elsewhere in this book, as it bears on ongoing advances in surgical and endovascular therapy and critical care, will further reduce mortality and morbidity from SAH. Those who survive will likely benefit from early rehabilitation.[73] Some studies showed an improvement in the functional independence measure (FIM) after an inpatient rehabilitation stay.[73,74] The quality of life of those who recover with minimal disability may still be impaired by cognitive, psychologic, and emotional sequelae. Recognition and intervention for these higher-functional deficits may further improve the quality of life of patients afflicted by this disease.[75]

The clinical outcome after SAH cannot be addressed at a single point in time, without regard to whether an aneurysm has been treated effectively. It is essential to note whether an aneurysm may still pose risk of future rupture and what additional follow-up and re-treatment may be indicated. It is essential that these questions of long-term durability of treatment, and the impact on quality of life and future risks, be considered when addressing the relative benefits of endovascular versus surgical interventions.

10.8 Future Directions

10.8.1 Endovascular Treatment of Aneurysms

Although the annual risk of rebleeding from partially coiled or recurrent aneurysms appears to be low in the ISAT, the rate of recanalization following endovascular aneurysm management remains a concern for treatment durability, especially in the real-world clinical practice. The endovascular field is witnessing major improvements and advances in aneurysm treatment.[58] For example, several modifications of bare platinum coils have been developed with the goal of facilitating the formation of thrombus within the aneurysm, thus reducing risk of recanalization. The Matrix coil (Siemens Healthineers) involves a platinum coil with an outer coating of a bioabsorbable polymeric material that has been shown in swine aneurysm models to accelerate aneurysm fibrosis and neointima formation, with increased neck tissue thickness but no parent artery stenosis, and has now been trialed in clinical trials.[76] A different bioactive coil technology, the Hydrocoil Embolic System (MicroVention), consists of a platinum coil coated with a polymer that "swells" upon contact with blood, increasing coil volume by 3- to 9-fold, but the clinical efficacy of these coils remains to be seen.[77] The future of bioactive endovascular technology will likely involve delivery of growth factors, gene therapies, or cellular substrates within the aneurysm that will regenerate an endothelial wall layer across the aneurysm neck.[78]

10.8.2 Vasospasm Management

A variety of calcium channel antagonists and other vasodilators have been studied via intrathecal, cisternal, and intra-arterial delivery,[58] but these approaches require further clinical validation. Future therapies for vasospasm will likely be aimed at improved delivery systems and development of biological agents that target the numerous cellular substrates responsible for vasospasm. However, one of the most important recent discoveries in vasospasm clinical trials was that medically reducing vasospasm does not necessarily translate to improved outcome.[79] Thus, it is likely that one direction in future studies will address mechanisms of poor outcome in aneurysmal SAH other than vasospasm.

References

[1] Connolly ES, Jr, Rabinstein AA, Carhuapoma JR, et al; American Heart Association Stroke Council. Council on Cardiovascular Radiology and Intervention. Council on Cardiovascular Nursing. Council on Cardiovascular Surgery and Anesthesia. Council on Clinical Cardiology. Guidelines for the management of aneurysmal subarachnoid hemorrhage: a guideline for healthcare professionals from the American Heart Association/American Stroke Association. Stroke. 2012; 43(6):1711–1737

[2] Vermeulen MJ, Schull MJ. Missed diagnosis of subarachnoid hemorrhage in the emergency department. Stroke. 2007; 38(4):1216–1221

[3] Raya AK, Diringer MN. Treatment of subarachnoid hemorrhage. Crit Care Clin. 2014; 30(4):719–733

[4] Edlow JA. Diagnosis of subarachnoid hemorrhage. Neurocrit Care. 2005; 2(2):99–109

[5] Agostoni E, Zagaria M, Longoni M. Headache in subarachnoid hemorrhage and headache attributed to intracranial endovascular procedures. Neurol Sci. 2015; 36(Suppl 1):67–70

[6] Beck J, Raabe A, Szelenyi A, et al. Sentinel headache and the risk of rebleeding after aneurysmal subarachnoid hemorrhage. Stroke. 2006; 37(11):2733–2737

[7] Report of World Federation of Neurological Surgeons Committee on a Universal Subarachnoid Hemorrhage Grading Scale. J Neurosurg. 1988; 68(6):985–986

[8] Hunt WE, Hess RM. Surgical risk as related to time of intervention in the repair of intracranial aneurysms. J Neurosurg. 1968; 28(1):14–20

[9] Chiang VL, Claus EB, Awad IA. Toward more rational prediction of outcome in patients with high-grade subarachnoid hemorrhage. Neurosurgery. 2000; 46(1):28–35, discussion 35–36

[10] Yoshikai S, Nagata S, Ohara S, Yuhi F, Sakata S, Matsuno H. [A retrospective analysis of the outcomes of patients with aneurysmal subarachnoid hemorrhages: a focus on the prognostic factors] No Shinkei Geka. 1996; 24(8):733–738

[11] van Donkelaar CE, Bakker NA, Veeger NJ, et al. Predictive factors for rebleeding after aneurysmal subarachnoid hemorrhage: rebleeding aneurysmal subarachnoid hemorrhage study. Stroke. 2015; 46(8):2100–2106

[12] Boesiger BM, Shiber JR. Subarachnoid hemorrhage diagnosis by computed tomography and lumbar puncture: are fifth generation CT scanners better at identifying subarachnoid hemorrhage? J Emerg Med. 2005; 29(1):23–27

[13] Szklener S, Melges A, Korchut A, et al. Predictive model for patients with poor-grade subarachnoid haemorrhage in 30-day observation: a 9-year cohort study. BMJ Open. 2015; 5(6):e007795

[14] Fink KR, Benjert JL. Imaging of nontraumatic neuroradiology emergencies. Radiol Clin North Am. 2015; 53(4):871–890, x

[15] Blok KM, Rinkel GJ, Majoie CB, et al. CT within 6 hours of headache onset to rule out subarachnoid hemorrhage in nonacademic hospitals. Neurology. 2015; 84(19):1927–1932

[16] Wiebers DO, Whisnant JP, Sundt TM, Jr, O'Fallon WM. The significance of unruptured intracranial saccular aneurysms. J Neurosurg. 1987; 66(1):23–29

[17] Wills S, Ronkainen A, van der Voet M, et al. Familial intracranial aneurysms: an analysis of 346 multiplex Finnish families. Stroke. 2003; 34(6):1370–1374

[18] Forget TR, Jr, Benitez R, Veznedaroglu E, et al. A review of size and location of ruptured intracranial aneurysms. Neurosurgery. 2001; 49(6):1322–1325, discussion 1325–1326

[19] Wiebers DO, Whisnant JP, Huston J, III, et al; International Study of Unruptured Intracranial Aneurysms Investigators. Unruptured intracranial aneurysms: natural history, clinical outcome, and risks of surgical and endovascular treatment. Lancet. 2003; 362(9378):103–110

[20] Kapadia A, Schweizer TA, Spears J, Cusimano M, Macdonald RL. Nonaneurysmal perimesencephalic subarachnoid hemorrhage: diagnosis, pathophysiology, clinical characteristics, and long-term outcome. World Neurosurg. 2014; 82(6):1131–1143

[21] Zoerle T, Lombardo A, Colombo A, et al. Intracranial pressure after subarachnoid hemorrhage. Crit Care Med. 2015; 43(1):168–176

[22] Pollack CV, Jr, Reilly PA, Eikelboom J, et al. Idarucizumab for dabigatran reversal. N Engl J Med. 2015; 373(6):511–520

[23] Lippi G, Sanchis-Gomar F, Favaloro EJ. Andexanet: effectively reversing anticoagulation. Trends Pharmacol Sci. 2016; 37(6):413–414

[24] Dewan MC, Mocco J. Current practice regarding seizure prophylaxis in aneurysmal subarachnoid hemorrhage across academic centers. J Neurointerv Surg. 2015; 7(2):146–149

[25] Raper DM, Starke RM, Komotar RJ, Allan R, Connolly ES, Jr. Seizures after aneurysmal subarachnoid hemorrhage: a systematic review of outcomes. World Neurosurg. 2013; 79(5–6):682–690

[26] De Marchis GM, Pugin D, Lantigua H, et al. Tonic-clonic activity at subarachnoid hemorrhage onset: impact on complications and outcome. PLoS ONE. 2013; 8(8):e71405

[27] Ibrahim GM, Fallah A, Macdonald RL. Clinical, laboratory, and radiographic predictors of the occurrence of seizures following aneurysmal subarachnoid hemorrhage. J Neurosurg. 2013; 119(2):347–352

[28] Chumnanvej S, Dunn IF, Kim DH. Three-day phenytoin prophylaxis is adequate after subarachnoid hemorrhage. Neurosurgery. 2007; 60(1):99–102, discussion 102–103

[29] Graff-Radford NR, Torner J, Adams HP, Jr, Kassell NF. Factors associated with hydrocephalus after subarachnoid hemorrhage. A report of the Cooperative Aneurysm Study. Arch Neurol. 1989; 46(7):744–752

[30] Hasan D, Vermeulen M, Wijdicks EF, Hijdra A, van Gijn J. Management problems in acute hydrocephalus after subarachnoid hemorrhage. Stroke. 1989; 20(6):747–753

[31] Roitberg BZ, Khan N, Alp MS, Hersonskey T, Charbel FT, Ausman JI. Bedside external ventricular drain placement for the treatment of acute hydrocephalus. Br J Neurosurg. 2001; 15(4):324–327

[32] Steinke D, Weir B, Disney L. Hydrocephalus following aneurysmal subarachnoid haemorrhage. Neurol Res. 1987; 9(1):3–9

[33] Ropper AH. Management of raised intracranial pressure and hyperosmolar therapy. Pract Neurol. 2014; 14(3):152–158

[34] Wybraniec MT, Mizia-Stec K, Krzych Ł. Neurocardiogenic injury in subarachnoid hemorrhage: a wide spectrum of catecholamine-mediated brain-heart interactions. Cardiol J. 2014; 21(3):220–228

[35] Wartenberg KE, Mayer SA. Medical complications after subarachnoid hemorrhage: new strategies for prevention and management. Curr Opin Crit Care. 2006; 12(2):78–84

[36] Kataoka H, Miyoshi T, Neki R, Yoshimatsu J, Ishibashi-Ueda H, Iihara K. Subarachnoid hemorrhage from intracranial aneurysms during pregnancy and the puerperium. Neurol Med Chir (Tokyo). 2013; 53(8):549–554

[37] Robba C, Bacigaluppi S, Bragazzi NL, et al. Aneurysmal subarachnoid hemorrhage in pregnancy—case series, review and pooled data analysis. World Neurosurg. 2016; 88:383–398

[38] Murthy SB, Moradiya Y, Shah S, Naval NS. In-hospital outcomes of aneurysmal subarachnoid hemorrhage associated with cocaine use in the USA. J Clin Neurosci. 2014; 21(12):2088–2091

[39] Oudshoorn SC, Rinkel GJ, Molyneux AJ, et al. Aneurysm treatment <24 versus 24–72 h after subarachnoid hemorrhage. Neurocrit Care. 2014; 21(1):4–13

[40] Perez-Barcena J, Llompart-Pou JA, O'Phelan KH. Intracranial pressure monitoring and management of intracranial hypertension. Crit Care Clin. 2014; 30(4):735–750

[41] Mak CH, Lu YY, Wong GK. Review and recommendations on management of refractory raised intracranial pressure in aneurysmal subarachnoid hemorrhage. Vasc Health Risk Manag. 2013; 9:353–359

[42] Humphreys H, Jenks PJ. Surveillance and management of ventriculitis following neurosurgery. J Hosp Infect. 2015; 89(4):281–286

[43] Zabramski JM, Whiting D, Darouiche RO, et al. Efficacy of antimicrobial-impregnated external ventricular drain catheters: a prospective, randomized, controlled trial. J Neurosurg. 2003; 98(4):725–730

[44] Hannon MJ, Behan LA, O'Brien MM, et al. Hyponatremia following mild/moderate subarachnoid hemorrhage is due to SIAD and glucocorticoid deficiency and not cerebral salt wasting. J Clin Endocrinol Metab. 2014; 99(1):291–298

[45] Hannon MJ, Thompson CJ. Neurosurgical hyponatremia. J Clin Med. 2014; 3(4):1084–1104

[46] McMahon AJ. Diabetes insipidus developing after subarachnoid haemorrhage from an anterior communicating artery aneurysm. Scott Med J. 1988; 33(1):208–209

[47] Nguyen BN, Yablon SA, Chen CY. Hypodipsic hypernatremia and diabetes insipidus following anterior communicating artery aneurysm clipping: diagnostic and therapeutic challenges in the amnestic rehabilitation patient. Brain Inj. 2001; 15(11):975–980

[48] Savin IA, Popugaev KA, Oshorov AV, et al. [Diabetes insipidus in acute subarachnoidal hemorrhage after clipping of aneurysm of the anterior cerebral artery and the anterior communicating artery] Anesteziol Reanimatol. 2007 ; Mar-Apr(2):56–59

[49] Lee Y, Zuckerman SL, Mocco J. Current controversies in the prediction, diagnosis, and management of cerebral vasospasm: where do we stand? Neurol Res Int. 2013; 2013:373458

[50] Dusick JR, Gonzalez NR. Management of arterial vasospasm following aneurysmal subarachnoid hemorrhage. Semin Neurol. 2013; 33(5):488–497

[51] Meyer R, Deem S, Yanez ND, Souter M, Lam A, Treggiari MM. Current practices of triple-H prophylaxis and therapy in patients with subarachnoid hemorrhage. Neurocrit Care. 2011; 14(1):24–36

[52] Chittiboina P, Conrad S, McCarthy P, Nanda A, Guthikonda B. The evolving role of hemodilution in treatment of cerebral vasospasm: a historical perspective. World Neurosurg. 2011; 75(5–6):660–664

[53] Dankbaar JW, Slooter AJ, Rinkel GJ, Schaaf IC. Effect of different components of triple-H therapy on cerebral perfusion in patients with aneurysmal subarachnoid haemorrhage: a systematic review. Crit Care. 2010; 14(1):R23

[54] Treggiari MM; Participants in the International Multi-disciplinary Consensus Conference on the Critical Care Management of Subarachnoid Hemorrhage. Hemodynamic management of subarachnoid hemorrhage. Neurocrit Care. 2011; 15(2):329–335

[55] Muench E, Horn P, Bauhuf C, et al. Effects of hypervolemia and hypertension on regional cerebral blood flow, intracranial pressure, and brain tissue oxygenation after subarachnoid hemorrhage. Crit Care Med. 2007; 35(8):1844–1851, quiz 1852

[56] Nakagawa I, Hironaka Y, Nishimura F, et al. Early inhibition of natriuresis suppresses symptomatic cerebral vasospasm in patients with aneurysmal subarachnoid hemorrhage. Cerebrovasc Dis. 2013; 35(2):131–137

[57] Suarez JI, Martin RH, Calvillo E, Bershad EM, Venkatasubba Rao CP. Effect of human albumin on TCD vasospasm, DCI, and cerebral infarction in subarachnoid hemorrhage: the ALISAH study. Acta Neurochir Suppl (Wien). 2015; 120:287–290

[58] Dabus G, Nogueira RG. Current options for the management of aneurysmal subarachnoid hemorrhage-induced cerebral vasospasm: a comprehensive review of the literature. Interv Neurol. 2013; 2(1):30–51

[59] Huttunen J, Kurki MI, von Und Zu Fraunberg M, et al. Epilepsy after aneurysmal subarachnoid hemorrhage: a population-based, long-term follow-up study. Neurology. 2015; 84(22):2229–2237

[60] Sorenson T, Lanzino G. Trials and tribulations: an evidence-based approach to aneurysm treatment. J Neurosurg Sci. 2016; 60(1):22–26

[61] Molyneux A, Kerr R, Stratton I, et al; International Subarachnoid Aneurysm Trial (ISAT) Collaborative Group. International Subarachnoid Aneurysm Trial (ISAT) of neurosurgical clipping versus endovascular coiling in 2143 patients with ruptured intracranial aneurysms: a randomized trial. J Stroke Cerebrovasc Dis. 2002; 11(6):304–314

[62] Molyneux AJ, Birks J, Clarke A, Sneade M, Kerr RS. The durability of endovascular coiling versus neurosurgical clipping of ruptured cerebral aneurysms: 18 year follow-up of the UK cohort of the International Subarachnoid Aneurysm Trial (ISAT). Lancet. 2015; 385(9969):691–697

[63] Hart Y, Sneade M, Birks J, Rischmiller J, Kerr R, Molyneux A. Epilepsy after subarachnoid hemorrhage: the frequency of seizures after clip occlusion or coil embolization of a ruptured cerebral aneurysm: results from the International Subarachnoid Aneurysm Trial. J Neurosurg. 2011; 115(6):1159–1168

[64] Scott RB, Eccles F, Molyneux AJ, Kerr RS, Rothwell PM, Carpenter K. Improved cognitive outcomes with endovascular coiling of ruptured intracranial aneurysms: neuropsychological outcomes from the International Subarachnoid Aneurysm Trial (ISAT). Stroke. 2010; 41(8):1743–1747

[65] Spetzler RF, McDougall CG, Zabramski JM, et al. The Barrow Ruptured Aneurysm Trial: 6-year results. J Neurosurg. 2015; 123(3):609–617

[66] Sturaitis MK, Rinne J, Chaloupka JC, Kaynar M, Lin Z, Awad IA. Impact of Guglielmi detachable coils on outcomes of patients with intracranial aneurysms treated by a multidisciplinary team at a single institution. J Neurosurg. 2000; 93(4):569–580

[67] Raper DM, Allan R. International subarachnoid trial in the long run: critical evaluation of the long-term follow-up data from the ISAT trial of clipping vs coiling for ruptured intracranial aneurysms. Neurosurgery. 2010; 66(6):1166–1169, discussion 1169

[68] Lee S, Huddle D, Awad IA. Which aneurysms should be referred for endovascular therapy? Clin Neurosurg. 2000; 47:188–220

[69] Jabbour P, Koebbe C, Veznedaroglu E, Benitez RP, Rosenwasser R. Stent-assisted coil placement for unruptured cerebral aneurysms. Neurosurg Focus. 2004; 17(5):E10

[70] Dabus G, Grossberg JA, Cawley CM, et al. Treatment of complex anterior cerebral artery aneurysms with Pipeline flow diversion: mid-term results. J Neurointerv Surg. 2016:neurintsurg-2016-012519

[71] Ng PY, Huddle D, Gunel M, Awad IA. Intraoperative endovascular treatment as an adjunct to microsurgical clipping of paraclinoid aneurysms. J Neurosurg. 2000; 93(4):554–560

[72] Abdulrauf SI, Furlan AJ, Awad I. Primary intracerebral hemorrhage and subarachnoid hemorrhage. J Stroke Cerebrovasc Dis. 1999; 8(3):146–150

[73] Saciri BM, Kos N. Aneurysmal subarachnoid haemorrhage: outcomes of early rehabilitation after surgical repair of ruptured intracranial aneurysms. J Neurol Neurosurg Psychiatry. 2002; 72(3):334–337

[74] O'Dell MW, Watanabe TK, De Roos ST, Kager C. Functional outcome after inpatient rehabilitation in persons with subarachnoid hemorrhage. Arch Phys Med Rehabil. 2002; 83(5):678–682

[75] Passier PE, Visser-Meily JM, Rinkel GJ, Lindeman E, Post MW. Determinants of health-related quality of life after aneurysmal subarachnoid hemorrhage: a systematic review. Qual Life Res. 2013; 22(5):1027–1043

[76] Ansari SA, Dueweke EJ, Kanaan Y, et al. Embolization of intracranial aneurysms with second-generation Matrix-2 detachable coils: mid-term and long-term results. J Neurointerv Surg. 2011; 3(4):324–330

[77] Poncyljusz W, Zarzycki A, Zwarzany Ł, Burke TH. Bare platinum coils vs. HydroCoil in the treatment of unruptured intracranial aneurysms—a single center randomized controlled study. Eur J Radiol. 2015; 84(2):261–265

[78] Lanzino G, Kanaan Y, Perrini P, Dayoub H, Fraser K. Emerging concepts in the treatment of intracranial aneurysms: stents, coated coils, and liquid embolic agents. Neurosurgery. 2005; 57(3):449–459, discussion 449–459

[79] Cossu G, Messerer M, Oddo M, Daniel RT. To look beyond vasospasm in aneurysmal subarachnoid haemorrhage. BioMed Res Int. 2014; 2014:628597

11 Chemical Thrombolysis and Mechanical Thrombectomy for Acute Ischemic Stroke

Michael Jones, Michael J. Schneck, William W. Ashley Jr., and Asterios Tsimpas

Abstract

Intravenous thrombolysis with alteplase (IV TPA) has been the "standard of care" for the treatment of acute ischemic stroke over the past two decades. Older mechanical thrombectomy devices (without IV TPA or with IV TPA as bridging therapy) failed to show benefit, as compared with IV TPA, in large vessel occlusive ischemic stroke. Recently, intra-arterial (IA) thrombo-embolectomy with stent retriever type devices, along with IV TPA as bridging therapy, was shown to be more effective than IV TPA alone for distal internal carotid artery and proximal middle cerebral artery occlusions. Future studies may demonstrate benefit for mechanical thrombectomy without prior bridging therapy. Randomized studies are also underway to confirm the benefit of IA thromboembolectomy in posterior circulation stroke. Better patient selection, with multimodality neuroimaging, may play a role in improved patient outcomes. To date, however, clinical assessment and rapid evaluation with computed tomography (and perhaps computed tomography angiography) appears sufficient for immediate evaluation of possible IA thromboembolectomy candidates.

Keywords: acute ischemic stroke, intra-arterial thrombolysis, IV TPA, mechanical thrombolysis, stent retrievers, thrombectomy/ thromboembolectomy

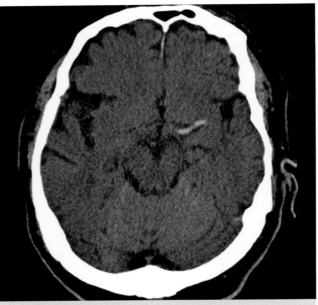

Fig. 11.1 Computed tomography scan of the brain demonstrating a left "dense" middle cerebral artery sign.

11.1 Introduction

Stroke is the leading cause of disability in the United States and the fifth leading cause of mortality, currently responsible for nearly eight hundred thousand deaths annually.[1] Approximately 87% of all strokes are ischemic in nature.[2] The location of the vascular occlusion can often be predicted with a detailed neurologic history and examination. The amount of time required to reestablish tissue perfusion is an important factor in determining outcome and recovery.[3] Although intravenous tissue plasminogen activator (IV tPA) remains the first-line treatment in restoring cerebral blood flow, its efficacy is limited. Endovascular approaches that lead to improved vascular recanalization rates are becoming a very attractive option for a select group of patients, particularly those with acute large vessel occlusion (LVO).[4]

11.2 Evaluation

A critical element of the evaluation of an acute ischemic stroke patient is the time of symptom onset, also known as the "ictus." It can often not be determined. In such cases, we rely on the last time the patient was seen to be normal. After airway, breathing, and circulation (ABCs) are secured, a neurologic examination should be rapidly performed that includes the National Institute of Health Stroke Scale (NIHSS). Other disease processes that can present with similar symptoms should be ruled out, such as hypoglycemia, migraine, seizure, and syncope. The initial work-up should include the patient's vital signs, as well as laboratory studies, such as blood glucose, complete blood count, cardiac enzymes, basic metabolic panel, and coagulation profile. In addition, an electrocardiogram and a noncontrast head computed tomography (CT) scan should be obtained promptly. A noncontrast head CT scan is performed to rule out an intracranial hemorrhage (ICH) (▶Table 11.1). Occasionally, a "dense middle cerebral artery (MCA) sign" can be seen, which typically indicates clot formation inside its M1 segment (▶Fig. 11.1).

Recent studies have advocated for emergent, noninvasive angiographic imaging, such as CT (CTA) or magnetic resonance (MRA) angiography with or without perfusion, to further select patients with LVO, who will benefit from endovascular therapy.[4,5,6,7,8] However, the optimal modalities are an area of ongoing investigation.[3]

11.3 Management

11.3.1 Intravenous Thrombolysis

The seminal National Institute of Neurological Disorders and Stroke (NINDS) IV tPA study, which involved 624 patients randomized to either IV tPA administration or placebo showed that systemic IV thrombolysis with tPA within 3 hours from the onset of symptoms can be an effective treatment of acute ischemic stroke.[9] The dose of IV tPA used was 0.9 mg/kg (maximum

Table 11.1 Emergency evaluation and initial management for a patient with suspected acute ischemic stroke

Initial evaluation and care

1. **Establishing last known well:** Treatment of acute stroke is time sensitive. Patients with symptoms consistent with acute ischemic stroke should be evaluated for acute reperfusion therapies. If presenting to the emergency department (ED), they should be triaged immediately
2. ED physician assessment upon arrival (if presenting to ED)
3. Stabilization of ABCs (airway, breathing, circulation)
4. Cardiac monitoring
5. SpO_2 monitoring and supplemental oxygen, if necessary, to maintain a SpO_2 above 94%
6. 2 large-bore peripheral IV access sites
7. Draw labs (as outlined below)
8. Obtain patient weight
9. Maintain NPO until dysphagia screening
10. NIHSS

Immediate diagnostic studies

1. Noncontrast brain CT/CTA or brain MRI/MRA to be available for review within 45 minutes from patient arrival
2. STAT labs including glucose, BMP*, CBC*, PT/INR*, PTT*, type and screen, and troponin to be completed and reported within 45 minutes from patient arrival
3. POC glucose and creatinine
4. ECG to be completed and available for review within 10 minutes from being ordered

*IV t-PA (Alteplase), thrombolytic therapy should not be delayed while awaiting results unless (1) there is clinical suspicion of a bleeding abnormality or thrombocytopenia; (2) the patient has received heparin, warfarin, or new oral anticoagulation (dabigatran, rivaroxaban, apixaban, edoxoban); or (3) use of anticoagulants is unknown.

Additional studies as indicated

1. CXR available for review within 45 minutes of order
2. Erythrocyte sedimentation rate
3. Liver function tests
4. Toxicology screen
5. Sickle cell screen
6. Blood alcohol level
7. Pregnancy test in women of childbearing age
8. Arterial blood gas
9. Lumbar puncture (if subarachnoid hemorrhage is suspected and CT scan is negative for blood)
10. Electroencephalogram (if seizures are suspected)

Abbreviations: BMP, basic metabolic panel CBC, complete blood count; CT, CTA, computed tomography, CT angiography; CXR, chest X-ray ECG, electrocardiogram; INR, international normalized ratio; MRA, MRI, magnetic resonance angiography, MR imaging; NPO, nil per os; POC, point of care PT, prothrombin time; PTT, partial thromboplastin time; SpO2, blood oxygen saturation; t-PA, tissue plasminogen activator.

dose 90 mg), with 10% of the dose given as an initial bolus over 1 minute and the remainder of the dose administered over an hour.[9] A pooled analysis of thrombolytic trials showed an adjusted odds ratio (OR) for favorable outcome of 2.81 at 90 minutes and 1.55 when administered between 91 and 180 minutes.[10] Nearly 30% of patients are likely to have minimal or no disability at 3 months. The risk of hemorrhagic complications was 6%. Achievement of these results with similarly low complication rates has been duplicated in a number of clinical series published since 1995.[8] This should be tempered, however, by understanding of an increased risk of complications in those patients with more severe strokes.[5,11] Predictors of favorable outcome included treatment within 90 minutes of symptom onset, "normal" baseline CT scan (no ICH or delineated infarct on initial imaging), milder baseline stroke severity, no history of diabetes mellitus, as well as normal pretreatment blood glucose level and blood pressure. Predictors of less favorable outcome and/or hemorrhagic conversion included extended hypodensity with mass effect or hypoattenuation in greater than a third of the MCA territory on pretreatment CT scan, increasing age, higher doses of IV tPA administered, pretreatment blood glucose level > 11 mmol/L, marked elevation of blood pressure (especially diastolic) before, during, and after treatment, hypertension requiring postrandomization antihypertensive treatment, severe pretreatment neurologic deficit, and protocol violations according to the NINDS study protocol.[5,9]

In 2008, the European Cooperative Acute Stroke Study III (ECASS III) trial was published, extending the treatment window to 4.5 hours for patients who meet the standard IV tPA criteria and who are less than 80 years of age, are not on any anticoagulation, and do not have a history of previous stroke and diabetes mellitus. More patients had a favorable outcome with IV tPA than placebo (52.4% vs. 45.2%). The incidence of ICH was higher with IV tPA than with placebo (for any ICH, 27.0% vs. 17.6%). Mortality did not differ significantly between the IV tPA and placebo groups (7.7% and 8.4%, respectively).[12] The caveats are that for the 3- to 4.5-hour window, in addition to the other IV TPA exclusion criteria of the 0- to 3-hour time window, patients above the age of 80, on anticoagulant therapy regardless of the measured international normalized ratio (INR), and with a history of both prior stroke and diabetes mellitus are not eligible for treatment within this time window.[3]

IV tPA is particularly effective when initiated early.[10] IV tPA given within 90 minutes has a more favorable outcome as compared with treatment initiated within the 91- to 180-minute window. In pooled analysis, the OR for favorable outcome beyond 3 hours was 1.4 when administered between 181 and 270 minutes and 1.15 when administered from 271 to 360 minutes.

Table 11.2 Inclusion and exclusion criteria for intravenous tPA administration

Intravenous t-PA evaluation guidelines
Stroke onset less than 3 hours ago

Indication:
   • Acute ischemic stroke with symptom onset of **less than 3 hours** in duration.
   • Head CT does *not* show hemorrhage.
   • Infusion must be initiated within **3 hours** of onset of stroke symptoms
Exclusion criteria:
  1. Stroke or serious head injury within 3 months
  2. Frank hypodensity on CT > 1/3 the MCA territory or evidence of intracranial hemorrhage
  3. Intracranial or intraspinal surgery within 3 months
  4. Persistent systolic BP ≥ 185 mm Hg or diastolic BP ≥ 110 mm Hg despite reasonable attempts to reduce
  5. Intracranial conditions that may increase bleeding risk, including some neoplasms, arteriovenous malformation, and aneurysm
  6. Active internal bleeding
  7. Arterial puncture at a noncompressible site in last 7 days
  8. Warfarin or heparin used within preceding 48 hours *and* elevated aPTT* or INR* ≥ 1.7. Other oral anticoagulant used within preceding 48 hours
  9. Platelet count* below 100,000/µL
 10. Blood glucose below 50 mg/dL
 11. Relative contraindications may include recent surgery, intracranial, GI, or urinary tract hemorrhage or major trauma, pregnancy, MI < 3 months, evidence of left heart thrombus, acute pericarditis, subacute bacterial endocarditis, or diabetic hemorrhagic retinopathy (or other hemorrhagic ophthalmic condition), significant hepatic dysfunction, and rapidly improving or minor neurologic deficits likely to result in minimal or no deficit
*In patients without a history of recent anticoagulant use, thrombocytopenia, or clinical suspicion of bleeding diathesis, t-PA may be initiated before the availability of corresponding laboratory test results.

Stroke onset 3 to 4.5 hours

Indication:
   • Acute ischemic stroke with symptom onset from **3 to 4.5 hours.**
   • Infusion must be initiated within **4.5 hours** of onset of stroke.
In addition to the above exclusion criteria, *all* exclusion criteria below must be considered:
  1. Patient 80 years of age or older
  2. Patient with a combination of previous stroke *and* diabetes mellitus
  3. Patient with NIHSS score above 25
  4. Patient using oral anticoagulants regardless of INR values

Abbreviations: aPTT, activated partial thromboplastin time; CT, computed tomography; GI, gastrointestinal; INR, international normalized ratio; MI, myocardial infarct; NIHSS, Institute of Health Stroke Scale; t-PA, tissue plasminogen activator.

The hazard ratio was around 1.0 for the 0–90-, 91–180-, and 181–270-minute intervals; it was, however, increased for the 271–360-minute interval at 0.45. The Cochrane review of thrombolytic trials reported an OR for fatal ICH of 3.60 with IV tPA, whereas the OR for symptomatic hemorrhage was 3.13.[13] In the pooled trials of IV tPA with a treatment window up to 6 hours, there was a nonsignificant increase in death equivalent to 19 excess deaths per 1,000 patients treated. Despite this, the OR for death or disability was only 0.80, which is equivalent to 55 more independent survivors per 1,000 treated.[10] The Cochrane meta-analysis of the IV tPA trials likely overstates the complication rate of IV tPA, as it includes trials that enrolled patients beyond the accepted 3-hour window. Strict adherence to a specified protocol with close attention to inclusion and exclusion criteria is therefore essential (►Table 11.2).

11.3.2 Intra-arterial Chemical Thrombolysis and Mechanical Thrombectomy

Many patients do not reach stroke centers within the time window that IV tPA can be administered. Intra-arterial (IA) thrombolysis became an attractive alternative that allows extension of the time window beyond 4.5 hours and might be particularly effective for proximal LVO, such as the basilar artery or proximal MCA.[14,15,16,17,18]

The Prolyse in Acute Cerebral Thromboembolism II (PROACT II) study showed that IA thrombolysis using a prodrug of urokinase in patients with large MCA occlusions, which were treated within 6 hours of symptom onset, resulted in greater likelihood of vessel recanalization and clinical improvement.[17] Prourokinase (proUK) was evaluated in this double-blind randomized trial of IA therapy for MCA occlusion in 180 patients who were randomized to IA proUK plus IV heparin or IV heparin only. Forty percent of the proUK versus 25% of control patients had good outcomes (modified Rankin score [mRS] ≤ 2; *p* = 0.04). The recanalization rate was 66% with proUK versus 18% for the control group (*p* < 0.001). ICH with neurologic deterioration within 24 hours occurred in 10% of proUK patients versus 2% of control patients (*p* = 0.06).[15]

The results of this randomized trial were insufficient for approval of this agent in the United States. Nevertheless, it stimulated the use of tPA, reteplase, and urokinase on an off-label basis in patients with acute ischemic stroke who were otherwise not eligible for IV thrombolysis. It is important to note that the actual time window for IA thrombolysis is not well established. In the PROACT II study, MCA occlusions were treated within 6 hours of symptom onset. However, some case series suggest that anterior circulation stroke might be treated up to 8 hours following symptom onset, and the window for posterior circulation occlusions is potentially longer, approaching 12 to 24 hours.[14,15,16,18] Chalela et al reported their experience for patients who underwent IA thrombolysis for stroke following surgical procedures such as coronary artery bypass grafting, with the total required dose ranging from 9 to 40 mg and a median dose of 21 mg.[19] The Ochsner Clinic reported their series of 11 patients who were not eligible for IV tPA and were given an average of 15.1 mg (± 8.0 mg) of IA tPA. Independence in activities of daily living at 30 days was achieved in 38% of patients.[20] These trials were mainly limited by challenges with patient enrollment and resultant small sample size, reflecting the available stroke system infrastructure of the previous decades.

The Emergency Management of Stroke (EMS) and Interventional Management of Stroke III (IMS III) bridging trial described the role of combined IV and IA thrombolytic strategies. Lewandowski and colleagues published a double-blind, randomized, placebo-controlled multicenter Phase I study of IV tPA versus placebo followed by immediate cerebral angiography and local IA administration of tPA. There was no difference in the 7- to 10-day and the 3-month outcomes, although there were more deaths in the IV/IA group. Recanalization was better in the IV/IA group, with Thrombolysis in Myocardial Infarction grade 3 (TIMI 3) flow in 6 of 11 IV/IA patients versus 1 of 10 placebo/IA patients ($p = 0.03$), and correlated with the total dose of tPA ($p = 0.05$). Life-threatening ICH occurred in two patients, both in the IV/IA group. Moderate to severe ICH-related complications occurred in two IV/IA patients and one placebo/IA patient.[21] In the more recent IMS III trial, Broderick et al reported the combined approach in 80 patients with NIHSS score > 10. They received lower dose IV tPA (0.6 mg/kg, 60 mg maximum dose over 30 minutes) within 3 hours of symptom onset, followed by IA tPA (22 mg maximum dose over 2 hours). The trial showed similar safety outcomes and no significant difference in functional independence with IA after IV tPA, as compared with IV tPA alone.[22]

Other than a more localized application of thrombolytic drugs that allowed treatment of surgical patients and a somewhat longer "window of opportunity," IA thrombolysis is still limited by most of the inclusion/exclusion criteria of systemic thrombolysis. Furthermore, the ICH rate is higher for IA versus IV thrombolysis, although this may also reflect the greater severity of strokes treated with endovascular methods, for which the baseline risk of hemorrhagic reperfusion injury is higher. As such, mechanical thrombectomy without thrombolytic drugs was proposed as an option. All kinds of devices have been investigated, including snares, baskets, aspiration devices, balloons, lasers, and intravascular ultrasonic devices.[23] The major advantage of mechanical thrombectomy in place of IA pharmacologic lysis is that it can be used for patients with elevated partial thromboplastin time (< 2 times normal), INR < 3.0, or platelet count < 30,000/µL that would otherwise preclude IA drug use.

The MERCI (Mechanical Embolus Removal in Cerebral Ischemia) clot retriever (Concentric Medical) was originally approved for clinical use (▶Fig. 11.2). The procedure involved inflation of a balloon-mounted guide catheter in the proximal internal carotid artery. A guidewire along with the MERCI microcatheter were then navigated through the guide catheter just beyond the clot, and the retriever device, shaped like a corkscrew, was used to trap the clot. The balloon was inflated to prevent forward blood flow, while the clot was withdrawn back into the guide catheter.[24,25,26] The approval of the device was based on the MERCI trial that reported an intracranial vascular

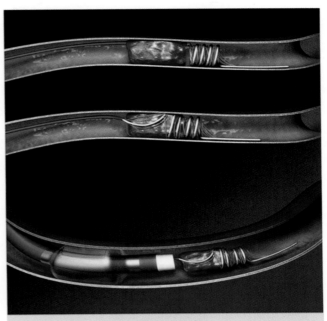

Fig. 11.2 The Concentric Medical MERCI device.

recanalization rate of 46% (69/151 patients) compared with an 18% recanalization rate in historical controls. The therapeutic window was extended to 8 hours post ictus. Good neurologic outcomes (mRS ≤ 2) were more frequent at 90 days in 46% of patients with successful recanalization compared with 10% patients with unsuccessful recanalization ($p = 0.0001$). Symptomatic ICH was described in 7.8% of cases. Mortality was also reduced in recanalized versus nonrecanalized patients (32% vs. 54%; $p = 0.01$).[27] The MERCI trial was a single-arm nonrandomized study, however, and the trial utilized historical controls from the PROACT II study as the placebo comparison. As such, there was only 27% mortality in the PROACT II placebo historical control arm, and the MCA recanalization rate of 46% in the MERCI trial compared unfavorably with the 66% recanalization rate in the proUK arm of PROACT II.[24,25]

The original MERCI trial was followed by the Multi MERCI trial 3 years later. Treatment with a newer version of the MERCI retriever resulted in successful recanalization in 57.3% of the cases without adjunctive therapy and in 69.5% of cases after adjunctive therapy with IA tPA. Favorable clinical outcomes (mRS ≤ 2) were achieved in 36% of the cases and mortality was 34%. Symptomatic ICH occurred in 9.8% of the patients.[28]

The MERCI device was quite cumbersome to use. In addition, many neurointerventionalists were not satisfied with the MERCI recanalization rates. As a "solution" to these problems, the Penumbra aspiration system was created. The system consisted of aspiration catheters, which could be combined in a coaxial fashion, and a separator wire, which had a teardrop-like tip. The catheter was navigated proximal to the clot, which was then aspirated. The separator wire had a dual purpose. It allowed maceration of the clot, which was then aspirated, and it cleaned the catheter tip of clot remnants that were too big for aspiration. The Penumbra Pivotal Stroke trial included 125 patients with NIHSS[3] score 8 who presented up to 8 hours after the onset of symptoms and were ineligible or refractory to IV tPA therapy.

Of the treated vessels, 81.6% were successfully revascularized to TIMI grade 2 or 3. Among the patients, 25% achieved an mRS score of ≤ 2; 28% of the patients were found to have an ICH on a 24-hour CT, of which 11.2% were symptomatic.[29]

The encouraging results of both aforementioned trials stimulated the use of mechanical thrombectomy devices for acute ischemic stroke. Nevertheless, randomized controlled trials (RCTs) using second-generation devices failed to show definitive benefits of IA pharmacologic thrombolysis or mechanical thrombectomy. Several major trials were published in the past few years, including the SYNTHESIS Expansion trial, the IMS III trial, and the MRRESCUE trial.[22,30,31] In all of these RCTs, endovascular therapy was not superior to IV tPA. Additionally, the MRRESCUE study could not demonstrate that perfusion imaging would identify a subset of patients for whom endovascular therapy was of particular benefit. Various reasons for the neutral results of these studies were proposed, including the relative delay in initiating IA treatment, absence of definitive inclusionary pretreatment imaging, and use of older-generation device technology. CTA was also far less developed, resulting in a large proportion of patients in these trials with unconfirmed proximal anterior artery occlusion.[22]

The most recent RCTs, published in 2015, have shown that newer-generation devices, used in combination with IV tPA, are superior to standard medical therapy with IV tPA alone in appropriately selected patients.[8] A more recent meta-analysis of eight trials, incorporating 2,423 patients, showed that functional independence (mRS = 0–2) at 90 days occurred in 44.6% of patients who underwent endovascular therapy, as compared with 31.8% in the patient who underwent standard medical care. Endovascular thrombectomy was associated with significantly higher rates of angiographic revascularization at 24 hours, when compared with standard medical care (75.8% vs. 34.1%; $p < 0.001$). Moreover, there was no significant difference in rates of symptomatic ICH within 90 days (5.7% vs. 5.1%; $p = 0.56$) or all-cause mortality at 90 days (15.8% vs. 17.8%; $p = 0.27$).[27]

MRCLEAN was the first of the new stent retriever trials to demonstrate a positive result for mechanical thrombectomy. In this trial, patients were selected to receive IA therapy, when they had an occlusive anterior circulation stroke, confirmed by arterial vascular imaging (CTA, MRA, or conventional angiography), with presentation and initiation of treatment within 6 hours of symptom onset. Eligible patients for thrombectomy included patients with occlusions of the distal internal carotid artery (ICA), M1 or M2 segments of the MCA, or anterior cerebral artery (ACA) branch. MRCLEAN reported that there was an absolute difference of 13.5% in the rate of functional independence (mRS = 0–2) in favor of the intervention (32.6% vs. 19.1%). There was no significant difference in mortality or symptomatic ICH rates.[4]

The MRCLEAN results were subsequently confirmed by the ESCAPE, SWIFT PRIME, EXTEND-IA, and REVASCAT trials, all of which incorporated the use of a stent retriever and a much more rapid intervention from time of symptom onset to intervention.[5,6,7,8] In the SWIFT PRIME trial, the median time from arrival to groin puncture was 90 minutes, with a goal of 70 minutes, whereas in the ESCAPE trial the median time from qualifying imaging to reperfusion was 84 minutes. This highlights the need for better systems of care to enhance the process of early stroke intervention.[8,32] Furthermore, the MRCLEAN investigators showed that combination of noncontrast CT and CTA was sufficient to identify those patients who might benefit from intervention. More recent studies have used the Alberta Stroke Program Early CT score (ASPECTS) methodology, which estimates the extent of salvageable tissue and the infarct core on the basis of noncontrast CT. ASPECTS is determined from evaluation of two standardized regions of the MCA territory: the basal ganglia level, where the thalamus, basal ganglia, and caudate are visible, and the supraganglionic level, which includes the corona radiata and centrum semiovale. A normal CT scan receives a score of 10, whereas a score of 0 indicates diffuse involvement throughout the MCA territory.[33]

Assessment of leptomeningeal collaterals has also been shown to predict outcome after endovascular treatment. Ideally, multiphase CTA is used to assess blood flow to brain tissue through pial arterial backfilling distal to the arterial obstruction.[34] Patients with poor collaterals are more likely to experience complications from endovascular treatment, whereas the presence of collaterals is associated with a smaller infarct volume and infarct expansion, as well as improved outcomes.[35,36] Recent trials have also incorporated MR diffusion-weighted imaging (DWI) and CT perfusion imaging, which both show promise as accurate predictors of positive outcome, following endovascular treatment. However, these imaging modalities require more time, additional radiation, and contrast exposure. As such, the relative utility of perfusion imaging remains unproven.[18,37] Selecting from the above imaging modalities, a balance will need to be struck between efficiency and accurate exclusion of patients who are unlikely to respond to endovascular treatment.

11.3.3 Tandem Occlusion

For patients who present with a proximal LVO, including the ICA, proximal MCA or ACA, and vertebral and basilar arteries, studies have found a high incidence of a second proximal LVO.[37,38] These tandem occlusions are associated to higher morbidity and mortality rates than isolated LVO, as well as lower rates of recanalization with IV tPA alone.[39,40] Similar to isolated occlusions of large vessels of the anterior circulation, endovascular treatment is thought to improve rates of recanalization and clinical outcomes compared with IV tPA alone, although the precise sequence and device for optimizing recanalization and clinical outcomes is a subject of much debate.[41] Some authors advocate recanalization of the ICA first, followed by recanalization of the distal occlusion.[42] Others argue for initial recanalization of the MCA or ACA occlusion, before the ICA occlusion is dealt with.[43,44,45] One recent study found that treatment of the distal occlusion reduced time to recanalization of dependent brain areas by close to 60 minutes,[46] whereas others have argued that the increased time is closer to 20 minutes.[47] Anterograde recanalization of the ICA, however, can improve collateral flow to the ischemic area. Furthermore, spontaneous recanalization has been observed in up to 50% of patients who underwent only recanalization of the more proximal ICA occlusion.[48] In addition, the possibility of distal embolism or recurrent embolization without treatment of the proximal ICA occlusion is a real concern.[46]

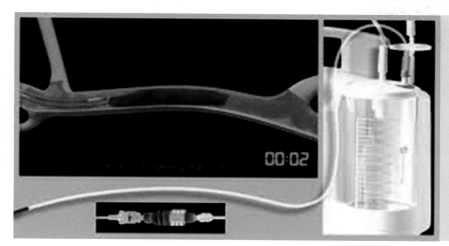

Fig. 11.3 The Penumbra 5Max ACE aspiration system in action.

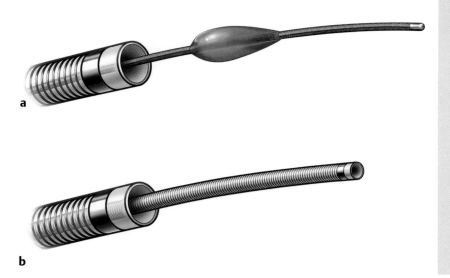

Fig. 11.4 The Penumbra 5Max ACE aspiration system with the separator (**a**) and over a microcatheter that can carry a stent retriever (**b**).

11.3.4 Procedural Details

At our institution, we advocate the use of conscious sedation instead of general anesthesia for stroke intervention, since patients treated under general anesthesia appear to have a higher chance of poor neurologic outcome and mortality.[49] An 8-French femoral arterial sheath is used for vascular access. This allows the use of a multiaxial system and placement of larger carotid stents, if the need arises. The use of an IV heparin bolus is operator dependent. An 8-French sheath is then navigated into the affected vessel. If a cervical carotid occlusion is identified, balloon angioplasty and stenting is performed first. Proximal protection is preferred over distal protection. If a carotid stent needs to be placed emergently, antiplatelet therapy is necessary. We use IV abciximab (0.25 mg/kg body weight), followed by 650 mg of aspirin and 600 of clopidogrel via a nasogastric tube. If a carotid stent is placed, the guide catheter is then used to cross the stent and advanced into the distal cervical ICA.

We want to avoid dragging a stent retriever through a newly placed carotid stent. An intermediate aspiration catheter, such as the Penumbra 5 MAX ACE (Penumbra Inc., Alameda, CA) (▶Fig. 11.3, ▶Fig. 11.4), is then navigated through the guide catheter at the proximal end of the clot. A microcatheter, such as the Marksman (Medtronic Neurovascular, Minneapolis, MN) or the Excelsior XT-27 (Stryker Neurovascular, Fremont, CA), is then used to cross the clot distally. A simultaneous contrast injection through the intermediate catheter and the microcatheter will delineate the extent of the clot. Once the clot is crossed, a stent retriever is then deployed from distal to proximal. It is important to use a stent that is long and wide enough, so the clot can be trapped within its struts. Most recent trials have advocated the use of either the Solitaire FR (Medtronic Neurovascular) (▶Fig. 11.5) or Trevo XP Provue (Stryker Neurovascular) (▶Fig. 11.6) stent retriever. The stent retriever is allowed to expand for 5 minutes. Suction is then applied through the intermediate catheter proximal to the clot, while the microcatheter

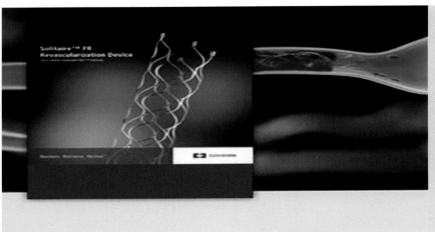

Fig. 11.5 The Solitaire FR stent retriever.

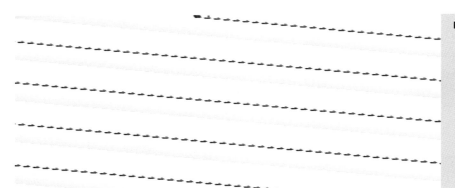

Fig. 11.6 The Trevo XP Provue stent retriever.

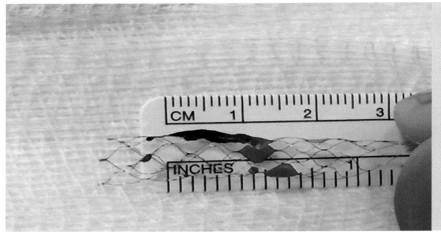

Fig. 11.7 Clot trapped inside the Solitaire FR stent retriever.

and stent are simultaneously removed under fluoroscopic visualization (▶Fig. 11.7, ▶Fig. 11.8). Angiographic runs are then obtained, and the result and revascularization can be assessed. The aforementioned maneuver can be repeated several times. If the clot is hard or calcified and cannot be trapped within the stent after several attempts, we sometimes use the wire separator (Penumbra) (▶Fig. 11.4) with good success. Occasionally, IA tPA is given to soften the clot. It should be used with caution though, especially in cases that a full dose of IV tPA had been administered. Assessment of revascularization can then be carried out, typically by using the Thrombolysis in Cerebral Infarction (TICI) scale.[50]

Until the occluded vessel is recanalized, we keep the mean arterial pressure on the higher side to allow perfusion of collateral vessels. However, immediately after the vessel is recanalized, the mean arterial pressure is dropped below 100, in order to avoid reperfusion injury. A CT scan is obtained shortly after the procedure to rule out reperfusion injury, followed by an MR imaging with diffusion sequence and apparent diffusion coefficient (ADC) map to identify the infarcted tissue. At our

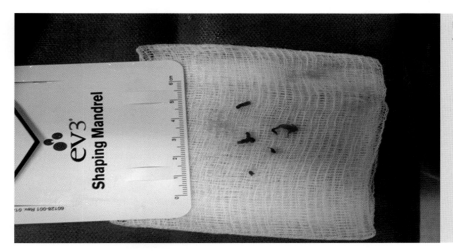

Fig. 11.8 Several pieces of clot removed from an occluded intracranial vessel.

institution, a repeat CT of the brain is obtained 24 hours after the procedure. If there are no signs of reperfusion injury, therapy with aspirin is initiated. A repeat NIHSS score is obtained 24 hours after the stroke intervention. Most studies objectively follow clinical outcomes with the mRS, which ranges from 0 (no impairment) to 6 (dead).[51]

11.4 Conclusion

After a long period in which IV tPA was the only proven thrombolytic therapy for acute ischemic stroke, mechanical thrombectomy with stent retrievers with or without aspiration catheters has been shown to have benefit for a selected subset of patients with acute ischemic stroke. Patients who present with LVO may be considered for endovascular intervention either following IV tPA or as monotherapy in those patients not eligible for IV tPA, if they meet specific selection criteria. Additional studies of pharmacologic and/or endovascular thrombolytic therapies may increase the numbers of patients eligible for recanalization therapies for acute ischemic stroke.

References

[1] Mozaffarian D, Benjamin EJ, Go AS, et al; American Heart Association Statistics Committee and Stroke Statistics Subcommittee. Heart disease and stroke statistics—2015 update: a report from the American Heart Association. Circulation. 2015; 131(4):e29–e322

[2] Caplan LR. Intracranial branch atheromatous disease: a neglected, understudied, and underused concept. Neurology. 1989; 39(9):1246–1250

[3] Jauch EC, Saver JL, Adams HP, Jr, et al; American Heart Association Stroke Council. Council on Cardiovascular Nursing. Council on Peripheral Vascular Disease. Council on Clinical Cardiology. Guidelines for the early management of patients with acute ischemic stroke: a guideline for healthcare professionals from the American Heart Association/American Stroke Association. Stroke. 2013; 44(3):870–947

[4] Berkhemer OA, Fransen PS, Beumer D, et al; MR CLEAN Investigators. A randomized trial of intraarterial treatment for acute ischemic stroke. N Engl J Med. 2015; 372(1):11–20

[5] Campbell BC, Mitchell PJ, Kleinig TJ, et al; EXTEND-IA Investigators. Endovascular therapy for ischemic stroke with perfusion-imaging selection. N Engl J Med. 2015; 372(11):1009–1018

[6] Goyal M, Demchuk AM, Menon BK, et al; ESCAPE Trial Investigators. Randomized assessment of rapid endovascular treatment of ischemic stroke. N Engl J Med. 2015; 372(11):1019–1030

[7] Molina CA, Chamorro A, Rovira À, et al. REVASCAT: a randomized trial of revascularization with SOLITAIRE FR device vs. best medical therapy in the treatment of acute stroke due to anterior circulation large vessel occlusion presenting within eight-hours of symptom onset. Int J Stroke. 2015; 10(4):619–626

[8] Saver JL, Goyal M, Bonafe A, et al; SWIFT PRIME Investigators. Stent-retriever thrombectomy after intravenous t-PA vs. t-PA alone in stroke. N Engl J Med. 2015; 372(24):2285–2295

[9] Molina CA. Futile recanalization in mechanical embolectomy trials: a call to improve selection of patients for revascularization. Stroke. 2010; 41(5):842–843

[10] Inoue M, Mlynash M, Straka M, et al. Patients with the malignant profile within 3 hours of symptom onset have very poor outcomes after intravenous tissue-type plasminogen activator therapy. Stroke. 2012; 43(9):2494–2496

[11] Hussein HM, Georgiadis AL, Vazquez G, et al. Occurrence and predictors of futile recanalization following endovascular treatment among patients with acute ischemic stroke: a multicenter study. AJNR Am J Neuroradiol. 2010; 31(3):454–458

[12] Hacke W, Kaste M, Bluhmki E, et al; ECASS Investigators. Thrombolysis with alteplase 3 to 4.5 hours after acute ischemic stroke. N Engl J Med. 2008; 359(13):1317–1329

[13] Bang OY, Saver JL, Kim SJ, et al. Collateral flow predicts response to endovascular therapy for acute ischemic stroke. Stroke. 2011; 42(3):693–699

[14] del Zoppo GJ, Higashida RT, Furlan AJ, Pessin MS, Rowley HA, Gent M. PROACT: a phase II randomized trial of recombinant pro-urokinase by direct arterial delivery in acute middle cerebral artery stroke. PROACT Investigators. Prolyse in Acute Cerebral Thromboembolism. Stroke. 1998; 29(1):4–11

[15] Furlan A, Higashida R, Wechsler L, et al. Intra-arterial prourokinase for acute ischemic stroke. The PROACT II study: a randomized controlled trial. Prolyse in Acute Cerebral Thromboembolism. JAMA. 1999; 282(21):2003–2011

[16] Ogawa A, Mori E, Minematsu K, et al; MELT Japan Study Group. Randomized trial of intraarterial infusion of urokinase within 6 hours of middle cerebral artery stroke: the Middle Cerebral Artery Embolism Local Fibrinolytic Intervention Trial (MELT) Japan. Stroke. 2007; 38(10):2633–2639

[17] Caplan LR. Caplan's Stroke: A Clinical Approach. 4th ed. Philadelphia, PA: Elsevier/Saunders; 2009

[18] Mozaffarian D, Benjamin EJ, Go AS, et al; American Heart Association Statistics Committee and Stroke Statistics Subcommittee. Heart disease and stroke statistics—2015 update: a report from the American Heart Association. Circulation. 2015; 131(4):e29–e322

[19] Chalela JA, Katzan I, Liebeskind DS, et al. Safety of intra-arterial thrombolysis in the postoperative period. Stroke. 2001; 32(6):1365–1369

[20] Ramee SR, Subramanian R, Felberg RA, et al. Catheter-based treatment for patients with acute ischemic stroke ineligible for intravenous thrombolysis. Stroke. 2004; 35(5):e109–e111

[21] Lewandowski CA, Frankel M, Tomsick TA, et al. Combined intravenous and intra-arterial r-TPA versus intra-arterial therapy of acute ischemic stroke: Emergency Management of Stroke (EMS) Bridging Trial. Stroke. 1999; 30(12):2598–2605

[22] Broderick JP, Palesch YY, Demchuk AM, et al; Interventional Management of Stroke (IMS) III Investigators. Endovascular therapy after intravenous t-PA versus t-PA alone for stroke. N Engl J Med. 2013; 368(10):893–903

[23] Nogueira RG, Lutsep HL, Gupta R, et al; TREVO 2 Trialists. Trevo versus Merci retrievers for thrombectomy revascularisation of large vessel occlusions in acute ischaemic stroke (TREVO 2): a randomised trial. Lancet. 2012; 380(9849):1231–1240

[24] Demchuk AM, Goyal M, Menon BK, et al; ESCAPE Trial Investigators. Endovascular treatment for Small Core and Anterior circulation Proximal occlusion with Emphasis on minimizing CT to recanalization times (ESCAPE) trial: methodology. Int J Stroke. 2015; 10(3):429–438

[25] Jovin TG, Chamorro A, Cobo E, et al; REVASCAT Trial Investigators. Thrombectomy within 8 hours after symptom onset in ischemic stroke. N Engl J Med. 2015; 372(24):2296–2306

[26] Song D, Cho AH. Previous and recent evidence of endovascular therapy in acute ischemic stroke. Neurointervention. 2015; 10(2):51–59

[27] Badhiwala JH, Nassiri F, Alhazzani W, et al. Endovascular thrombectomy for acute ischemic stroke: a meta-analysis. JAMA. 2015; 314(17):1832–1843

[28] Smith WS, Sung G, Saver J, et al; Multi MERCI Investigators. Mechanical thrombectomy for acute ischemic stroke: final results of the Multi MERCI trial. Stroke. 2008; 39(4):1205–1212

[29] Penumbra Pivotal Stroke Trial Investigators. The penumbra pivotal stroke trial: safety and effectiveness of a new generation of mechanical devices for clot removal in intracranial large vessel occlusive disease. Stroke. 2009; 40(8):2761–2768

[30] Ciccone A, Valvassori L, Nichelatti M, et al; SYNTHESIS Expansion Investigators. Endovascular treatment for acute ischemic stroke. N Engl J Med. 2013; 368(10):904–913

[31] Kidwell CS, Jahan R, Gornbein J, et al; MR RESCUE Investigators. A trial of imaging selection and endovascular treatment for ischemic stroke. N Engl J Med. 2013; 368(10):914–923

[32] Bradley EH, Curry LA, Webster TR, et al. Achieving rapid door-to-balloon times: how top hospitals improve complex clinical systems. Circulation. 2006; 113(8):1079–1085

[33] Pexman JH, Barber PA, Hill MD, et al. Use of the Alberta Stroke Program Early CT Score (ASPECTS) for assessing CT scans in patients with acute stroke. AJNR Am J Neuroradiol. 2001; 22(8):1534–1542

[34] Smit EJ, Vonken EJ, van Seeters T, et al. Timing-invariant imaging of collateral vessels in acute ischemic stroke. Stroke. 2013; 44(8):2194–2199

[35] Miteff F, Levi CR, Bateman GA, Spratt N, McElduff P, Parsons MW. The independent predictive utility of computed tomography angiographic collateral status in acute ischaemic stroke. Brain. 2009; 132(Pt 8):2231–2238

[36] Menon BK, Smith EE, Modi J, et al. Regional leptomeningeal score on CT angiography predicts clinical and imaging outcomes in patients with acute anterior circulation occlusions. AJNR Am J Neuroradiol. 2011; 32(9):1640–1645

[37] El-Mitwalli A, Saad M, Christou I, Malkoff M, Alexandrov AV. Clinical and sonographic patterns of tandem internal carotid artery/middle cerebral artery occlusion in tissue plasminogen activator-treated patients. Stroke. 2002; 33(1):99–102

[38] Christou I, Felberg RA, Demchuk AM, et al. Intravenous tissue plasminogen activator and flow improvement in acute ischemic stroke patients with internal carotid artery occlusion. J Neuroimaging. 2002; 12(2):119–123

[39] Rubiera M, Ribo M, Delgado-Mederos R, et al. Tandem internal carotid artery/middle cerebral artery occlusion: an independent predictor of poor outcome after systemic thrombolysis. Stroke. 2006; 37(9):2301–2305

[40] Saqqur M, Uchino K, Demchuk AM, et al; CLOTBUST Investigators. Site of arterial occlusion identified by transcranial Doppler predicts the response to intravenous thrombolysis for stroke. Stroke. 2007; 38(3):948–954

[41] Lavallée PC, Mazighi M, Saint-Maurice JP, et al. Stent-assisted endovascular thrombolysis versus intravenous thrombolysis in internal carotid artery dissection with tandem internal carotid and middle cerebral artery occlusion. Stroke. 2007; 38(8):2270–2274

[42] Dababneh H, Guerrero WR, Khanna A, Hoh BL, Mocco J. Management of tandem occlusion stroke with endovascular therapy. Neurosurg Focus. 2012; 32(5):E16

[43] Machi P, Lobotesis K, Maldonado IL, et al. Endovascular treatment of tandem occlusions of the anterior cerebral circulation with solitaire FR thrombectomy system. Initial experience. Eur J Radiol. 2012; 81(11):3479–3484

[44] Cohen JE, Gomori M, Rajz G, et al. Emergent stent-assisted angioplasty of extracranial internal carotid artery and intracranial stent-based thrombectomy in acute tandem occlusive disease: technical considerations. J Neurointerv Surg. 2013; 5(5):440–446

[45] Puri AS, Kühn AL, Kwon HJ, et al. Endovascular treatment of tandem vascular occlusions in acute ischemic stroke. J Neurointerv Surg. 2015; 7(3):158–163

[46] Lockau H, Liebig T, Henning T, et al. Mechanical thrombectomy in tandem occlusion: procedural considerations and clinical results. Neuroradiology. 2015; 57(6):589–598

[47] Stampfl S, Ringleb PA, Möhlenbruch M, et al. Emergency cervical internal carotid artery stenting in combination with intracranial thrombectomy in acute stroke. AJNR Am J Neuroradiol. 2014; 35(4):741–746

[48] Loh Y, Liebeskind DS, Shi ZS, et al. Partial recanalization of concomitant internal carotid-middle cerebral arterial occlusions promotes distal recanalization of residual thrombus within 24 h. J Neurointerv Surg. 2011; 3(1):38–42

[49] Abou-Chebl A, Lin R, Hussain MS, et al. Conscious sedation versus general anesthesia during endovascular therapy for acute anterior circulation stroke: preliminary results from a retrospective, multicenter study. Stroke. 2010; 41(6):1175–1179

[50] Higashida RT, Furlan AJ, Roberts H, et al; Technology Assessment Committee of the American Society of Interventional and Therapeutic Neuroradiology. Technology Assessment Committee of the Society of Interventional Radiology. Trial design and reporting standards for intra-arterial cerebral thrombolysis for acute ischemic stroke. Stroke. 2003; 34(8):e109–e137

[51] Farrell B, Godwin J, Richards S, Warlow C. The United Kingdom transient ischaemic attack (UK-TIA) aspirin trial: final results. J Neurol Neurosurg Psychiatry. 1991; 54(12):1044–1054

12 Surgical Interventions for Acute Ischemic Stroke

Michael J. Schneck and Christopher M. Loftus

Abstract

Management of acute ischemic stroke focuses on improving reperfusion and minimizing brain edema, recurrent stroke, and acute medical complications. Surgical interventions for acute ischemic stroke are centered on revascularization procedures to prevent recurrent stroke, and craniectomy to treat the complications of brain swelling post stroke. The specific timing of these procedures remains to be defined, but early and timely intervention is critical to prevent neurologic deterioration.

Keywords: acute ischemic stroke, carotid artery stenosis, carotid artery stenting (CAS), carotid endarterectomy (CEA), carotid occlusion, cerebellar stroke, decompressive hemicraniectomy, endovascular thrombectomy, middle cerebral artery (MCA) infarction, suboccipital craniectomy

12.1 Introduction

Most strokes are secondary to thromboembolic arterial occlusions.[1,2,3] A main goal of acute ischemic stroke therapy is to rapidly restore adequate blood flow so as to minimize tissue damage and thereby decrease neurologic morbidity and mortality, with resultant decreases in neurologic disability and improved quality of life. Current practice involves rapid reperfusion of tissue with thrombolytic therapies.[3,4] Recent clinical trials have established a role for endovascular mechanical thrombolysis, with stent retriever devices, alone or in conjunction with intravenous (IV) tissue plasminogen activator (tPA), for acute intracranial internal carotid artery (ICA) or middle cerebral artery (MCA) occlusions in eligible stroke patients.[4] Even in those instances where reperfusion cannot be fully reestablished in the core region of ischemia, mechanisms to salvage the surrounding tissue serve to minimize stroke severity. As such, the modern interventional paradigm for acute ischemic stroke is intended to promote rapid perfusion of brain tissue or treat the complications of brain swelling post stroke.[3]

12.2 General Management Principles

Rapid diagnosis of acute ischemic stroke is essential for patients to receive timely and appropriate treatment. In 1997, a National Institute of Neurological Disorders and Stroke (NINDS) conference highlighted the need for effective and organized stroke systems of care.[5] The conference recommendations emphasized the key factors for stroke systems, including early recognition of eligible stroke patients, early consideration for activation of a stroke team, and establishing standing orders for patients with stroke. Time frames were specified as targets for evaluation times of stroke patients, with the goal of optimization of the screening process to identify possible stroke thrombolysis candidates.

Certain basic principles apply to the immediate management of all stroke patients. These principles are well elucidated in two American Heart Association (AHA) guidelines on early management of acute ischemic stroke.[3,4] Rapid clinical assessment by physicians skilled in assessment of stroke patients is essential. The National Institutes of Health Stroke Scale (NIHSS) is used to clinically determine stroke severity.[6] The NIHSS is a useful and quick prognostic tool that is used by many US vascular neurology (stroke) specialists. Sixty percent to 70% of patients with a baseline NIHSS score < 10 will have a favorable outcome in 1 year, compared with only 4 to 16% of those with a score > 20.[3,6] Early imaging, using computed tomography (CT) or magnetic resonance imaging (MRI), to identify possible intracranial hemorrhage or signs of early cerebral ischemia, is mandatory. When available, MR diffusion-weighted imaging (DWI) and MR gradient echo imaging may be of particular utility in distinguishing acute ischemic strokes or hemorrhages. As noted in the AHA guidelines, relying on MRI availability, outside of clinical research studies, should not delay urgent systemic thrombolysis.

Treatment to lower arterial hypertension should be generally avoided in patients with acute ischemic stroke.[3] Current guidelines recommend no treatment of blood pressure (BP) for patients with systolic BP ≤ 220 mm Hg or diastolic BP ≤ 120 mm Hg unless there is evidence of other major end-organ damage such as aortic dissection, acute myocardial ischemia, pulmonary edema, or hypertensive encephalopathy. Physicians should only consider cautious BP reduction in acute stroke if a patient is otherwise eligible for thrombolytic therapy but has a systolic BP > 185 mm Hg or diastolic BP > 110 mm Hg. Volume expansion with IV fluids may be reasonable, but, as yet, drug-induced hypertension to improve cerebral blood flow is still unproven for acute ischemic stroke. Two pilot studies have described a role for drug-induced arterial hypertension, and phenylephrine was the preferred agent in both studies.[7,8] The titration BP goal was neurologic improvement, assessed by the NIHSS, or titration to a mean arterial BP of 130 mm Hg for the first study.[7] The other study aimed for a minimum systolic BP of 160 mm Hg or 20% above the admission systolic BP to a maximum of 200 mm Hg.[8]

Other important general principles in the care of acute ischemic stroke patients include admission to a stroke unit, a neurointensive care unit, or other monitored setting; aggressive management to maintain normothermia, normovolemia, and normoglycemia; and prevention of medical complications, including cardiac dysrhythmias, aspiration pneumonia, urinary tract infections, and deep venous thrombosis, along with early mobilization of patients through a comprehensive rehabilitation program.[3]

12.3 Revascularization Procedures

Surgical revascularization in ischemic cerebrovascular disease is predominantly a prophylactic measure to reduce the risk of initial or recurrent cerebral ischemic events.[9] Revascularization via extracranial to intracranial (EC–IC) bypass procedures for occlusive carotid disease fell out of favor with the publication of the randomized controlled trial (RCT) of the EC–IC Bypass Study in 1985.[10] The Carotid Occlusion Surgery Study (COSS) utilized stricter selection criteria and enrolled patients with hemispheric symptoms within 120 days or study enrollment, angiographic confirmation of carotid artery occlusion, and hemodynamic cerebral ischemia identified by ipsilateral increased oxygen extraction fraction measured by positron emission tomography(PET).[11] Of 195 patients, 97 were randomized to the surgery arm, and 98 to the nonsurgical arm of the study. Despite better selection criteria, this study also failed to show a benefit for EC–IC bypass. The study was stopped early for futility, with 2-year stroke or death event rates of 21.0% for the surgical group and 22.7% for the nonsurgical group. Variations of the EC–IC bypass procedure still have relevance in special clinical circumstances such as Moyamoya disease selected cases of chronic ischemic oculopathy.[12,13]

On the other hand, carotid endarterectomy (CEA) to prevent primary or recurrent ischemic events is a well-established procedure, based on a series of landmark trials for patients with symptomatic carotid artery disease.[9,14,15,16,17] In particular, the North American Symptomatic Carotid Endarterectomy Trial (NASCET) showed clear and convincing evidence that CEA was overwhelmingly superior to medical therapy for patients with 70 to 99% carotid artery stenosis, with a 16% absolute reduction in the risk of recurrent stroke.[14] The NASCET results were confirmed by the findings of the European Carotid Surgery Trial (ECST).[15] The NASCET group also reported a benefit for CEA versus medical therapy for patients with 50 to 69% carotid artery stenosis, but this benefit was much smaller, and subgroup analysis emphasized the need for careful risk assessment of patients in this intermediate-severity group prior to consideration of CEA.[16]

In the ensuing decade following the publication of the initial NASCET study, endovascular angioplasty and stenting (carotid artery stenting [CAS]) for revascularization of the cervicocerebral vessels began to take hold as an alternative to CEA or bypass procedures. Early trials comparing CAS with CEA suggested that surgery remained the preferred approach to carotid revascularization. The Boston Scientific/Schneider Wallstent study, one of the first RCTs of CAS versus CEA for symptomatic carotid artery stenosis, was stopped early when the morbidity and mortality rates were noted to be much higher in the stent arm of the study.[18,19] As operator experience with endovascular stents improved, however, morbidity and mortality rates began to approach those for CEA.

In 2004, the SAPPHIRE investigators reported results of an RCT of patients with carotid artery stenosis deemed to be at high risk for CEA encompassing those with > 80% asymptomatic carotid artery stenosis or > 50% symptomatic carotid artery stenosis.[20] One hundred fifty-one patients were randomized to CEA, and 159 were randomized to CAS. An additional 413 patients were followed in a registry of high-risk patients, with those patients in the registry deemed ineligible for randomization because the endovascular interventionalist or surgeon felt that the patient could not undergo one or the other procedure (406/413 patients underwent CAS). The primary end point was death, any stroke, or myocardial infarction (MI) at 30 days post procedure. High risk criteria included severe congestive heart failure, open heart surgery within the preceding 6 weeks, recent MI or unstable angina, severe pulmonary disease, contralateral carotid occlusion, contralateral laryngeal nerve palsy, radiation therapy to neck,

previous CEA with restenosis, and age above 80. Overall, the patients who underwent CAS had a statistically significant lower 30-day event rate versus CEA (4.4% vs. 9.9%, $p = 0.06$). At 1 year, the event rate was 12.2% for the stented patients and 20.1% for the surgical patients. The CAS and CEA outcome rates for symptomatic disease were 4.2% and 15.4%, respectively. For asymptomatic carotid artery stenosis, the outcome rates were 6.7% for the CAS arm and 11.2% for the CEA arm. At 30 days, there was no significant difference in the stroke rate, with the primary end point being driven mainly by the rate of predominantly non–Q wave MI. Using the more conventional end point of stroke or death at 30 days plus ipsilateral stroke or death up to 1 year, the differences for those treated by stenting versus surgery was 5% versus 7.5%, with $p = 0.4$. Also, of note, more than 70% of the patients in this trial fell into the asymptomatic group. The SAPPHIRE trial was also underpowered and generalizability is limited because 25% of cases were redo CEA for which the surgical risk is known to be increased. Furthermore, there were more patients in the registry arms of the trial than in the randomized arm, and patients in the registry did worse as compared with the randomized patients. The authors concluded that for high-risk patients, CAS compared favorably with CEA. A nuanced appraisal of this study would suggest that for asymptomatic disease in high-risk patients, medical therapy possibly may be equally or more appropriate than any intervention.

Subsequently, several European studies (SPACE, EVA-3S, and ICSS) failed to confirm a benefit for CAS.[21,22,23] Although these trials were criticized for problems of operator selection and training, and failure to procedurally deploy any embolic protection devices, the benefit of CAS remained to be proven until publication of the Carotid Revascularization Endarterectomy versus Stenting Trial (CREST). This was a large RCT of lower-risk carotid artery stenosis patients and only 47% of the enrolled subjects had asymptomatic carotid artery stenosis.[24] CREST found that the rate of stroke, MI, or death in the 30-day postprocedural period, or any ipsilateral stroke within 4 years after randomization, was a nonstatistically different 7.2% event rate for CAS and 6.8% event rate for CEA. The overall outcome of stroke and death favored CEA (4.7% vs. 6.4%, $p = 0.03$). The periprocedural stroke rate also favored CEA above CAS (2.3% vs. 4.1%, $p = 0.01$). The major stroke rates, however, were comparable between the surgical and stent groups. There was also a trend toward symptomatic patients faring better following CEA as opposed to CAS (6.0% CAS vs. 3.2% CEA; hazard ratio [HR] = 1.89, $p = 0.02$). Cranial nerve palsies were less frequent in the CAS arm. MI rates were also lower in the CAS arm; the periprocedural MI rate for CAS was 1.1% compared with 2.3% for CEA ($p = 0.03$). In the CREST study, patients in the 40- to 70-year age group had better outcomes following CAS, driven mainly by the MI rate, whereas patients in the 70- to 80-year age group had better outcomes following CEA, driven mainly by the stroke event rate. Whether these results are generalizable to the broader nonstudy population is unclear. Furthermore, the relative benefits of either stenting or surgery in the context of improved medical therapies that have developed since the publication of the symptomatic and asymptomatic CEA trials from 25 years ago may have lessened. This issue is under investigation in an ongoing clinical trial.[25]

In regard to CEA timing after acute stroke, there are no clear guidelines regarding when to perform surgery following stroke. Timing of carotid procedures had typically been delayed for up to 6 weeks because of concerns of reperfusion injury or worsening of stroke. CEA typically was not performed immediately post stroke, with early CEA being defined as any procedure occurring less than 2 weeks post event.[26,27] However, early surgery for stable lesions may be reasonable. Pooled data from ECST and NASCET demonstrated that benefits from surgery were greatest for men, patients aged 75 and older, and patients randomized within 2 weeks after the last ischemic event; the number needed to treat (NNT) benefit was 5 to 1 for those randomized within 2 weeks versus 125 to 1 for patients randomized after more than 12 weeks.[27] In a series of 228 patients who underwent CEA within 1 to 4 weeks of the event, there was an acceptable rate of perioperative permanent neurologic deficits of under 3.4%, with no difference between location or size of infarct and timing of surgery, and no worse outcome for those done within 1 week as compared with those who underwent CEA at a later date.[28] Only infarct size was predictive of the probability of neurologic deficit. In fact, functional outcomes actually appeared to be improved with earlier hospital discharge when CEA was performed within 7 days of stroke. In an early pilot study, Welsh et al suggested that, in the absence of randomized trials, data did not support a routine policy of CEA in the acute phase.[29] Other studies suggested, however, that in selected cases, urgent CEA was appropriate. Meyer et al described 34 patients with acute ICA occlusion at the time of emergency CEA. All of these patients had profound neurologic deficits, including hemiplegia and aphasia. There was a 94% success rate in restoring patency. In follow-up, 13 patients had no or minimal deficit, whereas 4 had severe hemiplegia and 7 patients died. The authors stated that these results were better than the "natural history" of nonoperated acute carotid occlusions at the time of the study.[30] Eckstein et al reported a series of 71 emergency CEAs performed between 1980 and 1998 for which they identified three groups: crescendo TIA ($n = 21$), evolving stroke ($n = 34$), and acute onset of severe stroke ($n = 16$).[31] Good outcome was assessed as modified Rankin score (mRS) of 0 to 3. For patients with acute severe stroke, 56.3% had a good outcome. A good outcome occurred in 76.4% of patients with evolving stroke and 80.9% of patients with crescendo TIA. Brandl et al noted, in a series of 233 symptomatic patients, that CEA was performed on 16 (3.8%) of patients within 4 to 24 hours of symptom onset.[32] Criteria for early surgery included crescendo TIA and fluctuating neurologic deficits. Nine of these patients had complete resolution of symptoms, four patients improved, and three remained unchanged or worsened. Findlay and Marchak described 13 patients with severe postoperative deficits; 5 had deficits upon awakening and 7 had deficits within 12 hours of surgery.[33] Of the five patients who underwent urgent reoperation, two had occlusions that were repaired and one had an intra-arterial injection of TPA. For seven patients who first underwent cerebral angiography, two instances of carotid occlusion and one instance of residual stenosis were identified. For the six patients who had revascularization, two of the four patients with occlusion and the one patient who received TPA, as well as the patient who had residual stenosis, improved. The authors noted that approximately one half of the strokes had an underlying correctable lesion of which one half improved early after reexploration. A meta-analysis of all published articles from 1994 to 2000 suggested that there was no excess risk for early versus late CEA in patients with stable symptoms.[26] The meta-analysis did note that the operative risk of stroke or death in patients operated for crescendo TIA or stroke-in-evolution was an unacceptably high 20% rate. A recent international multicenter study, however, of 165 patients with symptomatic carotid artery stenosis who underwent CEA within 1 week reported an acceptably low 5.5% combined outcome event rate of nonfatal stroke, MI, and death.[34] Urgent CEA was done in 20 (12%) of the cases, with no increase in adverse events. Furthermore, in this study, crescendo TIA, or contralateral ICA occlusion, was not associated with higher 30-day stroke rates.

Surgical intervention for "hyperacute" stroke, or crescendo TIA due to high-grade carotid artery stenosis or acute carotid occlusion has been superseded by mechanical embolectomy and/or carotid angioplasty plus stenting.[4] There have been several case series that have demonstrated a role for balloon angioplasty or stenting for patients with acute carotid occlusion, including those who experience perioperative neurologic complications following CEA,[35,36,37,38,39,40,41,42] and at this time, endovascular procedures for acute carotid occlusions are a preferred approach as compared with emergent CEA.

12.4 "Salvage" Procedures for Brain Swelling Post Stroke

12.4.1 Surgery for Cerebellar Infarctions

Cerebellar infarcts constitute about 3% of all ischemic strokes, but may be underdiagnosed, and can have potentially devastating outcome.[43,44] Acute cerebellar infarction or hemorrhage presents in a protean fashion.[43,44,45,4,6,47,48,49] This type of stroke may present with nonspecific ataxia, vertigo, nausea, vomiting, dysarthria, or just isolated severe headache. Focal findings are not common, and because cerebellar stroke may present with nonlocalizing symptoms, a stroke diagnosis may be initially missed.[43,44,45,46,47,48] Prognosis is worse for those presenting on admission with elevated systolic BP > 200 mm Hg, gaze paresis, a decreased level of consciousness, and CT evidence of midline lesion, fourth ventricle and basal cistern obstruction, signs of upward herniation, intraventricular blood, and/or hydrocephalus.[47] The initial CT is unremarkable in upwards of one fourth of cases. Initial infarct volume is one of the best predictors of worse outcome or deterioration.[50,51,52] Also, patients with infarcts > 3 cm in size are at significant risk of deterioration. Patients may present in stable fashion and only later rapidly deteriorate, as a result of brainstem compression or infarction, with hydrocephalus as a result of increased swelling of the infarcted cerebellum. Close to half of initially alert patients with cerebellar hemorrhage will deteriorate, especially those with midline vermian lesions.[47] These patients should be observed in a monitored intensive care setting for the first 3 to 5 days when cerebellar edema is at its maximum (see ►Fig. 12.1).

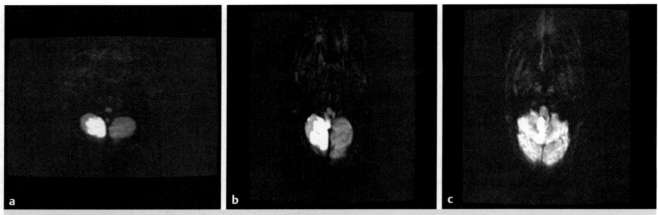

Fig. 12.1 (a–c) Magnetic resonance (MR) images of a 73-year-old woman who presented with headache, dizziness, and gait unsteadiness of 2 days' duration. Examination revealed minimal nystagmus, dysmetria, and gait unsteadiness. Diffusion-weighted MR images showed an acute posterior inferior cerebellar artery (PICA) territory infarction with compression of the fourth ventricle. This patient was observed in a monitored setting for 1 week and subsequently was sent to an acute rehabilitation unit and did well thereafter without need for surgical intervention.

Management of deteriorating stroke suggests that when deterioration is a result of brainstem direct compression as a result of mass effect, a suboccipital craniectomy with evacuation of infarcted tissue is indicated.[43,49] For patients in whom deterioration is related to hydrocephalus, particularly if older or with less rapid deterioration, ventriculostomy may be an alternative initial option, with definitive posterior fossa procedures indicated if there is no further improvement or continued deterioration.[43,49,53,54,55,56,57,58,59,60] There are no randomized or prospective series of expectant management versus early surgical intervention. Nor are there any prospective series of ventriculostomy versus craniectomy. In the German–Austrian cerebellar study of 84 patients with massive cerebellar infarction who underwent treatment according to preferences of the primary caregivers, 34 underwent craniectomy, 14 received ventriculostomy, and 36 were treated medically.[54] The main predictor of poor outcome was the level of consciousness following clinical deterioration (odds ratio [OR] = 2.88). Surgical treatment for massive cerebellar infarctions was not found superior to medical treatment, in either the awake/drowsy or somnolent/ stuporous patient subgroups, although a reasonable recovery was observed in about half the patients with massive infarction who underwent some sort of procedural intervention. Other small retrospective series have indeed suggested that surgery is associated with better outcome. Thus, for example, in a series of 53 patients on the Caribbean island of Martinique, Mostofi reported better survival and functional outcomes following surgery.[55] Even patients with decreased levels of consciousness or advanced age may benefit from surgical decompression of cerebellar infarction. There are case series, however, describing successful management of patients with ventriculostomy alone.[56,57,58] Raco et al described 44 cases of which 17 patients had surgery and 8 patients had ventriculostomy alone.[56] Overall mortality in their series was 13.6%; 89% of the conservatively treated patients had good outcome, with 10/17 patients taken to surgery experiencing a good outcome. Kirollos et al described a series of 50 cases and suggested a protocol based on level of alertness and appearance of the fourth ventricle. When the fourth ventricle was normal, patients were treated conservatively.[57] If the

patient's Glasgow Coma Scale (GCS) score then became worse, the patient underwent a ventriculostomy. When the fourth ventricle was compressed but not fully effaced, the patient was treated conservatively and only underwent ventricular drainage with deterioration of the GCS score, if hydrocephalus was present. In the absence of hydrocephalus, with deterioration of the GCS score and fourth ventricular compression, or if the patient did not improve despite ventricular drainage, the patient then underwent evacuation. For those patients with complete effacement of the fourth ventricle, the patients underwent early suboccipital craniectomy and ventricular drainage. Mortality in that series was high (40%), but 80% of survivors had a good outcome. Current recommendations from international societies are for patients who are not moribund; with any deterioration, suboccipital craniectomy is a preferred option[43,49]

12.4.2 Hemicraniectomy for "Malignant" Middle Cerebral Artery Infarctions

Massive hemispheric strokes due to MCA occlusion have a high mortality rate of > 50%.[61] MCA infarction is estimated to represent 5% of all strokes.[62] These large hemispheric strokes accounts for 10 to 15% of all supratentorial infarction and are typically associated with poor prognosis.[1,3,43,49,61,62,63,64,65,66,67] Approximately 13% of proximal MCA infarctions are associated with severe edema and herniation, with 7% of patients dying from brain swelling in the first week post stroke.[67] Kasner et al described 201 patients with large MCA strokes, of which 94 (47%) died from massive cerebral edema, 12 (6%) died from non-neurologic causes, and 95 (47%) survived to day 30.[62] Risk factors for fatal edema included history of arterial hypertension, history of congestive heart failure, elevated white blood cell count, > 50% MCA hypodensity, and additional infarct involvement of other cerebral blood vessel territories. Although the presenting level of consciousness, NIHSS score, early nausea and vomiting, and serum glucose were associated with neurologic death in univariate analyses, they were not significant

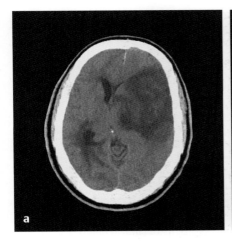 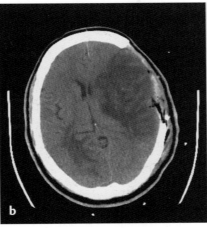

Fig. 12.2 Noncontrast head computed tomography **(a)** at day 7 following a left middle cerebral artery occlusive ischemic stroke. Patient had evidence of subfalcine and uncal herniation in the context of aphasia and left hemiplegia. **(b)** Day 8; status post left hemicraniectomy with improvement in level of consciousness; following some commands.

factors in multivariate analyses. Clinical manifestations reflect the hemisphere involved, and possible associated anterior cerebral artery (ACA) or posterior cerebral artery (PCA) infarctions. The semiology includes hemiplegia, hemianesthesia, hemianopia, aphasia (mainly in left, dominant hemispheric infarctions), hemineglect (typically in right, nondominant hemispheric infarction), forced gaze deviation, possible head deviation, and progressive deterioration in the level of consciousness. Hacke et al also reported that occlusion of the ICA or MCA and poor collateral flow were risk factors for poor outcome.[63] Other authors have also identified major CT hypodensity in the MCA territory as a significant risk factor.[65,68]

Imaging predictors of malignant cerebral edema due to MCA infarction include large cortical hypodensity on head CT, early involvement of more than one third of the MCA territory, and early midline shift of ≥ 2 mm.[65,68] Evidence of > 80 cm³ of cerebral ischemia by volumetric measurement of MR DWI done within 6 hours also predicts poor outcome, as well as MR DWI stroke volumes of ≥ 145 cm³ at 12 hours.[62,65,68,69,70] Mori et al noted that stroke volumes of > 240 cm³ predict a poor outcome in more than three quarters of cases.[70] Clinical factors remain more predictive of outcome than any imaging characteristics, with high NIHSS scores or alteration of level of consciousness as the most predictive of or poor outcome.

In the context of malignant MCA infarction, the assumption has been that clinical deterioration is due to enlargement of an ischemic swollen mass rather than global increases in intracranial pressure (ICP) and decreases in cerebral perfusion pressure (CPP).[61] The peak of cerebral edema is around 4 days (usually occurring around 3–7 days) and is the major cause of death in large strokes, but deterioration in massive MCA infarction may be more rapid than previously described.[61,62,63] A recent multicenter retrospective chart review of 53 cases not treated surgically reported that by 48 hours, two thirds of patients had clinical deterioration. Mortality was high in this population; 25/53 (47%) of the patients died in hospital, with most of the deaths occurring on day 3 post stroke.[66]

Approximately 13% of proximal MCA infarcts are associated with severe edema and herniation, with 7% of patients dying from brain swelling in the first week post stroke.[67] Traditional medical interventions to reduce ICP, including hyperventilation, ventricular drainage, and osmotic diuresis (i.e., with mannitol), have been utilized in malignant MCA infarction. The benefit of these therapies is unproven, however. Corticosteroids, used in the management of cerebral edema, do not increase poststroke survival.[71] Mannitol has been reported to decrease cerebral edema and infarction post stroke and has been widely used in acute stroke for control of malignant cerebral edema. Despite wide use of this agent, few randomized studies are available to support the use of mannitol, and its administration is based on clinical anecdote and animal studies at this time.[72]

A series of clinical trials over the past decade, have demonstrated that surgical intervention is a lifesaving procedure and will cut the mortality by half compared with medical therapy. Decompressive hemicraniectomy with durotomy is a lifesaving procedure for patients who have large MCA or carotid terminus strokes at high risk for malignant cerebral edema (▶Fig. 12.2). Hemicraniectomy will result in a 15% decrease in ICP, and when accompanied by durotomy, there is a significant 70% decrease in ICP.[73] The mechanism for benefit of hemicraniectomy has been mainly attributed to decompression with relief of pressure on noninfarcted brain tissue, but improved CPP also may account for some of the subsequent improvement observed after hemicraniectomy. Elevated ICP alone is not a clear indictor for intervention.[74]

Three European RCTs demonstrated benefit for hemicraniectomy when done within 96 hours (one trial) and preferably within 48 hours of symptoms onset: Hemicraniectomy after Middle cerebral artery infarction with Life-threatening Edema Trial (HAMLET; the Netherlands); DEcompressive Surgery for the Treatment of malignant INfarct of the middle cerebral arterY (DESTINY; Germany); and DEcompressive Craniectomy In Malignant middle cerebral artery infarcts (DECIMAL; France).[75,76,77] These studies, by intent, had similar designs and primary outcomes, and so the data were subsequently presented in a pooled analysis of patients with large strokes (NIHSS score > 15 and imaging that showed infarct volumes > 50% of the MCA territory) who were enrolled within 48 hours of symptoms onset.[78] Patients with life expectancy of less than 3 years, poor premorbid functional status, bilateral dilated pupils at time of enrollment, hemorrhagic transformation of stroke, or other areas of infarction outside of the affected MCA territory were excluded. The mRS was the primary outcome measure, and the analysis dichotomized patients into favorable (mRS = 0–4) and unfavorable groups (mRS = 5–6). In these clinical trials, patients were relatively young (< 60 years of age). There were 93 patients in the pooled analysis (52 surgical and 41 nonsurgical patients). At 1 year, 32/41 (78%) of patients in the nonsurgical arm and 13/52 (25%) of the patients in the surgical arm had an unfavorable outcome. The pooled analysis reported that there was no increase in the number of patients with severe disability, as opposed to death, in the surgical versus the nonsurgical group.

The Hemicraniectomy and Durotomy on Deterioration from Infarction Related Swelling Trial (HeADDFIRST) was a pilot study in which 26 patients were randomized, and there was a statistically nonsignificant reduction in mortality from 46% with medical therapy to 27% in the surgically treated group. A total of 4,909 patients were screened, but only 66 (1.3%) patients were eligible for the study, of which 40 were enrolled in the study. HeADDFIRST was initiated around the same time but was not published until well after the results of the European studies were available. The six month mortality was 40% (4/10) in the medical treatment only group and 36% (5/14) in the surgical group of the HeEADDFIRST study. Interestingly, mortality rates in the medical arm of this study were much lower in this study than in the European studies.[79]

The mortality benefit of hemicraniectomy is not restricted to young patients. DESTINY II demonstrated that early decompressive hemicraniectomy reduces mortality without increasing the risk of very severe disability in older patients.[80] The study enrolled 112 malignant MCA patients presenting within 48 hours of symptom onset, to either medical therapy or hemicraniectomy. Patients were 61 years of age or older (median: 70 years; range: 61–82 years). The primary outcome measure was survival without severe disability (mRS < 5) at 6 months; the proportion of patients who survived with mRS ≤ 4 was 38% in the surgery arm, as compared with 18% in the medical therapy arm (OR = 2.91). The results, however, were driven by lower mortality in the surgery arm (33% vs. 70%), and no patient had a favorable mRS of 0 to 2 (representing no or only mild disability).

In a subsequent Chinese hemicraniectomy RCT, Zhao et al described outcomes for patients aged 18 to 80, with the 6-month mRS as the primary outcome.[81] The study included a prespecified subgroup analysis of patients above age 60. The study was terminated early, with 47 subjects recruited (24 surgical; 23 medical). Surgery reduced significantly reduced mortality at 6 and 12 months (12.5% vs. 60.9%, p = 0.001 and 16.7% vs. 69.6%, p < 0.001, respectively), and significantly fewer patients had mRS > 4 after surgery (33.3 vs. 82.6%, p = 0.001). Similar results were present in the elderly subgroup as compared with the entire study population.

The results of a Cochrane meta-analysis of the initial European studies of patients under age 60 suggested improved survival, with no increase in patients with severe disability.[82] A subsequent meta-analysis of the six hemicraniectomy RCTs, including the elderly patients, observed, however, that hemicraniectomy was associated with decreased mortality but was associated with an increased proportion of patients who were left with "substantial" disability.[83] There was an OR of 0.19 for death at 6 months for decompressive surgery as compared with medical therapy alone. There was, however, a higher proportion of patients with mRS of 4 in the decompressive surgery group (OR = 3.29). On the other hand, there was a higher proportion of

patients in the long term with a relatively favorable mRS of 2 in the surgical group (OR = 4.51).

As an aside, the role of hypothermia for MCA infarction has not been established and is being investigated as part of a proposed trial of hemicraniectomy and hypothermia for malignant MCA infarction.[84] One recent study of hypothermia alone in 11 patients with MCA infarction (median age 76 years) who were deemed ineligible for hemicraniectomy suggested a favorable outcome, with an 18% mortality rate, although with a high 3-month posttreatment mRS of 4.9 ± 0.8[85]

A retrospective study at the Karolisnka Institute, investigating predictors of favorable outcome, defined using a dichotomized score on the mRS 3 months after surgery, with favorable outcome defined as mRS ≤ 4, demonstrated that preoperative GCS score, blood glucose, and involvement of basal ganglia tissue in the infarct were strong predictors of clinical outcome.[86] In a logistic regression analysis, the only statistically significant independent variable, however, was preoperative GCS score; there was a 59.6% increase in the probability of favorable outcome for every point gained in preoperative GCS score (p = 0.035) Thus, a better preoperative clinical state predicts an increased likelihood of favorable long-term functional outcomes.[86]

Retrospective series suggest that functional outcomes are related mainly to comorbidities.[87,88,89,90,91] In all of these retrospective series, and subsequent prospective RCTs, left versus right hemispheric stroke was not associated with differences in functional outcome. Furthermore, in both RCTs of elderly patients, as well as the retrospective cases series, age was in fact associated with poor functional outcomes.[80,81,87,88,89,90,91] Thus, although RCTs demonstrate improved survival, it is not surprising that Leonhardt et al noted that 4 of the 18 patients in their case series would not have consented again to the procedure because of poor postoperative quality of life.[91] The ethical implications of poor functional outcomes are certainly complex.[92,93] Despite poor functional outcomes from decompressive hemicraniectomy, many patients and families appear satisfied with their decision to proceed with surgery.[94] Medical professionals appear to have a different perspective, however. The ORACLE stroke study of 773 health care workers in Western Australia revealed that only a minority of those surveyed considered an mRS of 4 to 5 an acceptable outcome, and they felt that survival with major disability was unacceptable but would be willing to provide consent for hemicraniectomy with the hope of achieving functional independence.[95] Furthermore, DESTINY-S, a multicenter, international, cross-sectional survey of 1,860 physicians potentially involved in the treatment of malignant MCA infarction, reported that an mRS of 3 or less was considered acceptable by 79% of respondents, but an mRS of 4 was deemed acceptable only by 38% of respondents.[96] Despite the lack of differences in functional outcomes by involved hemisphere in randomized RCTs, 47% versus 73% of respondents stated that hemicraniectomy was preferred treatment for dominant versus nondominant hemisphere lesions. Significant differences were also found in acceptable disability and therapeutic choices among geographic regions, medical specialties, and respondents with different work experiences. In particular, neurosurgeons (65%) and physicians without stroke unit experience (60%) were more likely to deem dominant hemispheric involvement to be a major selection factor as compared with neurologists or those with stroke unit experience (48%).

Technically, decompressive hemicraniectomy is relative simple compared with other neurosurgical procedures: removal of the skull, durotomy and duraplasty to accommodate further swelling, and 3 to 6 months later re-placement of the stored cranium. Clinical trials have not demonstrated whether lobectomy should accompany hemicraniectomy, and removal of necrotic tissue is typically reserved for those few circumstances of severe temporal lobe swelling. A larger surgical resection may be associated with better outcome.[67] To date, there are no prospective data comparing early hemicraniectomy and duraplasty within 24 hours of infarction versus later intervention, or comparing hemicraniectomy and duraplasty with or without anterior temporal lobotomy.[61,67]

Demchuk describes the minimal adequate decompression with the following bony boundaries: interiorly frontal to the midpupillary line, posterior approximately 4 cm to the external auditory canal; superiorly to the saggital sinus; and inferiorly to the floor of the middle cranial fossa with a cruciate or circumferential durotomy over the entire region of bony decompression.[97] Current principles for case selection of hemicraniectomy patients, based on randomized trials and meta-analyses, includes recognition of high-risk patients. These include patients with high NIHSS scores (15 for right and 20 for left hemisphere lesions), early CT signs of > 50% MCA territory involvement, and high comorbidities. Patients should be rescanned early, within 6 to 12 hours after the initial scan, and consideration of hemicraniectomy may be appropriate if early signs of complete MCA, or MCA plus ACA or PCA infarcts with mass effect.[97] Otherwise, monitoring for an altered level of consciousness, and/or anisocoria, is warranted, and immediate CT scan if any change in neurologic status is further warranted. Additional evidence of right to left shift > 1 cm may then be an indicator for hemicraniectomy. Timely intervention is critical; when abnormal brainstem findings develop, the likelihood of any reasonable clinical outcome is poor, and patients are then probably not candidates for intervention.[74,98]

12.5 Conclusion

Surgical interventions for ischemic stroke are predominantly beneficial in the subacute setting, or as salvage procedures. With the advent of endovascular procedures for acute ischemic stroke, surgical intervention becomes more of a "rescue procedure" to prevent ongoing damage to normal brain tissue. Neurosurgeons will continue to play a significant role in the evaluation and management of acute stroke patients and should be familiar with current guidelines.[3,4,43,49,99] As previously stated by Loftus, "it behooves the neurosurgical practitioner to be aware of the strict and well defined indications for emergency surgical intervention in stroke patients and to be conversant with the surgical techniques involved."[35]

References

[1]   Fisher M, Ratan R. New perspectives on developing acute stroke therapy. Ann Neurol. 2003; 53(1):10–20

[2]   Dalal PM. Ischaemic strokes: management in first six hours. Neurol India. 2001; 49(2):104–115

[3]   Jauch EC, Saver J, Adams HR, Jr, et al; American Heart Association Stroke Council. Council on Cardiovascular Nursing. Council on Peripheral Vascular Disease. Council on Clinical Cardiology. Guidelines for the early management of patients with acute ischemic stroke: a guideline for healthcare professionals from the American Heart Association/American Stroke Association. Stroke. 2013; 44(3):870–947

[4]   Powers WJ, Derdeyn CP, Biller J, et al; American Heart Association Stroke Council. 2015 American Heart Association/American Stroke Association Focused Update of the 2013 Guidelines for the Early Management of Patients With Acute Ischemic Stroke Regarding Endovascular Treatment: a guideline for healthcare professionals from the American Heart Association/American Stroke Association. Stroke. 2015; 46(10):3020–3035

[5]   National Institute of Neurological Disorders and Stroke (NINDS). Proceedings of a National Symposium on Rapid Identification and Treatment of Acute Stroke. Bethesda, MD: NINDS. 1997. NIH Publication No. 97–4239

[6]   Brott T, Adams HP, Jr, Olinger CP, et al. Measurements of acute cerebral infarction: a clinical examination scale. Stroke. 1989; 20(7):864–870

[7]   Hillis AE, Ulatowski JA, Barker PB, et al. A pilot randomized trial of induced blood pressure elevation: effects on function and focal perfusion in acute and subacute stroke. Cerebrovasc Dis. 2003; 16(3):236–246

[8]   Rordorf G, Koroshetz WJ, Ezzeddine MA, Segal AZ, Buonanno FS. A pilot study of drug-induced hypertension for treatment of acute stroke. Neurology. 2001; 56(9):1210–1213

[9]   Loftus CM. Emergency surgery for stroke. In: Loftus CM, ed. Neurosurgical Emergencies. Vol. I. American Association of Neurosurgeons 1994;151–164

[10] The EC/IC Bypass Study Group. Failure of extracranial-intracranial arterial bypass to reduce the risk of ischemic stroke. Results of an international randomized trial. N Engl J Med. 1985; 313(19):1191–1200

[11] Powers WJ, Clarke WR, Grubb RL, Jr, Videen TO, Adams HP, Jr, Derdeyn CP; COSS Investigators. Extracranial-intracranial bypass surgery for stroke prevention in hemodynamic cerebral ischemia: the Carotid Occlusion Surgery Study randomized trial. JAMA. 2011; 306(18):1983–1992

[12] Grubb RL, Jr, Powers WJ. Risks of stroke and current indications for cerebral revascularization in patients with carotid occlusion. Neurosurg Clin N Am. 2001; 12(3):473–487, vii

[13] Barrall JL, Summers CG. Ocular ischemic syndrome in a child with moyamoya disease and neurofibromatosis. Surv Ophthalmol. 1996; 40(6):500–504

[14] North American Symptomatic Carotid Endarterectomy Trial Collaborators. Beneficial effect of carotid endarterectomy in symptomatic patients with high-grade carotid stenosis. N Engl J Med. 1991; 325(7):445–453

[15] European Carotid Surgery Trialist's Collaborative Group. Randomised trial of endarterectomy for recently symptomatic carotid stenosis: final results of the MRC European Carotid Surgery Trial (ECST) Lancet. 1998; 351(9113):1379–1387

[16] Barnett HJ, Taylor DW, Eliasziw M, et al. Benefit of carotid endarterectomy in patients with symptomatic moderate or severe stenosis. North American Symptomatic Carotid Endarterectomy Trial Collaborators. N Engl J Med. 1998; 339:1415–1425

[17] Rothwell PM, Eliasziw M, Gutnikov SA, et al; Carotid Endarterectomy Trialists' Collaboration. Analysis of pooled data from the randomised controlled trials of endarterectomy for symptomatic carotid stenosis. Lancet. 2003; 361(9352):107–116

[18] Alberts MJ, McCann R, Smith TP, et al. A randomized trial of carotid stenting versus endarterectomy in patients with symptomatic carotid stenosis: study design. J Neurovasc Dis. 1997; 2:228–234

[19] Alberts MJ. Results of a multicentre prospective randomized trial of carotid artery stenting vs. carotid endarterectomy. Stroke. 2001; 32:325

[20] Yadav JS, Wholey MH, Kuntz RE, et al; Stenting and Angioplasty with Protection in Patients at High Risk for Endarterectomy Investigators. Protected carotid-artery stenting versus endarterectomy in high-risk patients. N Engl J Med. 2004; 351(15):1493–1501

[21] Mas JL, Chatellier G, Beyssen B, et al; EVA-3S Investigators. Endarterectomy versus stenting in patients with symptomatic severe carotid stenosis. N Engl J Med. 2006; 355(16):1660–1671

[22] Ringleb PA, Allenberg J, Brückmann H, et al; SPACE Collaborative Group. 30 day results from the SPACE trial of stent-protected angioplasty versus carotid endarterectomy in symptomatic patients: a randomised non-inferiority trial. Lancet. 2006; 368(9543):1239–1247

[23] Ederle J, Dobson J, Featherstone RL, et al; International Carotid Stenting Study investigators. Carotid artery stenting compared with endarterectomy in patients with symptomatic carotid stenosis (International Carotid Stenting Study): an interim analysis of a randomised controlled trial. Lancet. 2010; 375(9719):985–997

[24] Brott TG, Hobson RW, II, Howard G, et al; CREST Investigators. Stenting versus endarterectomy for treatment of carotid-artery stenosis. N Engl J Med. 2010; 363(1):11–23

[25] Brott TG. Carotid revascularization and medical management for asymptomatic carotid stenosis trial (CREST II). https://clinicaltrials.gov/ct2/show/NCT02089217. Accessed March 2017

[26] Bond R, Rerkasem K, Rothwell PM. Systematic review of the risks of carotid endarterectomy in relation to the clinical indication for and timing of surgery. Stroke. 2003; 34(9):2290–2301

[27] Rothwell PM, Eliasziw M, Gutnikov SA, Warlow CP, Barnett HJ; Carotid Endarterectomy Trialists Collaboration. Endarterectomy for symptomatic carotid stenosis in relation to clinical subgroups and timing of surgery. Lancet. 2004; 363(9413):915–924

[28] Paty PS, Darling RC, III, Feustel PJ, et al. Early carotid endarterectomy after acute stroke. J Vasc Surg. 2004; 39(1):148–154

[29] Welsh S, Mead G, Chant H, Picton A, O'Neill PA, McCollum CN. Early carotid surgery in acute stroke: a multicentre randomised pilot study. Cerebrovasc Dis. 2004; 18(3):200–205

[30] Meyer FB, Sundt TM, Jr, Piepgras DG, Sandok BA, Forbes G. Emergency carotid endarterectomy for patients with acute carotid occlusion and profound neurological deficits. Ann Surg. 1986; 203(1):82–89

[31] Eckstein HH, Schumacher H, Klemm K, et al. Emergency carotid endarterectomy. Cerebrovasc Dis. 1999; 9(5):270–281

[32] Brandl R, Brauer RB, Maurer PC. Urgent carotid endarterectomy for stroke in evolution. Vasa. 2001; 30(2):115–121

[33] Findlay JM, Marchak BE. Reoperation for acute hemispheric stroke after carotid endarterectomy: is there any value? Neurosurgery. 2002; 50(3):486–492, discussion 492–493

[34] Tsivgoulis G, Krogias C, Georgiadis GS, et al. Safety of early endarterectomy in patients with symptomatic carotid artery stenosis: an international multicenter study. Eur J Neurol. 2014; 21(10):1251–1257, e75–e76

[35] Mori T, Kazita K, Mima T, Mori K. Balloon angioplasty for embolic total occlusion of the middle cerebral artery and ipsilateral carotid stenting in an acute stroke stage. AJNR Am J Neuroradiol. 1999; 20(8):1462–1464

[36] Anzuini A, Briguori C, Roubin GS, et al. Emergency stenting to treat neurological complications occurring after carotid endarterectomy. J Am Coll Cardiol. 2001; 37(8):2074–2079

[37] Hayashi K, Kitagawa N, Takahata H, et al. Endovascular treatment for cervical carotid artery stenosis presenting with progressing stroke: three case reports. Surg Neurol. 2002; 58(2):148–154, discussion 154

[38] Zaidat OO, Alexander MJ, Suarez JI, et al. Early carotid artery stenting and angioplasty in patients with acute ischemic stroke. Neurosurgery. 2004; 55(6):1237–1242, discussion 1242–1243

[39] Kim SH, Qureshi AI, Levy EI, Hanel RA, Siddiqui AM, Hopkins LN. Emergency stent placement for symptomatic acute carotid artery occlusion after endarterectomy. Case report. J Neurosurg. 2004; 101(1):151–153

[40] Ko JK, Choi CH, Lee SW, Lee TH. Emergency placement of stent-graft for symptomatic acute carotid artery occlusion after endarterectomy. BMJ Case Rep. 2015; 2015:bcr2014011553

[41] Paciaroni M, Inzitari D, Agnelli G, et al. Intravenous thrombolysis or endovascular therapy for acute ischemic stroke associated with cervical internal carotid artery occlusion: the ICARO-3 study. J Neurol. 2015; 262(2):459–468

[42] Son S, Choi DS, Oh MK, et al. Emergency carotid artery stenting in patients with acute ischemic stroke due to occlusion or stenosis of the proximal internal carotid artery: a single-center experience. J Neurointerv Surg. 2015; 7(4):238–244

[43] Wijdicks EF, Sheth KN, Carter BS, et al; American Heart Association Stroke Council. Recommendations for the management of cerebral and cerebellar infarction with swelling: a statement for healthcare professionals from the American Heart Association/American Stroke Association. Stroke. 2014; 45(4):1222–1238

[44] Edlow JA, Newman-Toker DE, Savitz SI. Diagnosis and initial management of cerebellar infarction. Lancet Neurol. 2008; 7(10):951–964

[45] Amarenco P. The spectrum of cerebellar infarctions. Neurology. 1991; 41(7):973–979

[46] Kase CS, Norrving B, Levine SR, et al. Cerebellar infarction. Clinical and anatomic observations in 66 cases. Stroke. 1993; 24(1):76–83

[47] Jensen MB, St Louis EK. Management of acute cerebellar stroke. Arch Neurol. 2005; 62(4):537–544

[48] Caplan LR. Cerebellar infarcts: key features. Rev Neurol Dis. 2005; 2(2):51–60

[49] Michel P, Arnold M, Hungerbühler HJ, et al; Swiss Working Group of Cerebrovascular Diseases with the Swiss Society of Neurosurgery and the Swiss Society of Intensive Care Medicine. Decompressive craniectomy for space occupying hemispheric and cerebellar ischemic strokes: Swiss recommendations. Int J Stroke. 2009; 4(3):218–223

[50] Hwang DY, Silva GS, Furie KL, Greer DM. Comparative sensitivity of computed tomography vs. magnetic resonance imaging for detecting acute posterior fossa infarct. J Emerg Med. 2012; 42(5):559–565

[51] Koh MG, Phan TG, Atkinson JL, Wijdicks EF. Neuroimaging in deteriorating patients with cerebellar infarcts and mass effect. Stroke. 2000; 31(9):2062–2067

[52] Tsitsopoulos PP, Tobieson L, Enblad P, Marklund N. Surgical treatment of patients with unilateral cerebellar infarcts: clinical outcome and prognostic factors. Acta Neurochir (Wien). 2011; 153(10):2075–2083

[53] Tchopev Z, Hiller M, Zhuo J, Betz J, Gullapalli R, Sheth KN. Prediction of poor outcome in cerebellar infarction by diffusion MRI. Neurocrit Care. 2013; 19(3):276–282

[54] Jauss M, Krieger D, Hornig C, Schramm J, Busse O. Surgical and medical management of patients with massive cerebellar infarctions: results of the German-Austrian Cerebellar Infarction Study. J Neurol. 1999; 246(4):257–264

[55] Mostofi K. Neurosurgical management of massive cerebellar infarct outcome in 53 patients. Surg Neurol Int. 2013; 4:28

[56] Raco A, Caroli E, Isidori A, Salvati M. Management of acute cerebellar infarction: one institution's experience. Neurosurgery. 2003; 53(5):1061–1065, discussion 1065–1066

[57] Kirollos RW, Tyagi AK, Ross SA, van Hille PT, Marks PV. Management of spontaneous cerebellar hematomas: a prospective treatment protocol. Neurosurgery. 2001; 49(6):1378–1386, discussion 1386–1387

[58] Kudo H, Kawaguchi T, Minami H, Kuwamura K, Miyata M, Kohmura E. Controversy of surgical treatment for severe cerebellar infarction. J Stroke Cerebrovasc Dis. 2007; 16(6):259–262

[59] Neugebauer H, Witsch J, Zweckberger K, Jüttler E. Space-occupying cerebellar infarction: complications, treatment, and outcome. Neurosurg Focus. 2013; 34(5):E8

[60] Pfefferkorn T, Eppinger U, Linn J, et al. Long-term outcome after suboccipital decompressive craniectomy for malignant cerebellar infarction. Stroke. 2009; 40(9):3045–3050

[61] Wijdicks EFM. Hemicraniotomy in massive hemispheric stroke: a stark perspective on a radical procedure. Can J Neurol Sci. 2000; 27(4):271–273

[62] Kasner SE, Demchuk AM, Berrouschot J, et al. Predictors of fatal brain edema in massive hemispheric ischemic stroke. Stroke. 2001; 32(9):2117–2123

[63] Hacke W, Schwab S, Horn M, Spranger M, De Georgia M, von Kummer R. 'Malignant' middle cerebral artery territory infarction: clinical course and prognostic signs. Arch Neurol. 1996; 53(4):309–315

[64] Wijdicks EF, Diringer MN. Middle cerebral artery territory infarction and early brain swelling: progression and effect of age on outcome. Mayo Clin Proc. 1998; 73(9):829–836

[65] Krieger DW, Demchuk AM, Kasner SE, Jauss M, Hantson L. Early clinical and radiological predictors of fatal brain swelling in ischemic stroke. Stroke. 1999; 30(2):287–292

[66] Qureshi AI, Suarez JI, Yahia AM, et al. Timing of neurologic deterioration in massive middle cerebral artery infarction: a multicenter review. Crit Care Med. 2003; 31(1):272–277

[67] Robertson SC, Lennarson P, Hasan DM, Traynelis VC. Clinical course and surgical management of massive cerebral infarction. Neurosurgery. 2004; 55(1):55–61, discussion 61–62

[68] von Kummer R, Meyding-Lamadé U, Forsting M, et al. Sensitivity and prognostic value of early CT in occlusion of the middle cerebral artery trunk. AJNR Am J Neuroradiol. 1994; 15(1):9–15, discussion 16–18

[69] Oppenheim C, Samson Y, Manaï R, et al. Prediction of malignant middle cerebral artery infarction by diffusion-weighted imaging. Stroke. 2000; 31(9):2175–2181

[70] Mori K, Aoki A, Yamamoto T, Horinaka N, Maeda M. Aggressive decompressive surgery in patients with massive hemispheric embolic cerebral infarction associated with severe brain swelling. Acta Neurochir (Wien). 2001; 143(5):483–491, discussion 491–492

[71] Qizilbash N, Lewington SL, Lopez-Arrieta JM. Corticosteroids for acute ischaemic stroke. Cochrane Database Syst Rev. 2000(2):CD000064

[72] Bereczki D, Liu M, Prado GF, Fekete I. Cochrane report: a systematic review of mannitol therapy for acute ischemic stroke and cerebral parenchymal hemorrhage. Stroke. 2000; 31(11):2719–2722

[73] Smith ER, Carter BS, Ogilvy CS. Proposed use of prophylactic decompressive craniectomy in poor-grade aneurysmal subarachnoid patients presenting with associated large sylvian hematomas. Neurosurgery. 2002; 51:117–124,– discussion 124

[74] Lanzino DJ, Lanzino G. Decompressive craniectomy for space-occupying supratentorial infarction: rationale, indications, and outcome. Neurosurg Focus. 2000; 8(5):e3

[75] Hofmeijer J, Kappelle LJ, Algra A, Amelink GJ, van Gijn J, van der Worp HB; HAMLET investigators. Surgical decompression for space-occupying cerebral infarction (the Hemicraniectomy After Middle Cerebral Artery infarction with Life-threatening Edema Trial [HAMLET]): a multicentre, open, randomised trial. Lancet Neurol. 2009; 8(4):326–333

[76] Jüttler E, Schwab S, Schmiedek P, et al; DESTINY Study Group. Decompressive Surgery for the Treatment of Malignant Infarction of the Middle Cerebral Artery (DESTINY): a randomized, controlled trial. Stroke. 2007; 38(9):2518–2525

[77] Vahedi K, Vicaut E, Mateo J, et al; DECIMAL Investigators. Sequential-design, multicenter, randomized, controlled trial of early decompressive craniectomy in malignant middle cerebral artery infarction (DECIMAL Trial). Stroke. 2007; 38(9):2506–2517

[78] Vahedi K, Hofmeijer J, Juettler E, et al; DECIMAL, DESTINY, and HAMLET investigators. Early decompressive surgery in malignant infarction of the middle cerebral artery: a pooled analysis of three randomised controlled trials. Lancet Neurol. 2007; 6(3):215–222

[79] Frank JI, Schumm LP, Wroblewski K, et al; HeADDFIRST Trialists. Hemicraniectomy and durotomy upon deterioration from infarction-related swelling trial: randomized pilot clinical trial. Stroke. 2014; 45(3):781–787

[80] Jüttler E, Unterberg A, Woitzik J, et al; DESTINY II Investigators. Hemicraniectomy in older patients with extensive middle-cerebral-artery stroke. N Engl J Med. 2014; 370(12):1091–1100

[81] Zhao J, Su YY, Zhang Y, et al. Decompressive hemicraniectomy in malignant middle cerebral artery infarct: a randomized controlled trial enrolling patients up to 80 years old. Neurocrit Care. 2012; 17(2):161–171

[82] Cruz-Flores S, Berge E, Whittle IR. Surgical decompression for cerebral oedema in acute ischaemic stroke. Cochrane Database Syst Rev. 2012; 1):CD003435

[83] Back L, Nagaraja V, Kapur A, Eslick GD. Role of decompressive hemicraniectomy in extensive middle cerebral artery strokes: a meta-analysis of randomised trials. Intern Med J. 2015; 45(7):711–717

[84] Neugebauer H, Kollmar R, Niesen WD, et al; DEPTH-SOS Study Group. IGNITE Study Group. DEcompressive surgery Plus hypoTHermia for Space-Occupying Stroke (DEPTH-SOS): a protocol of a multicenter randomized controlled clinical trial and a literature review. Int J Stroke. 2013; 8(5):383–387

[85] Jeong HY, Chang JY, Yum KS, et al. Extended use of hypothermia in elderly patients with malignant cerebral edema as an alternative to hemicraniectomy. J Stroke. 2016; 18(3):337–343

[86] von Olnhausen O, Thorén M, von Vogelsang AC, Svensson M, Schechtmann G. Predictive factors for decompressive hemicraniectomy in malignant middle cerebral artery infarction. Acta Neurochir (Wien). 2016; 158(5):865–872, discussion 873

[87] Kastrau F, Wolter M, Huber W, Block F. Recovery from aphasia after hemicraniectomy for infarction of the speech-dominant hemisphere. Stroke. 2005; 36(4):825–829

[88] Curry WT, Jr, Sethi MK, Ogilvy CS, Carter BS. Factors associated with outcome after hemicraniectomy for large middle cerebral artery territory infarction. Neurosurgery. 2005; 56(4):681–692, discussion 681–692

[89] Holtkamp M, Buchheim K, Unterberg A, et al. Hemicraniectomy in elderly patients with space occupying media infarction: improved survival but poor functional outcome. J Neurol Neurosurg Psychiatry. 2001; 70(2):226–228

[90] Kilincer C, Asil T, Utku U, et al. Factors affecting the outcome of decompressive craniectomy for large hemispheric infarctions: a prospective cohort study. Acta Neurochir (Wien). 2005; 147(6):587–594, discussion 594

[91] Leonhardt G, Wilhelm H, Doerfler A, et al. Clinical outcome and neuropsychological deficits after right decompressive hemicraniectomy in MCA infarction. J Neurol. 2002; 249(10):1433–1440

[92] Debiais S, Gaudron-Assor M, Sevin-Allouet M, de Toffol B, Lemoine M, Bonnaud I. Ethical considerations for craniectomy in malignant middle cerebral artery infarction: should we still deny our patient a life-saving procedure? Int J Stroke. 2015; 10(7):E71

[93] Honeybul S, Ho KM, Gillett G. Outcome following decompressive hemicraniectomy for malignant cerebral infarction: ethical considerations. Stroke. 2015; 46(9):2695–2698

[94] Rahme R, Zuccarello M, Kleindorfer D, Adeoye OM, Ringer AJ. Decompressive hemicraniectomy for malignant middle cerebral artery territory infarction: is life worth living? J Neurosurg. 2012; 117(4):749–754

[95] Honeybul S, Ho KM, Blacker DW. ORACLE Stroke Study: opinion regarding acceptable outcome following decompressive hemicraniectomy for ischemic stroke. Neurosurgery. 2016; 79(2):231–236

[96] Neugebauer H, Creutzfeldt CJ, Hemphill JC, III, Heuschmann PU, Jüttler E. DESTINY-S: attitudes of physicians toward disability and treatment in malignant MCA infarction. Neurocrit Care. 2014; 21(1):27–34

[97] Demchuk AM. Hemicraniectomy is a promising treatment in ischemic stroke. Can J Neurol Sci. 2000; 27(4):274–277

[98] Schwab S, Hacke W. Surgical decompression of patients with large middle cerebral artery infarcts is effective. Stroke. 2003; 34(9):2304–2305

[99] Kim DH, Ko SB, Cha JK, et al. Updated Korean clinical practice guidelines on decompressive surgery for malignant middle cerebral artery territory infarction. J Stroke. 2015; 17(3):369–376

13 Cerebral Venous Thrombosis

José M. Ferro and Diana Aguiar de Sousa

Abstract

Cerebral venous thrombosis (CVT) has a more diverse clinical presentation than other stroke types. The confirmation of the diagnosis of CVT relies on the demonstration of thrombi in the cerebral veins and/or sinuses by magnetic resonance imaging (MRI)/MR venography or computed tomography (CT) venography. The clinical presentation of CVT can be one of a venous infarction, an intracerebral hemorrhage, or rarely a subarachnoid hemorrhage or subdural hematoma. Head trauma and meningioma are well-known associated conditions for CVT. Diagnostics and treatment procedures (e.g., lumbar puncture, spinal anesthesia) that intentionally or accidentally pierce the dura are also risk factors for CVT, as well as insertion of central venous catheters. Some neurosurgical procedures, such as removal of meningiomas and other brain tumors, can be complicated by CVT. The prognosis of CVT is in general favorable, with about 4% mortality in the acute phase and a total of 15% of the patients remaining dependent or dying. The fundamental treatment in the acute phase is anticoagulation. In patients in severe condition on admission or who deteriorate despite anticoagulation, local thrombolysis or thrombectomy is an option. Decompressive hemicraniectomy is lifesaving in patients with large intracranial venous infarcts or hemorrhages and impending herniation. After the acute phase, patients should remain anticoagulated for a variable period of time, depending on their inherent thrombotic risk. A few patients develop a chronic syndrome of intracranial hypertension. In these patients, acetazolamide, repeated lumbar punctures, and eventually a lumboperitoneal drain or ventriculoperitoneal shunt may be used to ameliorate the symptoms. Exceptionally, a dural fistula may be a late complication of a permanent dural sinus occlusion.

Keywords: anticoagulation, brain lesion, cerebral venous thrombosis, decompressive surgery, differential diagnosis, intracerebral hemorrhage, subarachnoid hemorrhage

13.1 Introduction

Cerebral venous thrombosis (CVT) is a venous thrombosis of the dural sinus or cerebral veins. Similar to splanchnic, pelvic, and retinal venous thrombosis, CVT is considered a venous thrombosis at an unusual site,[1] much less frequent than deep venous thrombosis of the lower extremities. CVT is also less frequent than ischemic stroke or intracerebral hemorrhage (ICH). Nevertheless, its incidence is comparable to that of acute bacterial meningitis in adults.[2] CVT is more frequent in developing countries, with their attendant high pregnancy rates. CVT affects predominantly neonates, children, young adults, and females. Because of increased awareness for CVT and the use of magnetic resonance imaging (MRI) for investigating patients with acute and subacute headaches and new-onset seizures, CVT is now being diagnosed with higher frequency.

CVT has a more diverse clinical presentation than other stroke types and rarely presents as a stroke syndrome. The most frequent clinical presentations of CVT are isolated headache, intracranial hypertension syndrome, seizures, a focal lobar syndrome, and encephalopathy. The confirmation of the diagnosis of CVT relies on the demonstration of thrombi in the cerebral veins and/or sinuses by MRI/MR venography or computed tomography (CT) venography. There are many risk factors for CVT, which can be grouped in permanent or transient categories. The most frequent permanent risk factors are genetic prothrombotic disorders, diseases associated with a prothrombotic state, such as antiphospholipid syndrome, nephrotic syndrome, and cancer. Examples of transient risk factors are oral contraceptives, puerperium and pregnancy, infections, in particular mastoiditis, otitis, and sinusitis, and drugs with a prothrombotic action. The prognosis of CVT is in general favorable, with about 4% mortality in the acute phase and a total of 15% of the patients remaining dependent or dying. The fundamental treatment in the acute phase is anticoagulation with either low-molecular-weight or unfractionated heparin. In patients in severe condition on admission or who deteriorate despite anticoagulation, local thrombolysis or thrombectomy is an option. Decompressive hemicraniectomy is lifesaving in patients with large intracranial venous infarcts or hemorrhages. After the acute phase, patients should remain anticoagulated for a variable period of time, depending on their inherent thrombotic risk. CVT patients may experience recurrent seizures. Prophylaxis with antiepileptics is recommended after the first seizures, in particular in those with hemispheric hemorrhagic lesions. A few patients develop a chronic syndrome of intracranial hypertension. In these patients, acetazolamide, repeated lumbar punctures, and eventually a lumboperitoneal drain or ventriculoperitoneal shunt may be used to ameliorate the symptoms. If despite these measures, vision is threatened, optic nerve fenestration can prevent permanent visual loss, which is fortunately very rare nowadays. Exceptionally, a dural fistula may be a late complication of a permanent dural sinus occlusion. For reviews on CVT, see references.[3,4,5]

13.2 Cerebral Venous Thrombosis and the Neurosurgeon

The neurosurgeon can have an encounter with a patient with CVT in four different scenarios:

1. The clinical presentation of CVT mimics a neurosurgical condition (e.g., neoplasm).
2. A neurosurgical disease is a risk factor for CVT (e.g., head trauma, meningioma).
3. A neurosurgical procedure is a risk factor for CVT (e.g., parasagittal meningioma surgery).
4. CVT requires neurosurgical treatment (e.g., hematoma evacuation, decompressive hemicraniectomy, shunting).

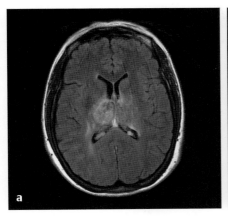
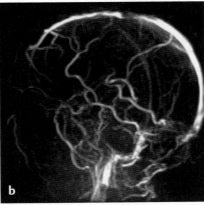

Fig. 13.1 A 39-year-old woman with progressive behavioral disturbances and impaired consciousness. **(a)** Axial fluid-attenuated inversion recovery (FLAIR) magnetic resonance (MR) image revealed a heterogeneous bilateral thalamic lesion, more prominent in the right side. **(b)** MR angiogram (time-of-flight) showed venous thrombosis with involvement of the deep system (internal cerebral vein, straight sinus, vein of Galen).

13.3 Cerebral Venous Thrombosis Mimicking a Neurosurgical Condition

The diagnosis of CVT can be a challenge. CVT patients usually show symptoms and signs related to increased intracranial pressure and/or focal brain injury. Some CVT clinical presentations may mimic neurosurgical conditions. Venous infarction and ICH associated with CVT are often difficult to differentiate from other types of stroke or neoplastic disorders. Because of their "malignant" appearance, lesions associated with CVT with mass effect and abnormal enhancement in CT or MRI may be unnecessarily biopsied.

13.3.1 Venous Infarction

CVT patients with venous infarction represent an intermediate group in clinical severity between patients without parenchymal lesions and those with ICH.[6] Most of the CVT patients with venous infarction present with a focal syndrome, defined as focal deficits (e.g., motor weakness, sensory deficit, aphasia, hemianopia) and/or partial seizures.[7,8] Bilateral motor signs may be noted in patients with bilateral parasagittal lesions due to sagittal sinus thrombosis or bithalamic involvement associated with thrombosis of the deep venous system (▶ Fig. 13.1a, b). Almost half of the patients with CVT and nonhemorrhagic brain lesion have seizures.[6] A subacute encephalopathy syndrome is also the presenting feature of CVT in some cases, when a decrease in mental status, progressive confusion, and impaired consciousness, with or without seizures, are major symptoms. Mental status disturbances are a presenting symptom in about 30% of the patients with venous infarction.[6] The progression of these symptoms is extremely variable, and neither the time of progression, which can range from a few hours to several days, nor the severity of the symptoms can distinguish CVT from other conditions. Only about one third of the CVT patients with nonhemorrhagic lesions have an acute onset, defined as the development of the full clinical picture in less than 4 days.[6]

The confirmation of the diagnosis of CVT is based in neuroimaging. Whenever CVT is clinically suspected, prompt investigation by noninvasive imaging should be done, as the positive findings of intraluminal thrombus are necessary to confirm the diagnosis of CVT. Anatomical variants of normal venous anatomy may mimic sinus thrombosis, such as sinus atresia/hypoplasia, asymmetrical sinus drainage, normal sinus filling defects related to prominent arachnoid granulations, and intrasinus septa; therefore, the diagnosis cannot rely only in CT or MR angiography. The occlusive thrombus may be detected on CT as a spontaneous hyperdensity in a venous structure, called "dense triangle" in the occlusion of the superior sagittal sinus and "cord" sign in vein thrombosis. However, it is only visible in about a quarter of the patients, disappears within 1 or 2 weeks, and is not specific, as it may be also seen in patients with high hematocrit, dehydration, or a subjacent subarachnoid or subdural hemorrhage.[9,10] MRI is very useful for detecting the thrombus in CVT. The signal also varies over time, and in the acute phase, because T1 and T2 can appear falsely reassuring, the use of sequences particularly sensitive to the susceptibility effects of iron atoms contained within hemosiderin (T2*-weighted gradient recalled echo or susceptibility-weighted imaging [SWI]) is recommended to improve diagnostic accuracy. Because cortical veins are variable in number and location and only the largest veins are detectable on MR or CT venography, the diagnosis in cases of isolated cortical vein thrombosis rests on the demonstration of a thrombosed cortical vein (▶ Fig. 13.2a, b). This should be evident in sequences identifying paramagnetic blood products (T2*/SWI) as a hypointense tubular sign.[11] Isolated cortical vein thrombosis is usually not associated with headache or other signs of increased intracranial hypertension but often results in brain parenchymal lesion,[12] leading to focal deficits and/or seizures.

Contrast injection in CT or MRI scans may reveal also the "empty delta sign," which represents the lumen of the thrombosed sinus with enhancement of its walls due to collateral circulation. This sign can disappear in chronic stages with the enhancement of the organized clot. False positives are also described, usually associated with a high or asymmetric bifurcation of the torcular herophili.[10] The high diagnostic accuracy associated with the current use of different sequences in MRI, particularly T2*/SWI, makes the need for conventional angiography nowadays very rare in the setting of CVT. The typical findings in direct cerebral venography include the failure of sinus appearance due to occlusion; venous congestion with dilated cortical, scalp, or facial veins; enlargement of typically diminutive veins from collateral drainage; reversal of venous flow; and delay in cerebral venous circulation.

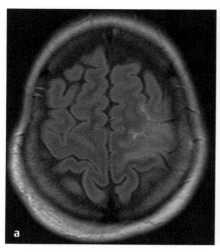
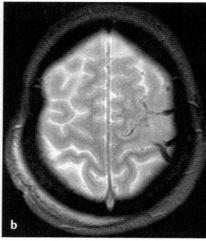

Fig. 13.2 Magnetic resonance imaging in a patient with left cortical vein thrombosis. **(b)** Cord-like hypointensities are evident in T2* gradient recalled echo (GRE) image. **(a, b)** The associated parenchymal brain lesion and a small convexity subarachnoid hemorrhage are also evident: as **(a)** sulcal hyperintensity in fluid-attenuated inversion recovery [FLAIR] image and **(b)** hypointensity in T2* GRE image.

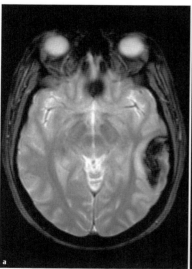
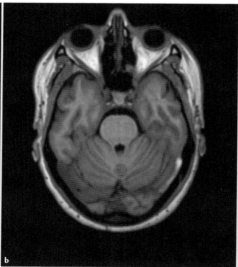

Fig. 13.3 (a) Temporal–parietal hemorrhagic venous infarct shown in T2* gradient recalled echo (GRE) image. **(b)** A hyperintense thrombus in the left transverse sinus is shown in the T1-weighted axial image.

Parenchymal changes associated with CVT share some characteristic patterns that may help in the differential diagnosis. The presence of an ischemic lesion that crosses usual arterial boundaries and often has an hemorrhagic component, particularly if it is close to a venous sinus, should raise suspicion of CVT. Lesions associated with thrombosis of specific sinus show a regional distribution, such as brain parenchymal changes in frontal, parietal, and occipital lobes usually corresponding to superior sagittal sinus thrombosis, temporal lobe parenchymal changes corresponding to transverse and sigmoid sinus thrombosis (▶Fig. 13.3a, b), and deep parenchymal abnormalities, including thalamic lesions, corresponding to thrombosis of the internal cerebral veins, vein of Galen, or straight sinus (▶Fig. 13.1a, b). Other features that differentiate venous lesions from other types of stroke are the early demarcation in CT and the presence of abnormal swelling, which is already evident within hours of onset of focal signs and is disproportionate to size of infarct or goes beyond the infarct boundaries (▶Table 13.1). The presence of bilateral parenchymal changes, which happens in about one third of the patients with nonhemorrhagic lesions associated with CVT, is also

suggestive.[6] Venous infarction rarely occurs in the posterior fossa because the infratentorial region has much more venous collateral circulation than the supratentorial. In a large cohort of CVT patients, only 8% of the nonhemorrhagic lesions were infratentorial.[6] MRI is more accurate than CT in the detection of brain lesions associated with CVT. Diffusion-weighted techniques allow further classification of the abnormalities as vasogenic edema or cytotoxic edema. An altered enhancement pattern suggestive of collateral flow or of venous congestion may be seen, including in the tentorium and falx.

13.3.2 Intracerebral Hemorrhage

Identification of CVT among patients with ICH is critical, given its potential treatment implications. Approximately 40% of CVT patients develop ICH.[8] A high index of clinical suspicion is needed to avoid misdiagnosing other conditions that may mimic ICH related to CVT, such as traumatic parenchymal contusions,[13,14,15] tumors,[16] and abscesses.[17]

Table 13.1 Imaging features suggestive of possible venous infarction/hemorrhage

Site	Not strictly arterial territory
	May involve both hemispheres
	Mainly supratentorial
	May be bilateral
Swelling	Early
	Disproportionate to size of infarct
	Beyond the infarct boundaries
Hemorrhage	Often present
	Spreading from the center to the periphery
	Finger-like appearance
Contrast enhancement	Present

Adapted from Bakaç and Warlaw 1997.[22]

There are some features suggestive of CVT as a cause of ICH, including history of prodromal headache, bilateral hemorrhages, combination of hemorrhagic and nonhemorrhagic lesions, and clinical evidence of a hypercoagulable state.[18] Presentation of CVT with ICH is usually associated with a more severe clinical picture. These patients are more likely to have an acute onset, coma, focal signs (aphasia, paresis), and seizures.[19,20] Headache alone, however, is not predictive of the presence of hemorrhage amongst patients with CVT.[21] Patients with CVT and ICH tend to be older and have higher blood pressure at admission.[20] CVT with ICH is associated with multiple sinus and vein involvement[20] and with a higher burden of brain lesions.[19] The distribution of blood in venous infarctions with a hemorrhagic component may also contribute to the diagnosis. Hemorrhage in venous infarcts tends to spread from the center to the periphery, sometimes with a finger-like appearance, whereas in arterial infarcts it is usually at the edges.[22] Besides, hemorrhages usually expand to the cortical surface, which may help in differentiating from the typical localization of parenchymal hypertensive bleeds (▶Table 13.1). As previously described for the nonhemorrhagic lesions associated with CVT, the lesion location is an important consideration in estimating the likelihood of CVT, as lesions associated with thrombosis of specific sinus show a regional distribution related to the known drainage territories of the involved venous structure. A highly suggestive pattern of ICH associated with CVT is the finding of bilateral parasagittal hemorrhages in combined superior sagittal sinus and cortical vein thrombosis or of temporal lobe hemorrhages in lateral sinus thrombosis (▶Fig. 13.3a, b).

ICH in the context of CVT is associated with poorer outcomes, with a higher proportion of patients experiencing neurologic worsening or dying in the acute phase and a worse functional outcome in survivors. In a large cohort of CVT patients with early ICH, older age, male gender, motor deficit, and involvement of the deep cerebral venous system or the right lateral sinus were predictors of death or dependency in the follow-up.[19]

As for all other CVT presentations, anticoagulation therapy is the recommended treatment for patients with ICH related to CVT. Endovascular treatments may be considered in patients with neurologic deterioration despite best medical treatment.

13.3.3 Subarachnoid Hemorrhage

Diffuse or convexity subarachnoid hemorrhage (SAH), isolated or in association with parenchymal brain lesions, is an uncommon presentation of CVT (1%).[8] The prevalence may be higher with the use of modern MRI standardized protocols.[23,24] The typical location of the SAH related to CVT is the cerebral convexity adjacent to a thrombosed sinus or vein, sparing the basal cisterns and skull base[23,24] (▶Fig. 13.2a, b), but more diffuse patterns mimicking aneurysmal rupture have been reported.[25]

Table 13.2 Summary of case series (> 5 operated patients) of decompressive surgery for cerebral venous thrombosis

Authors	Year	Country	No. operated patients	Median months of follow-up	Outcome				
					mRS = 0–1	MRS = 0–2	mRS = 3	mRS = 4–5	Death
Théaudin et al103	2010	France	8	23.1	6 (75%)	6 (75%)	1 (12.5%)	0	1 (12.5%)
Lath et al108	2010	India	11	7.4	7 (63.6%)	8 (72.7%)	0 (0%)	0 (0%)	3 (27.3%)
Ferro et al102	2011	Multicenter	69	12	26 (37.7%)	39 (56.5%)	15 (21.7%)	4 (5.8%)	11 (15.9%)
Systematic review102			31	12	14 (45.2%)	18 (58.1%)	8 (25.8%)	1 (3.2%)	4 (12.9%)
Registry			38	14.5	12 (31.6%)	21 (55.3%)	7 (18.4%)	3 (7.9%)	7 (18.4%)
Ferro et al104	2011	Multicenter	8	16	4 (50%)	4 (50%)	3 (37.5%)	1 (12.5%)	0 (0%)
Mohindra et al109	2011	India	13	35		5 (38.5%	6 (46.2%)		2 (15.4%)
Vivakaran et al110	2011	India	34	11.7	15 (44.1%)	26 (76.5%)	2 (5.9%)	0 (0%)	6 (17.6%)
Zuurbier et al111	2012	Netherlands	10	12	5 (50%)	6 (60%)	1 (10%)	1 (10%)	2 (20%)
Aaron et al112	2013	India	44	25.5		27 (61.4%)	1 (2.3%)	1 (2.3%)	9 (20.5%)
Raza et al113	2014	Pakistan	7	18		4 (22.2%)		1 (5.6%)	2 (11.1%)

Abbreviation: mRS, modified Rankin Scale score.

The exact cause of SAH associated with CVT is unknown, but it was hypothesized that it can be due to dilatation and rupture of the fragile cortical veins due to the increased venous pressure.[26,27] Alternatively, in cases with concomitant venous hemorrhagic infarction, SAH may be associated with secondary rupture of the hematoma into the subarachnoid space.

In a review of 26 case reports of SAH related to CVT, about two thirds of the patients had acute-onset severe headaches, one third presented with neck stiffness, and one third with seizures.[23] In a series of 22 patients, thunderclap headache was only reported in three patients. The involvement of the vein of Labbé together with the lateral sinus or of the frontal veins and the superior sagittal sinus were the most frequent patterns of venous thrombosis found in these patients.[24] MRI is more sensitive than CT, showing the typical finding of subarachnoid hyperintensity on fluid-attenuated inversion recovery (FLAIR) images. But the diagnosis is still challenging, particularly in patients with isolated cortical vein thrombosis.[24,28,29] Recent series suggest that most patients with CVT and SAH have associated cortical veins thrombosis, with or without sinus thrombosis.[11,28] Successful treatment with anticoagulation in cases of CVT with associated SAH has been reported in several cases and small series[26,28,30]

13.3.4 Subdural Hematoma

The earliest report of subdural hematoma (SDH) complicating CVT was published by Bucy and Lesemann in 1942.[31] Since then, several reports and some small case series of SDH in patients with CVT have been published.[32,33] In some reports, the causal association of CVT with SDH is controversial.[34,35] Intracranial hypotension may also be a confounding condition, as it is a risk factor for both CVT and SDH.[36] Nevertheless, this association was well established in several cases, being hypothesized that the SDH can be caused by rupture of small vessels due to the venous obstruction caused by thrombosis. Recurrence of the SDH after its successful treatment in patients in whom the underlying CVT is not recognized also supports this causal relationship.[32] Management of patients with SDH complicating CVT is complex because of the relative contraindications for anticoagulation in patients with symptomatic SDH, particularly if a surgical intervention is needed. Successful thrombectomy for the treatment of CVT in this setting was reported.[32]

13.4 Neurosurgical Diseases as a Risk Factor for Cerebral Venous Thrombosis

13.4.1 Head Trauma

The first descriptions of traumatic CVT were from soldiers wounded during World Wars I and II by tangential gunshots to the skull vertex. Some, but not all, patients had a depressed skull fracture. There was injury to the parietal lacunae, which receive the rolandic veins, leading to their thrombosis, which then propagated to the superior sagittal sinus and eventually to other cortical veins, causing a venous infarct. Patients had a unilateral or bilateral predominantly crural hemiparesis with immediate hypertonus, with loss of cortical sensation on the leg and foot and occasionally seizure and bladder incontinence.[37,38,39] CVT can also occur after closed head trauma.[40,41] In recent times, most cases of posttraumatic CVT are due to traffic accidents. In children, physical abuse should be suspected. Fractures over the dural sinus may predispose patients to CVT after blunt head trauma. In fact, more than 10% of skull fractures involve venous sinus.[42] CVT is a cause of secondary late neurologic deterioration after closed head trauma and is associated with uncontrollable intracranial hypertension and increased mortality. Several authors recommend a CT venogram as part of the initial trauma work-up,[42,43] as the frequency of CVT after head trauma in a series of patients examined with CT venography was 22%.[42,43] Anticoagulation can be safely used in the treatment of CVT associated with head trauma.[44,45]

13.4.2 Neoplasms

Meningiomas,[46,47] meningeomatosis,[48] and neoplasms of the meninges of the skull (sarcoma, Ewing's sarcoma, plasmocytoma, metastasis)[39] may cause direct tumoral thrombosis[49] or compression with subsequent thrombosis of the cortical veins or dural sinus.[50] Because the obstruction takes place slowly, there is time to develop collateral venous pathways, including dilated scalp veins, which can be easily visible. Individuals with brain tumors also have an increased risk of venous thromboembolism. The risk is higher in meningiomas.[51,52] Besides clinical factors such as hemiparesis and operating times, there is a subclinical prothrombotic state related to the release of brain-derived tissue factor, which may cause chronic, low-grade disseminated intravascular coagulation.[53]

13.4.3 Other Neurosurgical Conditions

Other neurosurgical conditions that have been associated with CVT are arteriovenous malformations and dural fistulae.[8,39]

13.5 Neurosurgical and Related Procedures as a Risk Factor for Cerebral Venous Thrombosis

In general, the diagnostic or therapeutic procedures that have been associated with CVT produce either a mechanical injury or a change of pressure on the dural sinus, cerebral veins, or meninges, or induce a transient prothrombotic state.

13.5.1 Lumbar Puncture, Epidural Anesthesia, and Related Procedures

Examination of the cerebrospinal fluid (CSF) by lumbar puncture (LP) is often included in the work-up of CVT patients to rule out/confirm meningitis or other intracranial infection.[4] There is clear evidence from large observational studies that LP can be safely performed in patients with acute CVT, as performing this diagnostic procedure is not associated with clinical worsening or unfavorable outcome.[54] On the other hand, it is well recognized that CVT is a possible, albeit rare, complication of diagnostic LP.[55] LP causes a craniospinal negative pressure gradient, a downward displacement of the brain, which eventually may cause traction on the sinus and bridging veins. A transcranial Doppler study performed before and after LP demonstrated that LP induces a decrease of 47% of the mean venous blood flow velocities in the straight sinus. This decrease in venous flow velocity is significant immediately at the end and also more than 6 hours after LP.[56] After LP, CVT (and also SDH) should be suspected if there is a changing pattern of post-LP headache. Post-LP headache losses its postural component, is not relieved by recumbence, and becomes constant. In this circumstance, neuroimaging should be performed to rule out CVT.[57]

CVT has been reported after diagnostic and therapeutic LP. Examples of the later are intrathecal[58] or epidural (with accidental dural puncture) corticosteroid infiltration for lumbar radicular pain.[59]

Spinal CVT has also been described after myelography with iopamidol,[60] after placement of a lumbar drain after spinal surgery,[61] and after epidural blood patch.[62,63]

Rarely, CVT has also been reported after epidural anesthesia, possibly due to accidental puncture of the dura. Over an 8-year period, three cases of CVT were diagnosed among 3,500 epidurals performed each year.[63] In most cases, the headache is initially a typical post-LP low-CSF-pressure headache.[64] The headache then changes its characteristics, becoming constant and severe and not improving with horizontal position. In some patients, drowsiness, seizures, or focal signs develop. In one report, CVT manifested as a SAH.[65] In several cases, besides epidural anesthesia, there were also other risk factors identified for CVT.[62,66]

13.5.2 Procedures on the Dural Sinus and Veins

Placement of diagnostic or therapeutic catheters in the dural sinuses or in the jugular or neighboring veins can produce CVT. Thrombosis begins at the tip of the cannula or at the local site of insertion and propagates through the vein. The first cases were reported in the 1980s following the insertion of long-term cannulas or catheters for administration of fluids, parenteral nutrition, and medications.[39]

The majority of these cases occurred after placement of a catheter in the jugular vein, but CVT has also been reported after implanted venous catheters in the brachial and subclavian veins[67] or the superior vena cava. Some of the patients had other risk factors for CVT.[68,69,70] Internal jugular and dural sinus thrombosis is one of the potential complications of jugular stenting.[71,72] Radical surgery of neck tumors and jugular ligation can also be complicated by CVT.

13.5.3 Neurosurgery

Neurosurgeons are well aware of the possibility of postoperative CVT after suboccipital,[73] transpetrosal,[73] and transcallosal[74] approaches. Nakase et al[75] reports an incidence of 0.3% (eight cases) of symptomatic CVT in patients who underwent neurosurgical interventions. Neurosurgery was performed for meningioma, acoustic neuroma, metastasis, cavernoma, dural fistulae, and trigeminal neuralgia. Ligation and division of the

anterior third of the superior sagittal sinus commonly used to approach the anterior fossa may cause sinus thrombosis with bifrontal venous infarcts.[76] Postoperative CVT can be divided into acute and chronic.[77] The acute form manifests during surgery and is in general quite severe, causing brain edema and venous infarcts. It is caused mainly by damage or ligation of the petrosal vein. The chronic form is milder, manifests one or a few days after surgery as headache, seizure, or focal deficits and is due to damage or sacrifice of the bridging cortical veins. Some patients may have previous thrombotic venous events and acquired (e.g., antiphospholipid syndrome) or genetic thrombophilia.[78]

Surgery of meningiomas has a 2 to 3% risk of CVT. The risk is higher (7%) in parasagittal meningiomas invading the superior sagittal sinus.[79] Besides location (parasagittal, convexity, falx), other risk factors for CVT are tumor size and perilesional edema. To prevent venous infarction, it is essential to maintain the intervening arachnoid plane as much as possible. The risk of CVT is reduced if an extended bifrontal surgical approach is used and if manipulation of the vascular structures is avoided.[79,80]

Lateral sinus thrombosis, most often asymptomatic, can follow posterior fossa surgery. Risk factors for CVT are history of deep venous thrombosis, oral contraceptives, midline surgical approach, and surgical exposure of the sinus.[81]

Two cases of CVT during and after placement of a ventriculoperitoneal shunt were reported,[82,83] attributed, respectively, to bipolar coagulation of a large paramedian cortical vein and compression of a cortical vein and coincidental protein C deficiency.

Two cases of CVT as a complication of spinal surgery were recently reported. One patient had a factor V Leiden mutation.[84] The other developed a CSF fistula after spinal surgery that was closed. CVT developed after closure of the fistulae.[85]

Thrombosis of the superior sagittal sinus thrombosis occurred as a complication of a craniotomy to reconstruct a complex craniofacial deformity, probably related to rapid brain expansion with obstruction of the venous outflow.[86]

Flowable topical hemostatic matrix is applied in neurosurgical procedures, to facilitate more rapid achievement of hemostasis. Iatrogenic cerebral venous occlusion induced by flowable topical hemostatic matrix occurred in 5 out of 651 infratentorial surgeries (0.8%), but in none of 3,318 supratentorial cases.[87]

CVT can also occur as a complication of the treatment of arteriovenous vascular malformations, either by endovascular or direct surgical procedures or by radiosurgery. The CVT can be asymptomatic and cause headache, seizures, or focal signs, or a massive sometimes fatal brain hemorrhage. It can also be a cause of delayed neurologic deterioration following treatment of arteriovenous malformations of the brain.

13.6 Neurosurgical Treatments for Cerebral Venous Thrombosis

13.6.1 Shunting

Shunting, either an external ventricular drain or ventriculo- or lumboperitoneal shunts, is a possible surgical intervention to decrease intracranial pressure in patients with CVT. We recently performed a systematic review of published cases of acute CVT patients treated with a shunt, excluding patients who were also treated by decompressive surgery. We found only case reports and small case series without controls. Overall, 15 patients, of whom 9 were included in the International Study on Cerebral Vein and Dural Sinus Thrombosis (ISCVT),[8] were treated with a shunt only. Types of shunting were as follows: external ventricular drain in six, ventriculoperitoneal shunt in eight, and unspecified type in one.[88] Shunted patients had a death rate of 26.7%, a death or dependency rate of 46.7%, and a severe dependency rate 13.3%. Three shunted patients had intracranial hypertension but no parenchymal lesions. They were treated with ventriculoperitoneal shunt and all regained independence.[88] Dramatic improvement after a lumboperitoneal shunt was recently reported in a case of CVT presenting as intracranial hypertension syndrome, no brain lesions or hydrocephalus, and extensive dural sinus thrombosis that was not improved with anticoagulation.[89]

A subgroup of CVT patients who could benefit from shunting are those with hydrocephalus. CVT rarely causes severe hydrocephalus.[90,91,92] However, milder forms of hydrocephalus are more frequent. Zuurbier et al[93] found hydrocephalus, defined as a bicaudate index larger than the 95th percentile for age and/or a radial width of the temporal horn 5 mm or greater, in 20% of acute CVT patients. Hydrocephalus in acute VT can be due to concomitant meningitis, intraventricular bleeding, compression, or distortion of the ventricular system by space-occupying hemispheric or cerebellar venous infarcts or hemorrhages. Hydrocephalus can also be found in thrombosis of the deep venous system because of thalamic edema and in the contralesional side in CVT complicated by large hemispherical lesions.[93] In the systematic review, four shunted patients had hydrocephalus: one became independent, two were dependent, and one died. In a recent case series of 14 CVT patients with acute hydrocephalus, only 1 patient had a shunt.[93] Despite shunting, the patient died.

When an indirect comparison is performed between the results of the systematic review of shunting in acute CVT[88] and those of a systematic review of decompressive surgery using the same methodology (see next section), the efficacy of shunting alone is inferior both for preventing death (38% deaths vs. 16%) and severe disability (25% vs. 6%). Therefore, shunting alone (without other surgical treatment) in patients with acute CVT and impending brain herniation due to parenchymal lesions should not be used because it does not prevent death. The efficacy of shunting to prevent death or improve outcome for patients with acute or recent CVT with symptomatic intracranial hypertension and no brain lesions or with hydrocephalus is uncertain.

A few patients who suffered a CVT developed a sustained clinical picture of intracranial hypertension with severe headaches or threatened vision. Management of these cases is similar to patients with idiopathic intracranial hypertension and includes weight controls, acetazolamide and other diuretics, topiramate, and repeated LPs.[94,95] In patients who do not improve with these interventions or have decreased visual acuity or increasing visual field defects, the consensus is that shunting is an option.[94,95] Either ventriculoperitoneal or lumboperitoneal shunts can be used. There are no randomized controlled studies comparing these two types of shunting. Descriptive series show that failure rates are higher for

ventriculoperitoneal shunts but revision rates are higher for lumboperitoneal shunts.[94] Stenting of the transverse sinus is an option in patients with bilateral transverse sinus stenosis and refractory symptoms and signs of intracranial hypertension who cannot undergo or have failed shunting. Both shunting and stenting in CVT patients are supported only by successful case reports and small case series.

13.6.2 Hematoma Evacuation and Decompressive Hemicraniectomy

Although most of the patients with CVT[8] have a favorable outcome, a few (4%)[96] may die in the acute phase. The main cause of death in acute CT is herniation due to unilateral mass effect produced by large edematous or hemorrhagic venous infarction. Fatal herniation can also be caused by multiple venous infarcts or bilateral massive brain edema.[96] Several recent randomized controlled trials[97,98,99] demonstrated that in malignant middle cerebral infarcts, decompressive hemicraniectomy reduces mortality and increases the number of patients with a favorable functional outcome (Fig 13.4).

The first decompressive hemicraniectomies for large space-occupying venous hemorrhagic infarcts were performed in the late 1990s.[100,101] The experience with decompressive surgery (hematoma evacuation or hemicraniectomy) in CVT is still limited. We recently upgraded our 2011 systematic review[102] and found only observational studies. Studies include case reports (39 patients), case series (166 patients), two systematic reviews, and two nonrandomized controlled studies (▶Table 13.2).

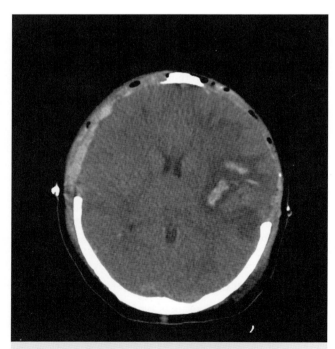

Fig. 13.4 Noncontrast computer tomography shows bilateral decompressive craniectomy in a young woman with extensive venous sinus thrombosis associated with bilateral parenchymal lesions (venous infarction and hemorrhage).

In observational studies, the average death rate among CVT patients treated with decompressive surgery (hemicraniectomy or hematoma evacuation) was 18.5%, the death or disability rate was 32.2%, the severe dependency rate only 3.4%, and the complete recovery rate 30.7%. The outcomes after decompressive surgery in CVT are much better than those observed in the pooled analysis of hemicraniectomy for ischemic arterial stroke, both in terms of mortality (22%), severe dependence (modified Rankin Scale score [mRS] = 4–5) (35%), and especially complete recovery (mRS = 0–1) (0%). The nonrandomized multicenter study performed in France[103] compared decompressive surgery with no surgery in 12 patients with "malignant CVT," of whom 8 were operated. All nonoperated patients died, in contrast with only one patient in the operated group ($p = 0.02$). One operated patient was alive with a mRS of 3, whereas four recovered completely. The other nonrandomized study had a "nested" design within the ISCVT cohort. The study compared patients included in ISCVT who were operated (8 patients) with three control groups of patients with parenchymal lesions > 5 cm and Glasgow Coma Scale (GCS) score < 14 (36 patients), or GCS score < 9 (9 patients), or clinical worsening attributable to mass effect and herniation (22 patients).[102,104] None of the operated patients died, whereas in the three control groups mortality rates were 19, 22, and 41%, respectively. Three operated patients had a mRS of 3, only one had a mRS of 4, and four did a complete recovery. Despite the low numbers, these figures indicate that decompressive surgery prevents death and does not result in an excess of severe disability.

In our systematic review and retrospective multicenter registry, results of decompressive surgery were similar after decompressive craniectomy, hematoma evacuation, or both interventions. Although the numbers were small, the outcome was very good for posterior fossa craniectomy, and independent survival was achieved in two patients who had bilateral cranial vault surgery. Practice did not seem to change the results of surgery significantly, as the outcomes were not influenced by the year when surgery was performed or by the number of operated patients reported. One third of the patients with bilateral fixed pupils before surgery recovered completely. Comatose patients and those with bilateral lesions were more likely to have an unfavorable outcome; nevertheless, complete recovery was observed in approximately one third of such patients. Aphasia did not influence outcome, or the interval between diagnosis and surgery.[102]

Operated patient needs close clinical and imaging monitoring. Decompressive surgery often has complications. These include seizures, sinking skin flap, paradoxical herniation, external brain tamponade, intracranial bleeding, intracranial or systemic infections, and pulmonary embolism, the frequency of which in this indication has not yet been described.

Anticoagulation has to be stopped before surgery but can be reassumed 12 hours later. There are a few case reports of combined use of endovascular thrombectomy and decompressive surgery with encouraging results. Sequential escalation of therapy in a case of fulminant CVT with intravenous heparin, local thrombolysis, and hemicraniectomy prevented death and resulted in an acceptable functional outcome (mRS = 3).[105] A good functional outcome (independence mRS = 2) resulted from the use of thrombosuction in a patient who did not improve after

decompressive hemicraniectomy.[106] Poulsen et al[107] described three patients who underwent decompressive hemicraniectomy for severe CVT causing coma, whose intracranial pressure remained elevated despite local thrombolysis/thrombectomy and neurointensive care treatment. One patient died but the other two recovered completely (mRS = 0 and 1).

The quality of evidence supporting routine use of decompressive surgery in "malignant" CVT with impending herniation is still low, but a randomized controlled trial is unlikely for ethical and feasibility reasons. Surgery saves lives and can lead to a complete recovery or produce acceptable sequels, as very few patients are left with severe dependency. This is particularly relevant considering the usual young age of CVT patients. These considerations support guideline recommendation of using decompressive surgery for patients with acute CVT and parenchymal lesion(s) with impending herniation to prevent death.[18]

All studies on decompressive surgery in CVT are retrospective. Retrospective design and publication bias may overestimate the effect of the intervention. To confirm the good results claimed by retrospective studies was the main reason that we designed and launched a prospective multicenter registry to describe the vital and functional outcomes of CVT patients treated by decompressive surgery and all complications of surgery. The second objective of the registry is to identify subgroups of CVT patients who benefit most from this surgery. The registry includes consecutive cases of CVT with parenchymal lesions treated by decompressive craniectomy or hematoma evacuation. Outcome is measured at discharge and at 6 and 12 months by an investigator not directly involved in the surgical intervention. The opinions of the patient and main caregiver concerning the results of surgery are also registered. Evaluation of cognition, mood, anxiety, quality of life, caregiver burden, and professional life is performed at 6- and 12-month follow-ups using the Mini-Mental State Examination (MMSE), Hospital Anxiety and Depression Scale (HADS), EuroQol questionnaire, Caregiver Strain Index Expanded, and Post Stroke Working Activity Questionnaires. We aim to collect 100 patients with the contribution of 80 recruiting centers. Inclusion started in January 2012; 66 centers are currently participating in the study and 32 patients are already included.

13.7 Conclusion

CVT can be challenging to diagnose; it can be misdiagnosed as a brain tumor or a SAH. Diagnostic and therapeutic procedures involving puncture of the spinal dural rarely can cause CVT, as well as some neurosurgical interventions, namely, meningioma surgery close to the dural sinus. Neurosurgeons have an important role in the treatment of severe CVT, with "malignant" large venous infarcts causing brain herniation. Decompressive surgery prevents death and often results in a complete functional recovery.

References

[1] Ageno W, Beyer-Westendorf J, Garcia DA, Lazo-Langner A, McBane RD, Paciaroni M. Guidance for the management of venous thrombosis in unusual sites. J Thromb Thrombolysis. 2016; 41(1):129–143

[2] Coutinho JM, Zuurbier SM, Aramideh M, Stam J. The incidence of cerebral venous thrombosis: a cross-sectional study. Stroke. 2012; 43(12):3375–3377

[3] Stam J. Thrombosis of the cerebral veins and sinuses. N Engl J Med. 2005; 352(17):1791–1798

[4] Bousser MG, Ferro JM. Cerebral venous thrombosis: an update. Lancet Neurol. 2007; 6(2):162–170

[5] Ferro JM, Canhão P. Cerebral venous sinus thrombosis: update on diagnosis and management. Curr Cardiol Rep. 2014; 16(9):523

[6] Ferro JM, Canhão P, Bousser MG, Stam J, Barinagarrementeria F, Stolz E; ISCVT Investigators. Cerebral venous thrombosis with nonhemorrhagic lesions: clinical correlates and prognosis. Cerebrovasc Dis. 2010; 29(5):440–445

[7] Preter M, Tzourio C, Ameri A, Bousser MG. Long-term prognosis in cerebral venous thrombosis. Follow-up of 77 patients. Stroke. 1996; 27(2):243–246

[8] Ferro JM, Canhão P, Stam J, Bousser MG, Barinagarrementeria F; ISCVT Investigators. Prognosis of cerebral vein and dural sinus thrombosis: results of the International Study on Cerebral Vein and Dural Sinus Thrombosis (ISCVT). Stroke. 2004; 35(3):664–670

[9] Virapongse C, Cazenave C, Quisling R, Sarwar M, Hunter S. The empty delta sign: frequency and significance in 76 cases of dural sinus thrombosis. Radiology. 1987; 162(3):779–785

[10] Leach JL, Fortuna RB, Jones BV, Gaskill-Shipley MF. Imaging of cerebral venous thrombosis: current techniques, spectrum of findings, and diagnostic pitfalls. Radiographics. 2006; 26(Suppl 1):S19–S41, discussion S42–S43

[11] Boukobza M, Crassard I, Bousser MG, Chabriat H. MR imaging features of isolated cortical vein thrombosis: diagnosis and follow-up. AJNR Am J Neuroradiol. 2009; 30(2):344–348

[12] Coutinho JM, Gerritsma JJ, Zuurbier SM, Stam J. Isolated cortical vein thrombosis: systematic review of case reports and case series. Stroke. 2014; 45(6):1836–1838

[13] Muthukumar N. Cerebral venous sinus thrombosis and thrombophilia presenting as pseudo-tumour syndrome following mild head injury. J Clin Neurosci. 2004; 11(8):924–927

[14] Zhao X, Rizzo A, Malek B, Fakhry S, Watson J. Basilar skull fracture: a risk factor for transverse/sigmoid venous sinus obstruction. J Neurotrauma. 2008; 25(2):104–111

[15] Krasnokutsky MV. Cerebral venous thrombosis: a potential mimic of primary traumatic brain injury in infants. AJR Am J Roentgenol. 2011; 197(3):W503–7

[16] Raizer JJ, DeAngelis LM. Cerebral sinus thrombosis diagnosed by MRI and MR venography in cancer patients. Neurology. 2000; 54(6):1222–1226

[17] Barua NU, Bradley M, Patel NR. Haemorrhagic infarction due to transverse sinus thrombosis mimicking cerebral abscesses. Annals of Neurosurgery.. 2008; 8(3):1–4

[18] Saposnik G, Barinagarrementeria F, Brown RD, Jr, et al; American Heart Association Stroke Council and the Council on Epidemiology and Prevention. Diagnosis and management of cerebral venous thrombosis: a statement for healthcare professionals from the American Heart Association/American Stroke Association. Stroke. 2011; 42(4):1158–1192

[19] Girot M, Ferro JM, Canhão P, et al; ISCVT Investigators. Predictors of outcome in patients with cerebral venous thrombosis and intracerebral hemorrhage. Stroke. 2007; 38(2):337–342

[20] Kumral E, Polat F, Uzunköprü C, Callı C, Kitiş Ö. The clinical spectrum of intracerebral hematoma, hemorrhagic infarct, non-hemorrhagic infarct, and non-lesional venous stroke in patients with cerebral sinus-venous thrombosis. Eur J Neurol. 2012; 19(4):537–543

[21] Wasay M, Kojan S, Dai AI, Bobustuc G, Sheikh Z. Headache in Cerebral Venous Thrombosis: incidence, pattern and location in 200 consecutive patients. J Headache Pain. 2010; 11(2):137–139

[22] Bakaç G, Wardlaw JM. Problems in the diagnosis of intracranial venous infarction. Neuroradiology. 1997; 39(8):566–570

[23] Benabu Y, Mark L, Daniel S, Glikstein R. Cerebral venous thrombosis presenting with subarachnoid hemorrhage. Case report and review. Am J Emerg Med. 2009; 27(1):96–106

[24] Boukobza M, Crassard I, Bousser MG, Chabriat H. Radiological findings in cerebral venous thrombosis presenting as subarachnoid hemorrhage: a series of 22 cases. Neuroradiology. 2016; 58(1):11–16

[25] Anderson B, Sabat S, Agarwal A, Thamburaj K. Diffuse subarachnoid hemorrhage secondary to cerebral venous sinus thrombosis. Pol J Radiol. 2015; 80:286–289

[26] Sztajzel R, Coeytaux A, Dehdashti AR, Delavelle J, Sinnreich M. Subarachnoid hemorrhage: a rare presentation of cerebral venous thrombosis. Headache. 2001; 41(9):889–892

[27] Kato Y, Takeda H, Furuya D, et al. Subarachnoid hemorrhage as the initial presentation of cerebral venous thrombosis. Intern Med. 2010; 49(5):467–470

[28] Chang R, Friedman DP. Isolated cortical venous thrombosis presenting as subarachnoid hemorrhage: a report of three cases. AJNR Am J Neuroradiol. 2004; 25(10):1676–1679

[29] Kim J, Huh C, Kim D, Jung C, Lee K, Kim H. Isolated cortical venous thrombosis as a mimic for cortical subarachnoid hemorrhage. World Neurosurg. 2016; 89:727.e5–727.e7

[30] Geraldes R, Sousa PR, Fonseca AC, Falcão F, Canhão P, Pinho e Melo T. Nontraumatic convexity subarachnoid hemorrhage: different etiologies and outcomes. J Stroke Cerebrovasc Dis. 2014; 23(1):e23–e30

[31] Bucy P, Lesemann F. Idiopathic recurrent thrombophlebitis—with cerebral venous thromboses and an acute subdural hematoma. JAMA. 1942; 119:402–405

[32] Akins PT, Axelrod YK, Ji C, et al. Cerebral venous sinus thrombosis complicated by subdural hematomas: case series and literature review. Surg Neurol Int. 2013; 4:85

[33] Chu K, Kang DW, Kim DE, Roh JK. Cerebral venous thrombosis associated with tentorial subdural hematoma during oxymetholone therapy. J Neurol Sci. 2001; 185(1):27–30

[34] Takamura Y, Morimoto S, Uede T, et al. Cerebral venous sinus thrombosis associated with systemic multiple hemangiomas manifesting as chronic subdural hematoma—case report. Neurol Med Chir (Tokyo). 1996; 36(9):650–653

[35] Singh S, Kumar S, Joseph M, Gnanamuthu C, Alexander M. Cerebral venous sinus thrombosis presenting as subdural haematoma. Australas Radiol. 2005; 49(2):101–103

[36] Mao YT, Dong Q, Fu JH. Delayed subdural hematoma and cerebral venous thrombosis in a patient with spontaneous intracranial hypotension. Neurol Sci. 2011; 32(5):981–983

[37] Holmes G, Sargent P. Injuries of the superior longitudinal sinus. BMJ. 1915; 2(2857):493–498

[38] Barker GB. Injuries to the superior longitudinal sinus. BMJ. 1949; 1(4616):1113–1116

[39] Bousser MG, Russel RR. Cerebral Venous Thrombosis. Vol. 33. London, UK: Saunders; 1997

[40] Hesselbrock R, Sawaya R, Tomsick T, Wadhwa S. Superior sagittal sinus thrombosis after closed head injury. Neurosurgery. 1985; 16(6):825–828

[41] Giladi O, Steinberg DM, Peleg K, et al. Head trauma is the major risk factor for cerebral sinus-vein thrombosis. Thromb Res. 2016; 137:26–29

[42] Rivkin MA, Saraiya PV, Woodrow SI. Sinovenous thrombosis associated with skull fracture in the setting of blunt head trauma. Acta Neurochir (Wien). 2014; 156(5):999–1007, discussion 1007

[43] Fujii Y, Tasaki O, Yoshiya K, et al. Evaluation of posttraumatic venous sinus occlusion with CT venography. J Trauma. 2009; 66(4):1002–1006, discussion 1006–1007

[44] Matsushige T, Nakaoka M, Kiya K, Takeda T, Kurisu K. Cerebral sinovenous thrombosis after closed head injury. J Trauma. 2009; 66(6):1599–1604

[45] Awad AW, Bhardwaj R. Acute posttraumatic pediatric cerebral venous thrombosis: case report and review of literature. Surg Neurol Int. 2014; 5:53

[46] DiMeco F, Li KW, Casali C, et al. Meningiomas invading the superior sagittal sinus: surgical experience in 108 cases. Neurosurgery. 2004; 55(6):1263–1272, discussion 1272–1274

[47] Mathiesen T, Pettersson-Segerlind J, Kihlström L, Ulfarsson E. Meningiomas engaging major venous sinuses. World Neurosurg. 2014; 81(1):116–124

[48] Acebes X, Arruga J, Acebes JJ, Majos C, Muñoz S, Valero IA. Intracranial meningiomatosis causing Foster Kennedy syndrome by unilateral optic nerve compression and blockage of the superior sagittal sinus. J Neuroophthalmol. 2009; 29(2):140–142

[49] Nadel L, Braun IF, Muizelaar JP, Laine FJ. Tumoral thrombosis of cerebral venous sinuses: preoperative diagnosis using magnetic resonance phase imaging. Surg Neurol. 1991; 35(3):189–195

[50] Wang S, Ying J, Wei L, Li S, Jing J. Guidance value of intracranial venous circulation evaluation to parasagittal meningioma operation. Int J Clin Exp Med. 2015; 8(8):13508–13515

[51] Gerber DE, Segal JB, Salhotra A, Olivi A, Grossman SA, Streiff MB. Venous thromboembolism occurs infrequently in meningioma patients receiving combined modality prophylaxis. Cancer. 2007; 109(2):300–305

[52] Sjavik K, Bartek J, Jr, Solheim O, et al. Venous thromboembolism prophylaxis in meningioma surgery—a population based comparative effectiveness study of routine mechanical prophylaxis with or without preoperative low-molecular-weight heparin. World Neurosurg. 2016; 88:320–326

[53] Sawaya R, Glas-Greenwalt P. Postoperative venous thromboembolism and brain tumors: part II. Hemostatic profile. J Neurooncol. 1992; 14(2):127–134

[54] Canhão P, Abreu LF, Ferro JM, et al; ISCVT Investigators. Safety of lumbar puncture in patients with cerebral venous thrombosis. Eur J Neurol. 2013; 20(7):1075–1080

[55] Albucher JF, Vuillemin-Azaïs C, Manelfe C, Clanet M, Guiraud-Chaumeil B, Chollet F. Cerebral thrombophlebitis in three patients with probable multiple sclerosis. Role of lumbar puncture or intravenous corticosteroid treatment. Cerebrovasc Dis. 1999; 9(5):298–303

[56] Canhão P, Batista P, Falcão F. Lumbar puncture and dural sinus thrombosis—a causal or casual association? Cerebrovasc Dis. 2005; 19(1):53–56

[57] Aidi S, Chaunu MP, Biousse V, Bousser MG. Changing pattern of headache pointing to cerebral venous thrombosis after lumbar puncture and intravenous high-dose corticosteroids. Headache. 1999; 39(8):559–564

[58] Ergan M, Hansen von Bünau F, Courthéoux P, Viader F, Prouzeau S, Marcelli C. Cerebral vein thrombosis after an intrathecal glucocorticoid injection. Rev Rhum Engl Ed. 1997; 64(7–9):513–516

[59] Milhaud D, Heroum C, Charif M, Saulnier P, Pages M, Blard JM. Dural puncture and corticotherapy as risks factors for cerebral venous sinus thrombosis. Eur J Neurol. 2000; 7(1):123–124

[60] Brugeilles H, Pénisson-Besnier I, Pasco A, Oillic P, Lejeune P, Mercier P. Cerebral venous thrombosis after myelography with iopamidol. Neuroradiology. 1996; 38(6):534–536

[61] Miglis MG, Levine DN. Intracranial venous thrombosis after placement of a lumbar drain. Neurocrit Care. 2010; 12(1):83–87

[62] Wilder-Smith E, Kothbauer-Margreiter I, Lämmle B, Sturzenegger M, Ozdoba C, Hauser SP. Dural puncture and activated protein C resistance: risk factors for cerebral venous sinus thrombosis. J Neurol Neurosurg Psychiatry. 1997; 63(3):351–356

[63] Mullane D, Tan T. Three cerebral venous sinus thromboses following inadvertent dural puncture: a case series over an eight-year period. Can J Anaesth. 2014; 61(12):1134–1135

[64] Ravindran RS, Zandstra GC. Cerebral venous thrombosis versus postlumbar puncture headache. Anesthesiology. 1989; 71(3):478–479

[65] Oz O, Akgun H, Yücel M, et al. Cerebral venous thrombosis presenting with subarachnoid hemorrhage after spinal anesthesia. Acta Neurol Belg. 2011; 111(3):237–240

[66] Kueper M, Goericke SL, Kastrup O. Cerebral venous thrombosis after epidural blood patch: coincidence or causal relation? A case report and review of the literature. Cephalalgia. 2008; 28(7):769–773

[67] Birdwell BG, Yeager R, Whitsett TL. Pseudotumor cerebri. A complication of catheter-induced subclavian vein thrombosis. Arch Intern Med. 1994; 154(7):808–811

[68] Holmes FA, Obbens EA, Griffin E, Lee YY. Cerebral venous sinus thrombosis in a patient receiving adjuvant chemotherapy for stage II breast cancer through an implanted central venous catheter. Am J Clin Oncol. 1987; 10(4):362–366

[69] Mazzoleni S, Putti MC, Simioni P, et al. Early cerebral sinovenous thrombosis in a child with acute lymphoblastic leukemia carrying the prothrombin G20210A variant: a case report and review of the literature. Blood Coagul Fibrinolysis. 2005; 16(1):43–49

[70] Souter RG, Mitchell A. Spreading cortical venous thrombosis due to infusion of hyperosmolar solution into the internal jugular vein. Br Med J (Clin Res Ed). 1982; 285(6346):935–936

[71] Thapar A, Lane TR, Pandey V, et al; Imperial College CCSVI Investigation Group. Internal jugular thrombosis post venoplasty for chronic cerebrospinal venous insufficiency. Phlebology. 2011; 26(6):254–256

[72] Burton JM, Alikhani K, Goyal M, et al. Complications in MS patients after CCSVI procedures abroad (Calgary, AB). Can J Neurol Sci. 2011; 38(5):741–746

[73] Keiper GL, Jr, Sherman JD, Tomsick TA, Tew JM, Jr. Dural sinus thrombosis and pseudotumor cerebri: unexpected complications of suboccipital craniotomy and translabyrinthine craniectomy. J Neurosurg. 1999; 91(2):192–197

[74] Garrido E, Fahs GR. Cerebral venous and sagittal sinus thrombosis after transcallosal removal of a colloid cyst of the third ventricle: case report. Neurosurgery. 1990; 26(3):540–542

[75] Nakase H, Shin Y, Nakagawa I, Kimura R, Sakaki T. Clinical features of postoperative cerebral venous infarction. Acta Neurochir (Wien). 2005; 147(6):621–626, discussion 626

[76] Salunke P, Sodhi HB, Aggarwal A, et al. Is ligation and division of anterior third of superior sagittal sinus really safe? Clin Neurol Neurosurg. 2013; 115(10):1998–2002

[77] Roberson JB, Jr, Brackmann DE, Fayad JN. Complications of venous insufficiency after neurotologic-skull base surgery. Am J Otol. 2000; 21(5):701–705

[78] Lega BC, Yoshor D. Postoperative dural sinus thrombosis in a patient in a hypercoagulable state. Case report. J Neurosurg. 2006; 105(5):772–774

[79] Raza SM, Gallia GL, Brem H, Weingart JD, Long DM, Olivi A. Perioperative and long-term outcomes from the management of parasagittal meningiomas invading the superior sagittal sinus. Neurosurgery. 2010; 67(4):885–893, discussion 893

[80] Jang WY, Jung S, Jung TY, Moon KS, Kim IY. Predictive factors related to symptomatic venous infarction after meningioma surgery. Br J Neurosurg. 2012; 26(5):705–709

[81] Apra C, Kotbi O, Turc G, et al. Presentation and management of lateral sinus thrombosis following posterior fossa surgery. J Neurosurg. 2017; 126:8–16

[82] Son WS, Park J. Cerebral venous thrombosis complicated by hemorrhagic infarction secondary to ventriculoperitoneal shunting. J Korean Neurosurg Soc. 2010; 48(4):357–359

[83] Matsubara T, Ayuzawa S, Aoki T, Ikeda G, Shiigai M, Matsumura A. Cerebral venous thrombosis after ventriculoperitoneal shunting: a case report. Neurol Med Chir (Tokyo). 2014; 54(7):554–557

[84] Yilmaz B, Eksi MS, Akakin A, Toktas ZO, Demir MK, Konya D. Cerebral venous thrombosis following spinal surgery in a patient with factor V Leiden mutation. Br J Neurosurg. 2016; 30(4):456–458

[85] Lourenço Costa B, Shamasna M, Nunes J, Magalhães F, Peliz AJ. Cerebral venous thrombosis: an unexpected complication from spinal surgery. Eur Spine J. 2014; 23(Suppl 2):253–256

[86] Ghizoni E, Raposo-Amaral CA, Mathias R, Denadai R, Raposo-Amaral CE. Superior sagittal sinus thrombosis as a treatment complication of nonsyndromic Kleeblattschädel. J Craniofac Surg. 2013; 24(6):2030–2033

[87] Singleton RH, Jankowitz BT, Wecht DA, Gardner PA. Iatrogenic cerebral venous sinus occlusion with flowable topical hemostatic matrix. J Neurosurg. 2011; 115(3):576–583

[88] Lobo S, Ferro JM, Barinagarrementeria F, Bousser MG, Canhão P, Stam J; ISCVT Investigators. Shunting in acute cerebral venous thrombosis: a systematic review. Cerebrovasc Dis. 2014; 37(1):38–42

[89] Torikoshi S, Akiyama Y. Report of dramatic improvement after a lumboperitoneal shunt procedure in a case of anticoagulation therapy-resistant cerebral venous thrombosis. J Stroke Cerebrovasc Dis. 2016; 25(2):e15–e19

[90] Stavrinou LC, Stranjalis G, Bouras T, Sakas DE. Transverse sinus thrombosis presenting with acute hydrocephalus: a case report. Headache. 2008; 48(2):290–292

[91] Mullen MT, Sansing LH, Hurst RW, Weigele JB, Polasani RS, Messé SR. Obstructive hydrocephalus from venous sinus thrombosis. Neurocrit Care. 2009; 10(3):359–362

[92] Leblebisatan G, Yiş U, Doğan M, Derundere U. Obstructive hydrocephalus resulting from cerebral venous thrombosis. J Pediatr Neurosci. 2011; 6(2):129–130

[93] Zuurbier SM, van den Berg R, Troost D, Majoie CB, Stam J, Coutinho JM. Hydrocephalus in cerebral venous thrombosis. J Neurol. 2015; 262(4):931–937

[94] Biousse V, Bruce BB, Newman NJ. Update on the pathophysiology and management of idiopathic intracranial hypertension. J Neurol Neurosurg Psychiatry. 2012; 83(5):488–494

[95] Batra R, Sinclair A. Idiopathic intracranial hypertension; research progress and emerging themes. J Neurol. 2014; 261(3):451–460

[96] Canhão P, Ferro JM, Lindgren AG, Bousser MG, Stam J, Barinagarrementeria F; ISCVT Investigators. Causes and predictors of death in cerebral venous thrombosis. Stroke. 2005; 36(8):1720–1725

[97] Vahedi K, Hofmeijer J, Juettler E, et al; DECIMAL, DESTINY, and HAMLET investigators. Early decompressive surgery in malignant infarction of the middle cerebral artery: a pooled analysis of three randomised controlled trials. Lancet Neurol. 2007; 6(3):215–222

[98] Hofmeijer J, Kappelle LJ, Algra A, Amelink GJ, van Gijn J, van der Worp HB; HAMLET investigators. Surgical decompression for space-occupying cerebral infarction (the Hemicraniectomy After Middle Cerebral Artery infarction with Life-threatening Edema Trial [HAMLET]): a multicentre, open, randomised trial. Lancet Neurol. 2009; 8(4):326–333

[99] Jüttler E, Unterberg A, Woitzik J, et al; DESTINY II Investigators. Hemicraniectomy in older patients with extensive middle-cerebral-artery stroke. N Engl J Med. 2014; 370(12):1091–1100

[100] Stefini R, Latronico N, Cornali C, Rasulo F, Bollati A. Emergent decompressive craniectomy in patients with fixed dilated pupils due to cerebral venous and dural sinus thrombosis: report of three cases. Neurosurgery. 1999; 45(3):626–629, discussion 629–630

[101] Kuroki K, Taguchi H, Sumida M, Onda J. Dural sinus thrombosis in a patient with protein S deficiency—case report. Neurol Med Chir (Tokyo). 1999; 39(13):928–931

[102] Ferro JM, Crassard I, Coutinho JM, et al; Second International Study on Cerebral Vein and Dural Sinus Thrombosis (ISCVT 2) Investigators. Decompressive surgery in cerebrovenous thrombosis: a multicenter registry and a systematic review of individual patient data. Stroke. 2011; 42(10):2825–2831

[103] Théaudin M, Crassard I, Bresson D, et al. Should decompressive surgery be performed in malignant cerebral venous thrombosis?: a series of 12 patients. Stroke. 2010; 41(4):727–731

[104] Ferro JM, Bousser MG, Canhão P, et al. A case-control study of decompressive surgery in cerebrovenous thrombosis. Cerebrovasc Dis. 2010; 29(Suppl 2):67

[105] Dohmen C, Galldiks N, Moeller-Hartmann W, Fink GR, Timmermann L. Sequential escalation of therapy in "malignant" cerebral venous and sinus thrombosis. Neurocrit Care. 2010; 12(1):98–102

[106] Coutinho JM, Hama-Amin AD, Vleggeert-Lankamp C, Reekers JA, Stam J, Wermer MJ. Decompressive hemicraniectomy followed by endovascular thrombosuction in a patient with cerebral venous thrombosis. J Neurol. 2012; 259(3):562–564

[107] Poulsen FR, Høgedal L, Stilling MV, Birkeland PF, Schultz MK, Rasmussen JN. Good clinical outcome after combined endovascular and neurosurgical treatment of cerebral venous sinus thrombosis. Dan Med J. 2013; 60(11):A4724

[108] Lath R, Kumar S, Reddy R, Boola GR, Ray A, Prabhakar S, Ranjan A. Decompressive surgery for severe cerebral venous sinus thrombosis. Neurol India. 2010; 58:392–397

[109] Mohindra S, Umredkar A, Singla N, Bal A, Gupta SK. Decompressive craniectomy for malignant cerebral oedema of cortical venous thrombosis: an analysis of 13 patients Br J Neurosurg. 2011; 25:422–429

[110] Vivakaran TT, Srinivas D, Kulkarni GB, Somanna S. The role of decompressive craniectomy in cerebral venous sinus thrombosis. J Neurosurg. 2012; 117:738–744

[111] Zuurbier SM, Coutinho JM, Majoie CB, Coert BA, van den Munckhof P, Stam J. Decompressive hemicraniectomy in severe cerebral venous thrombosis: a prospective case series. J Neurol. 2012; 259(6):1099–1105

[112] Aaron S, Alexander M, Moorthy RK, Mani S, Mathew V, Patil AK, Sivadasan A, Nair S, Joseph M, Thomas M, Prabhu K, Joseph BV, Rajshekhar V, Chacko AG. Decompressive craniectomy in cerebral venous thrombosis: a single centre experience J Neurol Neurosurg Psychiatry. 2013; 84:995–1000

[113] Raza E, Shamim MS, Wadiwala MF, Ahmed B, Kamal AK. Decompressive surgery for malignant cerebral venous sinus thrombosis: a retrospective case series from Pakistan and comparative literature review J Stroke Cerebrovasc Dis. 2014; 23:e13–22

14 Cerebral Infectious Processes

Alexa Bodman and Walter A. Hall

Abstract

The serious infectious processes encountered in neurosurgical practice require rapid identification and combined medical and surgical management. Bacterial, viral, fungal, and parasitic infections gain access to the central nervous system through hematogenous dissemination across the blood–brain barrier or by direct contiguous spread. Meningitis is common in the field of neurosurgery and was once associated with an extremely high mortality rate. Meningitis can occur after head trauma, systemic infections, and neurosurgical procedures and usually presents with distinct signs and symptoms that should be recognized before initiating treatment in order to lower neurologic morbidity and mortality. Encephalitis can be difficult to diagnose because of the variety of causative agents. Extracerebral infectious collections typically require emergent neurosurgical intervention for definitive diagnosis and treatment. Brain abscesses are usually managed surgically in the form of aspiration and drainage or through resection for diagnostic identification and to decompress neurologic tissue. Modern imaging of the central nervous system has aided in reducing the time to diagnosis and treatment in cerebral infectious processes in addition to improving the clinical outcomes for these potentially fatal conditions. An in-depth overview of each of these central nervous system infections is presented and discussed in this chapter.

Keywords: brain abscess, encephalitis, epidural abscess, meningitis, neurosurgical infections, subdural empyema

14.1 Introduction

Intracranial infections are frequently encountered by neurosurgeons, and their prompt recognition and treatment is essential. Meningitis, encephalitis, extra-axial abscesses, and brain abscesses develop once pathogens penetrate the blood–brain barrier (BBB), which can occur from hematologic spread or by direct invasion from a local infection. Identification of intracranial infections is often made by a combination of serum studies, cerebrospinal fluid (CSF) studies, and neuroimaging. After diagnosis, immediate treatment is required to minimize neurologic morbidity and mortality. This chapter focuses on the etiology, diagnosis, and both the medical and neurosurgical management of cerebral infectious processes.

14.2 Meningitis

Meningitis is a potentially life-threatening infection that requires prompt recognition and therapy. Bacterial meningitis is the most common form. The ability of a bacterium to cause an intracranial infection is determined by its virulence, the defenses of the host, and the inoculum size.[1] For each gram of tissue, roughly 100,000 bacteria are required for an infection to result.[1] Bacteria reach the meninges by either hematologic spread or from a local infection such as mastoiditis.[2] Anaerobic and gram-negative organisms can gain access to the brain through penetrating head trauma, whereas basilar skull fractures with

a CSF leak may give nasopharyngeal flora access to the central nervous system (CNS).[3] For hematologic spread, the bacteria must avoid phagocytosis to maintain bacteremia.[2] Considerable bacteremia is necessary for meningitis to develop.[4] Bacteria use several mechanisms, which may include the formation of a capsule or entering by neutrophils, to avoid the immune system while circulating in the bloodstream. In the CNS, the bacteria bind to extracellular matrix proteins. Once bound, the bacteria cross the BBB by a transcellular or paracellular process.[2] Pathogens may also enter the CNS by traveling within infected macrophages.[4] *Streptococcus pneumoniae* invades the brain parenchyma by both a transcellular and a paracellular process. This bacterium crosses the BBB through the cell by a receptor-mediated process and directly crosses the BBB by causing breakdown of endothelial cells. Once in the CNS, the bacterium replicates, during which process it releases components that cause a strong immune reaction leading to inflammation, neuronal death, and vasculitis.[2] Injury to the nervous tissue occurs from a combination of ischemia, increased intracranial pressure (ICP), apoptosis, and edema related to both the host's immune system and the bacterial toxins.[2] The CNS, isolated from the rest of the body by the BBB, has low levels of immunoglobulins and complement, which results in decreased host defenses when bacteria cross the BBB. Breaks in the BBB from trauma, tumor, inflammation, and surgery decrease the CNS's natural defenses against bacteria by allowing their entrance into the CNS.[1,3]

Meningitis is associated with a classic triad of symptoms, which includes stiff neck, fever, and altered mental status. Kernig's and Brudzinski's signs are also classic for meningitis.[3] The percentage of patients with meningitis presenting with all three symptoms of the classic triad is low; only 44% of patients in The Netherlands showed all three.[5] The most common presenting symptom is headache, followed by neck stiffness, fever, nausea, and altered mental status. Approximately one third of patients present with focal neurologic deficits. Seizures and hemiparesis can be present at initial evaluation but are uncommon.[5] At admission, older patients with meningitis are more likely to present with an abnormal neurologic examination.[6] Altered mentation, seizures, and hypotension on admission are associated with a worse clinical outcome.[7]

Initial laboratory values drawn in the evaluation of meningitis include a complete blood count (CBC) with differential, erythrocyte sedimentation rate (ESR), and C-reactive protein (CRP). Procalcitonin should also be tested, as this can be useful in differentiating between bacterial and viral meningitis in children.[8] Lumbar puncture (LP) should be performed as long as no contraindications exist, such as an intracranial mass that may lead to a herniation syndrome. CSF should be sent for protein, glucose, cell count, Gram stain, and culture and sensitivity.[3] Opening pressure on LP is often elevated to a range of 200 to 500 mm H_2O.[3,9] On cell count, white blood cells are elevated to usually greater than 100 cells/mm³. Glucose is markedly decreased, whereas the protein concentration is elevated. Gram stain identifies organisms in 60 to 90% of cases and cultures are positive in 70 to 85% of cases when CSF is sampled prior to antibiotic administration.[3,9]

Computed tomography (CT) of the head is usually not revealing—but it is usually performed in evaluating meningitis prior to LP, to evaluate for an intracranial mass.[10] Magnetic resonance imaging (MRI) is of limited use for the initial diagnosis of meningitis, with only about 50% of studies showing leptomeningeal enhancement, but it can be performed to evaluate for another underlying cause or for complications related to meningitis such as stroke, cerebritis, and venous sinus thrombosis.[10] MRI in infants with bacterial meningitis may aid in diagnosis of associated processes such as cerebritis (26%), subdural empyema (52%), infarction (43%), hydrocephalus (20%), and abscess (11%).[11] Extra-axial fluid collections can be seen in up to one third of patients with meningitis, which can represent either an effusion that will self-resolve or an empyema requiring surgical drainage.[10] Ventriculitis can also be associated with meningitis, and on MRI enhancement, thickening of the ependyma with T2 prolongation around the ventricles and fluid levels within the ventricles may be seen.[10,12]

The five most common organisms in the United States responsible for bacterial meningitis are *S. pneumoniae* (58%), group B *Streptococcus* (18%), *Neisseria meningitidis* (14%), *Haemophilus influenzae* (7%), and *Listeria monocytogenes* (3%).[13] In neonates, organisms common to the vaginal canal cause meningitis. The most common pathogens responsible for meningitis in this age group are group B *Streptococccus*, gram-negative bacteria, usually *Escherichia coli* and *L. monocytogenes*. In developing countries, *Klebsiella* spp., *Pseudomonas aeruginosa*, and *Salmonella* spp. are common causes of neonatal meningitis.[14] Human immunodeficiency virus (HIV)–infected patients are at a higher risk for developing bacterial meningitis.[15]

The incidence of meningitis in the United States has been falling since the introduction of the meningococcal (MCV) and pneumococcal (PCV) conjugate vaccines, MCV4 and PCV7, with *S. pneumoniae* falling to 0.3 cases per 100,000 people and *N. meningitidis* falling to 0.123 cases per 100,000 people in 2010.[16] This decrease in pneumococcal meningitis after the introduction of pneumococcal conjugate vaccination has also been seen in Germany.[17] PCV13, which replaced PCV7 in 2010 in the United States, has also been shown to decrease invasive pneumococcal disease.[18] Additionally, African countries have seen a decrease in *N. meningitidis* after widespread vaccination.[19] Mortality associated with pneumococcal meningitis has also fallen after the introduction of PCV7.[16] In The Netherlands, the meningococcal serogroup C conjugate vaccine showed a 99% decline in those eligible for the vaccine with evidence of herd immunity, as there was a 93% decline in the unvaccinated population as well.[20] *H. influenzae* was formerly a leading cause of meningitis in children. After the introduction of *H. influenzae* type b vaccine in 1990, rates of bacterial meningitis decreased by 55%.[21] These vaccines also increased the average age of meningitis, shifting the burden of meningitis to an older population.[13] Rates of group B streptococcal meningitis in neonates has also decreased, likely because of screening during pregnancy and the use of antibiotic prophylaxis.[22]

Meningitis may also occur after neurosurgical procedures. *Staphylococcus epidermidis* and *Staphylococcus aureus* are the most common causes of postneurosurgical meningitis, followed by gram-negative organisms.[23] Risk factors for developing meningitis after craniotomy include use of steroids, CSF leak, and presence of an external ventricular drain.[24] Gram-negative organisms are more prevalent in postcraniotomy meningitis; common pathogens include *Acinetobacter baumannii*, *Klebsiella pneumoniae*, *P. aeruginosa*, *Enterobacter cloacae*, and *Proteus mirabilis*. Antibiotic resistance can be high in postcraniotomy meningitis, and treatment should be tailored after sensitivities have been determined.[24] The most common bacterial causes of meningitis associated with CSF shunts include coagulase-negative staphylococci, *S. aureus*, and *P. aeruginosa*.[25,26,27] Gram-negative meningitis after neurosurgical procedures is associated with severe disease and a worse outcome; therefore, intraventricular antibiotics may be an option in these difficult-to-treat cases. Gentamicin and vancomycin are frequently used for intraventricular therapy and can aid in CSF sterilization.[28] If intraventricular antibiotics are administered, only preservative-free formulations should be used.[29]

S. epidermidis, *S. aureus*, and gram-negative organisms predominate infections associated with external ventricular drains (EVDs).[30] Routine analysis of the CSF has limited value in screening for bacterial meningitis in patients with EVDs.[31] Use of prophylactic antibiotics after EVD insertion and until removal does not lower the chance of an infection and may select for resistant pathogens.[32] Intraventricular hemorrhage, subarachnoid hemorrhage, basilar skull fractures, open depressed skull fracture, prior neurosurgery, irrigation of EVD, duration of the EVD, and a systemic infection are all factors associated with meningitis after EVD placement.[30]

Meningeal infections have significant morbidity and mortality rates. Until the discovery of antibiotics in the 1930s, the treatment of bacterial meningitis was severely limited.[3] Prior to the introduction of antibiotics, meningitis was associated with nearly 100% mortality when *S. pneumoniae* or *H. influenzae* was the underlying organism and greater than 75% mortality when *N. meningitidis* was the cause.[33] In recent years, the highest mortality rate is associated with *S. pneumoniae*, with mortality rates varying from 20 to 30%.[5,13] Bacterial meningitis can result in death and serious sequelae, including motor impairment, hearing impairment, and speech delay in children.[34] Stroke is a known complication of community-acquired bacterial meningitis, more common when *S. pneumoniae* is the causative pathogen, and is associated with a higher mortality in hospital and worse outcomes.[35] In children, group B *Streptococcus* is also known to cause ischemic stroke as well as cerebral venous sinus thrombosis, which can lead to neurologic deficits and seizures.[36]

As meningitis is associated with mortality and significant morbidities, prompt therapy is indicated. Empiric antibiotics for suspected bacterial meningitis in patients over 3 months of age should include a third-generation cephalosporin, cefotaxime or ceftriaxone, and vancomycin.[29,37] Delay in antibiotic administration should be avoided, since this is associated with a worse outcome.[7] Antibiotics should be administered within 3 hours of hospital admission.[29,37] Dexamethasone should also be given promptly because dexamethasone early in the course of acute bacterial meningitis improves that patient's outcome.[38] After speciation and antimicrobial sensitivities have returned, the antibiotic choice should be refined. Length of antibiotic treatment is organism dependent. Ampicillin should be added in patients over 50 years old and to patients who are immunocompromised to provide coverage for *L. monocytogenes*. In neonates, ampicillin and gentamicin are first-line agents in suspected bacterial meningitis.[29,37] Treatment of bacterial meningitis in neonates should not include intraventricular antibiotics, since a Cochrane review showed a 3-fold increased risk ratio for mortality in neonates receiving intraventricular antibiotics.[39]

Treatment of CNS infections can be difficult because of the BBB. Crossing the BBB is easier for small, lipophilic drugs compared with protein-bound drugs that are polarized and have more difficulty in passing through.[29] During the time of inflammation, the BBB may be easier to cross, leading to higher levels of antibiotics than when tissue is in its normal state.[29,40] Penicillin has poor CSF penetration because of the low pH of CSF in the setting of bacterial meningitis.[40] Resistant bacterial strains present challenges in the treatment of meningitis. Meropenem and fourth-generation cephalosporins such as cefepime have been used successfully to treat resistant strains. Daptomycin and linezolid are alternatives to vancomycin for penicillin-resistant gram-positive bacteria.[37]

Meningitis may also present in an insidious fashion. The most common causes of chronic meningitis are tuberculosis, *Cryptococcus* spp., and carcinoma.[41] Tuberculosis is the most common cause of meningitis in sub-Saharan Africa.[42] Diagnosis may be delayed because of the gradual onset of symptoms, beginning with fevers, weight loss, headaches, and vomiting.[42] Examination of CSF shows a low white blood cell count with predominantly lymphocytes, elevated protein levels, and typically a low glucose concentration.[42] Hydrocephalus, abnormal meningeal enhancement particularly in the basal cisterns, and complications from vascular involvement are commonly seen on MRI.[10] Vascular involvement is usually of the middle cerebral artery and lenticulostriate arteries, with infarction of their vascular territories being apparent on MRI and at autopsy.[10,43] Tuberculomas of the brain may also be seen on MRI and are more common in children than adults.[10] A tuberculin skin test that is positive or a chest X-ray that is consistent with tuberculosis supports the diagnosis, but they are not always available.[42] In suspected tuberculous meningitis, the initial treatment with isoniazid, rifampin, ethambutol, and pyrazinamide should be started.[29] Once the diagnosis is confirmed, this regimen should be continued for 2 months, followed by a continuation phase of at least 4 months on rifampin and isoniazid.[29,42]

Hydrocephalus from acute or tuberculous meningitis develops as a result of inflammation leading to fibrotic adhesions of the arachnoid villi, which in turn impairs CSF flow and can require ventriculoperitoneal shunt placement.[44] Predictors for the development of hydrocephalus during tuberculous meningitis include having basal exudates, cranial nerve involvement, and visual impairment.[45] Hydrocephalus can develop in the initial phase of tuberculous meningitis or can occur after treatment and may require ventriculoperitoneal shunt placement.[45] In tuberculous meningitis, enlarged ventricles do not always indicate increased ICP and may not require ventriculoperitoneal shunt placement.[44]

Cryptococcosis can begin as a pulmonary infection after inhalation of spores, which then travel to the CNS through the bloodstream.[46] *Cryptococcus neoformans* is the most common fungal cause of meningitis in HIV-infected patients.[47] The rates of cryptococcal meningitis are higher in Africa and Asia, with the rates in developed countries decreasing after the introduction of highly active anti retroviral therapy.[47] *Cryptococcal* meningitis usually presents with severe headache and malaise and can cause raised ICP, neurologic deficits, and hydrocephalus.

Cryptococcus gattii more commonly affects the immunocompetent population. After treatment, an immune reconstitution-like syndrome may occur in immunocompromised patients. Diagnosis of *Cryptococcus* spp. infection can be made by measuring cryptococcal antigen titers in the serum and CSF. India ink staining of the CSF and culture for *Cryptococcus* spp. can also be performed, but false-negative cultures are common.[48] Raised ICP in the setting of cryptococcal infection, which often does not show enlargement of the ventricles, may require external ventricular drainage, lumbar drainage, or serial lumbar punctures. Patients with persistent elevated ICP despite CSF drainage or serial lumbar punctures should have a ventriculoperitoneal shunt placed once their acute disease has been treated.[46,49] When cryptococcal infection is suspected, treatment with amphotericin B and flucytosine should be initiated. In patients with renal dysfunction, liposomal amphotericin B should be used. At least 2 weeks of amphotericin B should be administered before transitioning to oral agents.[46,47] Longer intravenous therapy may be needed in HIV-negative patients.[47] The patient may be transitioned to oral fluconazole for at least 8 weeks after initial treatment with amphotericin B if the fungal strain is sensitive.[46,47] Steroids may also be useful when a strong inflammatory reaction occurs.[46] Continued suppressive therapy is needed in patients who are HIV positive until their CD4 cell counts increase and are maintained.[47]

HIV infection can cause chronic aseptic meningitis. CSF abnormalities can be frequently found in HIV-infected patients.[50] This diagnosis is only made after exclusion of any opportunistic infections or neoplasms.[41] Acute meningitis related to *Treponema pallidum* can be seen in HIV-infected patients. In these patients, gummatas, also known as leptomeningeal granulomas, may be seen on MRI and can be mistaken for a primary brain tumor.[10] Neurosyphilis may also present in a chronic manner or even be asymptomatic. In evaluating for neurosyphilis, CSF venereal disease research laboratory (VDRL) test is carried out.[41]

In areas where it is endemic, *Coccidioides immitis* is a common cause of chronic meningitis.[47] The diagnosis of coccidioidomycosis can be made from a history of travel to an endemic area, the presence of basilar meningitis or hydrocephalus on brain imaging, and a positive serum antibody test.[47] This organism is typically treated with fluconazole, and the associated hydrocephalus may require a ventriculoperitoneal shunt.[47] The most common fungal pathogen in meningitis is *Candida albicans*.[47] Other fungal causes of meningitis include *Histoplasma capsulatum* and *Blastomyces dermatitidis*.[47]

14.3 Encephalitis

Patients with encephalitis can present with fever, headache, vomiting, seizures, personality changes, and altered mental status.[51] The diagnosis of encephalitis is based on several criteria, with the major one being altered mental status for greater than 24 hours without an alternative explanation. Minor criteria for the diagnosis of encephalitis include fever, new-onset seizures, new focal neurologic deficits, MRI findings suggestive of encephalitis, CSF leukocytosis, and an electroencephalogram (EEG) consistent with encephalitis without another causative explanation.[52] CT can initially show hypodense areas, particularly the temporal lobe in herpes simplex virus (HSV) infection, and later intraparenchymal hemorrhage may be evident.[51] All patients with suspected encephalitis should have blood cultures, treponemal testing, HIV testing, neuroimaging, chest X-ray, EEG, and an LP if not contraindicated because of the presence of an intracranial mass. Obtaining a careful patient history is important because recent and remote travel history and specific exposures, such as a recent animal bite, may also direct testing.[52] Polymerase chain reaction (PCR) of the CSF is used to screen for several pathogens, including HSV, varicella–zoster virus (VZV), cytomegalovirus (CMV), JC virus, toxoplasmosis, and tuberculosis.[51] HSV-1 and VZV are the most common viruses to cause encephalitis. The underlying cause of encephalitis varies greatly and may include viral, bacterial, fungal, parasitic, and prion diseases. Viral causes include dengue, Japanese encephalitis, West Nile, Eastern equine encephalitis, La Crosse encephalitis, St. Louis encephalitis, and rabies.[52] Epstein–Barr virus, CMV, JC virus, and human herpesvirus (HHV) 6/7 are potential causes of encephalitis in immunocompromised patients.[51,52] Creutzfeldt–Jakob disease caused by prions can present with unusual symptoms, such as a movement disorder or psychosis. Parasitic causes of encephalitis include malaria, toxoplasmosis, and amoebas. Initial management of encephalitis should include stabilizing the patient where impaired consciousness or status epilepticus may require intubation and mechanical ventilation of the patient. If cerebral edema is present with elevated ICP, the administration of mannitol or hypertonic saline may be indicated.[52] Severe cases of HSV encephalitis may require a decompressive hemicraniectomy.[53,54] Immunocompromised patients are at a higher risk for reactivation of HSV.[54] EEG should be obtained emergently to evaluate for underlying seizure activity and potential status epilepticus, which once discovered should be treated aggressively. Suspected HSV encephalitis should be treated empirically with acyclovir. If a bacterial source is suspected, broad-spectrum antibiotics should be initiated.[52] If there is a high suspicion for HSV encephalitis, treatment should be continued for the full 14- to 21-day course of therapy and a repeat LP should be performed because the PCR in HSV encephalitis may be negative for the first 3 days of infection.[29,55] In CMV encephalitis, ganciclovir and foscarnet should be started as treatment even though these drugs may have serious adverse effects.[29,56] Stereotactic brain biopsy may be required when the etiology of encephalitis remains unclear.[51]

Toxoplasmosis infections of the CNS are a frequent diagnosis in patients infected with HIV, with reports ranging from 3 to 50% of that population. Multiple intraparenchymal lesions may be seen on MRI, with hemorrhage occurring on occasion.[10] The incidence of toxoplasmosis in the CNS has decreased in HIV patients after the introduction of highly active antiretroviral therapy.[57]

CNS infection by amoebas causes a severe and usually fatal disease. The most common causes of amebic encephalitis are *Naegleria fowleri*, *Acanthamoeba* spp., and *Balmuthia mandrillaris*. *N. fowleri* causes a primary amebic meningoencephalitis (PAM) after accessing the CNS through the olfactory mucosa. In the brain, this amoeba causes cortical hemorrhage, cerebral edema, and necrosis of the olfactory bulbs, leading to coma and death over the course of a week. In the CSF, *N. fowleri* can usually be detected by PCR and can sometimes be seen on wet mount. *Acanthamoeba* spp. occurs in immunocompromised patients, and *B. mandrillaris* infections develop gradually, resulting in

granulomatous amebic encephalitis. These amoebas reach the brain through the bloodstream from the skin or lungs and once in the brain cause necrosis and formation of granulomas with associated cerebral edema. Brain biopsy is generally necessary for diagnosis.[58]

14.4 Extra-axial Abscesses

Extra-axial abscesses are neurosurgical emergencies that, once recognized, require urgent treatment. Extra-axial abscess includes subdural empyema (SDE) and cranial epidural abscess (CEA). CEAs are uncommon, one study showing them to be only 1.6% of intracranial infections. CEA forms in the potential space between the dura mater and the cranium.[51] Like SDE, they often develop in association with sinusitis and otitis media. Untreated complex skull fractures may also lead to the development of a CEA.[59,60] Patients on admission for a CEA often do not show a neurologic deficit.[59,60] Common signs and symptoms at presentation are Pott's puffy tumor, headaches, vomiting, and neck stiffness.[59,61] Pott's puffy tumor, the subperiosteal abscess with associated frontal osteomyelitis, may be misdiagnosed initially as a scalp abscess with superficial incision and drainage and treatment with antibiotics were carried out prior to being evaluated by a neurologic surgery service.[61] Bone removal may be necessary when significant osteomyelitis is present.[61] Prognosis after CEA is good, and full neurologic recovery is frequent in patients with epidural empyema.[59,61,62] *Streptococcus milleri* and *P. mirabilis* are common pathogens in CEA. Following trauma, *S. aureus* is the most common causative pathogen.[59] When associated with otitis media, abscesses frequently occur in the presence of cholesteatomas and are caused by gram-negative organisms.[63]

CT of the head with contrast can show an epidural collection with a hypodense center and peripheral enhancement.[51] T1-weighted images may show a hyperintense extra-axial collection with peripheral ring enhancement. On MRI, the abscess can be distinguished from a subdural abscess by its biconvex shape, ability to displace venous sinuses, and inability to cross suture lines.[10] An example of a CEA on MRI is shown in ▶ Fig. 14.1. Given the potential for clinical worsening, LP is not recommended in the setting of CEA.[51,59]

Broad-spectrum antibiotic therapy should be initiated that includes ceftriaxone, vancomycin, and metronidazole, with modification once organism speciation has resulted.[29] Urgent drainage is the definitive treatment in the vast majority of patients. Craniotomy or craniectomy is the preferred treatment, with débridement and irrigation of the infected space, but burr hole drainage is also utilized at times.[51,59] If CEA occurs after a neurosurgical procedure and there is osteomyelitis of the bone flap, the bone flap may need to be removed and discarded.[51] When necessary, otolaryngologic surgery for treating the primary infection can be performed concomitantly with drainage of the CEA.[59]

SDE presents with clinical symptoms that are more severe than those seen with an epidural abscess.[64] When compared with patients with epidural abscesses, patients with SDE have a lower Glasgow coma score on admission, have a longer duration of symptoms, are more likely to require multiple surgeries, have a longer length of stay and an increased morbidity, and are

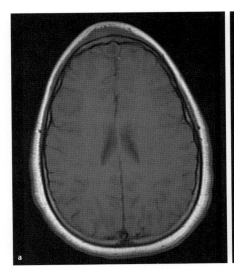
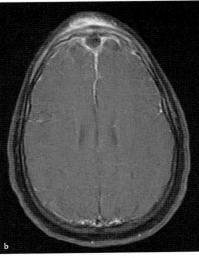

Fig. 14.1 Pediatric male with frontal epidural abscess and associated subgaleal edema on magnetic resonance imaging: **(a)** axial T1-weighted image without contrast; **(b)** axial T2-weighted image with contrast.

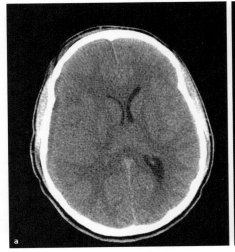
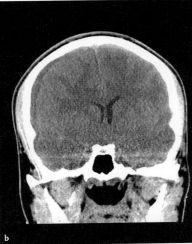

Fig. 14.2 Adolescent male with right-sided subdural empyema on computed tomography (CT) of the head without contrast: **(a)** axial CT image; **(b)** coronal CT image.

more likely to have seizures.[60] Fever, vomiting, headache, and altered mentation are the most common symptoms at presentation. The symptoms typically develop 2 or more weeks prior to presentation.[51] Males are affected more often than females.[51] Pott's puffy tumor is not unusual in patients with SDE.[65,66] In patients with sinusitis and frontal or periorbital swelling, the clinician should evaluate for potential SDE.[65] The most common cause of a SDE is a prior neurosurgical procedure, followed by sinusitis and an otogenic infectious source such as otitis media or, less commonly, mastoiditis.[67] In pediatric patients, the majority of spontaneous SDEs are associated with rhinogenic or otogenic sources.[64] Intracranial complications of sinusitis, otitis media, and mastoiditis have decreased with the introduction of broad-spectrum antibiotics.[63] In infants, subdural empyemas are typically related to bacterial meningitis.[64]

The most common pathogens in pediatric SDE are gram-positive cocci, with the *S. milleri* group being the most prevalent organism.[64] Bacteria enter the subdural space by two proposed mechanisms: direct contamination from osteomyelitis or by retrograde thrombophlebitis.[60,68] Retrograde thrombophlebitis is more common in sinusitis and direct extension is more common when the SDE has an otogenic origin.[68] In postoperative SDE, *S. aureus* is the most frequent organism cultured.[65]

CBC with differential, CRP, and ESR should be measured on admission. White blood cell count (WBC), CRP, and ESR are typically elevated.[64] Blood cultures should be obtained and may be positive.[51] LP is contraindicated in SDE and may cause neurologic decline.[66] On CT with contrast, a hypodense subdural collection with peripheral enhancement can be seen.[51] Fig. 14.2 is an example of a noncontrast CT of the head with a SDE. MRI may show an enhancing membrane around a subdural collection with decreased diffusion that shows hyperintensity on T1-weighted images.[10] Cerebritis of the adjacent brain parenchyma may be evident.[10] Cerebral thrombosis can occur with a SDE, and radiographic signs of this may be apparent on imaging.[64]

Urgent neurosurgical drainage is required for the majority of cases.[51,67] Burr hole drainage has a higher rate of recurrence when compared with a craniotomy for evacuation.[64] Decompressive craniectomy may be necessary in cases with extensive brain edema.[65] Infants with SDE, unlike older pediatric patients, can be successfully treated with burr hole drainage.[69] Screening

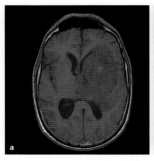 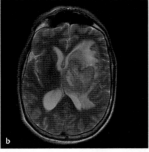 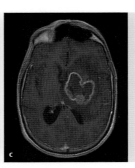

Fig. 14.3 Adult male with left-sided ring-enhancing lesion on magnetic resonance imaging of the brain: **(a)** axial T1-weighted image without contrast; **(b)** axial T2-weighted image; **(c)** axial T1-weighted image with contrast.

for recurrent SDE in infants may be accomplished with cranial ultrasound.[69] As with CEA, eradication of the primary infectious source by the otolaryngologic surgeons should be attempted at the time of SDE evacuation.[60,66]

An infratentorial location is a rare for SDE and requires rapid treatment. This location of SDE is associated with hydrocephalus in 77% of cases and a higher mortality rate (23%) than those in a supratentorial location.[70] These patients require urgent treatment of their hydrocephalus if present, along with a posterior fossa craniectomy for removal of the empyema. The most common source for an infratentorial empyema is otogenic in nature, with the majority of patients undergoing mastoidectomy for definitive treatment of their primary site of infection.[70]

The majority of patients with supratentorial SDE treated urgently and with appropriate antibiotic therapy have a good prognosis, with Glasgow outcome scores of 4 or 5.[66] Having significant neurologic signs at the time of presentation of SDE is associated with a worse outcome, and SDE generally has a worse prognosis than does epidural abscess.[60] Seizures are a common complication after SDE.[65,66]

14.5 Brain Abscess

Immunosuppressed patients, such as patients with neutropenia, on immunosuppressive therapy, and with HIV, are at a higher risk for the development of a brain abscess.[71] Brain abscesses can develop through contiguous spread from sinusitis and otitis media frequently being the primary infection site, or by hematogenous spread, with endocarditis and pulmonary infection frequently being the primary infections.[71] Penetrating head trauma is also a risk factor for the development of a brain abscess.[72] In pediatric patients, congenital heart disease that creates a right-to-left shunt is a common underlying source for a brain abscess.[51]

Patients with brain abscess can present with a variety of symptoms, which often include fever, headache, a focal neurologic deficit, altered mental status, seizures, and emesis.[71,73] CBC may show an elevated WBC, but this finding is unreliable. An elevated ESR and an increased CRP level can aid in the diagnosis of an infection and can be used to follow the response to treatment.[51] Diagnosis of a brain abscess is usually made on CT or MRI of the brain. LP is generally contraindicated because of the presence of mass effect from the lesion.[71]

Brain abscesses may be discovered during any of their four stages of development. The appearance of brain abscesses on imaging depends on the stage of the abscess. Four stages of

brain abscess can be seen on MRI. In the first 1 to 4 days, early cerebritis is present, followed by late cerebritis at 4 to 10 days, then early capsule formation is present at 11 to 14 days, and after 14 days there is late capsule formation.[12,74] On CT of the head, cerebritis appears as an area of hypodensity that after administration of contrast diffusely enhances, although the presence of enhancement is inconsistent.[12,51] In the cerebritis stage, little or no contrast enhancement may be found on MRI with prolongation on T1- and T2-weighted images. Once a capsule has formed, the lesion will be hyperintense on T1-weighted images, with peripheral ring enhancement that is hypointense on T2 with surrounding vasogenic edema (▶Fig. 14.3).[10] On CT, the encapsulated abscess shows as a ring-enhancing lesion with a hypodense surround. This appearance can be identical to malignant tumor, metastatic disease, resolving hematoma, radiation necrosis, or a stroke.[51] Diffusion-weighted imaging (DWI) can be useful in making the diagnosis, since abscesses show high signal intensity on DW images with reduced apparent diffusion coefficient (ADC) signal, whereas neoplasms usually have a low signal intensity on DW images and high signal intensity on ADC.[12] Magnetic resonance spectroscopy can also aid in diagnosis, as untreated abscesses can show the products of bacterial breakdown, including succinate, amino acids, acetate, and elevated lactate.[12,75] Brain abscesses can be associated with ventriculitis when they rupture into the ventricle, where the capsule surrounding the brain abscess is at its thinnest.[51]

In immunocompetent patients, brain abscesses usually have a bacterial origin and often more than one organism is identified.[71] The most common species identified is *Streptococcus*.[71,73] Sterile cultures can occur, typically after antibiotic administration occurs prior to drainage or biopsy.[71] The most common cause of cerebral abscess in HIV patients is *Toxoplasma gondii*. Other common pathogens for patients with immunosuppression include *C. neoformans*, mycobacteria, *L. monocytogenes*, *Nocardia asteroides*, *Aspergillus* spp., and *Candida* spp.[71] In patients who undergo bone marrow transplantation, a fungal organism is the most common cause of brain abscess, with *Aspergillus* spp. and *Candida* spp. being the most frequent infectious agents.[76] *Aspergillus* spp., albeit rare, can cause strokes from a cerebrovascular infection.[47]

Empiric therapy in a suspected bacterial brain abscess should include vancomycin, a third-generation cephalosporin such as ceftriaxone or cefotaxime, and metronidazole.[29,71] One should also consider the source of the infection and adjust empiric antibiotics accordingly.[71] In fungal abscesses, amphotericin B with flucytosine is often the initial therapy.[29] Surgical aspiration with CT or MRI guidance is often the procedure of choice in these patients, but it often needs to be repeated and carries the risk of abscess rupture into the ventricle. Open excision should be performed for lesions in the cerebellum, multiloculated lesions, fungal abscesses, and if a foreign body is present.[51] Stereotactic brain biopsy has been shown to have a high diagnostic yield with low morbidity and mortality rates.[77] In cases in the cerebritis stage and for deep collections, open excision should not be performed.[51] If surgery to aspirate, biopsy, or excise the abscess is planned urgently, antibiotics should be withheld until a sample is obtained. Imaging to evaluate medical treatment after surgery should be repeated on a weekly or biweekly basis through the duration of antibiotic therapy.[71] Imaging should be repeated again after medical therapy to evaluate for recurrence.[71] These patients should be followed for at least 1 year to monitor for recurrence. In lesions less than 2.5 cm in diameter in patients who are poor surgical candidates, medical treatment alone may be considered.[51] A common exception to biopsy and aspiration is in HIV patients who have a positive serum test for *T. gondii* and have lesions without significant mass effect. In these patients, antimicrobial therapy with pyrimethamine and sulfadiazine can be started and the response to therapy monitored with imaging.[71] With prompt treatment, mortality for brain abscesses is low. An exception to this is in patients who are immunosuppressed after bone marrow or solid organ transplantation where mortality rates remains high.[71,76]

Another consideration in the patient presenting with a brain abscess is a parasitic CNS infection. The most common parasite to infect the CNS is the larval form of *Taenia solium*, a pork tapeworm for which humans are the definitive host.[78] CNS involvement is common, with lesions occurring most frequently in the brain parenchyma and subarachnoid space.[78,79] Once in the CNS, the parasites go through several stages, beginning with the vesicular stage in which they can remain viable. Once degeneration begins, the cyst enters the colloidal stage, followed by the nodular–granular stage and finally the calcified stage.[78] Patients may present with seizures, as neurocysticercosis is a common cause of epilepsy in developing countries, symptoms of encephalitis, and increased ICP from hydrocephalus.[78,79] Hydrocephalus develops with fourth ventricular cysts that cause obstruction and may require emergent ventriculostomy and eventual ventriculoperitoneal shunting.[78,80] Serum, stool, and CSF tests are of limited value, but stool may be positive for *T. solium* eggs and CSF can show a low glucose level with eosinophilia.[78] Diagnosis is usually made on MRI or CT, with the appearance of the infection depending on the stage. Treatment with neuroendoscopy has been used for intraventicular cysts.[78,80] Albendazole is the antihelminthic drug of choice in neurocysticercosis, followed by praziquantel, and corticosteroids should be started prior to antihelminthic therapy.[78,80] Echinococcosis is another less common parasitic infection that can cause cerebral cysts requiring surgical intervention.[78]

14.6 Conclusion

Intracranial infections represent neurosurgical emergencies that require rapid diagnosis and immediate management. Advances in antimicrobial therapies have significantly improved the prognosis for meningitis, encephalitis, extra-axial abscesses, and brain abscesses. Even with improved medical management, many of these processes still require urgent neurosurgical intervention to lower neurologic morbidity and mortality rates.

References

[1] Borges LF. Infections in neurologic surgery. Host defenses. Neurosurg Clin N Am. 1992; 3(2):275–278

[2] Doran KS, Fulde M, Gratz N, et al. Host-pathogen interactions in bacterial meningitis. Acta Neuropathol. 2016; 131(2):185–209

[3] Hall WA. erebral infectious processes. In: Loftus CM, ed. Neurosurgical Emergencies. New York: Thieme Medical Publishers; 2008:115–124

[4] Kim KS. Mechanisms of microbial traversal of the blood-brain barrier. Nat Rev Microbiol. 2008; 6(8):625–634

[5] van de Beek D, de Gans J, Spanjaard L, Weisfelt M, Reitsma JB, Vermeulen M. Clinical features and prognostic factors in adults with bacterial meningitis. N Engl J Med. 2004; 351(18):1849–1859

[6] Wang AY, Machicado JD, Khoury NT, Wootton SH, Salazar L, Hasbun R. Community-acquired meningitis in older adults: clinical features, etiology, and prognostic factors. J Am Geriatr Soc. 2014; 62(11):2064–2070

[7] Aronin SI, Peduzzi P, Quagliarello VJ. Community-acquired bacterial meningitis: risk stratification for adverse clinical outcome and effect of antibiotic timing. Ann Intern Med. 1998; 129(11):862–869

[8] Henry BM, Roy J, Ramakrishnan PK, Vikse J, Tomaszewski KA, Walocha JA. Procalcitonin as a serum biomarker for differentiation of bacterial meningitis from viral meningitis in children: evidence from a meta-analysis. Clin Pediatr (Phila). 2016; 55(8):749–764

[9] Tunkel AR, Hartman BJ, Kaplan SL, et al. Practice guidelines for the management of bacterial meningitis. Clin Infect Dis. 2004; 39(9):1267–1284

[10] Hazany S, Go JL, Law M. Magnetic resonance imaging of infectious meningitis and ventriculitis in adults. Top Magn Reson Imaging. 2014; 23(5):315–325

[11] Oliveira CR, Morriss MC, Mistrot JG, Cantey JB, Doern CD, Sánchez PJ; MD CRO. Brain magnetic resonance imaging of infants with bacterial meningitis. J Pediatr. 2014; 165(1):134–139

[12] Foerster BR, Thurnher MM, Malani PN, Petrou M, Carets-Zumelzu F, Sundgren PC. Intracranial infections: clinical and imaging characteristics. Acta Radiol. 2007; 48(8):875–893

[13] Thigpen MC, Whitney CG, Messonnier NE, et al; Emerging Infections Programs Network. Bacterial meningitis in the United States, 1998–2007. N Engl J Med. 2011; 364(21):2016–2025

[14] Pong A, Bradley JS. Bacterial meningitis and the newborn infant. Infect Dis Clin North Am. 1999; 13(3):711–733, viii

[15] van Veen KEB, Brouwer MC, van der Ende A, van de Beek D. Bacterial meningitis in patients with HIV: a population-based prospective study. J Infect. 2016; 72(3):362–368

[16] Castelblanco RL, Lee M, Hasbun R; MD RLC. Epidemiology of bacterial meningitis in the USA from 1997 to 2010: a population-based observational study. Lancet Infect Dis. 2014; 14(9):813–819

[17] Imöhl M, Möller J, Reinert RR, Perniciaro S, van der Linden M, Aktas O. Pneumococcal meningitis and vaccine effects in the era of conjugate vaccination: results of 20 years of nationwide surveillance in Germany. BMC Infect Dis. 2015; 15:61

[18] Moore MR, Link-Gelles R, Schaffner W, et al. Effect of use of 13-valent pneumococcal conjugate vaccine in children on invasive pneumococcal disease in children and adults in the USA: analysis of multisite, population-based surveillance. Lancet Infect Dis. 2015; 15(3):301–309

[19] Kristiansen PA, Ba AK, Ouédraogo AS, et al. Persistent low carriage of serogroup A Neisseria meningitidis two years after mass vaccination with the meningococcal conjugate vaccine, MenAfriVac. BMC Infect Dis. 2014; 14:663

[20] Bijlsma MW, Brouwer MC, Spanjaard L, van de Beek D, van der Ende A. A decade of herd protection after introduction of meningococcal serogroup C conjugate vaccination. Clin Infect Dis. 2014; 59(9):1216–1221

[21] Schuchat A, Robinson K, Wenger JD, et al; Active Surveillance Team. Bacterial meningitis in the United States in 1995. N Engl J Med. 1997; 337(14):970–976

[22] Dery MA, Hasbun R. Changing epidemiology of bacterial meningitis. Curr Infect Dis Rep. 2007; 9(4):301–307

[23] Federico G, Tumbarello M, Spanu T, et al. Risk factors and prognostic indicators of bacterial meningitis in a cohort of 3580 postneurosurgical patients. Scand J Infect Dis. 2001; 33(7):533–537

[24] Kourbeti IS, Vakis AF, Ziakas P, et al. Infections in patients undergoing craniotomy: risk factors associated with post-craniotomy meningitis. J Neurosurg. 2015; 122(5):1113–1119

[25] Filka J, Huttova M, Tuharsky J, Sagat T, Kralinsky K, Krcmery V, Jr. Nosocomial meningitis in children after ventriculoperitoneal shunt insertion. Acta Paediatr. 1999; 88(5):576–578

[26] Turgut M, Alabaz D, Erbey F, et al. Cerebrospinal fluid shunt infections in children. Pediatr Neurosurg. 2005; 41(3):131–136

[27] Arnell K, Cesarini K, Lagerqvist-Widh A, Wester T, Sjölin J. Cerebrospinal fluid shunt infections in children over a 13-year period: anaerobic cultures and comparison of clinical signs of infection with Propionibacterium acnes and with other bacteria. J Neurosurg Pediatr. 2008; 1(5):366–372

[28] Remeš F, Tomáš R, Jindrák V, Vaniš V, Setlík M. Intraventricular and lumbar intrathecal administration of antibiotics in postneurosurgical patients with meningitis and/or ventriculitis in a serious clinical state. J Neurosurg. 2013; 119(6):1596–1602

[29] Ziai WC, Lewin JJ, III. Update in the diagnosis and management of central nervous system infections. Neurol Clin. 2008; 26(2):427–468, viii

[30] Lozier AP, Sciacca RR, Romagnoli MF, Connolly ES, Jr. Ventriculostomy-related infections: a critical review of the literature. Neurosurgery. 2002; 51(1):170–181, discussion 181–182

[31] Schade RP, Schinkel J, Roelandse FWC, et al. Lack of value of routine analysis of cerebrospinal fluid for prediction and diagnosis of external drainage-related bacterial meningitis. J Neurosurg. 2006; 104(1):101–108

[32] Alleyne CH, Jr, Hassan M, Zabramski JM. The efficacy and cost of prophylactic and periprocedural antibiotics in patients with external ventricular drains. Neurosurgery. 2000; 47(5):1124–1127, discussion 1127–1129

[33] Swartz MN. Bacterial meningitis—a view of the past 90 years. N Engl J Med. 2004; 351(18):1826–1828

[34] Klobassa DS, Zoehrer B, Paulke-Korinek M, et al. The burden of pneumococcal meningitis in Austrian children between 2001 and 2008. Eur J Pediatr. 2014; 173(7):871–878

[35] Bodilsen J, Dalager-Pedersen M, Schønheyder HC, Nielsen H. Stroke in community-acquired bacterial meningitis: a Danish population-based study. Int J Infect Dis. 2014; 20:18–22

[36] Tibussek D, Sinclair A, Yau I, et al. Late-onset group B streptococcal meningitis has cerebrovascular complications. J Pediatr. 2015; 166(5):1187–1192.e1

[37] Tan YC, Gill AK, Kim KS. Treatment strategies for central nervous system infections: an update. Expert Opin Pharmacother. 2015; 16(2):187–203

[38] de Gans J, van de Beek D; European Dexamethasone in Adulthood Bacterial Meningitis Study Investigators. Dexamethasone in adults with bacterial meningitis. N Engl J Med. 2002; 347(20):1549–1556

[39] Shah SS, Ohlsson A, Shah VS. Intraventricular antibiotics for bacterial meningitis in neonates. Cochrane Database Syst Rev. 2012; 7(7):CD004496

[40] Nau R, Sörgel F, Eiffert H. Penetration of drugs through the blood-cerebrospinal fluid/blood-brain barrier for treatment of central nervous system infections. Clin Microbiol Rev. 2010; 23(4):858–883

[41] Hildebrand J, Aoun M. Chronic meningitis: still a diagnostic challenge. J Neurol. 2003; 250(6):653–660

[42] Donald PR, Schoeman JF. Tuberculous meningitis. N Engl J Med. 2004; 351(17):1719–1720

[43] Chatterjee D, Radotra BD, Vasishta RK, Sharma K. Vascular complications of tuberculous meningitis: an autopsy study. Neurol India. 2015; 63(6):926–932

[44] Chatterjee S, Chatterjee U. Overview of post-infective hydrocephalus. Childs Nerv Syst. 2011; 27(10):1693–1698

[45] Raut T, Garg RK, Jain A, et al. Hydrocephalus in tuberculous meningitis: Incidence, its predictive factors and impact on the prognosis. J Infect. 2013; 66(4):330–337

[46] Franco-Paredes C, Womack T, Bohlmeyer T, et al. Management of Cryptococcus gattii meningoencephalitis. Lancet Infect Dis. 2015; 15(3):348–355

[47] Murthy JMK, Sundaram C. Fungal Infections of the Central Nervous System. Vol. 121. 1st ed. Amsterdam, the Netherlands: Elsevier B.V.; 2014:1383–1401. doi: 10.1016/B978-0-7020-4088-7.00095-X

[48] Chen SCA, Slavin MA, Heath CH, et al; Australia and New Zealand Mycoses Interest Group (ANZMIG)-Cryptococcus Study. Clinical manifestations of Cryptococcus gattii infection: determinants of neurological sequelae and death. Clin Infect Dis. 2012; 55(6):789–798

[49] Cherian J, Atmar RL, Gopinath SP. Shunting in cryptococcal meningitis. J Neurosurg. 2016; 125(1):177–186

[50] Marshall DW, Brey RL, Cahill WT, Houk RW, Zajac RA, Boswell RN. Spectrum of cerebrospinal fluid findings in various stages of human immunodeficiency virus infection. Arch Neurol. 1988; 45(9):954–958

[51] Hall WA, Truwit CL. The surgical management of infections involving the cerebrum. Neurosurgery. 2008; 62(Suppl 2):519–530, discussion 530–531

[52] Venkatesan A, Geocadin RG. Diagnosis and management of acute encephalitis: a practical approach. Neurol Clin Pract. 2014; 4(3):206–215

[53] Adamo MA, Deshaies EM. Emergency decompressive craniectomy for fulminating infectious encephalitis. J Neurosurg. 2008; 108(1):174–176

[54] Sánchez-Carpintero R, Aguilera S, Idoate M, Bejarano B. Temporal lobectomy in acute complicated herpes simplex encephalitis: technical case report. Neurosurgery. 2008; 62(5):E1174–E1175, discussion E1175

[55] De Tiège X, Héron B, Lebon P, Ponsot G, Rozenberg F. Limits of early diagnosis of herpes simplex encephalitis in children: a retrospective study of 38 cases. Clin Infect Dis. 2003; 36(10):1335–1339

[56] Anduze-Faris BM, Fillet AM, Gozlan J, et al. Induction and maintenance therapy of cytomegalovirus central nervous system infection in HIV-infected patients. AIDS. 2000; 14(5):517–524

[57] Mayor AM, Fernández Santos DM, Dworkin MS, Ríos-Olivares E, Hunter-Mellado RF. Toxoplasmic encephalitis in an AIDS cohort at Puerto Rico before and after highly active antiretroviral therapy (HAART). Am J Trop Med Hyg. 2011; 84(5):838–841

[58] Hall WA. Free-living amoebas: is it safe to go in the water? World Neurosurg. 2012; 78(6):610–611

[59] Nathoo N, Nadvi SS, van Dellen JR. Cranial extradural empyema in the era of computed tomography: a review of 82 cases. Neurosurgery. 1999; 44(4):748–753, discussion 753–754

[60] Patel AP, Masterson L, Deutsch CJ, Scoffings DJ, Fish BM. Management and outcomes in children with sinogenic intracranial abscesses. Int J Pediatr Otorhinolaryngol. 2015; 79(6):868–873

[61] Salomão JF, Cervante TP, Bellas AR, et al. Neurosurgical implications of Pott's puffy tumor in children and adolescents. Childs Nerv Syst. 2014; 30(9):1527–1534

[62] Kombogiorgas D, Solanki GA. The Pott puffy tumor revisited: neurosurgical implications of this unforgotten entity. Case report and review of the literature. J Neurosurg. 2006; 105(2, Suppl):143–149

[63] Migirov L, Duvdevani S, Kronenberg J. Otogenic intracranial complications: a review of 28 cases. Acta Otolaryngol. 2005; 125(8):819–822

[64] Legrand M, Roujeau T, Meyer P, Carli P, Orliaguet G, Blanot S. Paediatric intracranial empyema: differences according to age. Eur J Pediatr. 2009; 168(10):1235–1241

[65] Gupta S, Vachhrajani S, Kulkarni AV, et al. Neurosurgical management of extraaxial central nervous system infections in children. J Neurosurg Pediatr. 2011; 7(5):441–451

[66] Nathoo N, Nadvi SS, van Dellen JR, Gouws E. Intracranial subdural empyemas in the era of computed tomography: a review of 699 cases. Neurosurgery. 1999; 44(3):529–535, discussion 535–536

[67] French H, Schaefer N, Keijzers G, Barison D, Olson S. Intracranial subdural empyema: a 10-year case series. Ochsner J. 2014; 14(2):188–194

[68] Brook I. Microbiology and antimicrobial treatment of orbital and intracranial complications of sinusitis in children and their management. Int J Pediatr Otorhinolaryngol. 2009; 73(9):1183–1186

[69] Liu Z-H, Chen N-Y, Tu P-H, Lee S-T, Wu C-T. The treatment and outcome of postmeningitic subdural empyema in infants. J Neurosurg Pediatr. 2010; 6(1):38–42

[70] Nathoo N, Nadvi SS, van Dellen JR. Infratentorial empyema: analysis of 22 cases. Neurosurgery. 1997; 41(6):1263–1268, discussion 1268–1269

[71] Calfee DP, Wispelwey B. Brain abscess. Semin Neurol. 2000; 20(3):353–360

[72] Rish BL, Caveness WF, Dillon JD, Kistler JP, Mohr JP, Weiss GH. Analysis of brain abscess after penetrating craniocerebral injuries in Vietnam. Neurosurgery. 1981; 9(5):535–541

[73] Seydoux C, Francioli P. Bacterial brain abscesses: factors influencing mortality and sequelae. Clin Infect Dis. 1992; 15(3):394–401

[74] Haimes AB, Zimmerman RD, Morgello S, et al. MR imaging of brain abscesses. AJR Am J Roentgenol. 1989; 152(5):1073–1085

[75] Burtscher IM, Holtås S. In vivo proton MR spectroscopy of untreated and treated brain abscesses. AJNR Am J Neuroradiol. 1999; 20(6):1049–1053

[76] Hagensee ME, Bauwens JE, Kjos B, Bowden RA. Brain abscess following marrow transplantation: experience at the Fred Hutchinson Cancer Research Center, 1984–1992. Clin Infect Dis. 1994; 19(3):402–408

[77] Hall WA. The safety and efficacy of stereotactic biopsy for intracranial lesions. Cancer. 1998; 82(9):1749–1755

[78] Hall WA, Kim PD, eds. Parasitic infections of the central nervous system. In: Neurosurgical Infectious Disease. Surgical and Nonsurgical Management. New York, NY: Thieme Medical Publishers; 2013:81–94

[79] White AC, Jr. Neurocysticercosis: updates on epidemiology, pathogenesis, diagnosis, and management. Annu Rev Med. 2000; 51(1):187–206

[80] Sinha S, Sharma BS. Intraventricular neurocysticercosis: a review of current status and management issues. Br J Neurosurg. 2012; 26(3):305–309

15 Emergency Treatment of Brain Tumors

Pierpaolo Peruzzi and E. Antonio Chiocca

Abstract

It is unlikely for brain tumors to present as neurologic emergencies/urgencies. Most frequently, this is due to sudden hemorrhagic conversion of an otherwise already present lesion, obstructive hydrocephalus, and/or seizures that can precipitate the labile equilibrium between the tumor and the surrounding brain already compressed by the preexisting lesion. Melanoma, choriocarcinoma, and thyroid metastases account for the majority of intracranial tumors presenting with hemorrhage. In situations of rapid and progressive neurologic decline, surgical intervention is necessary and that should be guided only by a rapidly acquired noncontrast head computed tomography (CT) scan and possibly a CT angiography of the brain to rule out any underlying vascular lesions that would require a different surgical approach. When a large hemorrhage is visualized on CT, surgical intervention aimed at clot evacuation should be the priority. In cases of obstructive hydrocephalus, the placement of an external ventricular drain is a simple and safe procedure that usually takes care of the emergent setting and allows extra time to address the underlying lesion in a more controlled and less emergent scenario. When the degree of mass effect observed in the CT scan does not correlate with the clinical/neurologic presentation, ruling out seizures and effects from vasogenic edema is a fundamental next step before embarking in a premature surgical intervention. In such cases, an initial medical management with antiepileptic drugs, steroids, and hyperosmolar therapies should be favored as a first step, in order to gain some time for establishing the best surgical approach to the underlying tumor.

Keywords: brain imaging, brain tumor, edema, emergency, hemorrhage, hydrocephalus, mass effect

15.1 Introduction

The concept of emergency in neurosurgery applies to any situation whereby immediate intervention is necessary in order to restore or prevent further damage to critical neurologic functions caused by a sudden insult to the central nervous system. In neuro-oncology, these situations are generally caused by the mass effect exerted by the tumor on surrounding brain structures.

In fact, intracranial tumors can sometimes present with sudden neurologic deterioration requiring prompt intervention. Tumors, including the most malignant ones, do not grow fast enough to cause sudden, life-threatening symptoms just by virtue of their biological aggressiveness. Instead, they can present acutely, after a period of relatively asymptomatic growth, when they reach a critical mass and a situation of unstable equilibrium with the surrounding brain. Any minor acute changes, either within the tumor itself or involving the rest of the brain, can then precipitate an emergent situation. There are several different ways an intracranial tumor can acutely compromise neurologic functions, and it is important to realize that the response to these situations in the emergent setting is not necessarily uniform and must take into account the pathophysiology of the ongoing acute process.

15.2 Pathophysiology

The intracranial content is mainly made up by three different components: brain parenchyma, blood, and cerebrospinal fluid (CSF). In physiologic circumstances, these three volumes are constant. Any time there is an increase in any of the three components, the other two change accordingly, within certain limits, to maintain the total intracranial volume constant. When this compensatory mechanism is exhausted, the intracranial pressure (ICP) raises steadily to pathologic levels with any further increase of the intracranial volume (i.e., Monro–Kellie doctrine).[1,2] In an attempt to accommodate extra volume within the closed, inexpansible, intracranial space, the brain shifts, resulting in herniation through the foramen magnum or tentorial incisura. Such shifting can be tolerated to some degree by the brain as long as it happens in a slow and progressive fashion (as it happens with the growth of a tumor), but it is devastating when it happens suddenly, as in the case of large intracranial bleeding or acute hydrocephalus.

The pathophysiologic reasons for an emergent clinical deterioration of a neuro-oncologic patient can be broadly separated into *tumor specific* (mainly intratumoral hemorrhage or ischemia), *tumor associated* (mainly due to vasogenic edema or seizures), and *metabolic* (hyponatremia, hypocarbia). Regardless of the etiology, the acuity of the presentation is due to a sudden increase of mass effect that becomes symptomatic either as a direct and acute force against vital structures of the brain (e.g., the brainstem or the optic nerves) or as an obstruction to CSF flow, thus causing obstructive hydrocephalus.

15.2.1 Tumor-Associated Hemorrhage

Symptomatic spontaneous intracranial hemorrhage (ICH) has been reported to occur in 1.5 to 14.5% of all primary or metastatic intracranial tumors,[3,4,5] and up to 4.4% of ICH were found to be secondary to underlying brain tumors.[5] In a series of almost 300 patients, the hemorrhage volume was smaller than 5 mL in 45% of cases and thus the hemorrhage was usually treated conservatively.[6] Among the tumors with the highest propensity for bleeding, metastases and glioblastoma multiforme account for greater than 75% of total cases.[7] The bleeding rate for gliomas is about 3%.[8] Among metastases, choriocarcinoma thyroid carcinoma, hepatocellular carcinoma, melanoma, and renal cell carcinoma are by far the most prone to spontaneous hemorrhage,[9] although the first three are quite rare entities, so statistically the bulk of hemorrhagic metastases is caused by melanoma and kidney cancers. Risk factors leading to hemorrhagic presentation of brain tumors have been reported to be thrombocytopenia and chemotherapy.[10] Recent evidence suggests that the risk of hemorrhage is not significantly increased by concomitant use of therapeutic anticoagulation.[6,9]

Histologically, tumors tend to bleed because of tumor neoangiogenesis, i.e., the formation of new, immature, and fragile blood vessels to support neoplastic growth. In addition, as a consequence of radiation therapy, the small blood vessels within and around the tumor can undergo degenerative changes leading to rupture and hemorrhage.[11,12] Pathologically, tumor-associated hemorrhage can cause neurologic deficits by destroying neural tissue, or by exerting mass effect on the brain, or both.

15.2.2 Tumor-Associated Ischemia

Tumor-associated ischemia is much rarer than hemorrhage, but there are occasional reports in the literature of tumors presenting with acute neurologic deficits due to sudden cerebrovascular accidents. Generally, the mechanisms are invasion, compression, and encasement of cerebrovascular structures. Tumor-associated ischemia has been described sporadically with meningiomas,[13] epidermoid tumors,[14] and glioblastomas[15,16] that can affect the large arteries at the base of the brain and with dura-based metastases in the cerebral convexities, mainly due to infiltration through the Virchow–Robin spaces, resulting in local ischemia.[17] Overall, a retrospective analysis of ischemic strokes associated with skull base meningiomas reported an incidence of 0.2%.[13]

15.2.3 Tumor-Associated Edema

Different from hemorrhage, edema is not a sudden manifestation of brain tumors and temporally evolves with the lesion. Usually the amount of edema is proportional to the histologic grade and aggressiveness of the tumor itself. The edema associated with the tumor directly contributes to the creation of mass effect and, as such, constitutes a fundamental component of tumor pathophysiology. Moreover, edema, in contrast to the tumor, can progress rapidly, particularly in the presence of precipitating events, such as hyponatremia, thus contributing to rapid neurologic deterioration.

There are three different types of edema: interstitial, cytotoxic, and vasogenic.

The first is usually related to the transependymal influx of water molecules from the subarachnoid/intraventricular spaces into the parenchyma and is commonly observed in chronic hydrocephalus.[18] As such, it does not represent an acute or emergent feature associated with brain tumors.

Cytotoxic edema occurs as a consequence of toxic or metabolic insult to the cells and is associated with ischemia, drugs, or metabolite imbalances.[19] It involves failure of the cellular osmotic regulation caused by loss of function of the energy-dependent Na^+/K^+ transporters.[19] This results in net water intake into the cell, swelling, and loss of cellular function.[20] Significant mass effect can derive from parenchymal swelling.

Vasogenic edema is most relevant to brain neoplasia. It is caused by a "leak" of oncotic and osmotic molecules from abnormally permeable blood vessels into the interstitium, resulting in a net movement of water molecules from the intravascular into the interstitial/extracellular compartment. Vessel permeability is due to a combination of poorly functional tumor vessels and loosening of tight junctions of the vascular endothelium by tumor-induced inflammation.[21]

Regardless of the mechanism, brain edema contributes to the clinical presentation of the tumor by significantly worsening mass effect and by interfering with the normal function of the brain surrounding the tumor. Understanding the different pathophysiologies of brain edema is fundamental for its treatment, as each one of the three forms of edema responds to different interventions.

15.2.4 Seizures

Seizures have been associated with up to 60% of primary brain tumors and 25 to 35% of metastatic brain lesions.[22,23] Seizures result from irritation of the brain immediately surrounding the tumor (as in metastases) or from brain directly infiltrated by primary tumors. This explains why lower-grade, indolent lesions such as oligodendroglioma are usually more epileptogenic than rapidly destructive, mass-occupying, high-grade lesions such as glioblastomas.[22] Seizures are a rather benign neurologic manifestation, as long as they are controlled and short-lived. In contrast, prolonged "status epilepticus" is considered a real neurologic emergency, as it can be associated with brain damage, due to neuronal excitotoxicity. In the presence of a brain tumor, however, seizures can carry a much higher risk of causing unwanted neurologic consequences. This is particularly true for large tumors, or tumors associated with noticeable mass effect, which can be "tipped over" by the transient intracranial changes triggered by the ictal episode. In particular, generalized tonic–clonic seizures have been shown to transiently increase ICP,[24] possibly as a combination of cerebral hyperemia and hypermetabolism, muscle rigidity, and hypocapnia/hypercarbia.

15.2.5 Hydrocephalus

Cerebrospinal fluid dynamics can be altered by intracranial tumors by three different mechanisms: (1) CSF flow obstruction; (2) impaired CSF reabsorption; and (3) CSF overproduction. In the first case, the result is obstructive hydrocephalus, and among the three, it is usually the one presenting in the most acute fashion. Usually the obstruction is localized at specific anatomical points, including the foramen of Monro and the aqueduct of Sylvius/fourth ventricle. Tumors can cause obstruction either by arising in close proximity to these areas (such as colloid cysts of the lateral ventricle or fourth ventricular tumors such as ependymomas) or by mass effect resulting in distortion of brain anatomy and compression/obliteration of the ventricular system (▶ Fig. 15.1).

In contrast, impaired CSF resorption usually results in communicating hydrocephalus, and this is most commonly observed as a consequence of diffuse leptomeningeal carcinomatosis or occlusion of major intracranial venous drainage by tumor compression. In both cases, the ability of the venous system to drain CSF is impaired, resulting in CSF accumulation.

Finally, some intraventricular tumors, particularly choroid plexus tumors, can produce an excess of CSF, which thus accumulates as its production outpaces the brain's ability to dispose of it. Both communicating hydrocephalus and hydrocephalus resulting from CSF overproduction are rarely encountered as clinical emergencies, since they are associated with progressive, subacute/chronic headache, and worsening of neurologic functions.

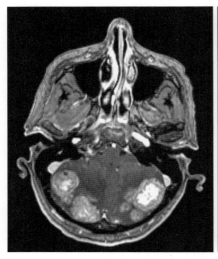
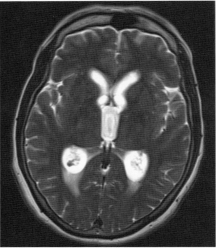

Fig. 15.1 This 57-year-old female with history of breast cancer presented with 2 days of progressive headaches and 24 hours of vomiting and lethargy. Brain imaging was obtained revealing diffuse intracranial metastatic disease, particularly in the posterior fossa, resulting in acute obstructive hydrocephalus by obliteration of the fourth ventricle (red arrow). Since the extent of the disease precluded a meaningful tumor resection, she underwent emergent placement of a ventriculoperitoneal shunt for palliation, and her examination improved to normal immediately after surgery.

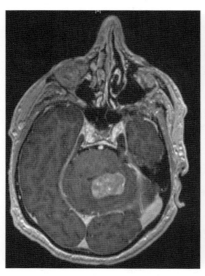
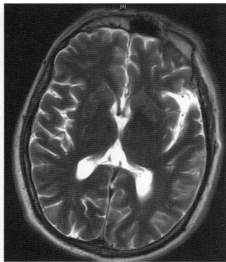

Fig. 15.2 This 58-year-old male with a newly diagnosed lung adenocarcinoma, presented with 1 week's history of subtle left dysmetria. Brain magnetic resonance imaging revealed a large posterior fossa mass critically distorting the fourth ventricle (red arrow), but no hydrocephalus was present yet. The patient was taken to the operating room for tumor resection within 48 hours, to prevent acute complications from impending obstructive hydrocephalus.

15.3 Tumor Location

Intracranial tumors can occur anywhere within the brain and its coverings. However, there are certain areas that are more prone than others to cause acute and severe complications. In particular, tumors arising in the posterior fossa, the anterior temporal lobe along the tentorial incisura, and the region of the foramen of Monro may be reasons for concern because of their location. These are locations where even a small, acute change in mass effect, by tumor growth, hemorrhage, or associated edema, could lead to significant consequences.

For instance, temporal tumors can suddenly expand to produce uncal herniation and compress the lateral brainstem and vessels in the perimesencephalic and ambient cisterns. Tumors of the foramen of Monro can suddenly occlude CSF flow from the lateral ventricles to the third ventricle, resulting in acute obstructive hydrocephalus. Finally, posterior fossa tumors can quickly cause obstructive hydrocephalus by closing the aqueduct of Sylvius. Moreover, they can exert direct mass effect on the brainstem with neurologic consequences. The authors

follow the rule of thumb that all tumors arising in these "sensitive areas" of the brain, even if asymptomatic, should be addressed quickly, as the best treatment of an emergency is to prevent it (▶Fig. 15.2).

15.4 Patient Evaluation

15.4.1 Presentation

It is crucial to rapidly understand if the symptoms and signs experienced by the patient constitute a temporal progression of preexisting complaints or if they are new and acute. This will help understand how rapidly the clinical situation has been evolving and what the next move should be.

As part of the fundamental initial evaluation, vital signs should be carefully analyzed for evidence of bradycardia associated with hypertension suggestive of brainstem compression. Similarly, a focused neurologic examination should quickly assess the patient's mental status, cranial nerve, and gross motor functions. This will provide some hints related to the location

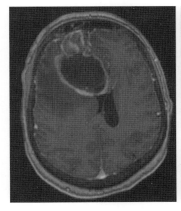
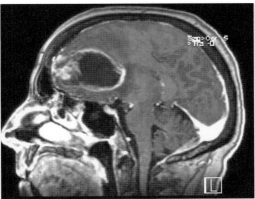

Fig. 15.3 This 70-year-old female with no significant medical history was found profoundly incoherent in the bathroom by her husband. She had been complaining of headaches the week prior. Magnetic resonance imaging upon admission revealed a large right fontal mass with vasogenic edema and profound mass effect on the forebrain and right thalamus. She progressed quickly to become unresponsive within a few hours after admission. She was taken to the operation room the same day for resection of the tumor (glioblastoma). She was discharged home 3 days after surgery with an intact neurologic examination.

of the lesion, but, most importantly, at this stage of assessment, it will help establish the level of urgency and create a baseline clinical and neurologic examination to be used to monitor for further deterioration of the clinical picture. A proper execution of these very preliminary steps is fundamental; in fact, recognizing a real emergency is vital, but it is almost as important trying not to make an emergency out of something that is not and which could be better addressed in a nonemergent fashion.

15.4.2 Imaging

In an emergent setting, a computed tomography of the head (HCT) without intravenous contrast is the imaging modality of choice, as it is fast, readily available, and devoid of major contraindications or side effects. The information obtained from a single HCT is fundamental to determining (1) the presence of an intracranial abnormality; (2) the location of the abnormality; (3) the nature of the abnormality (i.e., large intracranial mass vs. bleeding vs. edema); (4) the presence of hydrocephalus; and (5) the presence of mass effect.

As an only drawback, in the acute setting, HCT is not sensitive enough to detect ischemic strokes (at least not before 6–12 hours from their occurrence). Any evidence of edema surrounding an area of hyperacute or acute intracranial bleeding should raise suspicion for an underlying neoplastic lesion.

If the HCT is felt to be worrisome, together with a rapidly deteriorating neurologic status (such as impending clinical signs of herniation), usually it is all that is needed to guide the decision to proceed immediately with intervention. Even in real emergencies, it is, however, common practice to obtain a contrast HCT and/or a CT angiogram to better delineate the pathology and exclude any underlying vascular lesions.

On the contrary, if patient is clinically stable, the next step consists in obtaining a magnetic resonance imaging (MRI) with and without IV gadolinium. This imaging modality helps define the etiology of the intracranial process as well as its anatomy in relationship with the surrounding brain. For example, an intracerebral bleed seen on HCT might reveal an underlying tumor on a MRI. Obtaining this information is fundamental to planning surgery in order to treat the acute finding (hemorrhage, bleed) and to target the malignancy responsible for it.

15.4.3 Laboratory Work

During the first minutes spent assessing the patient, a baseline analysis of blood electrolytes, cell count, and coagulation should be obtained in order to uncover metabolic abnormalities that might account for the clinical presentation and to decide whether intervention is needed to correct abnormal values.

In particular, it is important to determine serum sodium levels, since hyponatremia (< 134 mEq/L) can precipitate brain edema, and severe hyponatremia (< 128 mEq/L) is a risk factor for seizures. Platelet counts and international normalized ratio (INR) values are also essential information to know, particularly in cases of intracranial hemorrhages.

It is important to remember that certain medications can impair coagulation and platelet function without reflection in laboratory values; for this reason, it is important to know if a patient has been regularly taking antiplatelet agents (aspirin or clopidogrel) or new-generation oral anticoagulant agents (NOAC), like dabigatran, a direct thrombin inhibitor, and rivaroxaban, a factor X inhibitor.

15.5 Intervention

After clinical assessment of the patient and review of the MRI, the most important decision is whether the next step should be medical or surgical management (with the understanding that the two approaches might coexist and do not exclude each other).

With the exception of a few straightforward situations, such as uncal herniation and severe hydrocephalus, there are, in fact, no rules or algorithms helping to decide when to operate, and the decision usually comes as a result of common sense and experience. In fact, preservation of neurologic function should remain the primary goal; however, in the presence of a brain tumor, it is also important to maximize the chances of obtaining a maximal resection by careful preoperative planning.

Our approach, thus, is to operate without hesitation in cases of real emergencies, but we prefer to delay surgery, when safe, in order to maximize the chances of a successful operation. Just a few additional hours might be all that is needed to obtain more brain imaging, setting up appropriate operative instrumentation, and medically optimize the patient for a safer surgery (▶ Fig. 15.3).

15.5.1 Medical Management

Stabilization of Vital Signs

Especially in the presence of an intracranial hemorrhage, it is important to prevent systolic blood pressure (SBP) to rise above 160 mm Hg, a value after which the chance for further bleeding increases greatly. Beta blockers and/or intravenous (IV) hydralazine as needed are the drugs of choice, but nicardipine or esmolol infusion might be necessary in refractory cases.

On the contrary, in cases associated with significant mass effect, it is important not to let SBP drop below 90 mm Hg, as this can increase the risk of poor parenchymal perfusion in areas of the brain constricted by the mass, resulting in ischemic strokes. It is thus important to make sure that 0.9% NaCl saline infusion is started promptly and titrated to 1 mL/kg/h. Occasionally, IV pressors (such as phenylephrine or norepinephrine) might be needed to sustain SBP to acceptable levels.

Cerebral Edema

Mannitol is the agent of choice when a quick decrease in brain edema is needed, regardless of its cause. It is usually given as a bolus of a 20% aqueous solution, within the span of 15 to 20 minutes. The standard initial dose range is usually 1 g per kilogram of body weight. Repeated administrations can be given, usually at the dose of 25 g every 6 hours. Mannitol works in the brain by increasing the osmotic gradient between the intravascular and the interstitial spaces, with a net movement of water molecules into the circulation and out from the brain parenchyma. Mannitol also has a profound diuretic effect, with resulting increased natremia and serum osmolality. In fact, it is important to monitor both values when using mannitol, as osmolality greater than 320 mOsm/kg is often associated with acute kidney failure. Loop diuretics (i.e., furosemide) are also commonly used to augment the effect of mannitol, by further stimulating diuresis and, to some extent, preventing hypernatremia, as loop diuretics induce a net loss of sodium by the kidneys. The dosage of furosemide is usually 0.3 mg/kg.

Corticosteroids are agents with antiedema properties and act by reducing vessel permeability associated with abnormal blood–brain barrier, as it is often encountered in tumors. In general, the agent of choice is dexamethasone (10 mg IV bolus, followed by 4–6 mg IV every 6 hours). It is important to stress that the effect of corticosteroids on brain edema is much slower than that of hyperosmolar therapy, and usually their effect does not become evident for 12 to 24 hours after administration.

After instituting hyperosmolar therapy, the goal should be to maintain serum sodium levels between 145 and 155 mEq/L. Normal saline should be used as maintenance IV fluid.

Seizures

If the patient is actively seizing at time of presentation, 2 mg IV lorazepam should be administered. If seizures persist after 1 minute, an additional 2 mg IV are given. The sequence can be repeated once if seizures persist for greater than 5 minutes. Concomitantly, the patient should receive a loading dose of IV fosphenytoin (20 mg/kg). If seizures continue, then the patient should be loaded with a bolus of 15 to 20 mg/kg phenobarbital. This can cause respiratory depression, so it is important to be prepared to mechanically ventilate the patient, if needed. For patients who are already intubated, refractory seizures can be treated with propofol infusion at a rate of 2 to 4 mg/kg/h or with midazolam (0.2–0.4 mg/kg/h). Finally, as a last resort for refractory status epilepticus, burst suppression can be achieved with a 5 mg/kg bolus of IV pentobarbital.[25]

For patients presenting after the ictal event, levetiracetam (Keppra, UCB, Inc.) 500 mg IV can be used to prevent further episodes. Keppra is preferred to fosphenytoin for its better safety profile, but it is not recommended during the ictal phase.

Optimization of Coagulation

It is imperative for patients presenting with tumor-associated hemorrhage to have their platelet count and INR checked and, if abnormal, corrected as needed. It is in fact not rare that patients with cancer have coagulation disorders, and many of them routinely use oral anticoagulants or antiplatelets.

An INR greater than 1.5 in the setting of acute intracranial bleeding needs to be addressed. Usually this is best achieved with transfusion of fresh frozen plasma if INR is between 1.6 and 2.5. For higher values, it is more effective and rapid to use concentrated clotting factors, usually in the form of Prothrombin Complex Concentrate (PCC), which is a combination of factors II, VII and IX. They usually normalize INR within 30 minutes from infusion, although it is not uncommon to observe a rebound increase in INR a few hours later, as the factors get metabolized. Newer oral NOAC anticoagulants are more difficult to deal with, since their activity is not reflected by a measurable laboratory value as INR is for warfarin (Coumadin, Bristol-Myers Squibb). In general, it is assumed that their anticoagulation effect is lost 24 hours from last administration. However, when reversal is needed, only dabigatran has an approved "antidote" (namely, idarucizumab).[26]

A platelet count less than 100,000/mL needs to be addressed with platelet transfusions. More complicated is when a patient is on aspirin or clopidogrel (Plavix), both of which are irreversible inhibitors of platelet aggregation. In these cases, platelet transfusion remains the first line of treatment, but transfused platelets might still become inactivated by the circulating drugs. In cases where bleeding persists despite platelet replenishment, desmopressin (DDAVP) 0.4 mg/kg can be considered.[27]

Further Bedside Maneuvers

In certain critical situations, particularly those with an extremely poor neurologic examination and evidence of severe mass effect at brain imaging, hyperventilation can be attempted as an extreme measure to decrease ICP. The fastest way to achieve this is to change the setting of the ventilator in order to lower the end-tidal partial pressure of carbon dioxide (pCO_2) to about 25 mm Hg, i.e., about 10 points lower than normal. This will cause some reactive vasoconstriction of cerebral blood flow, with resulting decrease production of CSF and decrease of the blood component. This procedure is only a temporary solution, usually to buy some time in preparation of a more definitive intervention, as ICP will rebound within 30 to 60 minutes after sustained hyperventilation.

15.5.2 Surgical Management

Hydrocephalus

Once it is demonstrated that hydrocephalus is acute, it represents a surgical emergency that needs to be addressed immediately, possibly even in the emergency department.

As described above, hydrocephalus can be caused by different mechanisms, and obstructive hydrocephalus should be regarded as the most worrisome.

In theory, the treatment of obstructive hydrocephalus should be aimed at removing the cause of obstruction when possible. However, in the majority of cases, obstructive hydrocephalus can be easily controlled with insertion of an external ventricular drain (EVD), a relatively easy and safe procedure that can be performed at the bedside. Our approach is to always attempt EVD insertion before operating on a patient with obstructive hydrocephalus: the first reason is that placement of a drain will buy time to plan surgery, in most cases transforming an emergent case in a semielective one. The second reason is that reduction of ICP by CSF egress improves the ease of surgery, reduces the need for brain retraction, and prevents brain herniation at the craniotomy site.

External ventricular drains are usually placed in the lateral ventricles by either a frontal approach (more commonly) or a posterior parietal approach. As a rule of thumb, for feasibility reasons, the most prominent ventricle should be cannulated, although there are exceptions to this: (1) if the ventricle is filled up by blood, it is usually better to target the contralateral one; and (2) in cases of major mass effect and brain shift, the biggest ventricle is usually the one contralateral to the lesion. In such cases, decompressing the ventricle might precipitate herniation even further.

When the obstruction is secondary to mass effect in the posterior fossa, EVD placement might be complicated by upward transtentorial herniation (UTH). This is caused by a sudden decrease of ICP in the supratentorial space due to the drain, and, as a consequence, the content of the posterior fossa tends to shift upwards through the tentorial incisura, resulting in distortion of the brainstem and obliteration of the perimesencephalic blood vessels with diffuse brainstem ischemia. This complication is rare, having been reported in about 1% of cases, but almost invariably lethal.[28] We think that the existence of this potential complication should always be entertained in the decision-making, but in general we believe that when meticulous care is taken not to overdrain CSF, the risk–benefit ratio is towards the latter. Brain imaging should always be obtained after placement of an EVD to confirm appropriate placement of the catheter, as well as to ascertain that no new acute changes have happened intracranially as a result of the procedure.

Hematoma Evacuation

Evidence of intracranial hemorrhage always leads to the decision of whether surgical evacuation is the best first step or if alternative actions can be taken instead. This determination is straightforward in cases where there is clear mass effect and midline shift associated with a poor neurologic examination. However, in situations where the hemorrhage can cause severe impairment of mental status and other neurologic functions without necessarily exerting major mass effect, the clinical picture might be the result of hematoma-related destruction of critical brain areas; in these cases, the role of surgery is much more controversial.

Once surgery has been decided, surgical planning should encompass the multiple goals of decompressing the brain, obtain tissue diagnosis, and possibly, as the presence of tumor is confirmed by intraoperative consultation with the pathologist, resection of the underlying lesion.

15.6 Summary

- Intracranial tumors can present acutely with hemorrhage, severe edema, hydrocephalus, and seizures.
- No matter how severe the clinical presentation, always perform an accurate neurologic examination and obtain a noncontrast HCT to guide further decisions. In a real emergent situation, consider obtaining a contrast HCT with CT angiogram. In all other cases, obtain an MRI with and without IV contrast.
- Decide whether the patient needs immediate surgical intervention or if medical treatment should be attempted first: always try to limit emergent surgeries only to true emergent situations.
- Regardless of surgical intervention, it is fundamental to optimize vital signs, electrolytes, and coagulation parameters.

References

[1]   Kellie G. An account with some reflections on the pathology of the brain. Edinburgh Med Chir Soc Trans.. 1824; 1:84–169

[2]   Monro A. Observations on the Structure and Function of the Nervous System. Edinburgh: Creech & Johnson; 1783

[3]   Iwama T, Ohkuma A, Miwa Y, et al. Brain tumors manifesting as intracranial hemorrhage. Neurol Med Chir (Tokyo). 1992; 32(3):130–135

[4]   Kondziolka D, Bernstein M, Resch L, et al. Significance of hemorrhage into brain tumors: clinicopathological study. J Neurosurg. 1987; 67(6):852–857

[5]   Licata B, Turazzi S. Bleeding cerebral neoplasms with symptomatic hematoma. J Neurosurg Sci. 2003; 47(4):201–210, discussion 210

[6]   Donato J, Campigotto F, Uhlmann EJ, et al. Intracranial hemorrhage in patients with brain metastases treated with therapeutic enoxaparin: a matched cohort study. Blood. 2015; 126(4):494–499

[7]   Schrader B, Barth H, Lang EW, et al. Spontaneous intracranial haematomas caused by neoplasms. Acta Neurochir (Wien). 2000; 142(9):979–985

[8]   Seidel C, Hentschel B, Simon M, et al. A comprehensive analysis of vascular complications in 3,889 glioma patients from the German Glioma Network. J Neurol. 2013; 260(3):847–855

[9]   Pan E, Tsai JS, Mitchell SB. Retrospective study of venous thromboembolic and intracerebral hemorrhagic events in glioblastoma patients. Anticancer Res. 2009; 29(10):4309–4313

[10] Galicich JH, Arbit E. Metastatic brain tumors. In: Youmans JR, ed. Neurological Surgery. 3rd ed. Philadelphia, PA: WB Saunders; 1990:3204–3222

[11] Chung E, Bodensteiner J, Hogg JP. Spontaneous intracerebral hemorrhage: a very late delayed effect of radiation therapy. J Child Neurol. 1992; 7(3):259–263

[12] Burger PC, Boyko OB. The pathology of central nervous system radiation injury. In: Gutin PH, Leibel SA, Sheline GE, eds. Radiation injury to the nervous system. New York: Raven Press; 1991:191–208

[13] Komotar RJ, Keswani SC, Wityk RJ. Meningioma presenting as stroke: report of two cases and estimation of incidence. J Neurol Neurosurg Psychiatry. 2003; 74(1):136–137

[14] Yilmazlar S, Kocaeli H, Cordan T. Brain stem stroke associated with epidermoid tumours: report of two cases. J Neurol Neurosurg Psychiatry. 2004; 75(9):1340–1342

[15] Aoki N, Sakai T, Oikawa A, Takizawa T, Koike M. Dissection of the middle cerebral artery caused by invasion of malignant glioma presenting as acute onset of hemiplegia. Acta Neurochir (Wien). 1999; 141(9):1005–1008

[16] Züchner S, Kawohl W, Sellhaus B, Mull M, Mayfrank L, Kosinski CM. A case of gliosarcoma appearing as ischaemic stroke. J Neurol Neurosurg Psychiatry. 2003; 74(3):364–366

[17] Rudolph J, Kats J. Cerebrovascular complication of malignancy. In: Newton HB, Malkin MG, eds. Neurologic Complication of Systemic Cancers and Antineoplastic Therapy. New York: Informa Healthcare; 2010:109–119

[18] Milhorat TH. Classification of the cerebral edemas with reference to hydrocephalus and pseudotumor cerebri. Childs Nerv Syst. 1992; 8(6):301–306

[19] Rama Rao KV, Jayakumar AR, Norenberg MD. Brain edema in acute liver failure: mechanisms and concepts. Metab Brain Dis. 2014; 29(4):927–936

[20] Simard JM, Sheth KN, Kimberly WT, et al. Glibenclamide in cerebral ischemia and stroke. Neurocrit Care. 2014; 20(2):319–333

[21] Gerstner ER, Duda DG, di Tomaso E, et al. VEGF inhibitors in the treatment of cerebral edema in patients with brain cancer. Nat Rev Clin Oncol. 2009; 6(4):229–236

[22] van Breemen MS, Wilms EB, Vecht CJ. Epilepsy in patients with brain tumours: epidemiology, mechanisms, and management. Lancet Neurol. 2007; 6(5):421–430

[23] Armstrong TS, Grant R, Gilbert MR, Lee JW, Norden AD. Epilepsy in glioma patients: mechanisms, management, and impact of anticonvulsant therapy. Neuro Oncol. 2016; 18(6):779–789

[24] Solheim O, Vik A, Gulati S, Eide PK. Rapid and severe rise in static and pulsatile intracranial pressures during a generalized epileptic seizure. Seizure. 2008; 17(8):740–743

[25] Al-Mufti F, Claassen J. Neurocritical care: status epilepticus review. Crit Care Clin. 2014; 30(4):751–764

[26] Abo-Salem E, Becker RC. Reversal of novel oral anticoagulants. Curr Opin Pharmacol. 2016; 27:86–91

[27] Frontera JA, Lewin JJ, III, Rabinstein AA, et al. Guideline for reversal of antithrombotics in intracranial hemorrhage: a statement for healthcare professionals from the Neurocritical Care Society and Society of Critical Care Medicine. Neurocrit Care. 2016; 24(1):6–46

[28] El-Gaidi MA, El-Nasr AH, Eissa EM. Infratentorial complications following preresection CSF diversion in children with posterior fossa tumors. J Neurosurg Pediatr. 2015; 15(1):4–11

16 Acute Bony Decompression of the Optic and Facial Nerves

Stephen J. Johans, Zach Fridirici, Jason Heth, Christine C. Nelson, H. Alexander Arts, Matthew Kircher, and Anand V. Germanwala

Abstract

Neurosurgical consideration of cranial nerve decompression following head and facial trauma arises primarily in the setting of optic (II) and facial (VII) nerve injury. The course of these cranial nerves through bony foramina in the frontal and temporal regions makes them particularly susceptible to compromise following fracture or deformation of the skull base. The role of surgical decompression in these injuries has been widely debated. The use of high-dose steroids has improved outcome without the need for surgical intervention in some cases. Management has been dictated by interpretation of retrospective data. Despite the increased push in medicine toward randomized trials and outcomes studies, prospective data regarding optimal treatment of traumatic optic and facial neuropathies have not been obtainable. Each surgeon's treatment of such neuropathies requires his or her best judgment in an analysis of the available retrospective data.

Keywords: facial nerve compression, nerve decompression, optic nerve compression, traumatic optic neuropathy

16.1 Traumatic Injury to the Optic Nerve

16.1.1 Introduction

Disturbances of the visual system have been described in 2 to 11% of patients with head injury[1,2,3,4,5,6] and in up to 67% of patients with facial fracture.[7] Indirect optic nerve injuries are estimated to occur in 0.5 to 1.5% of closed cranial trauma[8,9] and in up to 3% of patients with facial fractures.[7] Patients with orbital trauma may present with decreased or absent visual acuity, afferent pupillary defects, blindness and concomitant ophthalmoplegia (orbital apex syndrome), proptosis, mydriasis, and ptosis (superior orbital fissure syndrome).[10,11,12]

The optic nerve can be anatomically divided into four parts: intraocular, orbital, intracanalicular, and intracranial. The optic nerve is most susceptible to injury within rigid confines of the optic canal, where it is fixed to the meninges and periosteum.[13,14] Patients with immediate blindness following trauma are generally believed to have suffered avulsion of the optic nerve and have a dismal prognosis for return of visual acuity. Partial preservation of vision suggests compromise of the optic nerve without avulsion and a reasonable chance of maintaining vision in the injured eye. High-dose steroids are believed to improve the outcome of visual acuity in such patients.[15,16,17]

The role of surgical intervention for decompression of the optic nerve within its canal has been controversial. The clinical outcome following posttraumatic decompression of the optic nerve varies significantly.[18,19,20,21] The wide spectrum of injuries and pathophysiologic mechanisms that may produce optic nerve dysfunction further complicates the interpretation of these results. High-dose steroids are frequently administered as a first-line treatment.[22,23,24] Most authors agree that a documented decline in visual acuity following serious head injury or facial fracture warrants consideration of optic nerve decompression, particularly if there has been an initial improvement on high-dose steroids followed by further decline.[17,20,25] If surgery is undertaken, the approach is determined by the pathology of the lesion and associated injuries. Fronto-orbital,[17,20,25] lateral orbital,[26,27,28,29] and transethmoidal approaches[5,15,18,30,31,32,33] have all been described. There continue to be no large prospective clinical studies comparing surgical with nonsurgical management, and the surgeon confronted with a patient with declining visual acuity following head or facial injury is therefore best guided by a critical review of the available retrospective studies.

16.1.2 Pathophysiology of Optic Nerve Injury

Optic nerve compression may be associated with a variety of pathologic conditions. Most commonly, compression is associated with fractures of the orbital complex,[34] including the ethmoid bones, optic canal, frontal orbital plate, orbital floor, sphenoid bone, lateral orbital wall, and "blow-in" fractures of the orbit.[4,5,10,17,26,35,36,37,38] In some cases of posttraumatic optic nerve dysfunction, no fractures can be identified.[15,20] Many authors believe that compressive edema or vascular insufficiency is the most likely pathologic mechanism of posttraumatic optic neuropathy.[38,39] Hemorrhage[25,40,41,42] into the optic nerve sheath has been described, as well as laceration of the intracanalicular optic nerve by fracture fragments.[18,19] Walsh[25] classified optic nerve lesions occurring in conjunction with head injuries into primary and secondary insults. A primary insult refers to alterations that occur with impact forces, such as hemorrhage, shearing of nerve fibers, and contusion. Secondary insults represent the delayed effects of impact, such as edema, necrosis secondary to local vascular compromise, and infarction secondary to thrombosis of the ophthalmic artery.

Kline et al[20] described six categories of indirect optic nerve injury: laceration, bone deformation or fracture, vascular insufficiency, concussion, contusion, and hemorrhage. Lacerations or stretch avulsion injuries are usually seen in the area of the cranial opening of the optic canal and are most likely secondary to a tethering effect of the fixed intracanalicular portion and the relatively mobile brain and globe. Direct compression of the optic nerve by bony fragments, with subsequent visual improvement following decompression, has often been reported. Pathologic evidence of vascular insufficiency with resultant optic nerve infarction was reported by Hughes[38] and Ramsay,[39] supporting the explanation that the mechanism involved in indirect optic nerve injury is vascular compromise. Their findings were localized to the intracanalicular portion of the optic nerve, supporting the idea that this is the region susceptible to compressive ischemia following injury. Hemorrhage within the optic sheath or optic nerve has been detected intraoperatively

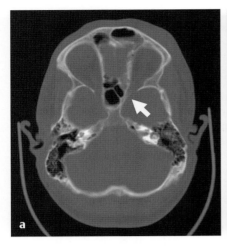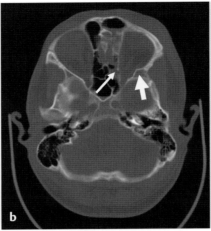

Fig. 16.1 Axial computed tomography images of a 24-year-old man who sustained orbital apex and optic foramen fractures. **(a)** Orbital apex fractures in region of optic foramen and superior orbital fissure (white arrow). **(b)** Fractures in medial (thin arrow) and lateral (large arrow) orbital wall fractures. The lateral orbital wall fracture is impinging the lateral rectus muscle.

and in postmortem studies by Pringle,[43] Walsh,[25] and Niho et al.[41] In the operative series reported by Hammer and Ambos,[40] four patients were noted with optic nerve sheath hematoma, all of which improved postoperatively, following evacuation of the blood clot.

16.1.3 Evaluation of Traumatic Optic Nerve Injury

Concomitant head and facial injuries often complicate the initial evaluation of visual acuity following trauma. Indirect injuries to the optic nerve can be classified into anterior and posterior types.[20] Visual acuity may be unavailable, absent, diminished, or preserved in either type of injury. Anterior injuries involving the intraocular portion of the optic nerve generally present with funduscopic abnormalities, including diffusely swollen optic disks, retinal edema secondary to central retinal artery disruption, and total avulsion of the optic nerve head. Posterior injuries are defined as optic nerve dysfunction in the absence of funduscopic abnormalities and are generally the result of insult to the optic nerve in the optic canal. Degenerative funduscopic abnormalities such as optic disk pallor and loss of the retinal nerve fiber layer are not apparent on initial evaluation but may be observed several weeks after injury. Although described separately, these two types of injury may occur in combination.

An initial assessment of visual acuity of each eye separately is critical, if possible. Ideally, this is accomplished using a formal acuity chart. The ability to read printed material, count fingers, or simply perceive light should be documented in each eye. In patients with a diminished level of consciousness, absence of an afferent pupillary defect and an aversive response to bright light suggest intact light perception. Documented progressive deterioration in visual acuity following head trauma should prompt consideration of optic nerve decompression.

Decreased direct pupillary response to light is cited as the most reliable index of optic nerve compromise, according to Edmund and Godtfredsen.[36] With unilateral optic nerve injury, the initial pupillary size is equal bilaterally; however, upon direct light stimulation of the impaired eye, pupillary constriction occurs more slowly and to a lesser degree—or not at all—than if the stimulus had been applied to the normal eye. This

difference in pupillary constriction, constituting a relative afferent pupillary defect (RAPD), carries the eponym the Marcus Gunn pupil.[44] It is important to note, however, that if bilateral optic nerve injury is present, an RAPD may be more subtle or not be present.

Assessment of the visual pathways is often difficult when the level of consciousness is decreased in patients with severe head injuries, as previously noted. Visual evoked responses and electroretinograms may provide additional information to guide long-term clinical management. From a practical standpoint, limited availability and technical difficulty associated with testing in the setting of acute trauma may limit the usefulness of monitoring visual evoked response and electroretinography. Good correlation between the initial visual evoked response and ultimate visual acuity has been described.[45,46,47] Furthermore, in some settings, the visual evoked response may be superior to clinical assessment in determining outcome of visual acuity. Greenberg et al[48] described a 90% predictive accuracy with visual evoked response testing, as opposed to 30% with clinical examination, in a series of patients with retrobulbar dysfunction examined within 3 days of insult and again at 3 months or longer.

16.1.4 Neuroimaging Assessment

The association of optic nerve injury with facial and orbital fractures and the reported cases of improvement following removal of compressive bony fragments mandates thorough neuroimaging investigation in cases of compromised visual acuity. The procedure of choice is thin-section computed tomography (CT), as it allows resolution of the bony detail of the orbital apex region (▶ Fig. 16.1).[13,49,50] Axial and coronal CT scans can be obtained, and these may demonstrate orbital fractures and bony fragments. Reconstructed images including three-dimensional views can also assist in detailed evaluation of facial and orbital injuries. It must be remembered, however, that it has been reported that compressive bony fragments not observed on preoperative CT imaging have been found at operation.[51] Magnetic resonance (MR) imaging may demonstrate soft-tissue injury and hemorrhage or hematoma within the dural sheath or optic nerve.

16.1.5 Management of Traumatic Optic Nerve Injury

Nonoperative Treatment and Comparisons with Operative Treatment

Corticosteroids have assumed a prominent role in the management of traumatic optic nerve injury. This occurred at the same time trials using corticosteroids in the management of spinal cord injury were suggesting a beneficial treatment effect. Although a range of dosages have been studied, the most common regimen calls for an initial loading dose of 30 mg/kg followed by 15 mg/kg infused every 6 hours for 3 days. Several series utilizing corticosteroids reported substantial improvement of visual acuity.[15,16,17,23,24,52,53,54] In one meta-analysis, any treatment (corticosteroids, extracranial decompression, or corticosteroids plus extracranial decompression) improved visual acuity more than observation alone.[52] No difference between treatment modalities could be found. In contrast, there are other series that do not show any benefit for steroids over observation, most prominently the report from the International Optic Nerve Trauma Study.[55] The International Optic Nerve Trauma Study was conceived to compare extracranial optic nerve decompressive surgery plus corticosteroids with corticosteroids alone. Unfortunately, enrollment of eligible patients was insufficient to provide statistical validity. The study was changed to an observational study. The results of this study suggest no differences in traumatic optic nerve injury outcome between observation, corticosteroid, and decompressive surgery groups. In 2011, a review was published in the *American Journal of Ophthalmology* that concluded that high-dose steroids could be harmful when given to head trauma patients for optic nerve injury. The review also concluded that surgery should be reserved for conscious patients with delayed visual loss, or whose vision does not improve in 4 days.[56]

Indications for Optic Nerve Decompression

An afferent pupillary defect with a normal funduscopic examination suggests injury to the optic nerve. Once the diagnosis of optic nerve compromise is made, decisions regarding appropriate management must be addressed. The time since injury and the degree of progression of visual deficit should be noted. Complete loss of vision immediately following injury generally carries a dismal prognosis, and, although cases of recovery have been described,[18,19] most authors advocate treatment with corticosteroids in these circumstances.[17,20,27] Several related but subtly different indications have been utilized for individuals with some degree of preserved vision. One of the more common indications recommends optic nerve decompression if visual function deteriorates during or after corticosteroid treatment. Others extend this indication by offering decompression if visual function does *not* improve during corticosteroid treatment. Still others advocate decompression if any optic nerve hematoma or orbital fracture causing an optic canal compressive fragment is discovered on imaging. Emanuelli and colleagues encountered 26 patients in a 10-year period with traumatic optic neuropathy. All patients were treated with system steroids. All patient required a surgical treatment, because of poor response to medical therapy; it consisted of an endonasal endoscopic decompression of the optic nerve. Improvement of visual acuity was achieved in 65% of the cases. No complications occurred with follow-up time of 41 months. An improvement in visual acuity was achieved, although very limited in some cases, when surgery was performed as close as possible to the traumatic event. They concluded that surgical decompression offers best outcome for patients if medical therapy failed and if surgery is done within 12 to 24 hours.[57]

Debate continues regarding the optimal time for decompression. Several reports document improved visual outcome for decompression performed within 7 days of injury compared with decompression performed after 7 days.[22,24,53] Others have not found this time period to be a significant factor in visual outcome.[51,58,59] Thakar and colleagues[60] reported improvements in visual function for patients undergoing decompression up to 1 year after injury and recommend decompression for patients with traumatic optic neuropathy with decreased vision persisting up to 1 year after injury. Another factor that may be important is the presence of orbital, orbital apex, or optic canal fractures. Again there is no agreement as to whether the presence of such fractures is prognostic of visual outcome. Some reports document worse visual outcomes in patients suffering orbital apex fractures,[22,24,59] whereas others find no difference in outcomes between patients with and without such fractures.[23,51,52,53,55] Some authors who found no difference admit that small sample sizes may have limited their power to detect a difference between the two groups.

Choice of Surgical Approach

When surgical intervention is considered, the approach is dictated by the mechanism and location of the insult, as well as associated injuries. Successful optic nerve decompression requires removal of one half of the circumference of the bone along the entire length of the optic canal. If a fracture is present, the approach is best selected on the basis of the type of fracture and the direction of compression, if this can be determined by preoperative radiologic studies. In the absence of clear pathology, adequate decompression of the canal should be possible regardless of the direction of approach. The intracranial frontal orbital approach to the optic canal, as described in 1922 by Dandy[61] for orbital tumors, is frequently utilized. This exposure is particularly useful when associated intracranial pathology requires surgical attention. The transethmoid approach, originally described in 1926 by Sewall[62] and popularized and modified by Niho et al,[41] Fukado,[19] Sofferman,[63] and others,[5] avoids a formal craniotomy and provides exposure of the medial orbital apex with minimal morbidity. When the compression is secondary to fractures of the lateral orbital wall, the lateral facial or lateral temporal approach has been successfully used to decompress the optic nerve and canal.[26,27,28,29] This approach provides wide access to the lateral orbit, including the region of the superior orbital fissure, with minimal retraction of the orbital contents.

Transfrontal Approach

The transfrontal approach to visualize the optic nerve and chiasm is very familiar to neurosurgeons (▶ Fig. 16.2). Access to

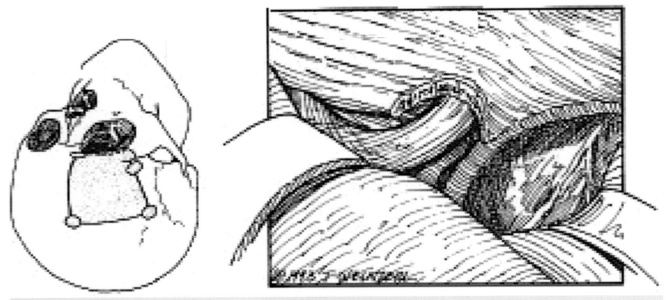

Fig. 16.2 Transfrontal optic nerve decompression via a right frontal craniotomy. The approach to the optic canal is shown. The frontal lobe has been retracted and a portion of the bony optic canal unroofed, allowing inspection of the optic nerve and dural sheath.

the optic chiasm, intracranial optic nerve, and posterior aspect of the optic canal allows direct inspection of these structures in cases of frontotemporal injury.[2,38,41,59] Dural tears and orbital plate fractures can be repaired, and associated intracranial pathology can be addressed concurrently. The optic canal can be unroofed and the dural sheath of the optic nerve incised to allow adequate decompression and inspection of the optic nerve. This technique has been described and utilized by many authors and has been labeled by Sofferman as "the standard surgical technique upon which virtually all reported series of optic nerve decompression are based."[63]

Transethmoidal Approach

Transethmoidal approaches to the optic canal have assumed a prominent role in optic nerve decompression for trauma. There are several reasons for this. Transethmoidal approaches obviate the need for craniotomy, which some surgeons feel carries a higher rate of risks. Transethmoidal approaches require less time in fashioning the approach and take less time to perform. Finally, these approaches tend to be less invasive, particularly when performed endoscopically,[64] and coincide with trends toward minimally invasive surgery. There are two particular drawbacks to these approaches, however. Foremost, the carotid artery travels near the optic nerve adjacent to the lateral wall of the sphenoid sinus (▶ Fig. 16.3). Removal of bone over the optic nerve must be meticulous to avoid injury to the carotid artery. Carotid artery laceration in this location may be a fatal event because there is no vascular control. Another risk in these approaches is cerebrospinal fluid (CSF) leak. This occurs through two primary events. First, any exposure or drilling that is too superior risks traversing the planum sphenoidale dura and can result in CSF rhinorrhea. Second, the optic nerve sheath may either be lacerated from the traumatic event or incised as part of the procedure. Such openings in the optic nerve sheath can also lead to CSF leak.

Transethmoidal approaches may be subdivided into transfacial, endoscopic transnasal, and transconjunctival. The transfacial transethmoidal approach to the medial aspect of the orbital apex includes a facial incision. A vertical incision is made just medial to the medial canthus of the eye (Lynch incision), dividing the medial palpebral ligament (▶ Fig. 16.4). An oval portion of bone (1 × 1.5 cm) near the junction of the maxillary, ethmoidal, and frontal bones is resected, exposing the ethmoidal sinus. After removal of the mucous membranes and bony septa of the sinus, the prominence of the optic canal is found deep in the lateral recess of the sinus. If the thin medial wall of the sinus has been fractured, the bony fragments are carefully removed. The optic canal is decompressed along its medial wall. There are no consistent recommendations regarding incision of the optic nerve sheath, with some authors incising the sheath,[33,51,63,65] some avoiding incision,[23,66] and others undecided.[24,30,67] This approach is hampered by limited visibility and a narrow angle of approach to the optic canal. A modified sphenoethmoid approach has been extensively described by Sofferman[63] to improve the angle of approach.

Endoscopic transnasal transethmoidal approaches begin with an endoscopic ethmoidectomy. Once the sphenoid sinus is identified, it is entered. The lateral wall of the sinus is examined to find the prominences overlying the optic nerve and carotid artery (▶ Fig. 16.3). Bone removal begins over the thin lamina papyracea and proceeds posteriorly. Drilling should occur under continuous irrigation to prevent thermal injury to the optic nerve. The bone should be drilled to a thin remnant, which is then carefully removed to prevent carotid artery injury. The optic nerve sheath may be incised, as previously discussed. Any evidence of CSF leak should be treated with any of many methods available (fibrin glue, dural substitutes, cadaveric fascia

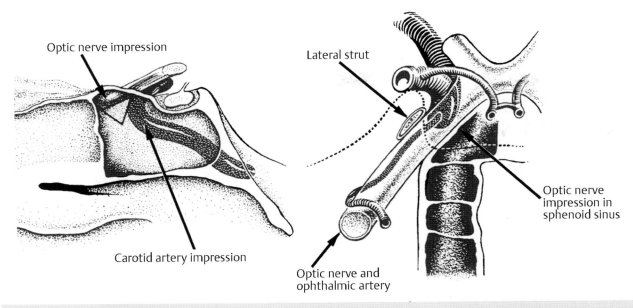

Fig. 16.3 The lateral wall of the sphenoid sinus. The optic nerve and carotid artery create impressions on the lateral wall. The carotid artery is posterior and inferior in relation to the optic nerve; therefore, optic nerve exposure should begin anterior and superior in relation to the optic nerve impression. (Adapted from Goldberg RA, Steinsapir KD. Extracranial optic canal decompression: indications and technique. Ophthal Plast Reconstr Surg 1996;12:163–170.)

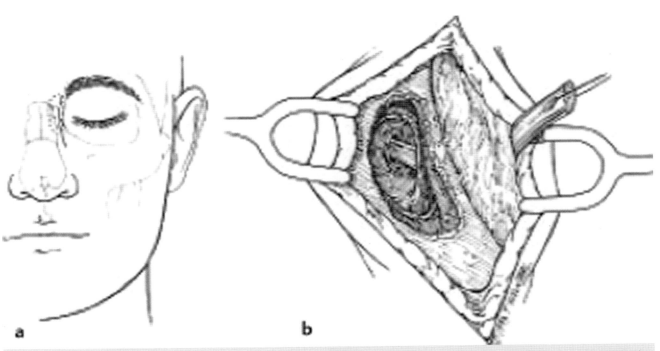

Fig. 16.4 A left transethmoid optic nerve decompression. **(a)** The incision and area of bone resection are outlined. **(b)** The contents of the ethmoid sinus are removed, and the optic canal is found passing obliquely in the lateral recess of the ethmoid sinus. A portion of the bony optic canal has been unroofed to allow inspection of the optic nerve and sheath. The divided medial palpebral ligament is retracted with a suture.

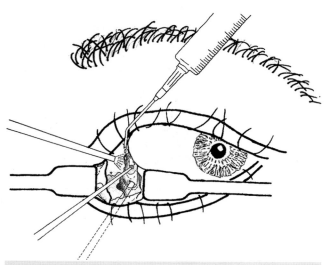

Fig. 16.5 An endoscopic assisted transorbital for optic nerve decompression. A conjunctival incision has been fashioned, the periorbita carefully dissected from the orbital walls, and the ethmoidal arteries cauterized and incised. The lamina papyracea has been removed, and drilling has begun to open the optic canal. A straight suction has been placed in the sphenoid sinus through the nose. (Adapted from Yang WG, Chen CT, Tsay PK, De Villa GF, Tsai YJ, Chen YR. Outcome for traumatic optic neuropathy—surgical versus nonsurgical treatment. Ann Plast Surg 2004;52:36–42.)

lata, etc.). Endoscopic approaches have also utilized transconjunctival exposure to increase the orbital exposure. Approaches through the orbit alone[24] (▶ Fig. 16.5) and through the orbit and nasal cavity together[32] have both been described as increasing visualization.

Lateral Approach

Lateral facial and lateral temporal approaches for orbital decompression have been utilized with success in the treatment of lateral orbital wall fractures.[26,27,28,29] A vertical or hemicoronal incision is made, and a limited anterior temporal craniectomy (with removal of the zygomatic process) is performed. This allows for extradural exposure of the anterior temporal lobe, the anterolateral frontal lobe, and the lateral aspect of the periorbita. Wide access to the lateral orbit is obtained with direct exposure of the contents of the superior orbital fissure and optic canal. The superior aspect of the optic canal can be decompressed, and the dural optic sheath can be inspected and incised. This technique has been criticized because it involves extensive exposure of the superior orbital fissure and a portion of the cavernous sinus, placing both at risk for injury.[63]

16.2 Traumatic Injury to the Facial Nerve: Overview

Posttraumatic facial nerve injuries have been described in 2% of all head injuries and is the second leading cause of facial paralysis in adults.[68,69] Among patients with skull fractures, 14 to 22% have temporal bone fractures, which can result in hearing

loss, CSF fistulas, and facial nerve palsy.[70,71] An appreciation of the anatomy of the facial nerve and the temporal bone allows localization of the lesion and aids in the selection of appropriate management.

Similar to the optic nerve, indications for surgical decompression of the facial nerve are still debated. In general, the decision to operate is dependent on the site of injury, the time course of facial palsy, radiographic evidence, and electrodiagnostic criteria. Immediate facial nerve paralysis associated with an extratemporal facial nerve trauma should be repaired within 72 hours of the injury.[72] Facial paralysis associated with temporal bone fractures are divided into immediate and delayed facial paralysis. Most authors advocate for early operation in temporal bone fractures with total facial paralysis and radiographic evidence of facial canal discontinuity or facial paralysis satisfying electrodiagnostic criteria after 3 days.[73] Patients with delayed-onset facial paralysis are generally believed to have a better prognosis, regardless of management, than those with immediate nerve dysfunction, although this has been challenged.[73] Up to 95% of patients with partial facial injury will improve without intervention. Thus, intervention is more controversial, with some authors favoring a more conservative approach. The technique and extent of facial nerve decompression is dependent on the site of the lesion and the patient's level of hearing.

16.3 Pathology of Temporal Bone Fractures

Fractures of the temporal bone tend to occur along points of weakness (foramina) and parallel to the traumatic force. Temporal bone fractures are classically described as longitudinal or transverse fractures in relationship to the long axis of the petrous pyramid.[72] However, this scheme has given way to a new classification based on the involvement of the otic capsule (bone encasing the cochlea and semicircular canal).

Fractures that spare the otic capsule are typically due to trauma in the temporoparietal region. These fractures tend to result in a mixed or conductive hearing loss and a lower rate of facial paralysis. Otic capsule disrupting fractures generally result from trauma to the occiput and are associated with sensorineural hearing loss and an increased risk of CSF fistula, meningitis, and facial nerve palsy.[74]

16.4 Anatomy of the Facial Nerve

The facial nerve is a mixed cranial nerve that contains 7,000 to 10,000 fibers. It arises as two roots from the lateral pontomedullary sulcus, just anterior to the vestibulocochlear nerve. The larger component is the motor facial nerve and is located anterior to the smaller nervus intermedius, which subserves sensory and preganglionic autonomic fibers. The facial nerve enters into the internal auditory canal (IAC), passing through the meatus with the cochlear and vestibular nerves, and lies along the anterosuperior quadrant within the canal. The nerve enters the fallopian canal through the meatal foramen at the lateral edge of the IAC above the transverse crest and anterior to the vertical crest (Bill's bar). This foramen is the narrowest segment of the facial canal and begins the labyrinthine segment of the facial nerve. Just distal to the labyrinthine segment the nerve is the geniculate ganglion, with branches extending as the greater petrosal nerve (providing preganglionic fibers to the pterygoid plexus for lacrimation), a branch to the tympanic plexus, and a branch to the sympathetic plexus of the middle meningeal artery. At the geniculate, the facial nerve turns abruptly posteriorly, passing just inferior to the prominence of the lateral semicircular canal in the aditus of the mastoid antrum. Just medial to the aditus, it again abruptly courses downward in a bony septum, splitting off to form the nerve to the stapedius muscle (which dampens motion of the stapes), the chorda tympani (which joins the lingual nerve to provide taste to the anterior two thirds of the tongue and parasympathetic fibers to the submandibular ganglion), and a communicating branch to the auricular component of the vagus (X) nerve (sensory fibers to external acoustic meatus) before emerging from the stylomastoid foramen. The nerve then courses anterolaterally between the styloid process and the posterior belly of the digastric muscle, innervating the digastric and the stylohyoid muscles, and giving off a posterior auricular branch that supplies the intrinsic and auricular muscles. The nerve enters the posteromedial surface of the parotid gland and divides it into its superficial and deep lobes as it branches to supply the muscles of facial expression.

16.4.1 Pathophysiology of Facial Nerve Injury

Injury to the facial nerve near the geniculate ganglion was first reported in 1926 by Ulrich.[75] Subsequent clinical studies support his observation that this represents the most frequent site of facial nerve injury in temporal bone trauma. Yanagihara[76] reported a fracture involving the geniculate ganglion in 55% of patients with facial palsy following head injury. Fisch[77,78] and Fisch and Esslen[79] reported a 93% incidence of intraoperative pathology in the labyrinthine segment (including the geniculate ganglion), with a second, less frequent focus in the descending tympanic segment (7%). The labyrinthine segment is pivotal to facial nerve injury because of its small diameter, constricting arachnoid band, and limited epineurium. As a result, any edema quickly uses up the little residual extraneural canalicular space; this is hypothesized to decrease nerve perfusion, which, in turn, causes more edema, setting off a downward spiral.

The histopathology of facial nerve injury secondary to temporal bone fracture has been described,[10,80,81,82,83,84,85,86,87] and the findings are consistent with those seen in other injuries to a proximal neural segment (i.e., marked distal degeneration, disorganized nerve bundles, and Schwann cell proliferation proximally and distally). Loss of myelination in the geniculate ganglion, with loss of ganglion cells and fibrosis in the perineurium and endoneurium, has been described, along with severe degeneration of nerve fibers and fibrosis extending into the tympanic and mastoid portions of the facial nerve.

16.4.2 Evaluation of Facial Nerve Injury

In the evaluation of facial nerve injury, it is important to document the time of onset, the site of injury, and the degree of functional deficit. Acute paralysis within the first 24 hours suggests a more severe injury, with mechanical disruption by stretching, tearing, or shearing of the nerve, and is associated with a poor prognosis for spontaneous recovery. Delayed paralysis, which can develop up to 2 weeks following injury, is secondary to compressive edema or hemorrhage within the fallopian canal and is generally felt to carry a better prognosis for spontaneous recovery.[73,88] The most common scale to evaluate facial function is the House–Brackmann facial nerve grading scale. The House–Brackmann grading scale uses six grades of increasing dysfunction, from grade 1 (normal) to grade 6 (total facial paralysis).

Facial nerve topography as well as nerve excitability testing (NET) has largely been replaced by more objective electrophysiologic testing.

Electroneurography (ENoG), effective from postinjury day 3 to 21, records facial muscle response at the nasolabial fold to supramaximal stimulation over the facial nerve as it exits the stylomastoid foramen.[70,89,90] Results are compared with the contralateral side and recorded as a percentage of deficit. Supramaximal stimulation is applied to ensure that every possible working nerve fiber is tested. Greater than 90% reduction in the first 1 to 2 weeks post injury is regarded as severe neuronal dysfunction and is a relative indication for facial nerve exploration.[70]

Electromyography (EMG) is different from ENoG in that no stimulation is performed. Intramuscular needle electrodes are placed, and recordings are made at baseline and during attempts at voluntary facial contractions. Maintenance or early return of voluntary motor unit potentials suggests at least partial continuity of the facial nerve. This finding has been reported to be predictive of return to good facial nerve function, even in the presence of ENoG demonstrating greater than 90% reduction on the affected side.[70,91,92] Development of fibrillation potentials at this time suggests severe denervation. Outside possible documentation of voluntary motor potentials at any time, EMG otherwise is not useful until 14 to 21 days post injury, as this is the period required for neural degeneration to become evident.

Electrophysiologic testing provides information relating to the extent of injury on the basis of denervation of the facial muscles and may be of benefit in patients with a decreased level of consciousness.[70,77,89,90,93,94,95,96] Electrophysiologic studies are a useful tool in the evaluation of facial nerve injury, although expert interpretation is essential.

16.4.3 Radiographic Assessment

The imaging modality of choice for the evaluation of the temporal bone is axial and coronal high-resolution CT scan (▶Fig. 16.6 and ▶Fig. 16.7).[71,72] Focused scans of the temporal bones can be obtained, following initial evaluation and management of intracranial pathology. Multiplanar reconstructions can be used to identify facial canal fractures or impingement.[97] The anatomy of the temporal bone and associated fractures as they appear on CT have been fully described.[97,98,99,100] Associated skull and facial fractures, ossicular disruption, hemorrhage in the middle ear or mastoid air cells, and potential injury to the carotid artery can also be appreciated with CT. Resnick and colleagues found an 18% incidence of carotid injury in patients with fractures through the carotid canal and a 5% incidence of carotid injury if the fracture did not.[101]

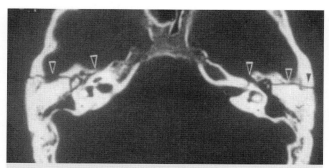

Fig. 16.6 Axial temporal bone computed tomography scan demonstrating bilateral longitudinal temporal bone fractures (arrowheads).

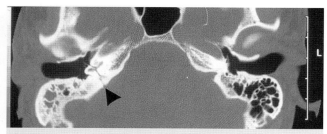

Fig. 16.7 Axial temporal bone computed tomography scan demonstrating a transverse temporal fracture on the right (arrowhead).

16.4.4 Management of Facial Nerve Injury

Indications for Facial Nerve Decompression

After identifying a facial nerve palsy and its severity, clinical management must be addressed.[80,85,94,102,103,104,105,106,107,108,109,110,111,112] Initially, protection of the cornea of the eye is paramount. Interventions include conservative measures such as lubricating ointments and intermittently taping the eye shut, as well as more invasive procedures such as upper eyelid gold weights and tarsorrhaphy. Short-term steroid administration is widely used. Although unproven, steroids are thought to improve outcomes, presumably by reducing nerve edema in patients managed conservatively.[73,108]

Patients with facial nerve paresis that has not progressed to complete paralysis are managed nonoperatively, as more than 95% of such patients will reach House–Brackman grades of 1 and 2. Patients with total facial paralysis of immediate onset and/or radiologic evidence of facial canal disruption are candidates for early operation. The management of patients with immediate-onset facial paralysis without evidence of fracture evokes debate. Most surgeons now tend to favor decompression based on electrophysiologic criteria. The most frequently cited criterion uses ENoG. After 72 hours, the patients are followed with serial ENoG up to 21 days. If degeneration reaches 90% or more,[70] and there are no volitional motor unit potentials seen on EMG, then surgical exploration may be warranted. Patients whose ENoG remains below 90% degeneration, or whose volitional motor unit potentials are seen on EMG, should be managed nonoperatively, as the prognosis is very good in these cases. Most authors recommend early decompression (within 1–3 weeks post injury) in an attempt to prevent ischemic injury, retrograde degeneration, and extensive fibrotic changes in the nerve. This is based on retrospective surgical series and postmortem examinations on patients failing to improve following decompressive procedures. In the series reported by Alford et al,[94] patients operated on after 48 hours had a worse outcome and a higher incidence of facial synkinesis. In contrast, others have found improvements in facial nerve function in facial nerve paralysis undergoing decompression in delayed fashion.[104,109] Thus, a delay in referral does not preclude a successful outcome in selected cases.

The role of surgical decompression in patients with a delayed facial paralysis is less clear, because it is generally held that the prognosis for delayed-onset facial paralysis is favorable regardless of management.[73,88] The delayed onset of the paralysis suggests continuity of the nerve with subsequent secondary edema or hematoma formation, leading to compression of the nerve within the facial canal, although this dictum has been questioned by Adegbite et al.[73] In reviewing 25 patients with immediate and delayed traumatic facial paralysis, they could not demonstrate a significant difference in outcome in patients with an immediate-onset versus delayed-onset deficit. These authors found that the degree of injury, rather than the time of onset, had significant predictive value in determining outcome. On the basis of partial recovery of function in 95% of those patients managed expectantly, a conservative approach was advocated. The finding in this study that, regardless of the time of onset, patients with complete paralysis have a poor prognosis when managed conservatively may support the role of early surgery to avoid irreparable damage.[110] Following that line of reasoning, some surgeons support decompression for delayed onset of paralysis if ENoG demonstrates 90% or greater degeneration, similar to acute-onset cases.

Choice of Surgical Approach

The choice of surgical approach is based on the site of the lesion as determined by physical examination, testing of facial nerve branch function, hearing status and audiometric data, and radiologic evaluation.[73,112] The choice of surgical approach should also be considered tentative, because exposure of the entire facial nerve may be required.

Lesions proximal to or involving the geniculate ganglion occur in 55 to 90% of cases and are best approached via an extradural middle cranial fossa craniotomy when hearing is preserved.[112] Although some authors report successful exposure of the geniculate ganglion via the transmastoid route,[85,103,105,106] this approach may lead to incomplete exposure of the geniculate ganglion or proximal labyrinthine portion of the facial nerve and cannot be done while maintaining good hearing. When there is complete loss of hearing, a translabyrinthine approach allows extensive exposure of the facial nerve for decompression and/or repair. The middle cranial fossa craniotomy is generally combined with a transmastoid decompression to ensure total decompression of the facial nerve, as 7 to 20% of patients will have a second focus of injury in the distal tympanic segment.[79,85,103] If the lesion is clearly

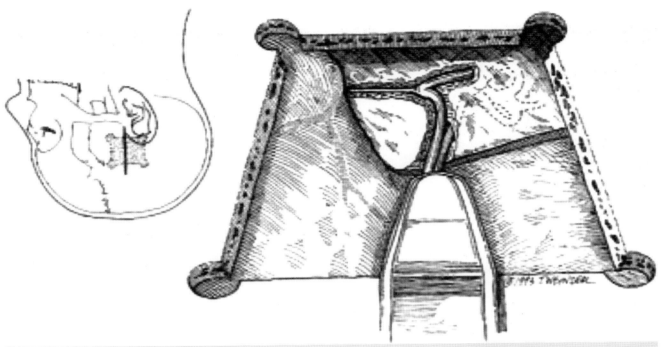

Fig. 16.8 A right middle cranial fossa approach for decompression of the facial nerve is shown. Through a small craniotomy, the dura of the middle cranial fossa is elevated to allow inspection of the floor of the middle cranial fossa. The facial nerve is identified either at the internal auditory meatus or by tracing the greater superficial petrosal nerve to the geniculate ganglion. The facial nerve can be decompressed from the internal auditory canal past the geniculate ganglion to the level of the cochleariform process. This technique is combined with a transmastoid decompression to allow total intratemporal decompression of the facial nerve.

distal to the geniculate ganglion and hearing is preserved, then a transmastoid decompression may suffice.

Middle Cranial Fossa Approach

The middle cranial fossa approach is generally performed through a linear vertical or temporal flap incision, extending from the root of the zygoma to the superior temporal line. A small craniotomy is fashioned, and the dura of the middle cranial fossa is elevated (►Fig. 16.8). Elevation of the dura must proceed with care, as the geniculate ganglion may have no bony covering in 16% of cases.[113] There are two well-known methods of identifying the geniculate ganglion and the facial nerve in the middle fossa approach. The first method utilizes the greater superficial petrosal nerve (GSPN) as a landmark. Drilling begins over the proximal GSPN and progresses posterolaterally until the geniculate ganglion is identified. Drilling continues to identify the meatal portions and IAC portions of the facial nerve. The second method utilizes landmarks on the floor of the middle fossa. An angle is envisioned between the long axis and the GSPN, which is ~120 degrees and opening medially. This angle is bisected, and this bisecting line approximates the location of the IAC. The IAC can then be unroofed first, followed by drilling laterally to identify the meatal segment, and eventually the geniculate ganglion. Once the geniculate ganglion has been identified, the tympanic portion of the facial nerve can be exposed to the level of the cochleariform process. This approach allows exposure of the most proximal portion of the intratemporal facial nerve, the labyrinthine segment, and full

exposure of the geniculate ganglion.[77,105,106,107] If the nerve is severed, direct repair or repair with an interpositional graft may be accomplished. The greater auricular nerve may be used as a donor, because it can be exposed in the field and its diameter approximates that of the facial nerve. Combined with a subsequent transmastoid approach, this technique allows total intratemporal exposure of the facial nerve. Reported complications of the middle fossa approach include sensorineural hearing loss and vestibular dysfunction (2.6–4%), CSF leak (2–5.1%), meningitis (2–2.6%), epidural hematoma (2.6%), and injury to the temporal cortex secondary to retraction.[111,112]

Transmastoid Approach

The transmastoid approach allows facial nerve exposure from the geniculate ganglion to the stylomastoid foramen. Although successfully described for exposure of the geniculate ganglion, some surgeons feel that inadequate proximal exposure is obtained and prefer combining the transmastoid and middle cranial fossa approaches for total exposure.[77,97]

A transcortical mastoidectomy can be performed through a retroauricular incision (►Fig. 16.9). The horizontal semicircular canal and short process of the incus are identified. An opening is created just inferior to the short process of the incus to enter the facial recess. Through the opening, the incudostapedial joint and second genu of the facial nerve are identified. The bone overlying the descending portion of the facial nerve is thinned and removed to the stylomastoid foramen. Additional exposure can be obtained to visualize the geniculate ganglion

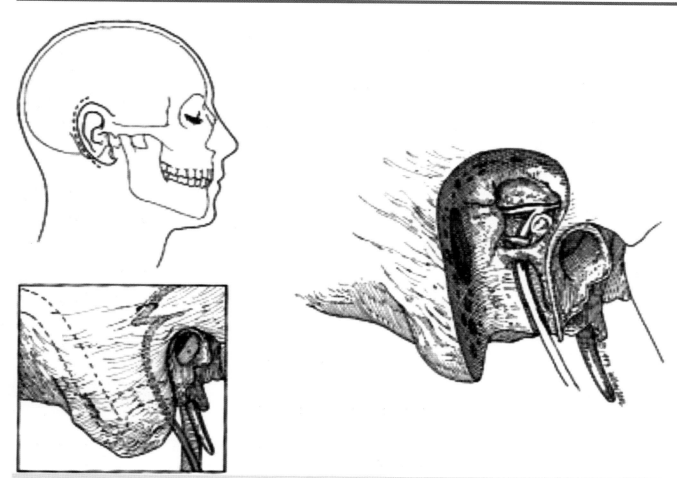

Fig. 16.9 A right transmastoid approach for decompression of the distal components of the facial nerve is shown. Following a transcortical mastoidectomy, the facial nerve is identified and traced proximal to the facial recess. The incus can be dislocated and rotated or removed to allow exposure of the second genu of the facial nerve and distal aspect of the geniculate ganglion. The facial nerve can then be decompressed in its bony canal from the level of the geniculate ganglion to the stylomastoid foramen.

by disarticulating and removing the incus, which causes conductive hearing loss. This conductive hearing loss can typically be corrected via an ossiculoplasty.

Translabyrinthine Approach

The translabyrinthine approach allows visualization from the IAC to the stylomastoid foramen for either decompression or for nerve repair. The greater auricular nerve is accessible for cable graft repair. The main condition for the use of the translabyrinthine approach is that hearing is completely lost.

A retroauricular incision is performed, and a total mastoidectomy is performed with a high-speed drill (►Fig. 16.10a). The drill is used to remove the bone over some of the posterior fossa dura posterior to the sigmoid sinus, the posterior fossa dura anteromedial to the sigmoid sinus, and the middle fossa. The facial nerve should be identified either inferior to the lateral semicircular canal or in the mastoid portion (►Fig. 16.10a). The labyrinthectomy is started by removing the lateral semicircular canal. The removal extends posteriorly, and the posterior semicircular canal is entered. The posterior semicircular canal is opened into the common crus, and the removal now is extended

to the superior semicircular canal. The bone is removed posterior to the IAC. The IAC dura should not be opened until all bone drilling is completed, to protect the nerves in the IAC. The facial nerve can be exposed from the IAC to the stylomastoid foramen at this point (►Fig. 16.10b).

16.5 Conclusion

The role of surgical decompression in both optic and facial nerve injuries remains controversial. Review of the available literature provides guidelines for the management of patients with such injuries, but randomized prospective trials are lacking. Most authors agree that a decline in visual acuity following head injury warrants optic nerve decompression, and that an immediate or early onset delayed posttraumatic facial paralysis, with 90% or greater degeneration by ENoG and absence of voluntary motor unit potentials, should undergo exploration. The role of surgical intervention in immediate posttraumatic blindness and delayed-onset facial paralysis is less clear. Although widely utilized, the role of steroids in the management of such patients is based on anecdotal evidence. A review of the literature on the

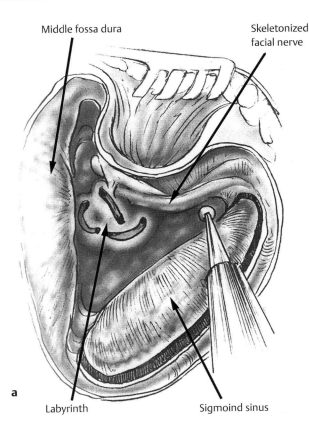

Middle fossa dura

Skeletonized facial nerve

a

Labyrinth

Sigmoind sinus

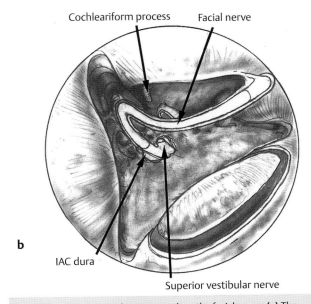

Cochleariform process

Facial nerve

b

IAC dura

Superior vestibular nerve

Fig. 16.10 Translabyrinthine approach to the facial nerve. **(a)** The mastoidectomy has been performed, and the facial canal has been identified from the lateral semicircular canal to the stylomastoid foramen. The bony labyrinth has begun to be opened. **(b)** The removal of the labyrinth and exposure of the facial nerve has been completed. The facial nerve has been exposed from the IAC to the stylomastoid foramen. IAC, internal acoustic canal. (Reproduced with permission of Elsevier from Brackman DE, Shelton C, Arriaga MA, eds. Translabyrinthine approach. In: Otologic Surgery. 2nd ed. St. Louis, MO: Elsevier; 2001:512, Copyright 2001.)

management of these lesions highlights the need for a systematic, controlled study to optimize management.

Many patients who have suffered injury to the facial or optic nerve or both are managed concurrently by neurosurgeons, ophthalmologists, and otolaryngologists. The role of the neurosurgeon in coordinating appropriate management among these disciplines requires a thorough knowledge of the natural history and available literature regarding optic and facial nerve injuries.

References

[1] Gjerris F. Traumatic lesions of the visual pathways. In: Vinken PJ, Bruyn GW, eds. Handbook of Clinical Neurology. Vol 24. New York: Elsevier; 1976:27–57

[2] Hooper RS. Orbital complications of head injury. Br J Surg. 1951; 39(154):126–138

[3] Ioannides C, Treffers W, Rutten M, Noverraz P. Ocular injuries associated with fractures involving the orbit. J Craniomaxillofac Surg. 1988; 16(4):157–159

[4] Nayak SR, Kirtane MV, Ingle MV. Fracture line in post head injury optic nerve damage. J Laryngol Otol. 1991; 105(3):203–204

[5] Nayak SR, Kirtane MV, Ingle MV. Transethmoid decompression of the optic nerve in head injuries: an update. J Laryngol Otol. 1991; 105(3):205–206

[6] Osguthorpe JD. Transethmoid decompression of the optic nerve. Otolaryngol Clin North Am. 1985; 18(1):125–137

[7] Holt GR, Holt JE. Incidence of eye injuries in facial fractures: an analysis of 727 cases. Otolaryngol Head Neck Surg. 1983; 91(3):276–279

[8] Brandle K. Post-traumatic optic nerve lesions (especially optic atrophy).. Confin Neurol. 1955; 15(3):169–208

[9] Turner JWA. Indirect injuries of the optic nerve. Brain. 1943; 66:140–151

[10] Ghobrial W, Amstutz S, Mathog RH. Fractures of the sphenoid bone. Head Neck Surg. 1986; 8(6):447–455

[11] Stuzin JM, Cutting CB, McCarthy JG, Dufresne CR. Radiographical documentation of direct injury of the intracanalicular segment of the optic nerve in the orbital apex syndrome. Ann Plast Surg. 1988; 20(4):368–373

[12] Zachariades N. The superior orbital fissure syndrome. Review of the literature and report of a case. Oral Surg Oral Med Oral Pathol. 1982; 53(3):237–240

[13] Manfredi SJ, Raji MR, Sprinkle PM, Weinstein GW, Minardi LM, Swanson TJ. Computerized tomographic scan findings in facial fractures associated with blindness. Plast Reconstr Surg. 1981; 68(4):479–490

[14] Tao H, Ma Z, Dai P, Jiang L. Computer-aided three-dimensional reconstruction and measurement of the optic canal and intracanalicular structures. Laryngoscope. 1999; 109(9):1499–1502

[15] Anderson RL, Panje WR, Gross CE. Optic nerve blindness following blunt forehead trauma. Ophthalmology. 1982; 89(5):445–455

[16] Krausen AS, Ogura JH, Burde RM, Ostrow DE. Emergency orbital decompression: a reprieve from blindness. Otolaryngol Head Neck Surg. 1981; 89(2):252–256

[17] Lipkin AF, Woodson GE, Miller RH. Visual loss due to orbital fracture. The role of early reduction. Arch Otolaryngol Head Neck Surg. 1987; 113(1):81–83

[18] Fukado Y. Results in 350 cases of surgical decompression of the optic nerve. Trans Ophthalmol Soc N Z. 1973; 25:96–99

[19] Fukado Y. Results in 400 cases of surgical decompression of the optic nerve. Mod Probl Ophthalmol. 1975; 14:474–481

[20] Kline LB, Morawetz RB, Swaid SN. Indirect injury of the optic nerve. Neurosurgery. 1984; 14(6):756–764

[21] Spoor TC, Mathog RH. Restoration of vision after optic canal decompression. Arch Ophthalmol. 1986; 104(6):804–806

[22] Rajiniganth MG, Gupta AK, Gupta A, Bapuraj JR. Traumatic optic neuropathy: visual outcome following combined therapy protocol. Arch Otolaryngol Head Neck Surg. 2003; 129(11):1203–1206

[23] Spoor TC, McHenry JG. Management of traumatic optic neuropathy. J Craniomaxillofac Trauma. 1996; 2(1):14–26, discussion 27

[24] Yang WG, Chen CT, Tsay PK, de Villa GH, Tsai YJ, Chen YR. Outcome for traumatic optic neuropathy—surgical versus nonsurgical treatment. Ann Plast Surg. 2004; 52(1):36–42

[25] Walsh FB. Pathological-clinical correlations. I. Indirect trauma to the optic nerves and chiasm. II. Certain cerebral involvements associated with defective blood supply. Invest Ophthalmol. 1966; 5(5):433–449

[26] Funk GF, Stanley RB, Jr, Becker TS. Reversible visual loss due to impacted lateral orbital wall fractures. Head Neck. 1989; 11(4):295–300

[27] Knox BE, Gates GA, Berry SM. Optic nerve decompression via the lateral facial approach. Laryngoscope. 1990; 100(5):458–462

[28] Obwegeser HL. Temporal approach to the TMJ, the orbit, and the retro-maxillary-infracranial region. Head Neck Surg. 1985; 7(3):185–199

[29] Stanley RB, Jr. The temporal approach to impacted lateral orbital wall fractures. Arch Otolaryngol Head Neck Surg. 1988; 114(5):550–553

[30] Goldberg RA, Steinsapir KD. Extracranial optic canal decompression: indications and technique. Ophthal Plast Reconstr Surg. 1996; 12(3):163–170

[31] Karnik PP, Maskati BT, Kirtane MV, Tonsekar KS. Optic nerve decompression in head injuries. J Laryngol Otol. 1981; 95(11):1135–1140

[32] Kuppersmith RB, Alford EL, Patrinely JR, Lee AG, Parke RB, Holds JB. Combined transconjunctival/intranasal endoscopic approach to the optic canal in traumatic optic neuropathy. Laryngoscope. 1997; 107(3):311–315

[33] Sofferman RA. Sphenoethmoid approach to the optic nerve. Laryngoscope. 1981; 91(2):184–196

[34] Romanes GJ. Cunningham's Textbook of Anatomy. New York: Oxford University Press; 1981

[35] Antonyshyn O, Gruss JS, Kassel EE. Blow-in fractures of the orbit. Plast Reconstr Surg. 1989; 84(1):10–20

[36] Edmund J, Godtfredsen E. Unilateral optic atrophy following head injury. Acta Ophthalmol (Copenh). 1963; 41:693–697

[37] Gonzalez MG, Santos-Oller JM, de Vicente Rodriguez JC, Lopez-Arranz JS. Optic nerve blindness following a malar fracture. J Craniomaxillofac Surg. 1990; 18(7):319–321

[38] Hughes B. Indirect injury of the optic nerves and chiasma. Bull Johns Hopkins Hosp. 1962; 111:98–126

[39] Ramsay JH. Optic nerve injury in fracture of the canal. Br J Ophthalmol. 1979; 63(9):607–610

[40] Hammer G, Ambos E. [Traumatic hematoma of the optic nerve sheath and the possibilities of its surgical treatment] [in German]. Klin Monatsbl Augenheilkd. 1971; 159(6):818–819

[41] Niho S, Niho M, Niho K. Decompression of the optic canal by the transethmoidal route and decompression of the superior orbital fissure. Can J Ophthalmol. 1970; 5(1):22–40

[42] Steinsapir KD, Goldberg RA. Traumatic optic neuropathies. In: Miller NR, Newman NJ, eds. Walsh and Hoyt's Clinical Neuro-Ophthalmology. Baltimore, MD: Williams and Wilkins; 1998:715–739

[43] Pringle JH. Atrophy of the optic nerve following diffuse violence to the skull. BMJ. 1922; 2:1156–1157

[44] Kestenbaum A. Clinical Methods of Neuro-ophthalmologic Examination. New York: Grune and Stratton; 1961

[45] Feinsod M, Selhorst JB, Hoyt WF, Wilson CB. Monitoring optic nerve function during craniotomy. J Neurosurg. 1976; 44(1):29–31

[46] Holmes MD, Sires BS. Flash visual evoked potentials predict visual outcome in traumatic optic neuropathy. Ophthal Plast Reconstr Surg. 2004; 20(5):342–346

[47] Mashima Y, Oguchi Y. Clinical study of the pattern electroretinogram in patients with optic nerve damage. Doc Ophthalmol. 1985; 61(1):91–96

[48] Greenberg RP, Becker DP, Miller JD, Mayer DJ. Evaluation of brain function in severe human head trauma with multimodality evoked potentials. Part 2: localization of brain dysfunction and correlation with post-traumatic neurological conditions. J Neurosurg. 1977; 47(2):163–177

[49] Avrahami E, Sperber F, Cohn DF. Computerized tomographic demonstration of intraorbital bone fragments caused by penetrating trauma. Ophthalmic Surg. 1986; 17(1):41–43

[50] Grove AS, Jr. Computed tomography in the management of orbital trauma. Ophthalmology. 1982; 89(5):433–440

[51] Wohlrab TM, Maas S, de Carpentier JP. Surgical decompression in traumatic optic neuropathy. Acta Ophthalmol Scand. 2002; 80(3):287–293

[52] Cook MW, Levin LA, Joseph MP, Pinczower EF. Traumatic optic neuropathy. A meta-analysis. Arch Otolaryngol Head Neck Surg. 1996; 122(4):389–392

[53] Mine S, Yamakami I, Yamaura A, et al. Outcome of traumatic optic neuropathy. Comparison between surgical and nonsurgical treatment. Acta Neurochir (Wien). 1999; 141(1):27–30

[54] Spoor TC, Hartel WC, Lensink DB, Wilkinson MJ. Treatment of traumatic optic neuropathy with corticosteroids. Am J Ophthalmol. 1990; 110(6):665–669

[55] Levin LA, Beck RW, Joseph MP, Seiff S, Kraker R. The treatment of traumatic optic neuropathy: the International Optic Nerve Trauma Study. Ophthalmology. 1999; 106(7):1268–1277

[56] Steinsapir KD, Goldberg RA. Traumatic optic neuropathy: an evolving understanding. Am J Ophthalmol. 2011; 151(6):928–933.e2

[57] Emanuelli E, Bignami M, Digilio E, Fusetti S, Volo T, Castelnuovo P. Post-traumatic optic neuropathy: our surgical and medical protocol. Eur Arch Otorhinolaryngol. 2015; 272(11):3301–3309

[58] Lübben B, Stoll W, Grenzebach U. Optic nerve decompression in the comatose and conscious patients after trauma. Laryngoscope. 2001; 111(2):320–328

[59] Wang BH, Robertson BC, Girotto JA, et al. Traumatic optic neuropathy: a review of 61 patients. Plast Reconstr Surg. 2001; 107(7):1655–1664

[60] Thakar A, Mahapatra AK, Tandon DA. Delayed optic nerve decompression for indirect optic nerve injury. Laryngoscope. 2003; 113(1):112–119

[61] Dandy WE. Prechiasmal intracranial tumors of the optic nerves. Am J Ophthalmol. 1922; 5(3):169–188

[62] Sewall EC. External operation on the ethmosphenoid-frontal group of sinuses under local anesthesia: technic for removal of part of optic foramen wall for relief of pressure on optic nerve. Arch Otolaryngol. 1926; 4(5):377–411

[63] Sofferman RA. Sphenoethmoid approach to the optic nerve. In: Schmidek HH, Sweet WH, eds. Operative Neurosurgical Techniques. Orlando, FL: Grune and Stratton; 1988:269–278

[64] Horiguchi K, Murai H, Hasegawa Y, Mine S, Yamakami I, Saeki N. Endoscopic endonasal trans-sphenoidal optic nerve decompression for traumatic optic neuropathy—technical note. Neurol Med Chir (Tokyo). 2010; 50(6):518–522

[65] De Ganseman A, Lasudry J, Choufani G, Daele J, Hassid S. Intranasal endoscopic surgery in traumatic optic neuropathy—the Belgian experience. Acta Otorhinolaryngol Belg. 2000; 54(2):175–177

[66] Jiang RS, Hsu CY, Shen BH. Endoscopic optic nerve decompression for the treatment of traumatic optic neuropathy. Rhinology. 2001; 39(2):71–74

[67] Kountakis SE, Maillard AA, El-Harazi SM, Longhini L, Urso RG. Endoscopic optic nerve decompression for traumatic blindness. Otolaryngol Head Neck Surg. 2000; 123(1 Pt 1):34–37

[68] Cannon CR, Jahrsdoerfer RA. Temporal bone fractures. Review of 90 cases. Arch Otolaryngol. 1983; 109(5):285–288

[69] Fisch U. Prognostic value of electrical tests in acute facial paralysis. Am J Otol. 1984; 5(6):494–498

[70] Nageris B, Hansen MC, Lavelle WG, Van Pelt FA. Temporal bone fractures. Am J Emerg Med. 1995; 13(2):211–214

[71] Hasso AN, Ledington JA. Traumatic injuries of the temporal bone. Otolaryngol Clin North Am. 1988; 21(2):295–316

[72] Gantz BJ. Traumatic facial paralysis. In: Gates GA, ed. Current therapy in otolaryngology head and neck surgery. Toronto, Canada: BC Decker; 1987:112–115

[73] Rhoton AL. The temporal bone and transtemporal approaches. In: Cranial Anatomy and Surgical Approaches. Philadelphia, PA: Lippincott Williams and Wilkins; 2003:643–698

[74] Vrabec JT. Otic capsule fracture with preservation of hearing and delayed-onset facial paralysis. Int J Pediatr Otorhinolaryngol. 2001; 58(2):173–177

[75] Ulrich K. Verletzungen des Gehororgans bei Schadelbasisfrakturen. Acta Otolaryngol Suppl (Helsingfors). 1926; 6:S1–S150

[76] Yanagihara N. Transmastoid decompression of the facial nerve in temporal bone fracture. Otolaryngol Head Neck Surg. 1982; 90(5):616–621

[77] Fisch U. Facial paralysis in fractures of the petrous bone. Laryngoscope. 1974; 84(12):2141–2154

[78] Fisch U. Management of intratemporal facial nerve injuries. J Laryngol Otol. 1980; 94(1):129–134

[79] Fisch U, Esslen E. Total intratemporal exposure of the facial nerve. Pathologic findings in Bell's palsy. Arch Otolaryngol. 1972; 95(4):335–341

[80] Curtin JM. Fracture of the skull and intratemporal lesions affecting the facial nerve. Adv Otorhinolaryngol. 1977; 22:202–206

[81] Eby TL, Pollak A, Fisch U. Histopathology of the facial nerve after longitudinal temporal bone fracture. Laryngoscope. 1988; 98(7):717–720

[82] Eby TL, Pollak A, Fisch U. Intratemporal facial nerve anastomosis: a temporal bone study. Laryngoscope. 1990; 100(6):623–626

[83] Felix H, Eby TL, Fisch U. New aspects of facial nerve pathology in temporal bone fractures. Acta Otolaryngol. 1991; 111(2):332–336

[84] Grobman LR, Pollak A, Fisch U. Entrapment injury of the facial nerve resulting from longitudinal fracture of the temporal bone. Otolaryngol Head Neck Surg. 1989; 101(3):404–408

[85] Lambert PR, Brackmann DE. Facial paralysis in longitudinal temporal bone fractures: a review of 26 cases. Laryngoscope. 1984; 94(8):1022–1026

[86] May M. Trauma to the facial nerve. Otolaryngol Clin North Am. 1983; 16(3):661–670

[87] Ylikoski J. Facial palsy after temporal bone fracture: (light and electron microscopic findings in two cases). J Laryngol Otol. 1988; 102(4):298–303

[88] Wilberger J, Chen DA. Management of head injury. The skull and meninges. Neurosurg Clin N Am. 1991; 2(2):341–350

[89] Gantz BJ, Gmuer AA, Holliday M, Fisch U. Electroneurographic evaluation of the facial nerve. Method and technical problems. Ann Otol Rhinol Laryngol. 1984; 93(4 Pt 1):394–398

[90] Gordon AS, Friedberg J. Current status of testing for seventh nerve lesions. Otolaryngol Clin North Am. 1978; 11(2):301–324

[91] Gantz BJ, Gmür A, Fisch U. Intraoperative evoked electromyography in Bell's palsy. Am J Otolaryngol. 1982; 3(4):273–278

[92] Sillman JS, Niparko JK, Lee SS, Kileny PR. Prognostic value of evoked and standard electromyography in acute facial paralysis. Otolaryngol Head Neck Surg. 1992; 107(3):377–381

[93] Alford BR. Electrodiagnostic studies in facial paralysis. Arch Otolaryngol. 1967; 85(3):259–264

[94] Alford BR, Sessions RB, Weber SC. Indications for surgical decompression of the facial nerve. Laryngoscope. 1971; 81(5):620–635

[95] May M, Harvey JE, Marovitz WF, Stroud M. The prognostic accuracy of the maximal stimulation test compared with that of the nerve excitability test in Bell's palsy. Laryngoscope. 1971; 81(6):931–938

[96] Silverstein H, McDaniel AB, Hyman SM. Evoked serial electromyography in the evaluation of the paralyzed face. Am J Otol. 1985(Suppl):80–87

[97] Murakami M, Ohtani I, Aikawa T, Anzai T. Temporal bone findings in two cases of head injury. J Laryngol Otol. 1990; 104(12):986–989

[98] Chakeres DW, Spiegel PK. A systematic technique for comprehensive evaluation of the temporal bone by computed tomography. Radiology. 1983; 146(1):97–106

[99] Ghorayeb BY, Yeakley JW, Hall JW, III, Jones BE. Unusual complications of temporal bone fractures. Arch Otolaryngol Head Neck Surg. 1987; 113(7):749–753

[100] Johnson DW, Hasso AN, Stewart CE, III, Thompson JR, Hinshaw DB, Jr. Temporal bone trauma: high-resolution computed tomographic evaluation. Radiology. 1984; 151(2):411–415

[101] Resnick DK, Subach BR, Marion DW. The significance of carotid canal involvement in basilar cranial fracture. Neurosurgery. 1997; 40(6):1177–1181

[102] Jackler RK. Facial, auditory, and vestibular nerve injuries associated with basilar skull fractures. In: Youmans JR, ed. Neurological Surgery. Vol 4. Philadelphia, PA: WB Saunders; 1990:2305–2316

[103] Adegbite AB, Khan MI, Tan L. Predicting recovery of facial nerve function following injury from a basilar skull fracture. J Neurosurg. 1991; 75(5):759–762

[104] Brodsky L, Eviatar A, Daniller A. Post-traumatic facial nerve paralysis: three cases of delayed temporal bone exploration with recovery. Laryngoscope. 1983; 93(12):1560–1565

[105] Coker NJ. Management of traumatic injuries to the facial nerve. Otolaryngol Clin North Am. 1991; 24(1):215–227

[106] Coker NJ, Kendall KA, Jenkins HA, Alford BR. Traumatic intratemporal facial nerve injury: management rationale for preservation of function. Otolaryngol Head Neck Surg. 1987; 97(3):262–269

[107] McCabe BF. Injuries to the facial nerve. Laryngoscope. 1972; 82(10):1891–1896

[108] Briggs M, Potter JM. Prevention of delayed traumatic facial palsy. BMJ. 1971; 3(5772):458–459

[109] Quaranta A, Campobasso G, Piazza F, Quaranta N, Salonna I. Facial nerve paralysis in temporal bone fractures: outcomes after late decompression surgery. Acta Otolaryngol. 2001; 121(5):652–655

[110] Gates GA. Facial nerve decompression following a basilar skull fracture. J Neurosurg. 1992; 77(2):332

[111] Bento RF, Pirana S, Sweet R, Castillo A, Brito Neto RV. The role of the middle fossa approach in the management of traumatic facial paralysis. Ear Nose Throat J. 2004; 83(12):817–823

[112] May M, Klein SR. Facial nerve decompression complications. Laryngoscope. 1983; 93(3):299–305

[113] Steenerson RL. Bilateral facial paralysis. Am J Otol. 1986; 7(2):99–103

17 Status Epilepticus

Aradia X. Fu and Lawrence J. Hirsch

Abstract

Status epilepticus (SE) is a common neurologic emergency that requires rapid assessment and early treatment in order to avoid pharmacoresistance, to prevent potential neuronal injury, and to reduce overall morbidity and mortality. In 2015, the International League Against Epilepsy redefined and classified the different types of SE. In 2016, the American Epilepsy Society published guidelines for SE, including a treatment algorithm. These and other guidelines agree on a 5-minute time point after which convulsive activity should be considered to be SE and requires treatment. For continuous nonconvulsive seizure (NCSz) activity on electroencephalography, guidelines use 5 or 10 minutes. Confirmation of termination of seizures via electroencephalography is crucial if the patient does not awaken rapidly. Over the years, there is increasing recognition for the urgency in treatment, as animal and human studies have demonstrated a plethora of evidence for the adverse effects of prolonged seizure activity, including NCSz (excluding absence SE). There have been numerous prospective randomized trials on antiepileptic drugs, although the best second- and third-line treatments remain debated. Prehospital and home treatment with parenteral benzodiazepines (especially nasal, buccal, and intramuscular) is showing promise for early seizure termination, prevention of SE, and reduction of its associated costs and morbidities. Although some forms of SE will have high mortality regardless of treatment, many will have excellent prognosis if one can make an early diagnosis and promptly implement the appropriate treatment.

Keywords: antiepileptic treatment, continuous EEG monitoring, convulsion, convulsive status epilepticus, nonconvulsive status epilepticus, seizure, status epilepticus

17.1 Introduction

Status epilepticus (SE) is a relatively common neurologic emergency with substantial morbidity and mortality and high economic burden on the health care system. In the United States, annual direct inpatient cost for SE is estimated to be \$4 billion.[1] A more recent study in Germany estimated €83 million annual inpatient cost for SE in the adult population alone.[2] With increasing clinical and basic science research and the growing use of continuous electroencephalography(cEEG) monitoring, there have been many advances in our understanding and management of SE in recent years. This chapter will review various aspects of SE, including the definition and newly proposed classification system of SE, urgency to early treatment, results of recent prospective trials, and highlights of a very recent treatment guideline for convulsive status epilepticus (CSE).

17.2 Definition and Classification

Historically, the International League Against Epilepsy (ILAE) and Epilepsy Foundation had defined SE as continuous seizure activity of at least 30 minutes in duration or repetitive seizure activity without complete recovery of consciousness between attacks.[3,4] However, with increasing recognition of the urgency for early termination of SE to prevent adverse consequences, ILAE has recently revised the definition of SE, and in this same publication, ILAE also proposed a new classification of SE.

17.2.1 Definition

According to the new definition per ILAE published in 2015, SE will be defined conceptually with two operational dimensions (t_1 and t_2): "Status epilepticus is a condition resulting either from the failure of the mechanisms responsible for seizure termination or from the initiation of mechanisms, which lead to abnormally, prolonged seizures (after time point t_1). It is a condition, which can have long-term consequences (after time point t_2), including neuronal death, neuronal injury, and alteration of neuronal networks, depending on the type and duration of seizures."[5] Time point t_1 denotes when treatment should be implemented, and time point t_2 indicates when long-term consequences may occur. On the basis of animal and clinical studies, ILAE concluded that t_1 and t_2 for CSE may be 5 minutes (time to treat) and 30 minutes (time to neuronal injury), respectively. Data for nonconvulsive status epilepticus (NCSE) is much more limited. Best estimated t_1 and t_2 for focal SE with impaired mental status are 10 minutes (time to treat) and > 60 minutes (time to potential neuronal injury). For absence of SE, these times are estimated at 10 to 15 minutes and unknown (no evidence of neuronal injury even if prolonged).

Other societies have also proposed similar definitions for SE. In the 2016 American Epilepsy Society (AES) treatment algorithm for CSE, a 5-minute definition for CSE was used; there was no particular mention of definition for NCSE.[6] In the 2013 Neurocritical Care Society treatment guideline for SE, CSE and NCSE were defined as "5 min or more of (i) continuous clinical and/or electrographic seizure activity or (ii) recurrent seizure activity without recovery (returning to baseline) between seizures."[7]

17.2.2 Classification

ILAE proposed that SE be classified in the following four axes[5]: semiology, etiology, EEG correlates, and age. Axis 1 (semiology; ▶Table 17.1) is the most important axis, and it is broadly divided into those with prominent motor symptoms (e.g., CSE, myoclonic SE, focal motor SE) and those without prominent motor symptoms (e.g., NCSE with coma, absence SE). Axis 2 (etiology; ▶Table 17.2) is categorized into those with "known" (i.e., "symptomatic") causes and those with "unknown" (i.e., "cryptogenic") causes. Axis 3 (EEG correlates; ▶Table 17.3) uses descriptors of EEG patterns in SE. Lastly, axis 4 defines age groups: neonatal (0 to 30 days), infancy (1 month to 2 years), childhood (>2 to 12 years), adolescence and adulthood (> 12 to 59 years), and elderly (≥ 60 years).

Table 17.1 Classification of status epilepticus: Axis 1 (semiology)

A. With prominent motor symptoms

A.1. Convulsive SE (CSE, synonym: tonic–clonic SE)

- A.1.a. Generalized convulsive

- A.1.b. Focal onset evolving into bilateral convulsive SE

- A.1.c. Unknown whether focal or generalized

A.2. Myoclonic SE (prominent epileptic myoclonic jerks)

- A.2.a. With coma

- A.2.b. Without coma

A.3. Focal motor

- A.3.a. Repeated focal motor seizures (jacksonian)

- A.3.b. Epilepsia partialis continua (EPC)

- A.3.c. Adversive status

- A.3.d. Oculoclonic status

- A.3.e. Ictal paresis (i.e., focal inhibitory SE)

A.4. Tonic status

A.5. Hyperkinetic SE

B. Without prominent motor symptoms (i.e., nonconvulsive SE, NCSE)

B.1. NCSE with coma (including so-called "subtle" SE)

B.2. NCSE without coma

- B.2.a. Generalized

- B.2.a.a. Typical absence status

- B.2.a.b. Atypical absence status

- B.2.a.c. Myoclonic absence status

- B.2.b. Focal

- B.2.b.a. Without impairment of consciousness (aura continua, with autonomic, sensory, visual olfactory, gustatory, emotional/psychic/experiential, or auditory symptoms)

- B.2.b.b. Aphasic status

- B.2.b.c. With impaired consciousness

- B.2.c. Unknown whether focal or generalized

- B.2.c.a. Autonomic SE

Abbreviation: SE, status epilepticus.

Reproduced with permission from Trinka E, Cock H, Hesdorffer D, et al. A definition and classification of status epilepticus—report of the ILAE Task Force on Classification of Status Epilepticus. Epilepsia 2015;56:1515–1523.

Table 17.2 Classification of status epilepticus: Axis 2 (etiology)

Known (i.e., symptomatic)

- Acute (e.g., stroke, intoxication, malaria, encephalitis, etc.)

- Remote e.g., posttraumatic, postencephalitic, poststroke, etc.)

- Progressive (e.g., brain tumor, Lafora's disease, and other PMEs, dementias)

- SE in defined electroclinical syndromes

Unknown (i.e., cryptogenic)

Abbreviations: PMEs, progressive myoclonic epilepsies; SE, status epilepticus.

Reproduced with permission from Trinka E, Cock H, Hesdorffer D, et al. A definition and classification of status epilepticus—report of the ILAE Task Force on Classification of Status Epilepticus. Epilepsia 2015;56:1515–1523.

17.3 Epidemiology, Etiology, and Outcome

17.3.1 Epidemiology

The incidence of SE in the United States increased from 3.5 to 12.5 per 100,000 population between 1979 and 2010, with a bimodal distribution with highest incidence in the first 10 years of life and after 50 years of age.[8] The main factors that contributed to the apparent increase in incidence rate were thought to be better recognition of NCSE with cEEG (especially in the critically ill patients), population longevity, modification of definition of time criteria for SE from 30 minutes to 5 minutes, and change in diagnostic codes for SE.[8,9,10] A similar phenomenon was also seen in Thailand: incidence rate of SE increased from 1.29/100,000 in 2004 to 5.20/100,000 in 2012.[11] Roughly 1/3 of SEs occur as first-time unprovoked seizures, 1/3 in patients with established epilepsy, and 1/3 in patients with no history of epilepsy.[12,13] Up to 1/3 of patients in the neurologic intensive care unit (ICU) have nonconvulsive seizure (NCSz), and the majority of those will be in NCSE.[14,15] Important risk factors for NCSz and NCSE include acute brain injuries (e.g., intracerebral hemorrhage, subarachnoid hemorrhage, traumatic brain jury, ischemic stroke, central nervous system infection) as well as past history of intracranial tumor, epilepsy, and presence of encephalomalacia on magnetic resonance imaging (MRI).[15,16,17] High prevalence of NCSz in medical and surgical ICUs have also been identified (11%), even in patients without any known acute neurologic illness.[18,19,20] Approximately 15% of patients with newly diagnosed epilepsy have SE as their first seizure episode. About 0.5 to 1.0% of patients with epilepsy will experience SE each year, and 10 to 20% of patients with epilepsy will experience SE at least once in their lifetime.[21]

17.3.2 Etiology and Outcome

In-hospital mortality for patients with CSE varies from 2.6% (< 10 years old) to 20% (> 80 years old).[8] Predictors of poor outcome include older age, acute symptomatic etiology, alteration of consciousness, 20% or higher per hour seizure burden, periodic epileptiform discharges or burst suppression on EEG, and complications such as respiratory failure and infection during SE.[8,22,23] Significant functional disability will be seen between 20 and 50% of survivors.[24] According to one study in adults, the most common acute etiology for SE is stroke (20.5% mortality), the most common chronic etiology for SE is history of epilepsy (usually due to low antiepileptic drug level; 2.38% mortality), and the worst outcome (42.4% mortality) in SE is when it is due to anoxia.[8] The most common etiologies in young children are cryptogenic and infection with fever, both of which have low mortality rates.[25,26] Some of the most frequently encountered etiologies for SE are listed in ▶ Table 17.4.

Table 17.3 Classification of status epilepticus: Axis 3 (EEG correlates)

1. Location: generalized (including bilateral synchronous patterns), lateralized, bilateral independent, multifocal

1. Name of the pattern: periodic discharges, rhythmic delta activity or spike-and-wave/sharp-and-wave plus subtypes

1. Morphology: sharpness, number of phases (e.g., triphasic morphology), absolute and relative amplitude, polarity

1. Time-related features: prevalence, frequency, duration, daily pattern duration and index, onset (sudden vs. gradual), and dynamics (evolving, fluctuating, or static)

1. Modulation: stimulus-induced vs. spontaneous

1. Effect of intervention (medication) on EEG

Abbreviation: EEG, electroemcephalogram.

Reproduced with permission from Trinka E, Cock H, Hesdorffer D, et al. A definition and classification of status epilepticus—report of the ILAE Task Force on Classification of Status Epilepticus. Epilepsia 2015;56:1515–1523.

Table 17.4 Etiologies of status epilepticus

A. Acute etiologies

1. Metabolic disturbances: e.g., hyponatremia, hypocalcemia, hypomagnesium, hypophosphatemia, high osmolality, hypoglycemia, uremia, hepatic failure

1. Sepsis

1. CNS infection: e.g., meningitis, encephalitis, abscess

1. Stroke: ischemic stroke, intracerebral hemorrhage, subarachnoid hemorrhage, cerebral sinus thrombosis

1. Head trauma with or without epidural or subdural hematoma

1. Noncompliance with AEDs

1. Withdrawal: e.g., opioid, benzodiazepine, barbiturate, alcohol, AED

1. Drug toxicity

a. Analgesics: meperidine, fentanyl, tramadol
b. Antiarrhythmics: mexiletine, lidocaine, digoxin
c. Antibiotics: β-lactams (e.g., benzylpenicillin > semisynthetic penicillin, cefepime, imipenem), quinolones, isoniazid (treat with pyridoxine), antimalarials (e.g., primaquine), metronidazole
d. Neuroleptics: especially clozapine, phenothiazines, haloperidol, buproprion
e. Chemotherapeutic agents: chlorambucin, busulfan, α-interferons, tacrolimus, mycophenolate mofetil
f. Multiple sclerosis medications: dalfampridine, 4-aminopyridine
g. Others: baclofen, lithium, theophylline, cyclosporine

1. Hypoxic or anoxic injury: e.g., cardiac arrest

1. Hypertensive encephalopathy, posterior reversible encephalopathy syndrome

1. Immunologic: autoimmune encephalitis (e.g., anti-NMDA receptor antibodies, anti- VGKC complex antibodies), paraneoplastic syndromes, Rasmussen's encephalitis, cerebral lupus, adult-onset Still's disease, Goodpasture's syndrome, thrombotic thrombocytopenic purpura, antibody-negative limbic encephalitis

1. Illicit drugs: e.g., cocaine; amphetamine; phencyclidine; case reports on synthetic cannabinoid ("spice"),[72] MDMA ("Ecstasy"),[73] synthetic cathinones ("bath salts")[74]

B. Chronic etiologies

1. Preexisting epilepsy: breakthrough seizures, discontinuation of AEDs

1. Chronic ethanol abuse in setting of ethanol intoxication or withdrawal

1. CNS tumors

1. Remote CNS pathology: e.g., stroke, abscess, traumatic brain injury, cortical dysplasia

C. Cryptogenic

Abbreviations: AED = antiepileptic drug; CNS = central nervous system; MDMA = 3,4-methylenedioxymethamphetamine; NMDA = N-methyl-D-aspartic acid; VGKC = voltage-gated potassium channel.

Reproduced with permission from Brophy GM, Bell R, Claassen J, et al. Guidelines for the evaluation and management of status epilepticus. Neurocrit Care 2012;17:3–23, with additional modifications and data from Trinka E, Hofler J, Zerbs A. Causes of status epilepticus. Epilepsia 2012;53(Suppl 4):127–138.

17.4 Clinical Features and Diagnosis

CSE is well recognized clinically because of prominent rhythmic motor activity. NCSE, on the other hand, may be much more subtle (►Table 17.5), usually having no clinical signs except for depressed mental status. The possibility of NCSz or NCSE should be considered in any neurosurgical patient with unexplained impairment of mental status (although it is also common when there is an explanation), fluctuating mental status, slow awakening after CSE (not awake 30–60 minutes post convulsion), or prolonged alteration in consciousness following an uncomplicated neurosurgical procedure. To properly diagnose subclinical or subtle clinical SE, EEG remains the single most useful tool. Routine EEGs, however, are inadequate for this purpose, and cEEG is strongly recommended. Routine EEGs, which are typically recorded for 30 to 60 minutes, will detect seizures in only about half the patients who are found to have NCSz on cEEG monitoring.[16,27] For noncomatose patients, a 24-hour EEG will detect the first seizure in greater than 90% of patients with NCSz, but 48 hours or more are sometimes needed in comatose patients.[16] Thus, a 24-hour screen is recommended for noncomatose patients and a 48-hour screen for those in coma.

17.5 Urgency to Treat Status Epilepticus

With increasing knowledge of the basic mechanism of and complications directly related to SE, there is no question that SE requires urgent treatment. Animal models have advanced our understanding of the time-dependent maladaptive changes of SE.[28] Within minutes to days after onset of SE, there are changes to ion channel kinetics, membrane depolarization, posttranscriptional regulation, and early gene activation. In the weeks following, further modification in protein function, neuronal death, and inflammation will lead to reorganization of neuronal networks. The cascade of events will result in epileptogenesis that ultimately generates spontaneous recurrent seizures and (potentially) pharmacoresistance to antiepileptic drugs. Another reason for promoting early termination of SE is that SE is an established independent predictor of poor outcome in many conditions.[15,20,29,30]

17.5.1 Changes on Molecular and Cellular Levels during Status Epilepticus

Neuropeptide Modulation in Self-sustaining Status Epilepticus and Pharmacoresistance

Time-dependent molecular changes initiate shortly after the onset of a single seizure and can begin to transform into self-sustaining SE if endogenous mechanisms or exogenous therapy (e.g., antiepileptic drugs) fail to disrupt the cascade. Within milliseconds to seconds after onset of seizure, protein phosphorylation, release of neurotransmitters, and ion channel opening and closing take place to prepare for potentially prolonged seizure activity.[31] Soon after, endocytosis of inhibitory γ-aminobutyric acid type A ($GABA_A$) receptors[32,33] and increase in excitatory α-amino-3-hydroxy-5-methyl-4-isoxazolepropionic acid (AMPA) and N-methyl-D-aspartate (NMDA) receptors[34] occur simultaneously. Decreased expression of $GABA_A$ receptors is believed to be the cause of progressive loss of antiepileptic potency of benzodiazepines (GABA agonists) with prolonged seizure activity[35]; potency reduction drops as much as 20 times within 30 minutes of self-sustained SE.[36] Within minutes to hours, maladaptive modulations in neuropeptides occur to increase the expression of excitatory neuropeptides[32,37] and decrease the expression of inhibitory neuropeptides.[38,39,40,41,42] In the days and weeks after SE, changes in regulation of DNA

Table 17.5 Possible presentations of nonconvulsive status epilepticus

Behavioral/cognitive/sensory	Autonomic/vegetative	Motor
Agitation/aggression	Abdominal sensation	Automatisms
Amnesia	Apnea/hyperventilation	Dystonic posturing
Anorexia	Brady- and tachyarrhythmia	Eye blinking
Aphasia/muteness	Chest pain	Eye deviation
Catatonia	Flushing	Facial twitching
Coma	Miosis/mydriasis/hippus	Finger twitching
Confusion/delirium	Nausea/vomiting	Nystagmus
Delusions/hallucinations		Tremulousness
Echolalia		
Laughter		
Lethargy		
Perseveration		
Personality change		
Psychosis		
Singing		

Reproduced with permission from Hirsch LJ, Gaspard N. Status epilepticus. Continuum (Minneap, Minn) 2013;19:767–794.

methylation and microRNA further contribute to epileptogenesis and neuronal injury and death.[43,44]

Neuronal Injury and Death

There are several pathophysiologic mechanisms that lead to neuronal injury and death in SE, including increased neuronal metabolic demand, initiation of inflammatory mechanisms, generation of reactive oxygen species, excitotoxicity caused by NMDA and non-NMDA glutamate receptor–mediated calcium entry, necrosis, apoptosis, and mitochondrial dysfunction.[45,46,47,48,49,50] Studies have found hippocampal edema after prolonged febrile seizure in children, which was confirmed by animal models that also associated degree of edema to severity of hippocampal volume loss.[46] NCSz due to traumatic brain injury also appears to be associated with long-term hippocampal atrophy ipsilateral to the NCSz.[51] Serum neuron-specific enolase, a marker of neuronal injury,[50] is elevated after SE.[52,53] SE induced neuronal injuries may be demonstrated by T2 hyperintensity and restricted diffusion on MRI[54,55], as well as its subsequent metabolic changes as measured by MR spectroscopy.[56] Neuronal damage is further aggravated by adverse systemic factors, especially hypoxia, hypotension, fever, hypo- and hyperglycemia, and other metabolic abnormalities. Although neuronal injury can be clearly demonstrated after 60 minutes of SE, it probably occurs much earlier in the presence of these ubiquitous exacerbating factors.

17.5.2 Clinical Complications of Status Epilepticus

Failure to promptly treat SE may lead to systemic and/or neurologic complications.[57] During seizures, intrinsic compensatory mechanisms are initiated to meet the increased metabolic demand. These mechanisms trigger catecholamine release that leads to tachycardia, hypertension, hyperpyrexia, hyperglycemia, and demargination of leukocytes. After 5 to 30 minutes of seizure activity, as in SE, multiorgan failure ensues as the body fails to maintenance homeostasis. The majority of the early systemic complications occur because of the aforementioned cascade of events. There are also multiple systemic complications related to the treatment of SE (e.g., adverse reactions to nonanesthetic and anesthetic drugs) and prolonged hospitalization in the ICU (e.g., pulmonary embolism, hospital-acquired infection, critical illness neuropathy). ▶Table 17.6 details some of these complications.

17.6 Treatment

17.6.1 General Principle

"Time is brain." Rapid treatment is of paramount importance in the treatment of SE given all the reasons mentioned above. Operatively, treatment should be started within 5 minutes of continuous seizure activity. In humans, first-line medications control SE in 80% of patients when initiated within 30 minutes, but only in 40% if started 2 hours after onset.[58,59] Fever, hypotension, hypoxia, hypo- and hyperglycemia, and other metabolic abnormalities must be treated simultaneously. For practical purposes, SE can be categorized into two large groups: CSE with prominent generalized shaking and NCSE without prominent generalized shaking. The proposed treatment algorithm by the AES, which will be discussed below, targets CSE. Treatment for NCSE will be similar but typically with less urgency and aggressiveness (especially with regard to anesthetic medications). One should always evaluate the benefit of aggressive treatment against the risks of intubation and sedation in NCSE. There is another caveat when treating NCSE. Certain antiepileptic drugs should be avoided in specific seizures: lamotrigine, carbamazepine, oxcarbazepine, eslicarbazepine, and phenytoin may worsen myoclonic seizures[60,61,62]; carbamazepine, oxcarbazepine, eslicarbazepine, and phenytoin may worsen absence seizure.[62,63] Lastly, keep in mind that there is a high probability of ongoing subclinical seizures or NCSE after cessation of clinical convulsions if the patient does not wake up promptly. One study found subclinical seizure activity in 48% of patients after control of CSE (during 24 hours of monitoring), with 14% in NCSE.[64]

17.6.2 Randomized Controlled Trials

Studies in Adult Patients

AES reviewed randomized controlled trials (RCTs) from 1940 to 2014. Nine RCTs were conducted in adult patients regarding efficacy of initial therapy that involved benzodiazepines, phenytoin, phenobarbital, valproic acid, and levetiracetam. It was concluded that "In adults, IM midazolam, IV lorazepam, IV diazepam (with or without phenytoin), and IV phenobarbital are established as efficacious at stopping seizures lasting at least 5 minutes … Intramuscular midazolam has superior effectiveness compared with IV lorazepam in adults with convulsive status epilepticus without established IV access … Intravenous lorazepam is more effective than IV phenytoin in stopping seizures lasting at least 10 minutes … There is no difference in efficacy between IV lorazepam followed by IV phenytoin, IV diazepam plus phenytoin followed by IV lorazepam, and IV phenobarbital followed by IV phenytoin … Intravenous valproic acid has similar efficacy to IV phenytoin or continuous IV diazepam as second therapy after failure of a benzodiazepine … Insufficient data exist in adults about the efficacy of levetiracetam as either initial or second therapy."[6] After those guidelines were completed, a few more prospective randomized trials were published: Chakravarthi et al found no significant difference in efficacy between IV levetiracetam versus IV phenytoin as second-line treatment of SE.[65] Mundlamuri et al determined that phenytoin, valproic acid, and levetiracetam were all equally efficacious and safe in management of CSE after failure of lorazepam; postictal psychosis was seen in 3/50 patients in the levetiracetam arm, but not in any patients in the other two arms.[66] Navarro et al found that adding levetiracetam to IV clonazepam for first-line treatment of SE provided no benefit.[67]

Studies in Pediatric Patients

Twenty-six RCTs were reviewed by the AES in pediatric patients regarding efficacy of initial therapy that involved benzodiazepines, phenytoin, phenobarbital, valproic acid, and levetiracetam. It was concluded that "In children, IV lorazepam and IV

Table 17.6 Systemic complications of status epilepticus

Early systemic complications	Complications relating to treatment	Complications of prolonged intensive care unit care
Acidosis (respiratory > metabolic) • Increased CO_2 production • Decreased CO_2 removal • Depletion of glycogen stores • Exacerbated by carbonic anhydrase inhibitors (e.g., topiramate, zonisamide, acetazolamide)	Nonanesthetic drugs • Benzodiazepine: respiratory depression, sedation • Valproic acid: platelet and clotting dysfunction, hyperammonemia • Fosphenytoin/phenytoin: cardiac arrhythmias, hypotension • Levetiracetam: psychosis • Lacosamide: PR prolongation	Venous thromboembolic disease • Pulmonary embolism • Deep venous thrombosis
Hypoxia • Apnea • Upper airway obstruction • Aspiration of gastric contents • Mucous plugging • Neurocardiogenic pulmonary edema	Propofol • Propofol infusion syndrome • Hypotension	Pulmonary complications • Recurrent mucous plugging • Pleural effusions • Atelectasis • Tracheostomy • Ventilator-associated pneumonia
Hyperadrenergic state • Hyperpyrexia • Hypertension • Tachycardia • Hyperglycemia • Peripheral leukocytosis	Midazolam • Accumulation of obesity and renal or hepatic dysfunction • Hypotension	Other infectious complications • Catheter-associated urinary tract infections • Sepsis • Bloodstream infections • Pseudomembranous colitis
Cardiac injury • Left ventricular stunning • Cardiac arrhythmias • Cardiac troponin elevations • Electrical conduction abnormalities • Cardiac contraction band necrosis/takotsubo cardiomyopathy	Barbiturates • Hypotension • Paralytic ileus • Increased risk of infection • Propylene glycol toxicity • Hepatic toxicity • Pancreatitis • Lingual edema	Skin complications • Skin breakdown • Yeast infections
Musculoskeletal injury • Tongue bites • Long bone fractures • Vertebral body compression fractures • Posterior shoulder dislocation	Ketamine • Tachyarrhythmias	Intensive care unit–acquired weakness • Critical illness myopathy • Critical illness neuropathy
Renal injury • Rhabdomyolysis and acute renal failure	Inhalational anesthetics • Hypotension • Increased risk of infection • Paralytic ileus	
	Hypothermia • Acid base and electrolyte disturbances • Coagulopathy • Impaired immunity • Cardiac arrhythmias • Paralytic ileus • Thrombosis	

Reproduced with permission and modification from Hocker S. Systemic complications of status epilepticus—an update. Epilepsy Behav 2015;49:83–87.

diazepam are established as efficacious ... at stopping seizures lasting at least 5 minutes ... Rectal diazepam, IM midazolam, intranasal midazolam, and buccal midazolam are probably effective at stopping seizures lasting at least 5 minutes ... Insufficient data exist in children about the efficacy of intranasal lorazepam, sublingual lorazepam, rectal lorazepam, valproic acid, levetiracetam, phenobarbital, and phenytoin as initial therapy ... Intravenous valproic acid has similar efficacy but better tolerability than IV phenobarbital ... as second therapy after failure of a benzodiazepine. Insufficient data exist in children regarding the efficacy of phenytoin or levetiracetam as second therapy after failure of a benzodiazepine...."[6]

Ongoing Trials

Multiple ongoing drug trials may lead to further improvement in management and treatment of SE.

"Established Status Epilepticus Treatment Trial" (ESETT; clinical trial identifier: NCT01960075) is an ongoing study that aims to determine which of the following—fosphenytoin, levetiracetam, or valproic acid—is the most effective treatment for refractory status epilepticus among patients older than 2 years.

"Treatment of Electroencephalographic Status Epilepticus After Cardiopulmonary Resuscitation" (TELSTAR; clinical trial identifier: NCT02056236) is another ongoing trial that compares the effect of antiepileptic drugs versus their absence on neurologic outcome in treatment of postanoxic comatose patients with electrographic SE or periodic discharges.

There are also several studies in progress in relation to treatment of refractory SE, including the "Levetiracetam, Lacosamide and Ketamine as Adjunctive Treatment of Refractory Status Epilepticus" (clinical trial identifier: NCT02726867), the "Ketogenic Diet for Refractory Status Epilepticus" trial (clinical trial identifier: NCT01796574), and the "Ketamine in Refractory Convulsive Status Epilepticus" trial (KETASER01; clinical trial identifier: NCT02431663).

17.6.3 Treatment Guideline

Below is the proposed treatment algorithm for CSE by the AES,[6] with three different phases of treatment (▶ Fig. 17.1).

AES Guideline for Treatment of CSE: Stabilization Phase (0–5 Minutes)

This phase mainly focuses on stabilizing the patient (e.g., airway, breathing, circulation), establishing intravenous (IV) access, and initiation of basic metabolic work-up to evaluate for etiology of SE.

AES Guideline for Treatment of CSE: Initial Therapy Phase (5–20 Minutes)

Once seizure duration reaches 5 minutes (if not earlier, in the opinion of the authors), a benzodiazepine is recommended as first therapy choice, particularly intramuscular (IM) midazolam, IV lorazepam, or IV diazepam. IV lorazepam: 0.1 mg/kg/dose, maximum 4 mg/dose, may repeat once. IM midazolam: 10 mg for > 40 kg body weight, 5 mg for 13 to 40 kg body weight, single dose. IV diazepam: 0.15 to 0.2 mg/kg/dose, maximum 10 mg/dose, may repeat once. If above not available, consider following: IV phenobarbital 15 mg/kg/dose, single dose; rectal diazepam 0.2 to 0.5 mg/kg, maximum 20 mg/dose, single dose; intranasal or buccal midazolam.

AES Guideline for Treatment of CSE: Second Therapy Phase (20–40 Minutes)

If seizure duration reaches 20 minutes [note: the authors of this chapter believe this timing is too slow and that the second therapy phase should be in the first 10-25 minutes; see below], treatment should escalate to second therapy phase, usually include drugs such as fosphenytoin, valproic acid, levetiracetam, and phenobarbital. No evidence of superiority of one over another. All following drugs should be given as a single dose: IV fosphenytoin 20 mg percutaneous (PE)/kg, maximum 1500 mg PE/dose; IV valproic acid 40 mg/kg, maximum 3000 mg/dose; IV levetiracetam 60 mg/kg, maximum 4500 mg/dose; phenobarbital 15 mg/kg (reserve as last option because of side effects and slow administration).

AES Guideline for Treatment of CSE: Third Therapy Phase (40–60 Minutes)

SE is considered as refractory SE if seizure duration exceeds 30 minutes because of failure to respond to first and second lines of therapies (35–40% of SE),[68] or superrefractory SE if persists or recurs 24 hours or more after initiation of anesthetic agent.[65] No clear evidence-based guide to therapy in this phase. Treatment includes either repeating second-line therapy or use of continuous infusion of anesthetic agents with cEEG. Always, however, weigh the risks and benefits of using anesthetic infusion, especially in NCSE, since infusion of anesthetics may lead to increased infection and higher risk of death.[69]

At this stage, consider the following anesthetic agents as per the Yale New Haven Hospital SE Protocol[70]: midazolam 0.2 mg/kg bolus IV, repeated 5 minutes until seizures stop (maximum of 10 boluses), then maintenance infusion of 0.1 to 2.9 mg/kg/h; propofol 1 to 2 mg/kg IV push, repeated every 3 to 5 minutes until seizures stop (maximum 10 mg/kg) followed by 33 µg/kg/min (1.98 mg/kg/h) initial IV infusion rate, maintenance dose of 17 to 250 µg/kg/min (1.02–15 mg/kg/h); barbiturate such as pentobarbital, loading dose 5 mg/kg IV and maintenance dose of 1 to 5 mg/kg/h; ketamine loading dose 1.5 mg/kg IV every 3 to 5 minutes until seizures stop (maximum 4.5 mg/kg), initial infusion 1.2 mg/kg/h, maintenance 0.3 to 7.5 mg/kg/h; lidocaine bolus 100 to 400 mg IV followed by 1 to 3 mg/kg, or a continuous 2 to 4 mg/kg/h infusion without bolus.[71]

Authors' Opinion Regarding the AES Treatment Guideline

Timeline for each of the therapy phases is too slow. We advocate for a more rapid course of action in treatment of SE. Consider initiating and completing first therapy phase (benzodiazepine) within 10 minutes (i.e., as soon as possible, instead of 5–20 minutes), second therapy phase within 10 to 25 minutes (instead of 20–40 minutes), and third therapy phase within 25+ minutes (instead of 40–60 minutes). The goal is to start anesthesia, if still convulsing, in under 30 minutes, when it is known that neuronal injury is likely if CSE continues.

17.7 Conclusion

SE is a neurologic emergency with multiple etiologies that contributes to the outcome of the disease. Rapid and focused

Time line   Interventions for emergency department, in-patient setting, in-patient setting, or prehospital setting with trained paramedics

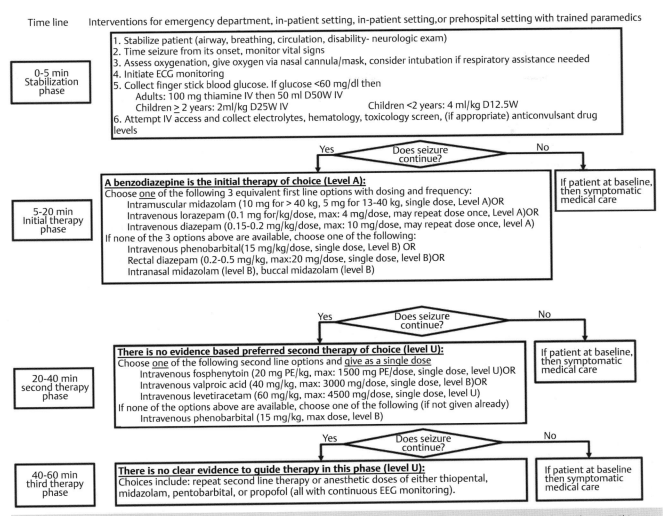

Fig. 17.1 Proposed treatment algorithm for status epilepticus by American Epilepsy Society.* (Reproduced with permission from Glauser T, Shinnar S, Gloss D, et al. Evidence-based guideline: treatment of convulsive status epilepticus in children and adults: report of the Guideline Committee of the American Epilepsy Society. Epilepsy Curr 2016;16:48–61.) *In the opinion of the authors of this chapter, the timing of the above phases is too slow and should be as follows: initial therapy phase within 0 to 10 minutes (rather than 5–20 minutes), second therapy phase within 10 to 25 minutes (rather than 20–40 minutes), and third therapy phase within 25+ minutes (rather than 40+ minutes).

assessment and treatment are the keys to better prognosis, as all forms of SE become increasingly refractory to treatment the longer they continue. The likelihood of a good outcome for a given etiology is inversely related to duration of seizure activity. Recognize that majority of seizures in critically ill patients are nonconvulsive. There should be a high suspicion for NCSE in patients with persistent or fluctuating altered mental status without a clear etiology or with an etiology that predisposes to seizures (such as any supratentorial injury, acute or chronic; prior epilepsy; or sepsis). Continuous EEG monitoring is highly recommended to evaluate for NCSz or NCSE. Technology is now available to study cerebral blood flow, brain tissue oxygen, brain metabolism and energy status, intracranial pressure, neuronal injury markers, and other parameters in these patients in detail. Research in these areas is progressing rapidly. In combination with research on neuroprotection and antiepileptogenesis, these advances will continue to improve our ability to recognize, treat, and prevent SE more effectively.

References

[1] Penberthy LT, Towne A, Garnett LK, Perlin JB, DeLorenzo RJ. Estimating the economic burden of status epilepticus to the health care system. Seizure. 2005; 14(1):46–51

[2] Strzelczyk A, Knake S, Oertel WH, Rosenow F, Hamer HM. Inpatient treatment costs of status epilepticus in adults in Germany. Seizure. 2013; 22(10):882–885

[3] Proposal for revised clinical and electroencephalographic classification of epileptic seizures. From the Commission on Classification and Terminology of the International League Against Epilepsy. Epilepsia. 1981; 22(4):489–501

[4] Treatment of convulsive status epilepticus. Recommendations of the Epilepsy Foundation of America's Working Group on Status Epilepticus. JAMA. 1993; 270(7):854–859

[5] Trinka E, Cock H, Hesdorffer D, et al. A definition and classification of status epilepticus—report of the ILAE Task Force on Classification of Status Epilepticus. Epilepsia. 2015; 56(10):1515–1523

[6] Glauser T, Shinnar S, Gloss D, et al. Evidence-based guideline: treatment of convulsive status epilepticus in children and adults: report of the Guideline Committee of the American Epilepsy Society. Epilepsy Curr. 2016; 16(1):48–61

[7] Brophy GM, Bell R, Claassen J, et al; Neurocritical Care Society Status Epilepticus Guideline Writing Committee. Guidelines for the evaluation and management of status epilepticus. Neurocrit Care. 2012; 17(1):3–23

[8] Dham BS, Hunter K, Rincon F. The epidemiology of status epilepticus in the United States. Neurocrit Care. 2014; 20(3):476–483

[9] Gilmore EJ, Hirsch LJ. Epilepsy: status epilepticus epidemiology—tracking a moving target. Nat Rev Neurol. 2015; 11(7):377–378

[10] Betjemann JP, Josephson SA, Lowenstein DH, Burke JF. Trends in status epilepticus-related hospitalizations and mortality: redefined in US practice over time. JAMA Neurol. 2015; 72(6):650–655

[11] Tiamkao S, Pranboon S, Thepsuthammarat K, Sawanyawisuth K. Incidences and outcomes of status epilepticus: a 9-year longitudinal national study. Epilepsy Behav. 2015; 49:135–137

[12] Hesdorffer DC, Logroscino G, Cascino G, Annegers JF, Hauser WA. Incidence of status epilepticus in Rochester, Minnesota, 1965–1984. Neurology. 1998; 50(3):735–741

[13] DeLorenzo RJ, Hauser WA, Towne AR, et al. A prospective, population-based epidemiologic study of status epilepticus in Richmond, Virginia. Neurology. 1996; 46(4):1029–1035

[14] Al-Mufti F, Claassen J. Neurocritical care: status epilepticus review. Crit Care Clin. 2014; 30(4):751–764

[15] Laccheo I, Sonmezturk H, Bhatt AB, et al. Non-convulsive status epilepticus and non-convulsive seizures in neurological ICU patients. Neurocrit Care. 2015; 22(2):202–211

[16] Claassen J, Mayer SA, Kowalski RG, Emerson RG, Hirsch LJ. Detection of electrographic seizures with continuous EEG monitoring in critically ill patients. Neurology. 2004; 62(10):1743–1748

[17] Carrera E, Claassen J, Oddo M, Emerson RG, Mayer SA, Hirsch LJ. Continuous electroencephalographic monitoring in critically ill patients with central nervous system infections. Arch Neurol. 2008; 65(12):1612–1618

[18] Kamel H, Betjemann JP, Navi BB, et al. Diagnostic yield of electroencephalography in the medical and surgical intensive care unit. Neurocrit Care. 2013; 19(3):336–341

[19] Gilmore EJ, Gaspard N, Choi HA, et al. Acute brain failure in severe sepsis: a prospective study in the medical intensive care unit utilizing continuous EEG monitoring. Intensive Care Med. 2015; 41(4):686–694

[20] Kurtz P, Gaspard N, Wahl AS, et al. Continuous electroencephalography in a surgical intensive care unit. Intensive Care Med. 2014; 40(2):228–234

[21] Hauser WA. Status epilepticus: frequency, etiology, and neurological sequelae. Adv Neurol. 1983; 34:3–14

[22] Sutter R, Kaplan PW, Rüegg S. Outcome predictors for status epilepticus—what really counts. Nat Rev Neurol. 2013; 9(9):525–534

[23] Payne ET, Zhao XY, Frndova H, et al. Seizure burden is independently associated with short term outcome in critically ill children. Brain. 2014; 137(Pt 5):1429–1438

[24] Claassen J, Lokin JK, Fitzsimmons BF, Mendelsohn FA, Mayer SA. Predictors of functional disability and mortality after status epilepticus. Neurology. 2002; 58(1):139–142

[25] Kravljanac R, Djuric M, Jankovic B, Pekmezovic T. Etiology, clinical course and response to the treatment of status epilepticus in children: a 16-year single-center experience based on 602 episodes of status epilepticus. Eur J Paediatr Neurol. 2015; 19(5):584–590

[26] Sahin S, Yazici MU, Ayar G, Karalok ZS, Arhan EP. Seizures in a pediatric intensive care unit: a prospective study. J Trop Pediatr. 2016; 62(2):94–100

[27] Pandian JD, Cascino GD, So EL, Manno E, Fulgham JR. Digital video-electroencephalographic monitoring in the neurological-neurosurgical intensive care unit: clinical features and outcome. Arch Neurol. 2004; 61(7):1090–1094

[28] Auvin S, Dupuis N. Outcome of status epilepticus. What do we learn from animal data? Epileptic Disord. 2014; 16(Spec No 1):S37–S43

[29] Herman ST, Abend NS, Bleck TP, et al; Critical Care Continuous EEG Task Force of the American Clinical Neurophysiology Society. Consensus statement on continuous EEG in critically ill adults and children, part I: indications. J Clin Neurophysiol. 2015; 32(2):87–95

[30] Hirsch LJ, Gaspard N. Status epilepticus. Continuum (Minneap Minn). 2013; 19(3 Epilepsy):767–794

[31] Chen JW, Wasterlain CG. Status epilepticus: pathophysiology and management in adults. Lancet Neurol. 2006; 5(3):246–256

[32] Naylor DE, Liu H, Wasterlain CG. Trafficking of GABA(A) receptors, loss of inhibition, and a mechanism for pharmacoresistance in status epilepticus. J Neurosci. 2005; 25(34):7724–7733

[33] Scharfman HE, Brooks-Kayal AR. Is plasticity of GABAergic mechanisms relevant to epileptogenesis? Adv Exp Med Biol. 2014; 813:133–150

[34] Naylor DE, Liu H, Niquet J, Wasterlain CG. Rapid surface accumulation of NMDA receptors increases glutamatergic excitation during status epilepticus. Neurobiol Dis. 2013; 54:225–238

[35] Wasterlain CG, Liu H, Naylor DE, et al. Molecular basis of self-sustaining seizures and pharmacoresistance during status epilepticus: the receptor trafficking hypothesis revisited. Epilepsia. 2009; 50(Suppl 12):16–18

[36] Treiman DM, Walton NY, Kendrick C. A progressive sequence of electroencephalographic changes during generalized convulsive status epilepticus. Epilepsy Res. 1990; 5(1):49–60

[37] Liu H, Mazarati AM, Katsumori H, Sankar R, Wasterlain CG. Substance P is expressed in hippocampal principal neurons during status epilepticus and plays a critical role in the maintenance of status epilepticus. Proc Natl Acad Sci U S A. 1999; 96(9):5286–5291

[38] Sloviter RS. Decreased hippocampal inhibition and a selective loss of interneurons in experimental epilepsy. Science. 1987; 235(4784):73–76

[39] Vezzani A, Sperk G, Colmers WF. Neuropeptide Y: emerging evidence for a functional role in seizure modulation. Trends Neurosci. 1999; 22(1):25–30

[40] Sperk G, Wieser R, Widmann R, Singer EA. Kainic acid induced seizures: changes in somatostatin, substance P and neurotensin. Neuroscience. 1986; 17(4):1117–1126

[41] Mazarati AM, Liu H, Soomets U, et al. Galanin modulation of seizures and seizure modulation of hippocampal galanin in animal models of status epilepticus. J Neurosci. 1998; 18(23):10070–10077

[42] Mazarati A, Liu H, Wasterlain C. Opioid peptide pharmacology and immunocytochemistry in an animal model of self-sustaining status epilepticus. Neuroscience. 1999; 89(1):167–173

[43] Jimenez-Mateos EM, Henshall DC. Epilepsy and microRNA. Neuroscience. 2013; 238:218–229

[44] Miller-Delaney SF, Das S, Sano T, et al. Differential DNA methylation patterns define status epilepticus and epileptic tolerance. J Neurosci. 2012; 32(5):1577–1588

[45] Lopez-Meraz ML, Niquet J, Wasterlain CG. Distinct caspase pathways mediate necrosis and apoptosis in subpopulations of hippocampal neurons after status epilepticus. Epilepsia. 2010; 51(Suppl 3):56–60

[46] Scott RC. What are the effects of prolonged seizures in the brain? Epileptic Disord. 2014; 16(Spec No 1):S6–S11

[47] Torolira D, Suchomelova L, Wasterlain CG, Niquet J. Widespread neuronal injury in a model of cholinergic status epilepticus in postnatal day 7 rat pups. Epilepsy Res. 2016; 120:47–54

[48] Wang C, Xie N, Wang Y, Li Y, Ge X, Wang M. Role of the mitochondrial calcium uniporter in rat hippocampal neuronal death after pilocarpine-induced status epilepticus. Neurochem Res. 2015; 40(8):1739–1746

[49] Williams S, Hamil N, Abramov AY, Walker MC, Kovac S. Status epilepticus results in persistent overproduction of reactive oxygen species, inhibition of which is neuroprotective. Neuroscience. 2015; 303:160–165

[50] Johnson EA, Guignet MA, Dao TL, Hamilton TA, Kan RK. Interleukin-18 expression increases in response to neurovascular damage following soman-induced status epilepticus in rats. J Inflamm (Lond). 2015; 12:43

[51] Vespa PM, McArthur DL, Xu Y, et al. Nonconvulsive seizures after traumatic brain injury are associated with hippocampal atrophy. Neurology. 2010; 75(9):792–798

[52] Rabinowicz AL, Correale JD, Bracht KA, Smith TD, DeGiorgio CM. Neuron-specific enolase is increased after nonconvulsive status epilepticus. Epilepsia. 1995; 36(5):475–479

[53] DeGiorgio CM, Gott PS, Rabinowicz AL, Heck CN, Smith TD, Correale JD. Neuron-specific enolase, a marker of acute neuronal injury, is increased in complex partial status epilepticus. Epilepsia. 1996; 37(7):606–609

[54] Cianfoni A, Caulo M, Cerase A, et al. Seizure-induced brain lesions: a wide spectrum of variably reversible MRI abnormalities. Eur J Radiol. 2013; 82(11):1964–1972

[55] Cartagena AM, Young GB, Lee DH, Mirsattari SM. Reversible and irreversible cranial MRI findings associated with status epilepticus. Epilepsy Behav. 2014; 33:24–30

[56] Wu Y, Pearce PS, Rapuano A, Hitchens TK, de Lanerolle NC, Pan JW. Metabolic changes in early poststatus epilepticus measured by MR spectroscopy in rats. J Cereb Blood Flow Metab. 2015; 35(11):1862–1870

[57] Hocker S. Systemic complications of status epilepticus—an update. Epilepsy Behav. 2015; 49:83–87

[58] Lowenstein DH, Alldredge BK. Status epilepticus at an urban public hospital in the 1980s. Neurology. 1993; 43(3 Pt 1):483–488

[59]   Lowenstein DH, Alldredge BK. Status epilepticus. N Engl J Med. 1998; 338(14):970–976

[60]   Genton P, Gelisse P, Crespel A. Lack of efficacy and potential aggravation of myoclonus with lamotrigine in Unverricht-Lundborg disease. Epilepsia. 2006; 47(12):2083–2085

[61]   Larch J, Unterberger I, Bauer G, Reichsoellner J, Kuchukhidze G, Trinka E. Myoclonic status epilepticus in juvenile myoclonic epilepsy. Epileptic Disord. 2009; 11(4):309–314

[62]   Thomas P, Valton L, Genton P. Absence and myoclonic status epilepticus precipitated by antiepileptic drugs in idiopathic generalized epilepsy. Brain. 2006; 129(Pt 5):1281–1292

[63]   Osorio I, Reed RC, Peltzer JN. Refractory idiopathic absence status epilepticus: a probable paradoxical effect of phenytoin and carbamazepine. Epilepsia. 2000; 41(7):887–894

[64]   DeLorenzo RJ, Waterhouse EJ, Towne AR, et al. Persistent nonconvulsive status epilepticus after the control of convulsive status epilepticus. Epilepsia. 1998; 39(8):833–840

[65]   Chakravarthi S, Goyal MK, Modi M, Bhalla A, Singh P. Levetiracetam versus phenytoin in management of status epilepticus. J Clin Neurosci. 2015; 22(6):959–963

[66]   Mundlamuri RC, Sinha S, Subbakrishna DK, et al. Management of generalised convulsive status epilepticus (SE): a prospective randomised controlled study of combined treatment with intravenous lorazepam with either phenytoin, sodium valproate or levetiracetam—pilot study. Epilepsy Res. 2015; 114:52–58

[67]   Navarro V, Dagron C, Elie C, et al; SAMUKeppra investigators. Prehospital treatment with levetiracetam plus clonazepam or placebo plus clonazepam in status epilepticus (SAMUKeppra): a randomised, double-blind, phase 3 trial. Lancet Neurol. 2016; 15(1):47–55

[68]   Shorvon S, Ferlisi M. The treatment of super-refractory status epilepticus: a critical review of available therapies and a clinical treatment protocol. Brain. 2011; 134(Pt 10):2802–2818

[69]   Sutter R, Marsch S, Fuhr P, Kaplan PW, Rüegg S. Anesthetic drugs in status epilepticus: risk or rescue? A 6-year cohort study. Neurology. 2014; 82(8):656–664

[70]   Grover EH, Nazzal Y, Hirsch LJ. Treatment of convulsive status epilepticus. Curr Treat Options Neurol. 2016; 18(3):11

[71]   Zeiler FA, Zeiler KJ, Kazina CJ, Teitelbaum J, Gillman LM, West M. Lidocaine for status epilepticus in adults. Seizure. 2015; 31:41–48

[72]   de Havenon A, Chin B, Thomas KC, Afra P. The secret "spice": an undetectable toxic cause of seizure. Neurohospitalist. 2011; 1(4):182–186

[73]   Armenian P, Mamantov TM, Tsutaoka BT, et al. Multiple MDMA (Ecstasy) overdoses at a rave event: a case series. J Intensive Care Med. 2013; 28(4):252–258

[74]   Gerona RR, Wu AH. Bath salts. Clin Lab Med. 2012; 32(3):415–427

18 The Evaluation and Management of Combined Cranial, Spinal, and Multisystem Trauma

Daphne D. Li, Hieu H. Ton-That, G. Alexander Jones, Paolo Nucifora, and Vikram C. Prabhu

Abstract

Injuries to the cranial and spinal regions are a significant cause of trauma-related morbidity and mortality. They may also occur with traumatic injuries to appendicular skeleton or viscera, in the context of multisystem trauma (MST). The most frequent cause of MST is high-velocity falls or motor vehicle accidents. Physicians involved in the care of MST must maintain a high index of suspicion for remote injuries, and close communication between emergency on-scene personnel, trauma surgeons, orthopedic surgeons, and neurosurgeons is critical. This chapter delineates the epidemiology, mechanisms, evaluation, and management of MST, with particular emphasis on the radiologic studies essential to diagnose injuries in the setting of acute trauma and the expedient management of these conditions to facilitate the best possible outcome.

Keywords: head injury, multisystem trauma, polytrauma, spinal cord injury

18.1 Introduction

Injuries to the cranial and spinal regions are a significant cause of trauma-related morbidity and mortality. They may occur individually but also frequently occur together; at times, they occur along with traumatic injuries to appendicular skeleton or viscera, compounding the problem. The most frequent cause of this is high-velocity injuries, such as those resulting from a pedestrian struck by a vehicle, a motor vehicle accident, or fall from a significant height. These traumatic episodes, due to a combination of forces, predispose to extensive multisystem trauma (MST). Multisystem trauma is generally defined as major trauma involving two or more body systems, and physicians involved in the care of these patients must maintain a high index of suspicion for remote injuries. Close communication between emergency on-scene personnel, trauma surgeons, orthopedic surgeons, and neurosurgeons involved in the care of patients with cranial and spinal injuries is essential, as is the appropriate prioritization of injury management.

In general, the surgical trauma attending physician assumes the role of team leader; this is a critical role that allows multidisciplinary input and care in a methodical fashion from the scene of the accident until the patient is adequately treated and stabilized and safely ensconced in the surgical intensive care unit (ICU). The purpose of this chapter is to address cranial and spinal trauma in the context of a patient with MST, with a focus on the evaluation and management of these complex patients.

18.2 Epidemiology

Epidemiologic data on the incidence of MST is not forthcoming simply because it is generally categorized under the different body systems rather than as a separate database. However, some general information is available that sheds light on the topic of MST. Trauma is the leading cause of death for Americans in the first five decades of life and accounts for almost half of all deaths in this age group; this far exceeds the mortality associated with cancer or heart disease.[1,2,3,4] Across all ages, trauma is the third leading cause of death and a substantial proportion of trauma-related mortality involves traumatic brain injury (TBI).[1,2,3,4] Statistics from the National Trauma Institute (NTI) indicate that each year trauma accounts for 41 million emergency department (ED) visits and 2.3 million hospital admissions (NTI, accessed August 27, 2016). Young males are the demographic group disproportionately represented here, especially with motor vehicle accidents (MVAs). Adolescents (ages 15–19 years) and older adults (ages 65 years and older) are more likely to sustain falls.

Although minor TBI is frequent and accounts for about 2.5 million ED visits in the United States each year, it tends to occur in isolation rather than in the context of MST. Similarly, minor injuries to the vertebral column are frequent but may not be accompanied by significant injury to other organ systems. On the other hand, severe TBI is commonly associated with craniofacial, orthopedic, and systemic or thoracoabdominal injuries.[5] Anatomical proximity can determine system involvement; severe TBI patients with a lower Glasgow Coma Scale (GCS) score and facial fractures are at high risk for injuries involving the craniovertebral junction and cervical spine; on the other hand, thoracolumbar spine injuries may be associated with injury to thoracoabdominal viscera or vascular structures.[6,7,8,9,10]

18.3 Mechanism of Injury

High-velocity trauma predisposes to severe cranial or spinal injuries. Patients with severe TBI or multilevel spinal fractures are at high risk for MST.[11] The mechanism of injury varies; blunt trauma and penetrating injuries can cause MST, as can acceleration/deceleration injuries. The severity of MST varies depending on several factors: the force and extent of blunt trauma or the force and trajectory of a penetrating injury or the speed of the acceleration/deceleration injury.[7] High speed (> 35 miles/hour) MVAs, particularly involving ejection, pedestrians struck by motor vehicles, or falls from a height greater than 10 feet or high-energy falls are the primary mechanisms underlying combined head and spine trauma with or without associated skeletal or visceral injuries.[5,6] Acceleration/deceleration forces, linear and rotational, are known to be involved in TBI and spine injuries and can also cause thoracic and abdominal organ injuries. For example, aortic injury may occur because of acceleration/deceleration forces that cause tears at fixed, immobile areas of the thoracic aorta (▶Fig. 18.1). Similar mechanisms are at play with "seat belt" injuries, which are associated with abdominal wall, colon, small bowel, mesenteric, intraperitoneal, and retroperitoneal solid organ injuries, as well as vertebral column injury. Combined craniofacial trauma involving the facial structures, calvarium, and brain are also

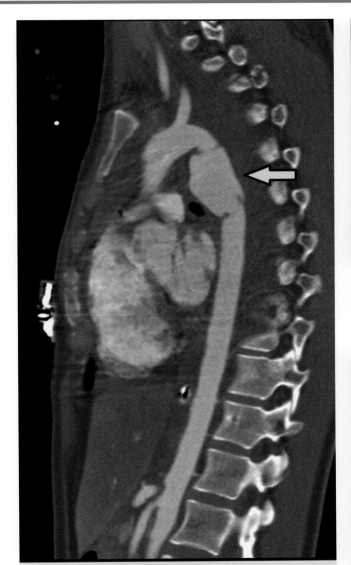

Fig. 18.1 Sagittal image of the aorta from contrast-enhanced computed tomography scan of the chest. Dilation of the descending thoracic aorta with intimal flaps is consistent with traumatic aortic dissection.

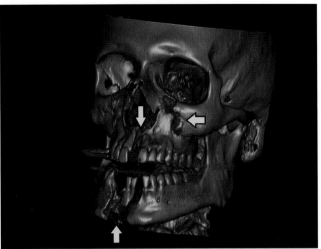

Fig. 18.2 Three-dimensional reconstruction of the maxilla and mandible from computed tomography scan of the facial bones. There are multiple acute facial fractures, including a midline mandibular fracture, a fracture of the hard palate, and a Le Fort type II fracture.

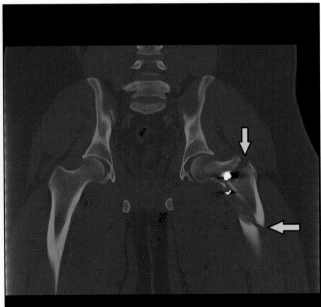

Fig. 18.3 Coronal image of the femoral necks, reformatted from computed tomography angiography of the lower extremities. There is a comminuted fracture of the femoral neck, with bullet fragments visible at the fracture site.

commonly seen with severe high-velocity MVAs, falls, or direct blows to the face. The fracture–collapse of the facial skeleton and paranasal sinuses at times dissipates the force transmitted to the brain and may in fact ameliorate the extent of the intracranial injury (▶ Fig. 18.2).

The specific mechanisms of injuries of the vertebral column structures are complex, varied, and frequently overlapping. Direct forces inflict injury when an object comes into direct contact with the spine; this frequently results in fractures of the vertebral arches or spinous processes. Penetrating trauma, such as gunshot wounds, may result in fractures along the trajectory of the foreign object (▶ Fig. 18.3); if severe, violation of the thecal sac and spinal cord injury may be seen along with visceral injuries. Indirect forces, on the other hand, inflict injury by causing movements that extend beyond the normal physiologic range for that segment of the spine.

Anatomical factors, including mobility and the orientation of the facet joints, predispose the cervical spine to frequent injury. By contrast, the thoracolumbar spine is able to resist translational forces because of the coronal orientation of the facet joints and the protective effect of the thoracic cage.[12,13] The lumbar spine has larger vertebral bodies that can sustain greater axial loads but is more vulnerable to injury than the thoracic spine because of the more sagittal orientation of its facet joints that results in more translational mobility.[14,15] The amount of injury force required to cause a thoracolumbar fracture increases the risk of accompanying neurologic injury and injury to the adjacent visceral and vascular structures.[16,17]

The force vectors placed on the vertebral column can be predictive of the type of injury. Excessive axial loading can result in compression fractures of the vertebral body (generally involving the anterior column) or burst fractures (involving both anterior and middle columns), compromising spinal stability. Burst fractures, or Chance fractures that involve the middle and posterior columns, are more frequently associated with neurologic injuries (▶ Fig. 18.4). Flexion injures may cause ligamentous disruption without associated bone fracture and can also lead to facet joint disruption and dislocation. Combined flexion–compression injuries can occur as well—the classic "teardrop" fracture in the cervical spine, and these are associated with a high rate of neurologic injury. Flexion–distraction injuries can result in ligamentous disruption or facet joint disruption; a rotational component may result in unilateral jumped facets. Extension injuries often result in laminar fractures or spinous process fractures. Fracture–dislocation injuries are three-column injuries involving multiple different forces—compression of the anterior column, distraction of the middle/posterior columns, and often association with a rotational or shearing force. These injuries most commonly occur at the thoracolumbar junction and are extremely unstable. The majority are associated with spinal cord injury and require surgical intervention.

18.4 Clinical Assessment

18.4.1 Primary Survey

The initial field assessment and management of a patient who has suffered MST is critical and occurs simultaneously, which could be the key difference between death and/or disability or recovery. The nature of the process is rapid, with essential smooth transition between on-site and ED care that overlaps and is complementary. A rapid primary survey should assess and address the following: airway, breathing, and circulation. Stabilization of vitals with adherence to principles of the basic life support (BLS) and advanced cardiac life support (ACLS) and placement of the patient in a cervical collar on a long backboard for transportation are rapidly performed.[18]

Airway control is the first priority. Patients with MST, particularly those with severe TBI and spinal cord injury, are at risk for airway compromise that may be due to mechanical (laryngeal or tracheal trauma, foreign body obstruction) or neurologic (hypotonia or muscle weakness, decreased level of consciousness) factors. The initial vital signs provide rapid clues and guide management; cyanosis or apnea, or a rapid and shallow breathing pattern with limited chest excursions that suggests thoracic injury such as a pneumothorax or flail chest, is noted. In an obtunded patient, the most basic maneuver includes a chin-lift and jaw-thrust maneuver to move the tongue anteriorly and open the upper airway.[18] The oropharynx is inspected and cleared of any foreign material. Awake and alert patients who are hemodynamically stable and vocalizing and breathing normally do not require intubation; all other patients require airway protection. Placement of an oropharyngeal or nasopharyngeal tube is a first measure, but endotracheal intubation is

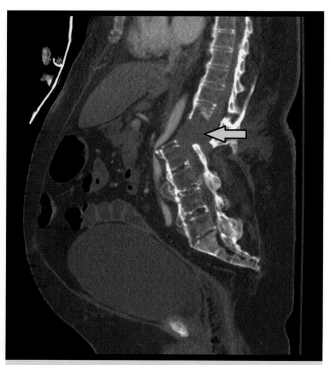

Fig. 18.4 Sagittal image of the lumbar spine, reformatted from contrast-enhanced computed tomography scan of the pelvis. There is an acute Chance fracture of L1, with marked distraction of the lumbar spine.

done promptly if required to avoid prolonged periods of hypoxia.[18] Administration of oxygen to maintain oxygen saturation above 95% as monitored by pulse oximetry is routine. In rare circumstances, anatomical or trauma-related factors may preclude establishment of an endotracheal or nasotracheal airway; in these circumstances, an emergency cricothyroidotomy is performed. Absolute in-line cervical immobilization throughout the process cannot be stressed enough, especially in the field. Lack of knowledge of the extent of a cervical injury can have devastating consequences of the patient's neurologic outcome.

Adequacy of ventilation is determined by observation of chest movements, by absence of hypoxia and cyanosis, and by chest auscultation to determine equal and normal breath sounds. Any asymmetry of breath sounds or hyperresonance or dullness to chest percussion in a persistently hypoxic, cyanotic, or hypotensive patient should raise concerns for a pneumothorax or hemothorax that may require emergent needle thoracocentesis, even prior to X-ray confirmation if in the field. Patients with MST or an injury to the craniospinal axis present special challenges; a depressed level of consciousness precludes a reliable history or complaints that can focus the examination. Sensory loss from a spinal cord injury may mask the symptoms of lower extremity or abdominal trauma. These patients are also at risk for apnea and/or aspiration.

Adequate circulation is the next priority. A strong radial pulse, warm skin, and capillary refill less than 2 seconds suggest adequate perfusion. On the other hand, an absence of these parameters should raise concern for hypoperfusion, which is most commonly due to large-volume hemorrhage in MST.

Hypotensive shock also compromises cerebral circulation and causes a depressed level of consciousness.[18] A minimum of two large-bore peripheral intravenous (IV) lines are placed (for children < 6 years, intraosseous access allows fluid administration); it is better to avoid IV access in limbs that are severely injured. Central venous access may be required, as hypotension can make peripheral cannulation difficult, but when possible, this is reserved for the ED and should always be followed by a chest radiograph to rule out an iatrogenic pneumothorax. Vital signs may be deceptive; a young patient may mount a robust sympathetic vasoconstrictive response to hypovolemia that manifests as tachycardia with normal or even slightly elevated blood pressure.[18] Eventually, tachycardia and hypotension will imply a hypovolemic state. On the other hand, bradycardia and hypotension may imply a spinal cord injury and neurogenic shock rather than hypovolemia, especially for spinal cord injury above the T5 level. The former is managed with rapid fluid resuscitation and control of the bleeding site, whereas the latter is managed with vasopressor agents and atropine, if required for profound bradycardia (heart rate < 50 beats/minute).

The complexity of MST precludes further detailed management at the scene, and patients should be rapidly evacuated to a trauma center. The primary Advanced Trauma Life Support (ATLS) survey developed by the American College of Surgeons (ACS), which all incoming surgical residents learn, primarily focuses on the first "golden hour" during which continuous rapid assessments and resuscitations are performed.[19] The primary survey focuses on five key areas: airway, breathing, circulation, disability, and exposure. In addition, blood is drawn for a complete blood count, metabolic panel, toxicology screen, coagulation parameters, and cross-matching; blood bank availability of 4 to 10 units of universal emergency transfusion blood type O is ensured while the patient's own blood type is determined. Massive crystalloid or colloid infusions or blood transfusions risk hypothermia in MST patients, and procedures for warming both the patient and these solutions must be rapidly instituted.[18]

These patients have a dynamic disease state and decision-making must be fluid, with input from various consulting services; life-threatening injuries are prioritized and immediately treated even as the initial evaluation proceeds. A spinal cord injury can impact ventilation because of neurologic or mechanical factors. High cervical or brainstem injuries can compromise respiratory drive, whereas midcervical cord injuries can cause phrenic and hence diaphragmatic paralysis. Thoracic cord injuries result in respiratory muscle paralysis. With spinal cord injury, the resultant ileus increases the risk of aspiration and placement of an orogastric or nasogastric tube is important. A poor cough reflex is also another risk factor for aspiration. Mechanical injuries such as fractured ribs or sternum and hemothorax or pneumothorax may also accompany thoracic spine injuries and result in ventilatory problems.

The usual major sources of hemorrhage are pelvic and extremity fractures, and occult injuries within the thorax and abdomen. These are assessed by direct inspection and radiographic imaging, but diagnostic peritoneal lavage, laparotomy, or thoracotomy may be performed as the situation indicates. Total exposure of the patient from head to toe is essential, and the patient is log-rolled to examine the back. The chest is examined for contusions, lacerations, or rib deformity and auscultated for differences in breath sounds and palpated for the crepitus associated with subcutaneous air that suggest a rib injury. In the abdominal survey, particular attention is paid to external signs such as contusions and lacerations or pathognomic marks such as a "seat belt sign." Pain, distension, tenderness, guarding, and abdominal rigidity, or a lack of bowel sounds suggesting ileus, are all concerning for abdominal trauma, but significant abdominal trauma or bleeding can also frequently go undetected, or be masked by associated injuries, particularly of the craniospinal axis. The characteristic signs of intra-abdominal bleeding: Cullen's sign (periumbilical ecchymosis) or Grey Turner's sign (ecchymosis over the flanks), are delayed in presentation and not evident during the primary survey unless a substantial amount of time has passed since the initial trauma.

Evaluation of the extremities is performed with attention to diminished or uneven pulses, ecchymosis or bleeding, deformity, and swelling. Orthopedic injuries are rapidly assessed; bone deformity and neurovascular integrity of the limb are key elements and reduction of a fracture and immobilization is performed rapidly. Limb ischemia may occur with vascular compromise or uncontrolled hemorrhage and other complications, including rhabdomyolysis and compartment syndrome. Hence, early involvement of the orthopedic trauma surgeons is essential. Obvious extremity fractures may be splinted temporarily and tourniquet or occlusive dressings applied to control significant uncontrollable bleeding while the patient is stabilized and the full extent of these injuries is assessed.

18.4.2 Evaluation of Cranial and Spinal Injuries

The presence of cranial and spinal injuries may obscure the clinical presentation of other injuries. Similarly, visceral or orthopedic injuries may mask injuries to the craniospinal axis, and a high index of suspicion when initially encountering a MST patient, especially those with altered consciousness, is essential to avoid a delay in diagnosis and treatment.[20] A quick survey of the scalp and face detects contusions, lacerations, or injuries to the craniofacial skeleton. Active facial or scalp bleeding and leakage of cerebrospinal fluid (CSF) or brain tissue are looked for. Patients are next evaluated using the Glasgow Coma Scale (GCS) and pupil size and reactivity. The GCS assigns a patient a numerical score on a scale that ranges from 3 to 15. Patients are graded on three categories: eye opening, verbal ability, and motor function (▶ Table 18.1). For intubated patients, the verbal score is supplanted by a 1T. A GCS score less than 8 implies a severe head injury, 9 to 12 implies a moderate head injury, and 13 to 15 implies a mild head injury. Pupil size, reactivity, and symmetry is important: a nonreactive dilated pupil in a patient with a normal GCS score suggests a traumatic oculomotor nerve injury, whereas the same finding in an obtunded patient or one with altered mentation may suggest uncal herniation with compromise of the third nerve in the ambient cistern. The risk of hypoxia, hypercarbia, or pulmonary aspiration is significant in patients with severe head injury (GCS score < 8), and airway protection and adequate ventilation are essential in these patients.[21,22] The focused neurologic examination should occur after the airway, breathing, and circulation have been stabilized.

Table 18.1 Glasgow Coma Scale

Points	Eye opening response	Verbal response	Motor response
6			Obeys commands
5		Oriented	Localizes to painful stimulus
4	Spontaneous	Confused conversation	Withdraws in response to pain
3	To verbal stimuli	Inappropriate words	Flexion in response to pain (decorticate posturing)
2	To pain only	Incomprehensible speech	Extension in response to pain (decerebrate posturing)
1	No response	No response	No response

Source: Glasgow Coma Scale. Centers for Disease Control and Prevention Web site. http://www.cdc.gov/masstrauma/resources/gcs.pdf. Accessed September 22, 2016.

Table 18.2 American Spinal Injury Association (ASIA) impairment scale

Grade	Spinal cord injury	Description
A	Complete	No sensory or motor function is preserved in the sacral segments S4–S5
B	Sensory incomplete	Sensory, but not motor, function is preserved below the neurologic level and includes the sacral segments S4–S5 (light touch, pin prick at S4–S5, or deep anal pressure [DAP]), AND no motor function is preserved > 3 levels below the motor level on either side of the body
C	Motor incomplete	Motor function is preserved below the neurologic level**, and more than half of the key muscle functions below the single neurologic level of injury (NLI) have a muscle grade of < 3
D	Motor incomplete	Motor function is preserved below the neurologic level**, and *at least half* of key muscle functions below the NLI have a muscle grade of ≥ 3
E	Normal	If sensation and motor function as tested are graded as normal in all segments and the patient had prior deficits

Source: Standard Neurological Classification of Spinal Cord Injury. American Spinal Injury Association and International Spinal Cord Society (ISCoS). http://asia-spinalinjury.org/wp-content/uploads/2016/02/International_Stds_Diagram_Worksheet.pdf. Archived from the original on June 18, 2011. Accessed 22 September 22, 2016.

**To receive a grade of C or D, patient must have (1) voluntary anal sphincter contraction or (2) sacral sensory sparing with of motor function > 3 levels below the motor level for that side of the body.

Among patients who present with a spine fracture, 20% have a concomitant TBI.[23] The cervical spine is most frequently involved in vertebral column and spinal cord injuries and is also the segment most commonly associated with TBI[24,25]; 2 to 6% of patients admitted with altered consciousness or with a TBI have an associated cervical spine injury,[23,24,25,26,27,28] hence the emphasis on the detection and appropriate management of the cervical spine in all trauma. The remainder of the spine is also important, as almost 20% of patients have more than one vertebral column injury; hence, clinical evaluation and imaging clearance of the remainder of the spine are also performed. Because of the potential for neurologic injury from a missed injury, some authors suggest the thoracolumbar spine be imaged in all patients with MST.[15] The thoracolumbar spine is more frequently injured in blunt trauma patients and is associated with abdominal or pelvic injuries in 7 to 9% of patients.[29] Furthermore, approximately 14% of patients with chest trauma have accompanying abdominal or pelvic injuries.[5] Visceral injuries may mask spine injuries; almost 20% of thoracolumbar fractures are diagnosed in a delayed fashion, with an average delay in diagnosis of 48 hours after presentation.[30] This delay is frequently due to resuscitation efforts or acute surgical intervention for higher-priority visceral or vascular injuries, but in some instances, the delay in diagnosis may be due to lack of clinical suspicion.[30]

All patients who have suffered a significant trauma are assumed to have a spine injury until proven otherwise, and spinal immobilization is maintained in a hard cervical collar and long backboard. On arrival in the ED and after a rapid primary survey, a patient may be carefully log-rolled and the long backboard removed. During this maneuver, the patient's back is examined for trauma debris, skin lacerations, or contusions, and palpated for deformity; an awake and alert patient is queried on the presence of tenderness, and the paraspinal muscles are checked for spasm. The spine trauma neurologic examination rapidly assesses key myotomes in the upper and lower extremities, along with a sensory examination and assessment of sensation in the perineal region and rectal tone. Key reflexes are the bulbocavernosus, cremasteric, and anal wink reflexes. The rectal examination assesses rectal tone and the presence of frank or occult blood in the lower gastrointestinal tract. If spinal cord injury (SCI) is suspected, the American Spinal Injury Association (ASIA) impairment scale may be employed. This scale assigns a letter (A–E) to a patient on the basis of the severity of their spinal cord injury: A being a complete injury and E representing a normal examination (▶Table 18.2).

Certain clinical findings in a trauma victim, especially one with a depressed level of consciousness, raise suspicion for the presence of spinal cord injury[26,31,32]: hypotensive shock in association with bradycardia; paradoxical breathing; pronounced contraction of diaphragm without proportional movement of chest wall; priapism or involuntary erection; flaccid paralysis of the arms and legs in the absence of paralytic administration, or asymmetric weakness of the arms legs, absence of response to painful stimuli, or only by facial grimacing; or the presence of a Horner's syndrome. Beevor's sign is an upward deflection of the umbilicus upon flexion of the neck in patients with a spinal cord injury at or below the T9 level due to partial paralysis of the rectus abdominis muscle.[33]

18.5 Imaging Evaluation

18.5.1 General Imaging Studies

At our institution, a large tertiary care center, patients undergo an initial evaluation with plain radiographs of the chest and pelvis. Trauma to the extremities, if present, is also initially evaluated by plain radiographs. This is typically followed by a "trauma protocol" for MST patients, which includes unenhanced head and cervical spine computed tomography (CT) and contrast enhanced CT of the chest, abdomen, and pelvis.[34] The goal is to efficiently localize potentially life-threatening conditions. On a chest X-ray, pneumothorax and hemothorax are easily demonstrated. Other injuries, including diaphragmatic rupture, pneumomediastinum, pneumopericardium, and mediastinal hematoma, may also be detected by a simple chest X-ray, but a CT scan may be more accurate. The pelvic films show fractures of the pelvic ring, acetabulum, or proximal femurs, as well as femoral head dislocations. Pelvic fractures can be a source of hemodynamically threatening hemorrhage and bladder and urethral injuries. The Focused Assessment with Sonography for Trauma (FAST) survey allows detection of hemopericardium and hemoperitoneum, using a series of four standard views of the heart, left and right upper quadrants, and pelvis. It is dependable, rapid, painless, and easily repeated at intervals if necessary. However, it is less sensitive for solid organ injury and suspicion of which should prompt CT scanning to more completely define the areas.[35,36] CT scanning with IV contrast of the chest, abdomen, and pelvis identifies the majority of solid organ injuries (▶ Fig. 18.5).

Intrathoracic pathology is identified by CT scanning with IV contrast. This allows excellent visualization of mediastinal structures, particularly the great vessels, as well as the trachea and lungs. It also identifies pulmonary contusions and lacerations, smaller pneumothorax or hemothorax, or foreign bodies, and severe injuries such as a traumatic aortic disruption (▶ Fig. 18.1). If there is suspicion of injury to smaller vessels, CT angiography should be obtained. Conventional angiography remains the reference standard for vascular injury and can provide time-resolved images that are useful in localizing the source of extravasation. For abdominal and pelvic injuries, once again, CT scans are sensitive for solid organ injuries to the liver, spleen, and kidneys. Multichannel scanners allow imaging of the chest, abdomen, and pelvis in an uninterrupted acquisition with a single contrast bolus. Reconstructions may also be performed for acetabular and pelvic fractures, complex vascular injuries, or thoracolumbar spine injuries, allowing appropriate decision-making regarding management of these injuries.[37,38] Reconstruction of the spine can often be performed a day or more after initial an trauma CT is performed, reducing the need for multiple imaging sessions.

A weakness of CT scans is in the detection of hollow viscus and diaphragmatic injuries. In the setting of trauma, sensitivity for esophageal or bowel injury is further limited by the inability

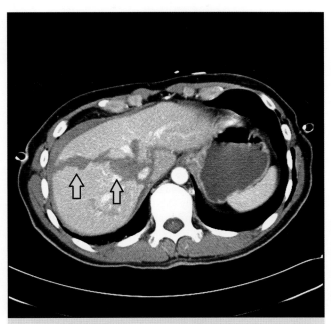

Fig. 18.5 Axial image of the liver, from contrast-enhanced computed tomography scan of the abdomen. There is a large hepatic laceration and surrounding hemoperitoneum.

to use oral contrast. Signs of bowel injury include intraperitoneal air or contrast leak, bowel wall thickening or discontinuity, free fluid in the absence of solid organ injury, mesenteric thickening, and hematoma. These signs are fairly insensitive, and CT has up to a 25% false-negative rate in detecting diaphragmatic injuries. Fluoroscopy can provide greater diagnostic certainty when evaluating these structures, particularly the esophagus.[39,40] If suspected, laparoscopy, video-assisted thoracoscopy, and laparotomy are considerations for further evaluation.[41,42] CT imaging accurately diagnoses renal contusions and lacerations, and simultaneous CT and IV pyelogram is typically adequate for ureteral injury screening. CT cystogram is also suitable and can be done along with the initial CT evaluation of the abdomen and pelvis.[43,44] If questions exist regarding urethral integrity, a bedside retrograde urethrogram may be obtained by instilling contrast into the urethral meatus, using an Angiocath or Foley catheter, and using anteroposterior (AP) and oblique plain films to demonstrate extravasation.

Most long-bone injuries, even in obtunded patients, are evident on initial physical examination. More subtle fractures, however, may be difficult to discern. Accordingly, any areas with deformity, pain on examination, or stigmata of trauma (contusion, abrasion, or swelling) should be imaged in at least two views with plain films. Any known injury should also include films of the joints and regions above and below the fracture. Any fracture or dislocation should also prompt a careful neurovascular examination; diminished or asymmetric pulses should prompt further work-up with conventional angiogram or CTA given their high association with vascular injury requiring repair.[45] Major extremity injuries should be detected initially on physical examination, with plain films targeted for fractures and consideration of CTA or formal angiography for vascular abnormalities.

CT requires the administration of IV contrast; the occurrence of true IV contrast allergies is relatively uncommon, but premedication with IV steroids (100 mg methylprednisolone), IV diphenhydramine chloride, and an IV histamine 2 (H$_2$) blocker is typically adequate to prevent reactions other than anaphylaxis. A longer course of premedication with multiple steroid doses if time permits can be used for prophylaxis.[46] The second concern with IV contrast is renal injury. This also appears to be less frequent than initially believed, and several studies have supported its use even in renal insufficiency. As with most cases, the maintenance of renal perfusion with adequate hydration and blood flow is essential to preventing an injury.[47,48] If necessary, an alternative such as magnetic resonance imaging/magnetic resonance angiography (MRI/MRA) may be considered.

Pregnancy is another condition worthy of particular consideration. Because fetal mortality is markedly increased by maternal shock, the trauma work-up should not be delayed, and necessary radiographic studies should be performed. However, the risks of radiation exposure should always be weighed against the potential benefit to the patient, particularly when multiple studies are contemplated. It is debatable whether any radiation dose is safe, and it is worth considering that the radiation dose from a single full-body CT far exceeds the annual occupational dose limit for pregnant CT technologists, angiographers, and other radiation workers. Because the radiation doses used in CT are high, the fetus must be shielded when imaging outside the pelvis. Note that this will only partly protect the fetus, since most of the dose it absorbs is indirect (scattered from solid organs). Ultrasound and unenhanced MRI are not associated with known adverse fetal effects at any state in pregnancy. Both should be strongly considered as an alternative to CT when possible.[49]

18.5.2 Craniospinal Axis Imaging

Cranial CT imaging rapidly detects scalp, calvarial bone, and intracranial injuries in most patients (▶ Fig. 18.6). The location, size and extent, and degree of mass effect of intracranial pathology, such as epidural or subdural hematomas, or intracerebral contusion or hemorrhage, are noted. Key elements to note are the degree of shift of midline structures to the side opposite the hematoma and the effacement of the basal cisterns that surround the brainstem. Excess shift of midline structures due to mass effect from a lesion can also efface the lateral and third ventricles and occlude the foramen of Monro, causing further ventricular dilatation. The presence of uncal, subfalcine, or tonsillar herniation is critical finding that influences the rapidity of surgical intervention. Calvarial bone fractures may be simple linear, nondisplaced fractures that require no surgical intervention or complex, depressed skull fractures that may require surgical intervention. The association of a scalp laceration over the depressed skull fracture, intracranial pneumocephalus or hemorrhage, and violation of the walls of the frontal sinus are key elements that influence surgical decision-making.

The presence of spine trauma may complicate intubation and operative treatment of other associated systemic injuries. Hence, rapid appropriate imaging studies are imperative to comprehensively evaluate the vertebral column. The role of plain films in evaluation of the cervical spine is controversial,

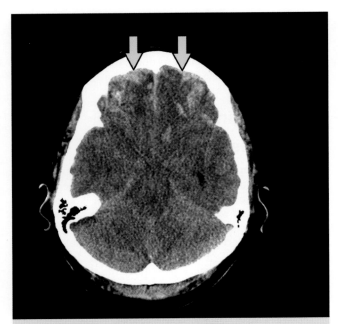

Fig. 18.6 Axial image of the inferior frontal lobes, from computed tomography scan of the head. There is a multicompartmental intracranial hemorrhage, with bifrontal hemorrhagic contusions.

but an emerging consensus suggests that unenhanced CT is a more appropriate initial imaging evaluation, given the high rate of false negatives in spine radiography (▶ Fig. 18.4).[25,50,51,52,53,54,55,56,57,58,59] The applicability of MRI in the acute settings of the ED and ICU to rule out osteoligamentous spine injuries is not well defined. When done within 48 hours of injury and findings are negative, MRI is helpful, but many soft-tissue findings seen on T2-weighted images may be clinically insignificant.[60,61] In Benzel et al's study, only 1 of 62 patients with discoligamentous injuries in a series of 174 patients with blunt trauma and without clinical or radiographic evidence of disruption of spinal integrity needed surgical fusion.[60] D'Alise et al studied 121 high-risk, intubated, obtunded/comatose patients with nonrevealing cervical spine radiographs. These investigators discovered 31 patients (25.6%) with disk, ligamentous, or bony cervical spine injuries. Eight of these 31 patients needed surgical intervention. Ninety of 121 patients were considered to have no cervical spine injuries and were thus cleared.[61] MRI is not particularly helpful in cervical spine fractures. Klein et al studied 32 patients with 75 known fractures. The sensitivity levels of MRI to detect posterior and anterior spinal fractures were 11.5% and 36.7%, respectively. Negative predictive values in this group of patients were 46% and 64%, respectively.[62]

Radiologic evaluation of the thoracic and lumbar spine should be performed in all MST patients with localized pain or other evidence of acute spinal injury. Plain radiographs have been criticized for the lack of sensitivity, diagnostic inaccuracies, and the amount of time required for adequate views. This becomes more difficult in the uncooperative head-injured patient.[54,58] With the widespread adoption of multiplanar reformation after routine CT of the chest, abdomen, and pelvis, CT is becoming the primary means of evaluating the thoracolumbar spine (▶ Fig. 18.4). In addition to ease of acquisition, CT offers increased diagnostic efficiency and accuracy compared with radiography.[12,52,53,54,57,58] Brown et al evaluated 3,537 blunt trauma patients who presented to their trauma center. In this population, there were 112 patients with lumbar fractures, 66 with thoracic fractures, and 45 with multilevel fractures. Sensitivity levels for plain radiographs in identifying thoracic and lumbar fractures were 64% and 69%, respectively. The sensitivity for dedicated CT of the spine was 98.5% in the thoracic and 100% in the lumbar spine. CT identified 99.3% of all fractures of the spine. The missed fracture was a thoracic compression fracture that was seen only with plain X-ray radiographs in a patient who had no neurologic injury and required no treatment. They concluded that CT and not routine plain radiographs was the radiographic study of choice in the evaluation of blunt trauma patients.[58]

In a prospective study of 222 trauma patients, Hauser et al compared CT scanning of the chest/abdomen/pelvis (CAP) with plain radiographs in identifying thoracolumbar fractures. In this study, the accuracy of CAP CT was 99%, compared with plain radiographs, which had an accuracy of 87%. Misclassification by plain radiographs was 12.6% compared with 1.4% for CT. Neither modality missed an unstable fracture.[54] Wintermark et al also evaluated thoracolumbar CT as a replacement for conventional radiographs in 100 consecutive blunt trauma patients. Twenty-six patients were identified with a total of 67 thoracolumbar fractures. Sensitivity and interobserver agreement for fractures were 32.0% and 0.661 for conventional radiography and 78.1% and 0.787 at multidetector-row CT. No false positives occurred with either X-ray or CT, so specificity was 100% for both. Twelve patients had unstable spine fractures. Sensitivity and interobserver agreement for these fractures were 33.3% and 0.368 with X-ray and 97.2% and 0.951 with CT. Eight patients appeared to have no fracture or no unstable fracture with X-ray but were found to have unstable fractures on CT. Identification errors regarding fracture level were observed in 13% of cases with X-ray, none with CT.[63]

Sheridan et al reported a prospective evaluation of patients with thoracic and lumbar spine fractures admitted over a 12-month period. Nineteen patients had thoracic spine fractures that underwent both X-ray evaluation and reformatted CT scanning. There was one (5%) fracture, a T8 compression fracture that was diagnosed by X-ray and missed by CT, and eight fractures (42%) diagnosed by CT that were missed by X-ray. Many of these missed fractures were transverse and spinous process fractures but did include two body fractures and a compression fracture. The sensitivity of CT for identifying thoracic fractures was 97% compared with 62% for X-ray. There were 27 patients with lumbar fractures that underwent both X-ray and reformatted abdominal CT scanning. There was one fracture (L5 transverse process) missed by both studies that was identified only on a dedicated lumbar spine CT. Three patients (11%) had fractures that were diagnosed by CT and missed by X-ray (L3 burst and two patients with multiple transverse process fractures). Two patients were read as having stable fractures on X-ray that were determined to be unstable on CT. The sensitivity of X-ray in the lumbar spine was 86%, whereas for CT it was 95%.[57]

In addition to improved accuracy, CT provides a single imaging modality to screen for brain, visceral, and spine injuries for a more efficient use of diagnostic time. To this end, Brandt et al found that for 50 patients undergoing radiographic evaluation of the thoracolumbar spine, plain radiographs took twice as long to perform compared with a CT of the CAP.[52] Wintermark et al reported that 9% of the thoracolumbar films had to be retaken because of insufficient quality. The average time needed to perform conventional X-ray of the entire spine in their study was 33 minutes, with 70% (23/33 minutes) devoted to imaging the thoracolumbar spine. The median time to perform a CT to include thoracic/abdominal/cranial and cervical spine was 40 minutes, including 7 minutes for the technologists to perform reformatting and reconstructions of the films.[63] The incidence of blunt cerebrovascular injuries detected by high-resolution CT and CT angiography (CTA) is 1 to 3% but with a high mortality of 10 to 40%.[64,65] An alternative to CTA is magnetic resonance angiography (MRA).[66] However, this is more time consuming and the patient is not readily accessible; thus, this is not as frequently employed in the acute setting.[67]

18.6 Management

A significant proportion of patients with severe MST succumb to their injuries at the scene of the accident; this is usually due to severe TBI or spinal cord injury or severe systemic injuries such as rupture of cardiac, aortic, or other large intrathoracic vessels.[18] The initial stabilization at the scene is critical along with rapid transport to an appropriate trauma hospital. On arrival of the patient in the ED trauma bay, the immediate interventions are under the purview of the surgical trauma service; early involvement of neurologic and orthopedic surgeons is essential and simultaneous activation of trauma pager codes ensures availability of all consulting services. This is the second period of vulnerability, and mortality during this phase is related to hypoxia or hypotension due to airway compromise or tension pneumothorax, hypovolemic shock, or cardiac tamponade, respectively.[18] This is the second time period during which rapid intervention is lifesaving. A trauma nurse or physician maintains a flow chart of all vital signs, evaluations, interventions, and consultations, and administration of medications are carefully recorded; tetanus toxoid administration is performed as well if the status of this is unknown.

Immediate assessment and establishment of airway patency is of paramount importance. Cervical and thoracolumbar spine precautions must be maintained during this period for all patients until spine injury is excluded.[68] In fact, patients with head and spinal cord injuries are at high risk for airway and breathing problems; 95% of patients with high spinal cord injury require intubation within the first 24 hours of hospitalization, and patients with cervical spinal cord injury above the fifth cervical vertebra are at particular risk for respiratory failure.[69] Orotracheal intubation, with an appropriately sized endotracheal tube, is by far the most common method of obtaining a definitive airway in these patients. Surgical airways, such as emergency cricothyroidotomy or tracheotomy, may be necessary in patients where the orotracheal route is not available. If an artificial airway is needed, it is established while maintaining cervical spine precautions; all these patients are presumed to have a spine injury until proven otherwise and immobilization in a cervical collar and long backboard maintaining the spine in a neutral position is essential.

With the airway protected, adequate ventilation and oxygenation is the next priority. Identification of severe life-threatening thoracic injuries is important, as patients with TBI or spinal cord injury are at particular risk of developing tension pneumothorax, hemothorax, or a flail chest. Similarly, a diaphragmatic rupture with or without migration of abdominal viscera into the thoracic cavity may compromise respiration. Following airway control, a rapid search should be made for these conditions, and they should be expeditiously treated if present. Strategies and modes for mechanical ventilation vary according to practitioner's resources, as well as the patient's pulmonary status and concomitant injuries. Standard volume-cycled modes of ventilation are commonly used, but other modes may be useful in settings of acute lung injury. In patients with head injury, avoidance of hypercarbia—elevated partial pressure of carbon dioxide (pCO_2) greater than 40 mm Hg—should be avoided to help maintain normal intracranial pressures and avoid secondary brain injury.

Assessing the adequacy of circulation and treating hemorrhage are the next priorities. In addition to external bleeding, there are certain body cavities into which a patient can lose significant amounts of blood: the abdomen, chest, thigh, pelvis, and retroperitoneum. A combination of physical examination and radiographic studies, such as a chest radiograph or a Focused Assessment with Sonography in Trauma (FAST), are adequate initially to detect a hematoma in these body cavities. Precise localization of the bleeding source requires more detailed imaging such as CT or MRI or angiography. Hemorrhage control and rapid resuscitation are essential to prevent shock and acidosis; this is particularly important in patients with TBI because hypotension markedly worsens outcome by potentiating secondary brain injury.[21,22] In addition to this, patients with cervical spinal cord injury may be hypotensive from neurogenic shock, compounding the deleterious effects of low intravascular pressures on cerebral function and recovery. Special consideration must be given to patients with severe TBI and elevated intracranial pressure (ICP), as the positioning and fluid administration during thoracic, abdominal, or orthopedic operations may lead to unwanted elevations in ICP.

Nasogastric tube placement allows decompression of the gastric contents but is contraindicated in patients with a cribriform plate fracture; this may be difficult to ascertain in a MST patient but intracranial pneumocephalus or blood, especially in the anterior cranial fossa, or a frank leakage of CSF from the nares are indicators of this. Under these circumstances, an orogastric tube is the best option. Vigorous orotracheal suction should be avoided in cervical cord injuries, as increased and unopposed vagal tone can result in cardiac arrest. A transurethral Foley catheter is essential for monitoring of urinary output unless contraindicated by a urethral injury, which may be seen in patients with severe pelvis, perineal, penile, or scrotal injuries; under these circumstances, urologic consultation as well as a urethrogram is needed prior to cannulation.[18]

18.6.1 Head Injury Management

Rapid clinical and radiographic assessment as detailed above provide clear delineation of most cranial injuries, and algorithms exist to provide reasonably clear guidelines as to the management of these patients. Patients with MST are at risk for coagulopathy, and correction of abnormal coagulation parameters is a prerequisite to any cranial intervention. Most patients are treated with rapid-reversal agents such as fresh frozen plasma and factor VII concentrates; the salutary effects of vitamin K administration on coagulation parameters manifest after approximately 12 hours and require normal liver function.

Patients with a GCS score 8 or lower, hypotension, or an abnormal motor examination require placement of an intracranial pressure monitor. Either intraparenchymal or intraventricular monitors are acceptable. The latter has the advantage of permitting CSF drainage as needed to treat intracranial pressure elevations. However, the intraparenchymal monitor is easier to insert; placement of an intraventricular catheter can be difficult in patients with small ventricles and a swollen brain. Intracranial pressure elevations are treated with simple measures such as head elevation, maintenance of normothermia or mild hypothermia, euvolemia, and a combination of carefully titrated analgesics, sedatives, and paralytics. Intractable intracranial hypertension is treated with intravenous barbiturate infusion titrated to achieve burst suppression on continuous bedside electroencephalogram monitoring or by a decompressive craniectomy that encompasses the frontal, temporal, and parietal regions of the calvarium, supplemented by a loose patulous duraplasty. Cases of intracranial pathology associated with significant mass effect and concordant with elevated intracranial pressure or a focal neurologic deficit, such as an epidural or a subdural hematoma or intraparenchymal hematoma, are taken to surgery for evacuation following stabilization of the patient's hemodynamic status.

After initial stabilization of the MST patient and assessment of the extent of TBI, the key goal is to prevent or ameliorate secondary brain injury. This is usually due to hypotension and hypoxia; hence, maintaining euvolemia, normotension, and normal oxygen saturation is essential. The administration of diuretic agents such as mannitol and hypertonic saline to treat intracranial pressure elevations is carefully balanced against the risk of hypotension and hypovolemia. Similarly, hyperventilation to induce hypocarbia may be used briefly to treat intracranial hypertension but runs the risk of aggravating cerebral ischemia in injured cerebral tissue.

18.6.2 Evaluation of Cervical Spine Injuries in Patients with Altered Mental Status

Evaluation of cervical spine injuries in the obtunded trauma patient remains a challenge. In the awake, asymptomatic patient, without significant distracting injuries, cervical spine injuries can generally be ruled out on the basis of clinical examination. For awake patients with significant neck pain, or obtunded patients, radiographic investigation should be carried out. In

2013, the Joint Section on Disorders of the Spine and Peripheral Nerves, comprising members of the American Association of Neurological Surgeons and the Congress of Neurological Surgeons, released revised guidelines for the management of acute cervical spine and spinal cord injuries.[70]

When cervical spine imaging is required, as in the case of an obtunded trauma patient, high-quality CT is recommended as the imaging study of choice. Plain three-view radiographs are not recommended if CT is available; they are, however, recommended if CT is unavailable. These recommendations are supported by high-quality research studies.[71] In the setting of a normal CT scan in an obtunded patient, the best course of action is less clear. Neurosurgical guidelines offer several options: continue cervical immobilization until asymptomatic; discontinue immobilization on the basis of a normal MRI scan obtained with 48 hours of injury (although the evidence for this is limited and conflicting); or discontinue the collar at the discretion of the treating physician. In this setting, dynamic imaging (i.e., flexion–extension radiographs) are of limited value and are not recommended.[71] Clearly, the circumstance requires the judgment of the treating physician, who must take into account such factors as the mechanism of injury (including the energy transfer), the patient's physiologic stability with regard to other injuries, the risk of complications from extended bracing such as decubitus ulcers, and the overall prognosis for recovery.

18.6.3 Management of Spinal Column Injuries

The general principles of spine fracture management are to realign the vertebral column, decompress any compromised neural elements, and stabilize segments determined to be at risk for injury within the range of normal physiologic motion.[72] Various scoring systems have been developed to grade the severity and guide management of both subaxial cervical spine injury and thoracolumbar spine injury. For both scales, an injury severity score (ISS) ≤ 3 may be managed nonoperatively, and an ISS ≥ to 5 indicates the need for operative intervention (▶Table 18.3, ▶Table 18.4). The use of intravenous high-dose steroids for spinal cord injury is no longer recommended. In general, therefore, any spine fracture requiring surgical stabilization should be treated as soon as the patient's medical condition allows. The patient's neurologic function also has an influence on the timing of surgical intervention. Patients with a complete spinal cord injury can be addressed in an elective manner with optimization of hemodynamic and nutritional parameters. On the other hand, patients with an incomplete spinal cord injury that can be attributed to a radiographic evidence of injury, such as dislocated facets or significant canal compromise, are treated in a more urgent manner; emergent surgical decompression is recommended for patients with a progressive neurologic deficit, or injuries that make a progressive deficit likely.

Spine or orthopedic fractures that are deemed nonemergent are addressed once the patient has been adequately resuscitated and hemodynamic stability can be assured throughout the operative procedure. Other injuries, such as acute respiratory distress syndrome (ARDS), may preclude operation if the patient cannot be safely placed under anesthesia and positioned

Table 18.3 Subaxial cervical spine injury classification scoring system

Injury morphology	Score
No abnormality	0
Compression	1
• Burst (extension through posterior wall, including vertical fracture, "teardrop" fracture)	+1
Distraction	3
• Perched facets, or bilateral widened facets (not jumped)	
• Hyperextension injury (torn anterior longitudinal ligament + disk)	
Rotation/translation (greater than 11 degrees or translation of 3.5 mm)	4
• Facet dislocation, unstable "teardrop"	
• Bilateral pedicle fracture, floating lateral mass	
Discoligamentous complex	
Intact	0
Indeterminate	1
• Interspinous widening, or MR STIR signal only	
Disrupted	3
• Widened disc space, perched or dislocated facets	
Neurologic status	
Intact	0
• Root injury	1
• Complete cord injury (ASIA A)	2
• Incomplete cord injury (ASIA B, C, and D)	3
• Continuous cord compression with neurologic deficit (modifier)	+1

Abbreviations: ASIA, American Spinal Injury Association; MR, magnetic resonance; STIR, Short tau inversion recovery.

Source: Vaccaro AR. The subaxial cervical spine injury classification system. Spine 2007;32;2365–2374.

for the procedure. Early surgical intervention, preferably within 72 hours of the initial injury, is increasingly recommended for patients with nonemergent spinal injuries. Delayed surgery, on the other hand, has been associated with longer hospital stay, skin breakdown, sepsis, pulmonary complications, and deep venous thrombosis.[73,74,75,76]Patient mobilization following surgical stabilization provides a good defense against these complications and is one of the major arguments in favor of early operation. Other advantages include pain control, improved neurologic outcomes, protection against progressive deformity (especially kyphosis), and increased freedom of positioning in the hospital bed.

In all of these cases, the treating neurosurgeon or orthopedic spine surgeon must work in conjunction with the trauma surgeon and anesthesiologist, to continually reevaluate the patient's clinical progress and the feasibility of operative fixation of a spine fracture. Although the initial management of trauma has become much more standardized in recent decades, treatment decisions further downstream from the initial trauma, including management of polytrauma patients with concurrent brain and spine injuries, must necessarily be individualized to the particular patient.

Table 18.4 Thoracolumbar injury classification and severity score

Injury morphology	Score
Compression	1
• Axial compression or burst	
• Flexion compression, flexion burst, burst with posterior elements distracted	
• Lateral compression, lateral burst	
Burst fractures (of any kind) (modifier)	+1
Translation/rotation	3
• Translation/rotation +/− compression or burst	
• Uni or bilateral facet dislocation +/− compression or burst	
Distraction	4
• Flexion–distraction +/− compression or burst	
• Extension–distraction	
Posterior ligamentous complex	
Intact	0
Suspected or indeterminate injury	2
• Injured	3
• Neurologic status	
• Intact	0
Nerve root injury	2
• Complete cord injury (ASIA A)	2
• Incomplete cord injury (ASIA B, C, and D)	3
• Cauda equina injury	3

Source: Vaccaro AR. A new classification of thoracolumbar injuries. Spine 2005;30;2325–2333.

18.7 Conclusion

Evaluation and management of patients with MST is complex and multidisciplinary. Close communication between consulting services, keen awareness of overlapping morbidities or the effects of therapeutic interventions, and a high index of suspicion for undetected injuries are essential. Cranial and spinal injuries, in particular, can complicate the management of MST patients, and there is a risk of secondary deterioration in these patients if inappropriately managed. The potential for a new or worsening neurologic injury from an undiagnosed fracture or worsening cerebral edema from injudicious fluid administration are examples of this. Rapid and precise radiographic imaging studies with careful interpretation cannot be emphasized enough. The seamless transition from on-scene care to in-hospital assessment and management is the critical element that determines the outcome for many patients. In the end, this serves also as an excellent paradigm for close cooperation between consulting physicians and services and the trauma team that is the hallmark of a high-quality trauma facility.

References

[1] World Health Organization. Injuries and Violence: The Facts. http://apps.who.int/iris/bitstream/10665/149798/1/9789241508018_eng.pdf?ua=1&ua=1. Published 2014. Accessed September 22, 2016

[2] Centers for Disease Control and Prevention, National Center for Injury Prevention and Control. Web-based Injury Statistics Query and Reporting System (WISQARS). https://www.cdc.gov/injury/wisqars/. Accessed June 19, 2016

[3] National Trauma Institute. Trauma statistics. http://www.nationaltraumainstitute.org/home/trauma_statistics.html. Published 2014. Accessed September 22, 2016

[4] Faul M, Xu L, Wald MM, Coronado VG. Traumatic Brain Injury in the United States: Emergency Department Visits, Hospitalizations, and Deaths. Atlanta, GA: Centers for Disease Control and Prevention, National Center for Injury Prevention and Control; 2010

[5] Cooper C, Dunham CM, Rodriguez A. Falls and major injuries are risk factors for thoracolumbar fractures: cognitive impairment and multiple injuries impede the detection of back pain and tenderness. J Trauma. 1995; 38(5):692–696

[6] Hanson JA, Blackmore CC, Mann FA, Wilson AJ. Cervical spine injury: a clinical decision rule to identify high-risk patients for helical CT screening. AJR Am J Roentgenol. 2000; 174(3):713–717

[7] Kaups KL, Davis JW. Patients with gunshot wounds to the head do not require cervical spine immobilization and evaluation. J Trauma. 1998; 44(5):865–867

[8] Patton JH, Kralovich KA, Cuschieri J, Gasparri M. Clearing the cervical spine in victims of blunt assault to the head and neck: what is necessary? Am Surg. 2000; 66(4):326–330, discussion 330–331

[9] Holly LT, Kelly DF, Counelis GJ, Blinman T, McArthur DL, Cryer HG. Cervical spine trauma associated with moderate and severe head injury: incidence, risk factors, and injury characteristics. J Neurosurg. 2002; 96(3, Suppl):285–291

[10] Iida H, Tachibana S, Kitahara T, Horiike S, Ohwada T, Fujii K. Association of head trauma with cervical spine injury, spinal cord injury, or both. J Trauma. 1999; 46(3):450–452

[11] Leucht P, Fischer K, Muhr G, Mueller EJ. Epidemiology of traumatic spine fractures. Injury. 2009; 40(2):166–172

[12] Post MJ, Green BA. The use of computed tomography in spinal trauma. Radiol Clin North Am. 1983; 21(2):327–375

[13] el-Khoury GY, Whitten CG. Trauma to the upper thoracic spine: anatomy, biomechanics, and unique imaging features. AJR Am J Roentgenol. 1993; 160(1):95–102

[14] Kaye JJ, Nance EP, Jr. Thoracic and lumbar spine trauma. Radiol Clin North Am. 1990; 28(2):361–377

[15] Brandser EA, el-Khoury GY. Thoracic and lumbar spine trauma. Radiol Clin North Am. 1997; 35(3):533–557

[16] Reid DC, Henderson R, Saboe L, Miller JD. Etiology and clinical course of missed spine fractures. J Trauma. 1987; 27(9):980–986

[17] Buduhan G, McRitchie DI. Missed injuries in patients with multiple trauma. J Trauma. 2000; 49(4):600–605

[18] Ali J. Priorities in multisystem trauma. In: Hall JB, Schmidt GA, Wood LH, eds. Principles of Critical Care. 3rd ed.; 2005:. http://accesssurgery.mhmedical.com/content.aspx?bookid=361&Sectionid=39866466. Published 2005. Accessed September 22, 2016

[19] American College of Surgeons Committee on Trauma. Advanced Trauma Life Support (ATLS) Student Course Manual. 9th ed. Chicago, IL: American College of Surgeons; 2012

[20] Lee WC, Chen CW, Lin YK, et al. Association of head, thoracic and abdominal trauma with delayed diagnosis of co-existing injuries in critical trauma patients. Injury. 2014; 45(9):1429–1434

[21] Chesnut RM. The management of severe traumatic brain injury. Emerg Med Clin North Am. 1997; 15(3):581–604

[22] Chesnut RM, Marshall SB, Piek J, Blunt BA, Klauber MR, Marshall LF. Early and late systemic hypotension as a frequent and fundamental source of cerebral ischemia following severe brain injury in the Traumatic Coma Data Bank. Acta Neurochir Suppl (Wien). 1993; 59:121–125

[23] Hoffman JR, Wolfson AB, Todd K, Mower WR. Selective cervical spine radiography in blunt trauma: methodology of the National Emergency X-Radiography Utilization Study (NEXUS). Ann Emerg Med. 1998; 32(4):461–469

[24] Roth BJ, Martin RR, Foley K, Barcia PJ, Kennedy P. Roentgenographic evaluation of the cervical spine. A selective approach. Arch Surg. 1994; 129(6):643–645

[25] Chiu WC, Haan JM, Cushing BM, Kramer ME, Scalea TM. Ligamentous injuries of the cervical spine in unreliable blunt trauma patients: incidence, evaluation, and outcome. J Trauma. 2001; 50(3):457–463, discussion 464

[26] Hasler RM, Exadaktylos AK, Bouamra O, et al. Epidemiology and predictors of cervical spine injury in adult major trauma patients: a multicenter cohort study. J Trauma Acute Care Surg. 2012; 72(4):975–981

[27] Hoffman JR, Mower WR, Wolfson AB, Todd KH, Zucker MI; National Emergency X-Radiography Utilization Study Group. Validity of a set of clinical criteria to rule out injury to the cervical spine in patients with blunt trauma. N Engl J Med. 2000; 343(2):94–99

[28] Hoffman JR, Schriger DL, Mower W, Luo JS, Zucker M. Low-risk criteria for cervical-spine radiography in blunt trauma: a prospective study. Ann Emerg Med. 1992; 21(12):1454–1460

[29] Katsuura Y, Osborn JM, Cason GW. The epidemiology of thoracolumbar trauma: a meta-analysis. J Orthop. 2016; 13(4):383–388

[30] Dai LY, Yao WF, Cui YM, Zhou Q. Thoracolumbar fractures in patients with multiple injuries: diagnosis and treatment—a review of 147 cases. J Trauma. 2004; 56(2):348–355

[31] Stephan K, Huber S, Häberle S, et al; TraumaRegister DGU. Spinal cord injury—incidence, prognosis, and outcome: an analysis of the TraumaRegister DGU. Spine J. 2015; 15(9):1994–2001

[32] Varma A, Hill EG, Nicholas J, Selassie A. Predictors of early mortality after traumatic spinal cord injury: a population-based study. Spine. 2010; 35(7):778–783

[33] Desai JD. Beevor's sign. Ann Indian Acad Neurol. 2012; 15(2):94–95

[34] Blackwood GA, Blackmore CC, Mann MD, et al. The importance of trauma series radiographs: have we forgotten the ABC's? Presented at the 13th Annual Scientific Meeting of the American Society of Emergency Radiology, March 13–20, 2002, Orlando, Florida

[35] Ballard RB, Rozycki GS, Knudson MM, Pennington SD. The surgeon's use of ultrasound in the acute setting. Surg Clin North Am. 1998; 78(2):337–364

[36] Shackford SR, Rogers FB, Osler TM, Trabulsy ME, Clauss DW, Vane DW. Focused abdominal sonogram for trauma: the learning curve of non-radiologist clinicians in detecting hemoperitoneum. J Trauma. 1999; 46(4):553–562, discussion 562–564

[37] Hoff WS, Holevar M, Nagy KK, et al; Eastern Asociation for the Surgery of Trauma. Practice management guidelines for the evaluation of blunt abdominal trauma: the East practice management guidelines work group. J Trauma. 2002; 53(3):602–615

[38] Miller LA, Shanmuganathan K. Multidetector CT evaluation of abdominal trauma. Radiol Clin North Am. 2005; 43(6):1079–1095, viii

[39] Fakhry SM, Watts DD, Luchette FA; EAST Multi-Institutional Hollow Viscus Injury Research Group. Current diagnostic approaches lack sensitivity in the diagnosis of perforated blunt small bowel injury: analysis from 275,557 trauma admissions from the EAST multi-institutional HVI trial. J Trauma. 2003; 54(2):295–306

[40] Menegaux F, Trésallet C, Gosgnach M, Nguyen-Thanh Q, Langeron O, Riou B. Diagnosis of bowel and mesenteric injuries in blunt abdominal trauma: a prospective study. Am J Emerg Med. 2006; 24(1):19–24

[41] Friese RS, Coln CE, Gentilello LM. Laparoscopy is sufficient to exclude occult diaphragm injury after penetrating abdominal trauma. J Trauma. 2005; 58(4):789–792

[42] Sliker CW. Imaging of diaphragm injuries. Radiol Clin North Am. 2006; 44(2):199–211, vii

[43] Deck AJ, Shaves S, Talner L, Porter JR. Computerized tomography cystography for the diagnosis of traumatic bladder rupture. J Urol. 2000; 164(1):43–46

[44] Quagliano PV, Delair SM, Malhotra AK. Diagnosis of blunt bladder injury: a prospective comparative study of computed tomography cystography and conventional retrograde cystography. J Trauma. 2006; 61(2):410–421, discussion 421–422

[45] Peng PD, Spain DA, Tataria M, Hellinger JC, Rubin GD, Brundage SI. CT angiography effectively evaluates extremity vascular trauma. Am Surg. 2008; 74(2):103–107

[46] Hagan JB. Anaphylactoid and adverse reactions to radiocontrast agents. Immunol Allergy Clin North Am. 2004; 24(3):507–519, vii–viii

[47] Kandzari DE, Rebeiz AG, Wang A, Sketch MH, Jr. Contrast nephropathy: an evidence-based approach to prevention. Am J Cardiovasc Drugs. 2003; 3(6):395–405

[48] Tremblay LN, Tien H, Hamilton P, et al. Risk and benefit of intravenous contrast in trauma patients with an elevated serum creatinine. J Trauma. 2005; 59(5):1162–1166, discussion 1166–1167

[49] Barraco RD, Chiu WC, Clancy TV, et al. Practice Management Guidelines for the Diagnosis and Management of Injury in the Pregnant Patient. EAST Practice Management Guidelines Work Group; 2005

[50] Berne JD, Velmahos GC, El-Tawil Q, et al. Value of complete cervical helical computed tomographic scanning in identifying cervical spine injury in the unevaluable blunt trauma patient with multiple injuries: a prospective study. J Trauma. 1999; 47(5):896–902, discussion 902–903

[51] Blackmore CC, Ramsey SD, Mann FA, Deyo RA. Cervical spine screening with CT in trauma patients: a cost-effectiveness analysis. Radiology. 1999; 212(1):117–125

[52] Brandt MM, Wahl WL, Yeom K, Kazerooni E, Wang SC. Computed tomographic scanning reduces cost and time of complete spine evaluation. J Trauma. 2004; 56(5):1022–1026, discussion 1026–1028

[53] Gestring ML, Gracias VH, Feliciano MA, et al. Evaluation of the lower spine after blunt trauma using abdominal computed tomographic scanning supplemented with lateral scanograms. J Trauma. 2002; 53(1):9–14

[54] Hauser CJ, Visvikis G, Hinrichs C, et al. Prospective validation of computed tomographic screening of the thoracolumbar spine in trauma. J Trauma. 2003; 55(2):228–234, discussion 234–235

[55] Holmes JF, Akkinepalli R. Computed tomography versus plain radiography to screen for cervical spine injury: a meta-analysis. J Trauma. 2005; 58(5):902–905

[56] Schenarts PJ, Diaz J, Kaiser C, Carrillo Y, Eddy V, Morris JA, Jr. Prospective comparison of admission computed tomographic scan and plain films of the upper cervical spine in trauma patients with altered mental status. J Trauma. 2001; 51(4):663–668, discussion 668–669

[57] Sheridan R, Peralta R, Rhea J, Ptak T, Novelline R. Reformatted visceral protocol helical computed tomographic scanning allows conventional radiographs of the thoracic and lumbar spine to be eliminated in the evaluation of blunt trauma patients. J Trauma. 2003; 55(4):665–669

[58] Brown CV, Antevil JL, Sise MJ, Sack DI. Spiral computed tomography for the diagnosis of cervical, thoracic, and lumbar spine fractures: its time has come. J Trauma. 2005; 58(5):890–895, discussion 895–896

[59] Diaz JJ, Jr, Gillman C, Morris JA, Jr, May AK, Carrillo YM, Guy J. Are five-view plain films of the cervical spine unreliable? A prospective evaluation in blunt trauma patients with altered mental status. J Trauma. 2003; 55(4):658–663, discussion 663–664

[60] Benzel EC, Hart BL, Ball PA, Baldwin NG, Orrison WW, Espinosa MC. Magnetic resonance imaging for the evaluation of patients with occult cervical spine injury. J Neurosurg. 1996; 85(5):824–829

[61] D'Alise MD, Benzel EC, Hart BL. Magnetic resonance imaging evaluation of the cervical spine in the comatose or obtunded trauma patient. J Neurosurg. 1999; 91(1, Suppl):54–59

[62] Klein GR, Vaccaro AR, Albert TJ, et al. Efficacy of magnetic resonance imaging in the evaluation of posterior cervical spine fractures. Spine. 1999; 24(8):771–774

[63] Wintermark M, Mouhsine E, Theumann N, et al. Thoracolumbar spine fractures in patients who have sustained severe trauma: depiction with multi-detector row CT. Radiology. 2003; 227(3):681–689

[64] Schneidereit NP, Simons R, Nicolaou S, et al. Utility of screening for blunt vascular neck injuries with computed tomographic angiography. J Trauma. 2006; 60(1):209–215, discussion 215–216

[65] Stallmeyer MJ, Morales RE, Flanders AE. Imaging of traumatic neurovascular injury. Radiol Clin North Am. 2006; 44(1):13–39, vii

[66] Bok AP, Peter JC. Carotid and vertebral artery occlusion after blunt cervical injury: the role of MR angiography in early diagnosis. J Trauma. 1996; 40(6):968–972

[67] Bromberg WJ, Collier BC, Diebel LN, et al. Blunt cerebrovascular injury practice management guidelines: the Eastern Association for the Surgery of Trauma. J Trauma. 2010; 68(2):471–477

[68] Stuke LE, Pons PT, Guy JS, Chapleau WP, Butler FK, McSwain NE. Prehospital spine immobilization for penetrating trauma—review and recommendations from the Prehospital Trauma Life Support Executive Committee. J Trauma. 2011; 71(3):763–769, discussion 769–770

[69] Como JJ, Sutton ER, McCunn M, et al. Characterizing the need for mechanical ventilation following cervical spinal cord injury with neurologic deficit. J Trauma. 2005; 59(4):912–916, discussion 916

[70] Walters BC. Methodology of the guidelines for the management of acute cervical spine and spinal cord injuries. Neurosurgery. 2013; 72(Suppl 2):17–21

[71] Ryken TC, Hadley MN, Walters BC, et al. Radiographic assessment. Neurosurgery. 2013; 72(Suppl 2):54–72

[72] Dimar JR, Carreon LY, Riina J, Schwartz DG, Harris MB. Early versus late stabilization of the spine in the polytrauma patient. Spine. 2010; 35(21, Suppl):S187–S192

[73] Cengiz SL, Kalkan E, Bayir A, Ilik K, Basefer A. Timing of thoracolomber spine stabilization in trauma patients; impact on neurological outcome and clinical course. A real prospective (rct) randomized controlled study. Arch Orthop Trauma Surg. 2008; 128(9):959–966

[74] Vallier HA, Moore TA, Como JJ, et al. Complications are reduced with a protocol to standardize timing of fixation based on response to resuscitation. J Orthop Surg. 2015; 10:155

[75] Kerwin AJ, Griffen MM, Tepas JJ, III, Schinco MA, Devin T, Frykberg ER. Best practice determination of timing of spinal fracture fixation as defined by analysis of the National Trauma Data Bank. J Trauma. 2008; 65(4):824–830, discussion 830–831

[76] Frangen TM, Ruppert S, Muhr G, Schinkel C. The beneficial effects of early stabilization of thoracic spine fractures depend on trauma severity. J Trauma. 2010; 68(5):1208–1212

19 Summary and Synopsis of The Brain Trauma Foundation Head Injury Guidelines

Courtney Pendleton and Jack Jallo

Abstract

Traumatic brain injury (TBI) remains a common cause of morbidity and mortality among Americans. The guidelines developed by the Brain Trauma Foundation and the American Association of Neurological Surgeons for management of severe traumatic head injury offer recommendations for optimal management of adult and pediatric patients in the prehospital and acute inpatient settings. Separate guidelines serve to optimize management strategies for combat-related TBI, but those are beyond the scope of this chapter. One key topic in these guidelines remains the recommendation that patients with TBI receive streamlined care through an established trauma center capable of providing multidisciplinary management of complex traumatic injuries in the adult or pediatric population. In-hospital management guidelines are largely level II and III recommendations, whereas the only level I recommendations are to avoid prophylactic steroid use in TBI patients. Overall, these recommendations help codify management of TBI patients across the United States, providing optimized evidence-based strategies for inpatient care.

Keywords: critical care, evidence-based medicine, guidelines, trauma, traumatic brain injury

19.1 Introduction

Of the 1 million Americans evaluated in emergency rooms for traumatic brain injury (TBI) annually, nearly one quarter require inpatient care. Of the 150,000 deaths due to trauma each year, one third are secondary to head injuries. Although difficult to calculate, the annual net cost of trauma to society is estimated at just under $40 billion. To this end, guidelines have been developed to assist in optimizing the multidisciplinary health care teams treating TBI patients.

The following guidelines are adapted from the recommendations developed jointly by the Brain Trauma Foundation (BTF) and the American Association of Neurological Surgeons for the management of severe traumatic head injury. This review of the guidelines is divided into three sections: general adult trauma management, surgical management of traumatic lesions, and general pediatric trauma management.

The third edition of the BTF guidelines changes the previous classification method of standards, guidelines, and options to the new system of level I, II, and III recommendations. The new classification system parallels the study group classification of evidence according to standard class I, II, and II data. Briefly, level I recommendations reflect the most certainty and are based on class I data, whereas level III recommendations have the least certainty and are most likely to be based on class II and III data. Class I data consist of good-quality prospective randomized studies. Class II data include moderate-quality randomized studies and good-quality retrospective analyses, such as cohort and case–control studies. Class III data are based on less reliable randomized and retrospective analyses, as well as case studies, databases, and patient registries.

With limited prospective data available, the guidelines leave much discretion to the clinician and individual patient circumstances. This chapter summarizes the pediatric and adult guidelines for the management of severe TBI and describes the surgical guidelines for the management of traumatic lesions.

19.2 Prehospital Guidelines

19.2.1 Trauma Systems

Multiple studies noted significant drops in mortality (50% and 20%, respectively) when organized trauma systems were put into place,[1,2] and the guidelines recommend all regions have an organized trauma care system. Although the system structure is not explicitly defined, several important considerations are discussed, including the role of the neurosurgeon in developing TBI management protocols, the need for 24-hour availability of trauma and neurosurgery teams, and the infrastructure to provide evaluation, monitoring, and management according to the guidelines. In particular, it is recommended that when available, pediatric patients be brought by emergency medical service (EMS) to a certified pediatric trauma center for definitive management. Data appear to support the conclusion that pediatric patients with severe TBI are more likely to survive if treated in pediatric trauma centers, or adult trauma centers with added qualifications in pediatrics rather than in a level I or level II adult trauma center, and that pediatric patients with severe TBI who require neurosurgical procedures have a low chance of survival in a level II adult trauma center as compared with the other centers.[3] Additionally, in metropolitan areas, direct transport to a pediatric trauma center appears to increase survival rate overall.[4]

19.2.2 Medical Optimization

It is known that hypoxemia in the prehospital setting is associated with worse outcomes in TBI patients.[5] Additionally, several studies have suggested that hypoxia during the prehospital care of pediatric patients with TBI is common. As many as nearly a third of pediatric patients with severe TBI are hypoxic on arrival to the emergency department.[6] Therefore, it may be tempting to advocate immediate endotracheal intubation for all pediatric patients with severe TBI and signs of hypoxia in the field. However, two large, randomized, prospective studies, including one using the National Pediatric Trauma Registry, demonstrated no significant difference in outcome among those managed with endotracheal intubation and those treated with bag mask ventilation in the field.[7] A smaller study of 16 pediatric patients intubated in the field demonstrated four deaths related to "major airway mishaps."[8] Although there is clear evidence that hypoxemia leads to poorer neurologic outcome in both pediatric and adult TBI patients, and that hypoxia frequently occurs in the prehospital setting in this patient population, there is also evidence that successful prehospital intubation of infants and children requires specialized training, and that success rates are in general lower than in adults.

Multiple studies have demonstrated the negative outcomes related to hypoxia and hypotension in both the adult and the pediatric population with TBI. One study by Pigula et al analyzed the influence of hypoxia and hypotension on mortality from severe TBI.[9] They reported an 18% incidence of hypotension on arrival at the emergency department. A mortality rate of 61% was associated with hypotension on admission versus 22% among patients without hypotension. When hypotension was combined with hypoxia, the mortality rate was 85%.[9]

The adult neurosurgical literature traditionally defines hypotension as systolic blood pressure less than 90 mm Hg. In pediatric patients, hypotension is defined as less than the 5th percentile of normal systolic blood pressure for age. In children, however, hypotension is a late sign of shock. Pediatric patients may maintain their blood pressure despite significant hypovolemia and clinical signs of shock. Signs of diminished perfusion include tachycardia, loss of central pulses, diminished urine output to less than 1 mL/kg/h, and increased capillary filling time more than 2 seconds. Fluid resuscitation is indicated in children for clinical signs of decreased perfusion even when an adequate blood pressure is observed. Fluid restriction to avoid cerebral edema or exacerbating cerebral edema is contraindicated in the management of the TBI pediatric patient in shock.[10]

19.3 General Adult Trauma Management Guidelines

▶Table 19.1 summarizes the guidelines for in-hospital management of adult TBI.

19.3.1 Resuscitation of Blood Pressure and Oxygenation

Hypoxemia and hypotension have been documented to cause worse outcomes in head injury patients.[6,11,12] Studies reveal that hypoxemia commonly affects TBI patients, up to 44% in one study,[13] occurring in the field or during transportation.

There is a level II recommendation to monitor blood pressure and avoid hypotension (systolic blood pressure < 90 mm Hg). There is a level III recommendation to monitor oxygenation and avoid hypoxia (partial arterial pressure of oxygen [PaO_2] < 60 mm Hg or O_2 saturation < 90%)

It is recommended that the clinician maintain an appropriate blood pressure so that an adequate cerebral perfusion pressure (CPP), defined as 50 to 70 mm Hg, can be achieved. For patients who remain hypoxemic, particularly in those with a Glasgow Coma Scale (GCS) score of less than 9, endotracheal intubation is strongly recommended.

The Traumatic Coma Data Bank (TCDB) provides prospectively collected data, which demonstrated the presence of either or both hypotension and hypoxemia was among the most important predictors of poor outcome.[5,14] Hypotension was found to double mortality and increase morbidity when compared with normotensive patients.

Although the American College of Surgeons (ACS) recommends that crystalloid be rapidly administered to trauma patients, the Advanced Trauma Life Support (ATLS) cautions that fluids may inadvertently exacerbate cerebral edema and elevate intracranial pressures (ICPs). Of note, one study showed no correlation between ICPs and the amount of fluid or blood administered.[15] Hypertonic saline has been demonstrated as a viable option for volume resuscitation in TBI patients: ICPs were found to be reduced in TBI patients,[16] and a meta-analysis[17] showed a doubling of survival in those patients receiving hypertonic saline.

19.3.2 Hyperosmolar Therapy

There are level II recommendations for using mannitol, with doses from 0.25 to 1 g/kg for the treatment of elevated ICPs in patients with existing ICP monitors. Level III recommendations are for the use of mannitol in patients without ICP monitoring who exhibit clinical decline. These recommendations were made on the basis of the data previously used for the second edition of the BTF guidelines; no new studies met the inclusion criteria during the updated literature review.

Mannitol is commonly used in the treatment of TBI, with multiple studies documenting its positive influence on a variety of parameters, including ICP and CPP. It most likely acts through both an immediate and a delayed mechanism. Within several minutes of being given as a bolus, mannitol can reduce ICP. This occurs because the intravascular volume is increased, diluting the hematocrit and subsequently decreasing blood viscosity. The result is an increase in CPP and cerebral blood flow (CBF).

The delayed effect of mannitol occurs after approximately 20 minutes, during which time gradients between the plasma and cells have developed, and this osmotic effect may last up to 6 hours. Its risks include precipitating acute renal failure and inadvertently increasing ICP. Risk factors for renal failure include a serum osmolarity above 320 mOsm and the presence of renal disease.

Although the BTF guidelines describe the common use of hypertonic saline both for ICP management and volume resuscitation in the neurotrauma population, insufficient quality studies were available in the adult population to make recommendations

19.3.3 Prophylactic Hypothermia

Given the controversy surrounding this intervention, the BTF performed its own meta-analysis of existing class II data to determine the appropriate level of recommendation for the use of prophylactic hypothermia.[18,19,20,21,22] The included studies were considered of sufficiently quality for level III recommendations, namely, that prophylactic hypothermia does not clearly reduce mortality, but survival benefit increases when hypothermia maintained for more than 48 hours, and there was a significant improvement in overall good outcome (GCS score 4 or 5) in TBI patients treated with prophylactic hypothermia

Table 19.1 Summary of adult trauma management guidelines

Topic	Guidelines
Blood pressure and oxygenation	Level I—Insufficient data Level II—Monitor blood pressure, avoid hypotension (SBP < 90 mm Hg) Level III—Monitor oxygenation, avoid hypoxia (PaO$_2$ < 60 mm Hg or O$_2$ saturation < 90%)
Hyperosmolar therapy	Level I—Insufficient data Level II—Mannitol may effectively control elevated ICP; dosing at 0.25 to 1 g/kg. Avoid SBP < 90 mm Hg Level III—Minimize use of mannitol in patients without ICP monitoring; use in unmonitored patients with clinical signs of neurologic deterioration or herniation
Prophylactic hypothermia	Level I—Insufficient data Level II—Insufficient data Level III—Based on BTF meta-analysis. Decrease in mortality when temperature maintained for > 48 h. Associated with improved GCS outcome
Infection prophylaxis	Level I—Insufficient data Level II—Antibiotics during intubation reduce pneumonia risk, without altering length of stay or mortality. Early tracheostomy is recommended, but does not affect mortality Level III—Early extubation in patients who meet clinical criteria does not affect pneumonia risk. Antibiotics during ventriculostomy placement are not recommended
DVT prophylaxis	Level I—Insufficient data Level II—Insufficient data Level III—Mechanical prophylaxis with compression stockings or pneumatic compression devices recommended until patients are ambulatory. Chemical prophylaxis is recommended, but carries a risk of expanding intracranial hemorrhage
Indications for intracranial pressure monitoring	Level I—Insufficient data Level II—ICP monitoring for TBI patients with a GCS score of 3–8 and presence of an intracranial contusion, hematoma, edema, or effacement of basal cisterns on head CT Level III—ICP monitoring in TBI patients with GC 3–8 and normal head CT if two or more of these criteria are met: > 40 years, unilateral or bilateral posturing, SBP > 90 mm Hg
Intracranial pressure monitoring technology	The ventricular catheter is considered to be the most cost-efficient and accurate means for monitoring ICP
Intracranial pressure threshold	Level I—Insufficient data Level II—Begin treatment when ICP > 20 mm Hg Level III—Management of ICPs requires evaluation of clinical examination, ICP measurement, and imaging findings
Cerebral perfusion thresholds	Level I—Insufficient data Level II—Avoid aggressively maintaining CPP > 70 mm Hg to minimize risk of ARDS Level III—Maintain CPP 50–70 mm Hg
Brain oxygen monitoring thresholds	Level I—Insufficient data Level II—Insufficient data Level III—Treat for jugular venous saturation < 50% or brain tissue oxygen < 15 mm Hg
Anesthetics, analgesics, sedatives	Level I—Insufficient data Level II—Prophylactic burst suppression with barbiturates not recommended. Avoid high-dose barbiturate management of ICPs Propofol is recommended for ICP management, but high doses should be avoided
Nutrition	Level I—Insufficient data Level II—Goal of full caloric provision by day 7
Antiseizure prophylaxis	Level I—Insufficient data Level II—Phenytoin and valproate not recommended for prevention of late posttraumatic seizures
Hyperventilation	Level I—Insufficient data Level II—Prophylactic hyperventilation (PaCO$_2$ < 25 mm Hg) is not recommended Level III—Hyperventilation may serve as a temporizing measure; it is not recommended within the first 24 h of injury. Monitoring jugular venous oxygen saturation or brain oxygen tension is recommended
Steroids	Level I—Not recommended for managing outcome or ICP

Abbreviations: BTF, Brain Trauma Foundation; CPP, cerebral perfusion pressure; CT, computed tomography; DVT, deep vein thrombosis; GCS, Glasgow Coma Scale; ICP, intracranial pressure; PaCO$_2$, partial arterial pressure of carbon dioxide; PaO$_2$, partial arterial pressure of oxygen; SBP, systolic blood pressure; TBI, traumatic brain injury.

19.3.4 Infection Prophylaxis

The main sources of infection in TBI patients addressed by the BTF guidelines are ventricular catheter/ICP monitor infections and ventilator-associated pneumonia

There are level III recommendations for infection prophylaxis in patients with ventricular catheters of ICP monitors. There is no evidence to recommend routine antibiotic prophylaxis in patients with such devices in place, and routine exchange of ventricular catheters is not recommended. Although a single study demonstrated reduction in infection and colonization in patients with antibiotic impregnated ventricular catheters,[23] the data were not compelling enough for the BTF to make formal recommendations; however, the guidelines emphasize that this is an area where additional clinical research would be beneficial

There are level II recommendations to provide a short course of periprocedural antibiotics to minimize the risk of pneumonia, although this does not reduce overall length of stay. Additional level II recommendations are to pursue early tracheostomy to reduce the days of mechanical ventilation, but this does not affect mortality or risk of pneumonia. There are level III recommendations to pursue extubation in patients who meet respiratory criteria and have intact cough/gag reflex

19.3.5 Deep Vein Thrombosis Prophylaxis

A level III recommendation is made for mechanical prophylaxis with graduated compression stockings or intermittent pneumatic compression devices until patients are ambulatory. A level III recommendation is made for chemical prophylaxis with low-molecular-weight or unfractionated heparin, in conjunction with mechanical prophylaxis.

A review of the National Trauma Databank demonstrated that patients with TBI are at increased risk of venous thromboembolic events, including deep vein thrombosis (DVT) and pulmonary embolism (PE).[24] Management of PEs in critically ill patients may be complicated, particularly in the neurosurgical and neurotrauma population, where the use of anticoagulation carries high risk of intracranial hemorrhage

Mechanical prophylaxis has been demonstrated to reduce the risk of symptomatic venous thromboembolism (VTE) as well as asymptomatic VTE found on routine screening (i.e., lower extremity Doppler ultrasounds).[25,26] Prophylaxis with low-molecular-weight or unfractionated heparin has been demonstrated to reduce the risk of VTE in TBI patients, but two studies demonstrated a 3% risk of new or evolving intracranial hemorrhage in TBI patients.[27,28]

19.3.6 Indications for Intracranial Pressure Monitoring

A level II recommendation is ICP monitoring for patients with a GCS score of 3 to 8 and a computed tomography (CT) scan with an acute intracranial abnormality. A level III recommendation is ICP monitoring in patients with a normal head CT who have any two of the following: age > 40, systolic blood pressure < 90 mm Hg, or unilateral or bilateral posturing.

Normal ICP is considered to be 0 to 10 mm Hg, with most citing 20 mm Hg as the upper limit of normal. Either systemic hypotension or intracranial hypertension may have a deleterious effect on TBI patients by reducing the CPP, which is defined as the difference between the mean arterial pressure and ICP. Ongoing monitoring allows the clinician to evaluate and maintain adequate cerebral perfusion by providing greater control over ICP management.

In TBI patients with a GCS score of less than 8, intracranial hypertension developed in 53 to 63% of patients with an abnormal CT as compared with 13% in those with a normal CT.[29]

An ICP monitor's most important role may be for evaluating and guiding intervention for management of elevated ICPs. Indications for the use and efficacy of treatment modalities, including hyperventilation, mannitol, sedation, and paralysis, are often guided by the values provided by the ICP monitor. In addition, multiple studies have ascertained that ICP values can determine outcome, with lower ICPs often equating with better outcomes.

One important concern in TBI patients is to monitor for changes in ICP during the immediate postinjury period, as patients' injuries may evolve, and patients with normal admission imaging may develop radiographically and clinically significant intracranial findings. In one study, 15% of TBI patients with normal admission head CT scans developed intracranial hemorrhage.[30]

Multiple studies appear to show a reduction in mortality and morbidity when an ICP monitor is used, both for ICP monitoring and for cerebrospinal fluid (CSF) drainage.[31,32]

The BTF guidelines point out the difficulty in creating an ethical construct for a randomized controlled study regarding the benefit of ICP monitoring with and without treatment of increased ICP in TBI patients, but the guidelines suggest that further research regarding the subset of patients with evolving or new intracranial pathology in the postinjury period may assist in selecting patients who will benefit most from ICP monitoring and treatment.

The BEST TRIP trial performed a randomized controlled study of two investigative protocols, one utilizing ICP monitors and one using current standard of care clinical observation and CT imaging in multiple hospitals in Latin America. The results of the study showed no significant differences in mortality or long-term functional outcome between the two groups.[33] Although the study has remained controversial,[34] the authors have addressed criticisms[35] and released a consensus analysis emphasizing the study's goals and advocating for further randomized controlled trial (RCT) of ICP monitoring, particularly in North American/European trauma centers where clinical observation and serial imaging remains the standard of care.[36]

19.3.7 Intracranial Pressure Monitoring Technology

No formal recommendations are made by the BTF guidelines. The ventricular catheter, with its ability to transduce ICPs and drain CSF, is considered the most effective means for monitoring a patient's ICPs. Transducing ICPs with a parenchymal monitor initially may be as accurate as a ventricular catheter but is prone to measurement drift. In addition, parenchymal monitors cannot be re-zeroed after placement, and if ongoing ICP monitoring is necessary, the monitor must be replaced.

There are data that appear to show a discrepancy between values read on a subdural or parenchymal monitor and true ventricular pressures.[37] Considering that most studies regarding ICP monitoring are based on ventricular pressures, these monitors have the potential to inadvertently cause mismanagement of a patient's ICPs.

Complications related to ICP monitors are uncommon and rarely cause long-term sequelae. The overall incidence of hematomas secondary to monitor placement was 1.4%,[29,38] with 0.5% requiring surgical intervention.[29] Rates of malfunction or obstruction vary greatly from 6.3% for ventricular catheters to as high as 40% in some studies for parenchymal monitors.[39,40]

19.3.8 Intracranial Pressure Treatment Threshold

The level II recommendation is that intervention for elevated ICPs should begin after a threshold of 20 mm Hg. The largest study, using prospective nonrandomized data, found that 20 mm Hg was the most predictive ICP value for outcome,[14] although additional studies show 20 versus 25 mm Hg to have no significant difference in outcomes.[41] The level III recommendation is that, as patients may herniated at ICP < 20 mm Hg, and others may tolerate ICPs > 20 mm Hg without clinical changes, data from ICP monitoring be used in conjunction with clinical examination and neuroimaging findings to determine the best course of management.

19.3.9 Cerebral Perfusion Thresholds

Cerebral perfusion pressure is the difference between the mean arterial pressure and ICP. Intravascular depletion with hypotension, loss of autoregulation, and posttraumatic vasospasm, as well as elevated ICP can significantly reduce CPP and lead to cerebral ischemia. Maintaining CPP > 60 mm Hg may significantly reduce the morbidity and mortality in TBI patients. In an early study, McGraw found an increase in mortality of 20% for each 10 mm Hg that the CPP was lowered; the difference is stark, with a mortality of 35 to 40% for patients with a CPP > 80 mm Hg and 95% when below 60 mm Hg for more than one third of their admission.[41] Of note, although this study establishes maintaining CPP as a key component of TBI management, it did not analyze CPP management independent of ICP monitoring and targeted therapy. There are level III recommendations to maintain CPP > 50 mm Hg in TBI patients.

Equally as detrimental as a low CPP is aggressively maintaining the CPP > 70 mm Hg, which is associated with the development of acute respiratory distress syndrome.[42,43] There is a level II recommendation to avoid aggressively maintaining the CPP > 70 mm Hg.

19.3.10 Brain Oxygenation Monitoring and Thresholds

This is a new category of recommendations in the updated BTF guidelines. There is level III recommendations to intervene if jugular venous saturation (SJO_2) < 50% or brain tissue oxygen tension ($PBrO_2$) < 15%.

Oxygenation of brain parenchymal is dependent on cerebral blood flow and oxygenation of hemoglobin in the blood. The importance of avoiding hypoxemia is more thoroughly addressed in the guidelines for prehospital airway management. Immediately following TBI, CBF appears to be significantly below normal, predisposing patients to cerebral ischemia. Unlike CPP or ICP, no consensus regarding a numerical value above which CBF should be maintained has been established.

SJO_2 is used as a proxy for brain parenchymal oxygen extraction, and high saturation has been correlated with poor outcome.[43] Conversely, extremely low SJO_2 is also correlated with poor patient outcome.[44,45]

Decreased $PBrO_2$ has been demonstrated to directly correlate with patient mortality, with one study showing an increased risk of mortality proportionate to the amount of time the $PBrO_2$ < 15 mm Hg.[46] Another study demonstrated a 50% mortality risk in patients with $PBrO_2$ < 15 mm Hg for longer than 4 hours.[47]

19.3.11 Anesthetics, Analgesics, Sedation

It is a level II recommendation that barbiturates be used for management of ICP refractory to all other available medical and surgical interventions. It is recommended that prophylactic barbiturates for burst suppression be avoided. Since 1979, several studies have documented increases in survival because barbiturate-induced coma was able to lower otherwise intractable elevations in ICP. In one study, 19 of the 25 patients treated with barbiturates had ICPs reduced, with 50% having a good recovery, whereas 83% of those who did not respond died.[48] A randomized trial by Eisenberg et al found that the barbiturate-treated group had at least twice the likelihood of their ICP being lowered. Ninety-two percent of those who responded were alive at 1 month compared with 17% for those who did not. Ninety percent of those whose ICP did not respond were dead or vegetative at 6 months compared with 36% for those who did. A randomized controlled trial found no difference in outcome between one group treated prophylactically and the other without and noted that the barbiturate group was nearly 8 times more likely to develop hypotension,[49] supporting the recommendation that barbiturates be used only to manage refractory ICP, rather than as prophylaxis in TBI patients. The Cochrane review determined that hypotension occurred in nearly 25% of patients treated with barbiturates, which led to decreases in the CPP that might offset any benefit seen in ICP reduction.[50]

Other sedatives and analgesics have been studied for the management of ICP. One study compared propofol and morphine as means of controlling ICP in TBI patients and found no significant difference in mortality or outcome as determined by GCS score.[51] However, long-term use of propofol, particularly in high doses, carries the risk of propofol infusion syndrome. There is a level III recommendation that propofol be used for ICP management, with the note that it is not associated with reduction in mortality and may carry significant morbidity at high doses.

19.3.12 Nutrition

The level III recommendation is that full nutritional replacement should begin by the seventh day after injury. Using either enteral or parenteral means, 140% of patients' metabolic needs should be replaced if they are not paralyzed, and 100% if they are. Metabolic needs increase an average of 60% in head injury patients without paralytics, and 20 to 30% in those with paralytics, indicating that increased muscle tone accounts for much of the increase in caloric needs. The caloric needs for a 25-year-old male, at 70 kg, is considered to be 1,700 kcal for 24 hours, which would make needs after injury approximately 2,400 kcal. Without nutrition, head injury patients lose approximately 15% of body weight per week, primarily in the form of nitrogen (protein). Mortality increases after loss of 30% body weight. Recommendations include that 15% of the calories replaced should be provided as protein. One study found an increase in mortality for patients with undernourishment for 2 weeks after injury.[52]

Enteral feeds are preferred over the parenteral route for several reasons, including a reduced likelihood of hyperglycemia and infection, and cost-effectiveness. Hyperglycemia is associated with exacerbation of hypoxic ischemic brain injury and may lead to worse outcomes overall.[53,54] More insulin is required to maintain a normal blood glucose level with parenteral feedings as compared with enteral, making another compelling argument for the early use of enteral feedings in TBI patients.[55] A single small study suggested that zinc supplementation may improve GCS motor score outcomes in TBI patients,[56] but further data are needed before recommendations regarding specific micronutrient supplementation can be made.

19.3.13 The Role of Antiseizure Prophylaxis Following Head Injury

Posttraumatic seizures (PTS) are categorized as early or late, with the dividing point being less than or more than 7 days post injury, respectively. PTS occur in up to 42% of patients up to 36 months after a head injury. Seizures may precipitate elevations in ICP, hemodynamic instability, and reductions in cerebral oxygenation, causing further decline in the clinical status of TBI patients.

There is a level II recommendation that antiepileptics should be used for early seizure prophylaxis, with the caveat that early PTS are not associated with worse outcome. There is also a level II recommendation that phenytoin or valproate not be used for prevention of late PTS.

Given the potential side effects, ranging from behavioral changes to Stevens–Johnson syndrome, antiepileptics should be limited to the patients most at risk for developing PTS. Studies have found certain intracranial lesions, such as intracerebral as well as extra-axial hematomas, depressed skull fractures, and low GCS score (< 10) predispose patients to developing seizures.[57,58] These patients, then, are most likely to benefit from prophylactic antiepileptics.

Phenytoin was one of the first medications found to be beneficial in reducing the development of PTS. In the largest randomized prospective trial, 404 patients were analyzed and phenytoin reduced early seizures but was of no benefit in reducing late seizures.[59] Notably, no difference in survival between the two treatment groups was seen.

A prospective study compared the efficacy of phenytoin and valproate in preventing seizures.[60] The medications appeared to be equally effective in reducing early seizures, although valproate was associated with a higher mortality rate.

19.3.14 Hyperventilation

Two important findings speak to the difficulty in determining when hyperventilation for TBI patients should be implemented: research indicating 40% of TBI patients develop brain swelling and consequently elevated ICP,[61] and studies showing that CBF is one half of normal 1 day after injury.[62] Although it may stem the devastating effects of uncontrolled ICP, by inducing cerebral vasoconstriction, hyperventilation may inadvertently exacerbate cerebral ischemia.

A level II recommendation is to avoid prophylactic hyperventilation ($PaCO_2$ < 25 mm Hg). It is a level III recommendation that prophylactic hyperventilation be particularly avoided, during the first 24 hours after injury, as CBF is often already compromised in this time period. An additional level III recommendation is that hyperventilation may be used as a temporizing measure in cases of refractory ICP crises. If used, monitoring for cerebral ischemia, utilizing brain tissue oxygen monitoring, for example, should be considered.

CBF drops precipitously following injury, falling as low as 20 mL/100 g/min in the hours immediately afterward. The relationship between decreased CBF and brain oxygenation, measured by SJO_2 or $PBrO_2$, is not entirely clear.[63,64,65] One randomized prospective trial demonstrated that patients undergoing hyperventilation therapy had lower GCS motor outcomes at multiple follow-up points, although the difference was not sustained in long-term follow-up.[66]

19.3.15 The Role of Steroids

There is a level I recommendation to avoid the use of steroids in the management of TBI patients, as it provides no clear benefit in ICP management and may increase the risk of mortality. Although steroids were successfully used to reduce cerebral edema in patients with brain tumors,[67] multiple studies since the 1970s have shown that steroids provide no clear improvement in outcomes, ICP management, or mortality.[68,69]

A meta-analysis completed in 1997 concluded that there was no improvement in outcome with steroid use in TBI patients.[70] Furthermore, the CRASH trial completed in 2004 found a higher mortality in head injury patients treated with methylprednisolone as compared with the group treated with placebo.[71]

Table 19.2

Surgical lesion	Guidelines
Acute epidural hematoma	Serial head CT and clinical examination: • EDH < 30 cm³, clot thickness < 15 mm, midline shift < 5 mm, GCS score > 8, and without focal neurologic deficit Emergent surgical evacuation: • All EDH > 30 cm³, GCS score < 9 with anisocoria
Acute subdural hematoma	ICP monitoring: • GCS score < 9 Emergent surgical evacuation: • SDH of > 10 mm thickness, or with > 5 mm MLS • GCS score < 9, and a SDH of < 10 mm thickness and < 5 mm MLS, if GCS score decreased by > 2, if ICP > 20 mm Hg, or if anisocoric
Traumatic parenchymal lesions	Close observation: • Neurologically stable without midline shift, mass effect, elevated ICP Emergent surgical intervention: • Neurologic deficit/decline, mass effect, or intractable ICP • GCS score 6–8 with frontal or temporal IPH > 20 cm³ and either > 5 mm MLS or cistern compression on head CT • IPH > 50 cm³
Posterior fossa mass lesion	Observation: • Patients without mass effect or neurologic deficit Emergent operative intervention: • Patients with mass effect or neurologic deficit
Depressed skull fractures	Observation: • < 1 cm depression, no dural tear, large hematoma, frontal sinus involvement, pneumocephalus, or wound infection/contamination Operative intervention: • Open fractures displaced greater than the thickness of the skull should undergo surgery

Abbreviations: CT, computed tomography; GCS, Glasgow Coma Scale; ICP, intracranial pressure; IPH, intraparenchymal hemorrhage; MLS, midline shift; SDH, acute subdural hematoma.

19.4 Surgical Management of Traumatic Lesions

▶ Table 19.2 summarizes the guidelines for surgical management of traumatic brain injuries.

19.4.1 Surgical Management of Acute Epidural Hematomas

Surgical evacuation of an acute epidural hematoma (EDH) is dependent on the patient's neurologic status and size of the hematoma. The recommendations are to surgically evacuate all EDHs > 30 cm³, regardless of neurologic status. Conservative management with serial head CT scans and clinical examination may be considered for patients who meet all of the following criteria: EDH < 30 cm³, clot thickness < 15 mm, midline shift < 5 mm, GCS score > 8, and without focal neurologic deficit. Regarding surgical timing, the guidelines specifically emphasize that patients with a GCS score < 9 and anisocoria on examination should undergo surgical evacuation urgently.

EDHs are found in up to 4% of TBI patients[65,66] and 9% of patients who present in a coma.[72,73] Classically, the source of

bleeding is considered to be the middle meningeal artery, but in a recent study this was identified as the source in only 36% of adults and 18% of children.[74] Other sources include the venous sinuses and diploic veins. The mechanism of injury associated with EDHs predisposes patients to extracranial injuries and has been noted in several studies. Although the data are inconsistent regarding their impact on outcome, skull fractures have been reported in up to 95% of patients with EDHs.

Patients with an EDH may present with a spectrum of findings, ranging from no deficits to comatose. A little under half (47%) present with the classic "lucid interval," whereas up to 27% present neurologically intact.[75,76]

Mortality is approximately 10% in adults and 5% in the pediatric population. Multiple factors, including the patient's age and GCS score, affect the outcome for patients with an EDH. Several studies have found that GCS score at presentation is the single most important factor in determining a patient's outcome. Gennarelli et al showed that patients with EDHs and a presenting GCS score of 6 to 8 had a mortality of 9% compared with 36% when the GCS score was 3 to 5.[77]

Although nonoperative management in patients with a GCS score greater than 12 has been documented, for those patients who require operative management, expedited surgery is imperative.[78]

Although studies have shown that the interval from onset of neurologic symptoms to operative evacuation is important in overall outcome,[77,78,79] there are not sufficient data available to comment on the relative effectiveness of emergent nonneurosurgical evacuation at the initial hospital, versus neurosurgical evacuation after transfer to a more specialized center.

19.4.2 Surgical Management of Acute Subdural Hematomas

It is recommended that all patients with acute subdural hematomas (SDHs) of > 10 mm thickness, or with > 5 mm midline shift (MLS) on head CT, undergo operative evacuation, independent of the patients' GCS score. In patients with a GCS score < 9, ICP monitoring is recommended. In patients with GCS score < 9, and a SDH of < 10 mm thickness and < 5 mm MLS, operative evacuation is recommended in the following circumstances: if the GCS score decreased by 2 or more points from the time of injury to arrival, if ICP > 20 mm Hg, or if anisocoria or fixed pupils are present on arrival.

In patients with a GCS score < 9 undergoing operative SDH evacuation, the guidelines recommend evacuation with craniotomy and duraplasty; use of a craniectomy is left to clinician discretion. No recommendations regarding SDH removal technique are made for those patients with a GCS score > 9 requiring operative intervention.

Acute SDHs occur in up to 29% of TBI patients, with the majority in males aged 31 to 47. The cause is more likely motor vehicle accidents in younger patients and falls in patients over age 65. The mortality from SDHs requiring surgery, regardless of GCS score at presentation, is between 40 and 60%.[80,81]

Several studies have documented a worsening prognosis with increasing age, with most studies finding an increased likelihood of poor outcome in patients over age 65.[82,83] As might be expected, increasing age with lower GCS scores correlated with worsening outcomes as well. Hatashita et al documented a 75% mortality rate in patients older than 65 who initially presented with a GCS score of 4 to 6 and underwent surgery; the rate was 34% in patients aged 19 to 40.[83]

Most studies support an improved outcome for patients who undergo early evacuation of acute SDHs. A large study by Haselsberger et al noted a mortality of 80% in comatose patients who underwent surgery more than 2 hours after the onset of clinical decline compared with a mortality rate of 47% for those operated on within 2 hours.[76] Likewise, Seelig et al documented 90% mortality for those undergoing surgery more than 4 hours after an injury compared with 30% for those operated on within 4 hours.[84]

Few studies evaluated the impact of differing surgical techniques such as burr hole trephination and craniotomy on outcome. For patients with GCS scores of 4 to 6, burr hole trephination was associated with a much higher rate of mortality as compared with those undergoing craniotomy in a study by Hatashita et al.[83]

For those patients who do require surgery, 60% or more have associated intracranial and extracranial lesions, and these are more commonly seen in patients presenting with a GCS score less than 10. For this reason, the guidelines considered salvageability when creating recommendations, recognizing that in some multisystem trauma patients, SDH evacuation may not affect the morbidity and mortality related to extensive non-neurologic injury.

19.4.3 Surgical Management of Traumatic Parenchymal Lesions

It is recommended that all patients with neurologic deficit/decline, mass effect on head CT, or intractable ICP undergo operative intervention. Surgical management is also recommended for patients with a GCS score of 6 to 8 with frontal or temporal intraparenchymal hemorrhage (IPH) > 20 cm^3 and either > 5 mm MLS or cistern compression on head CT, or any patient with an IPH > 50 cm^3. Conservative management with serial imaging and clinical examinations is recommended for patients with no neurologic deficits, midline shift, or ICP crises.

For patients undergoing surgical treatment, the recommendation is craniotomy and evacuation of mass lesion. Decompressive craniectomies remain options for patients with intractable ICP and diffuse intracranial injury. Specifically, bifrontal craniectomies are offered as an option within 48 hours of injury for patients with diffuse parenchymal injury.

Traumatic parenchymal lesions, broadly defined, occur in a little over one third of all TBI patients and represent approximately one fifth of head injury patients requiring surgical intervention. Radiographic findings, clinical status and course, and associated injuries, in addition to the evaluation of the parenchymal lesion, should be taken into account when deciding between surgical and medical management.

Parenchymal lesions may be focal or diffuse and include hematomas, contusions, and infarcts and diffuse cerebral edema. Regardless of type, parenchymal injuries can result in mass effect, midline shift, elevated ICPs, and herniation.

Studies have noted a negative correlation between nonoperative management and multiple findings. These include hypoxia, effacement of the cisterns, presence of subarachnoid hemorrhage (SAH), and intracranial hypertension. Bullock et al, in an attempt to determine the need for surgery, evaluated patients with ICP monitoring.[80,85] Although unable to predict clinical decline over a longer time frame, the study did find a positive correlation between peak ICP and the need for surgical evacuation.

The recommendation for considering clinical examination findings in addition to neuroimaging in determining the role of surgery stems in part from the static nature of imaging modalities and the fluid nature of intraparenchymal lesions. Yamaki et al showed that only 80% of intraparenchymal bleeds reached their maximal volume within 12 hours of the initial injury.[86] Conventionally, delayed traumatic intracerebral hematoma (DTICH) occurs in portions of initially unremarkable brain in patients with abnormal CT scans and has been correlated with poor outcome.[86,87]

19.4.4 Surgical Management of Posterior Fossa Mass Lesions

Although traumatic injuries of the posterior fossa (PF) make up a limited number of all head injuries (< 3%), the small volume

Table 19.3 Summary of general pediatric trauma management guidelines

Treatment	Guidelines
Indications for intracranial pressure monitoring	Level I, Level II—Insufficient data Level III—ICP monitoring may be considered in infants and children with TBI
Intracranial pressure treatment threshold	Level I, Level II—Insufficient data Level III—Treatment may be considered for ICP > 20 mm Hg
Cerebral perfusion pressure thresholds	Level I, Level II—Insufficient data Level III—Consider a minimum CPP 40 mm Hg, with a range of 40–50 mm Hg; infants may be at the low end, with older children at the higher end
Neuromonitoring	Level I, Level II—Insufficient data Level III—If brain oxygenation is monitored, $PBrO_2$ > 10 mm Hg may be considered
Neuroimaging	Level I, Level II—Insufficient data Level III—Routine head CT < 24 h after initial and follow-up imaging may not be necessary in the absence of clinical deterioration or ICP crises
Hyperosmolar therapy	Level I—Insufficient data Level II—Hypertonic saline should be considered for elevated ICP; dosing is 6.5–10 mL/kg Options—Hypertonic saline (3% at 0.1–1.0 mL/kg bw/h) can be effective in managing elevated ICP, using the minimum dose for ICP < 20 mm Hg. Maintain serum osmolarity < 360 mOsm/L
Temperature control	Level I—Insufficient data Level II—Moderate hypothermia (32–33°C) should be avoided if the course of treatment will be < 24 h. In patients within 8 h of injury, moderate hypothermia may be considered for a duration of treatment up to 48 h. Avoid rewarming faster than 0.5°C/h. Level III—Early moderate hypothermia for 48 h duration may be considered.
CSF drainage	Level I, Level II—Insufficient data Level III—CSF drainage through a ventriculostomy may be considered. A lumbar drain may be used in patients with a functional ventriculostomy and refractory ICP
Barbiturates	Level I, Level II—Insufficient data Level III—High-dose barbiturates may be used for refractory ICP. Should be accompanied by arterial blood pressure monitoring and maintenance of adequate CPP
Decompressive craniectomy	Level I, Level II—Insufficient data Level III—Decompressive craniectomy with duraplasty may be considered for refractory intracranial hypertension during early treatment course
Hyperventilation	Level I, Level II—Insufficient data Level III—Avoid prophylactic hyperventilation ($PaCO_2$ < 30 mm Hg) in first 48 h. If hyperventilation used to treat ICP, consider neuromonitoring
Corticosteroids	Level I—Insufficient data Level II—Corticosteroid use not recommended
Analgesics, sedatives, neuromuscular blockade	Level I, Level II—Insufficient data Level III—Etomidate may be considered; carries risk of adrenal suppression. Thiopental may be considered
Glucose and nutrition	Level I—Insufficient data Level II—No evidence for immune-modulating diet Level III—Without outcome data, the approach to glycemic control is left to clinician discretion
Antiseizure prophylaxis	Level I, Level II—Insufficient data Level III—Phenytoin may be considered for early seizure prophylaxis

Abbreviations: bw, body weight; CPP, cerebral perfusion pressure; CSF, cerebrospinal fluid; ICP, intracranial pressure; $PaCO_2$, partial arterial pressure of carbon dioxide; $PBrO_2$, brain tissue oxygen tension; TBI, traumatic brain injury.

of the PF predisposes the patient to the rapid development of hydrocephalus, mass effect, and neurologic decline.

It is recommended that patients with mass effect (effacement or obliteration of the fourth ventricle/cisterns, signs of hydrocephalus) or focal neurologic deficit undergo operative intervention. In patients without mass effect or neurologic deficit, observation is recommended. Given the propensity for these patients to rapidly deteriorate, urgent or emergent surgery is recommended for all operative candidates. Suboccipital craniectomy is the recommended surgical technique. Although conservative management is possible, it must be used in a carefully selected patient population to avoid clinical decline and poor overall outcomes.[88]

19.4.5 Surgical Management of Depressed Skull Fractures

It is recommended that patients with compound depressed skull fractures undergo operative treatment if the fracture is depressed greater than the thickness of the calvarium. In patients managed operatively, expeditious surgical intervention is recommended to minimize the risk of infection.

Conservative management is recommended in patients with compound depressed skull fractures with less than 1 cm depression, no evidence of dural tear, large hematoma, frontal sinus involvement, pneumocephalus, wound infection, or gross contamination. It is recommended that both operative and non-operative management include antibiotics.

The presence of depressed skull fractures, found in approximately 6% of TBI cases, exposes the patient to multiple complications. Open skull fractures account for the vast majority of these (up to 90%). The danger of open skull fractures is not only infection (found in up to 10.6% of patients) but also the development of late-onset epilepsy (in up to 15%) and increased neurologic morbidity (11% of patients) and mortality (19%).[89,90,91]

19.5 General Pediatric Trauma Management Guidelines

The pediatric neurotrauma guidelines are similar to those for adults with TBI, although the data available in the pediatric population are frequently insufficient to provide level I or level II recommendations. Therefore, the majority of pediatric TBI management guidelines are level III recommendations. The guidelines are summarized in ▶Table 19.3; here we discuss those guidelines that differ from the adult counterparts described in detail previously.

19.5.1 Indications for Intracranial Pressure Monitoring

There is a high incidence of elevated ICP in pediatric TBI patients,[92,93,94,95] with multiple studies demonstrating an association between ICP and overall outcome.[96] Furthermore, evidence shows that management of elevated ICP leads to improved outcome.[97,98]

Although GCS scores and the neurologic examination remain the standards for clinical evaluation of patients with TBI, these are less sensitive in infants and young children. Imaging correlates of intracranial hypertension, such as effacement of the basal cisterns of CT, can be misleading in children. The clinical evaluation of infants with TBI can be difficult, and a negative initial head CT does not exclude the possibility of increased ICP. The presence of open fontanels and sutures in an infant with severe TBI does not preclude the development of intracranial hypertension or negate the utility of ICP monitoring.

19.5.2 Cerebral Perfusion Pressure Thresholds

Similar to the adult guidelines, the pediatric guidelines specify a range of acceptable CPP, supported by data that consistent values less than 40 mm Hg are associated with increased mortality, independent of age.[99,100] No study demonstrates that active maintenance of CPP above any target threshold in pediatric TBI is responsible for improved mortality or morbidity.

19.5.3 Neuroimaging

There is no correlate in the adult TBI guidelines. The pediatric recommendations are based on a single retrospective study of 40 children,[101] which concluded that imaging obtained to evaluate clinical examination changes or ICP crises was more likely to provide new information requiring intervention (i.e., surgical treatment).

19.5.4 Cerebrospinal Fluid Drainage

The recommendations are based on four studies, two demonstrating the use of external ventricular drains in pediatric TBI patients, and two describing the use of lumbar drains to treat continued ICP crises in patients with functional ventriculostomies.[98,102,103,106] In children with severe TBI and intracranial hypertension, ventricular CSF drainage is a commonly employed therapeutic modality in conjunction with ICP monitoring. The role of CSF drainage is to reduce intracranial fluid volume and thereby lower ICP. With the use of a ventriculostomy as a common means of measuring the ICP of patients with TBI, the potential therapeutic benefits of CSF drainage became of interest. However, CSF drainage is not limited to the ventricular route. Controlled lumbar drainage has resulted in improved outcomes in the pediatric population with severe TBI and intracranial hypertension.[102,103]

In summary, ventricular CSF drainage in severe pediatric TBI is supported as a treatment option in the setting of refractory intracranial hypertension, and the addition of lumbar drainage in patients showing open cisterns on imaging and without major mass lesions or shift is also supported.

19.5.5 Hyperosmolar Therapy

Whereas the adult guidelines make recommendations regarding the use of mannitol, the pediatric guidelines have recommendations only for the use of hypertonic saline in the management of ICP. Although the guideline authors comment that mannitol is commonly used in pediatric TBI, there were no studies meeting inclusion criteria upon which to base any recommendations

Like mannitol, hypertonic saline provides osmolar gradient effects that reduce ICP. Hypertonic saline also exhibits several theoretical beneficial effects, including restoration of normal cellar resting membrane potential and cell volume,[104] stimulation of atrial natriuretic peptide release,[105] inhibition of inflammation, and enhancement of cardiac output. Possible side effects of hypertonic saline include a rebound in ICP, central pontine myelinolysis, and SAH. Effective doses as a continuous infusion of 3% saline range between 0.1 and 1 mL/kg of body weight per hour, administered on a sliding scale. The minimum dose needed to maintain ICP < 20 mm Hg should be used, and serum osmolarity should be kept at < 360 mOsm/L.

19.5.6 Temperature Control

If hypothermia is used prophylactically, it is recommended that it be done within 8 hours of arrival, with intervention lasting for up to 48 hours. Prophylactic hypothermia in the early period with treatment duration less than 24 hours should be avoided.

19.5.7 Barbituates

The use of barbiturates to treat elevated ICP in children with severe head injury has been reported since the 1970s[48] however, only two studies in pediatric populations were used to formulate the guidelines. Both studies correlated with adult studies showing that barbiturates were effective at reducing ICP, and that this was associated with improved overall outcome.[107,108]

Small studies of high-dose barbiturate therapy suggest that barbiturates are effective in lowering ICP in selected cases of refractory intracranial hypertension in children with severe TBI. However, use of barbiturates is associated with myocardial depression, risk of hypotension, and need for blood pressure support with intravascular fluids and inotropic agents. Therefore, use should be limited to critical care providers utilizing appropriate systemic monitoring to avoid and rapidly treat hemodynamic instability.

19.5.8 Analgesics, Sedatives, and Neuromuscular Blockade

Despite the common use of sedatives, analgesics, and neuromuscular blocking agents in pediatric patients with severe TBI both for emergency intubation and for management, including control of ICP, there has been little formal clinical investigation performed regarding these practices. In the pediatric population, etomidate[109] and thiopental[110] were shown to reduce ICP. Although propofol is recommended in the adult population, the Food and Drug Administration (FDA) does not recommend propofol infusions in pediatric patients.

19.5.9 The Role of Antiseizure Prophylaxis Following Severe Traumatic Brain Injury

Late PTS development has been found to occur in 7 to 12% of children following TBI compared with 9 to 13% of adults,[111,112] although no correlation between age, as in early PTS development, and late seizure development has been made. In attempting to correlate the presence of skull fractures and the development of late seizures, one study noted a significant difference based on age: 12% of children under the age of 5, 20% of children aged 5 to 16, and 9% of patients over 16 developing late PTS.[91] Another study noted that 12% of TBI patients under the age of 3 who developed early PTS also developed late PTS.[113] Young et al's randomized study found, although statistically insignificant, a slightly higher rate of late PTS development in the treatment group as compared with the placebo group (12% vs. 6%).[112] The study was marred by poor compliance.

Lewis et al's study, reviewing prophylactic treatment for early PTS development, found 53% of children who were not given medication developed seizures as compared with 15% of those who were treated.[114]

19.5.10 Surgical Treatment of Pediatric Intracranial Hypertension

As described in the surgical treatment guidelines, decompressive craniectomy with duraplasty is an option for addressing focal or diffuse intracranial injury leading to elevated ICP. Polin et al completed a case–control study where 35 TBI patients, both adult and pediatric, were treated for uncontrolled intracranial hypertension with bifrontal decompressive craniectomies.[115] In an evaluation of children with TBI secondary to abuse, Cho et al found that in patients with ICPs greater than 30 mm Hg, there was a significant improvement in outcome for those who received surgery as well as medical management compared with those treated with medical management only.[116] In the majority of cases, surgery was completed within 1 day of the injury.

References

[1] Mullins RJ, Veum-Stone J, Hedges JR, et al. Influence of a statewide trauma system on location of hospitalization and outcome of injured patients. J Trauma. 1996; 40(4):536–545, discussion 545–546

[2] Sampalis JS, Lavoie A, Boukas S, et al. Trauma center designation: initial impact on trauma-related mortality. J Trauma. 1995; 39(2):232–237, discussion 237–239

[3] Potoka DA, Schall LC, Gardner MJ, Stafford PW, Peitzman AB, Ford HR. Impact of pediatric trauma centers on mortality in a statewide system. J Trauma. 2000; 49(2):237–245

[4] Johnson DL, Krishnamurthy S. Send severely head-injured children to a pediatric trauma center. Pediatr Neurosurg. 1996; 25(6):309–314

[5] Chesnut RM, Marshall LF, Klauber MR, et al. The role of secondary brain injury in determining outcome from severe head injury. J Trauma. 1993; 34(2):216–222

[6] Cooke RS, McNicholl BP, Byrnes DP. Early management of severe head injury in Northern Ireland. Injury. 1995; 26(6):395–397

[7] Gausche M, Lewis RJ, Stratton SJ, et al. Effect of out-of-hospital pediatric endotracheal intubation on survival and neurological outcome: a controlled clinical trial. JAMA. 2000; 283(6):783–790

[8] Nakayama DK, Gardner MJ, Rowe MI. Emergency endotracheal intubation in pediatric trauma. Ann Surg. 1990; 211(2):218–223

[9] Pigula FA, Wald SL, Shackford SR, Vane DW. The effect of hypotension and hypoxia on children with severe head injuries. J Pediatr Surg. 1993; 28(3):310–314, discussion 315–316

[10] Armstrong PF. Initial management of the multiply injured child: the ABC's. Instr Course Lect. 1992; 41:347–350

[11] Manley G, Knudson MM, Morabito D, Damron S, Erickson V, Pitts L. Hypotension, hypoxia, and head injury: frequency, duration, and consequences. Arch Surg. 2001; 136(10):1118–1123

[12] Stocchetti N, Furlan A, Volta F. Hypoxemia and arterial hypotension at the accident scene in head injury. J Trauma. 1996; 40(5):764–767

[13] Silverston P. Pulse oximetry at the roadside: a study of pulse oximetry in immediate care. BMJ. 1989; 298(6675):711–713

[14] Marmarou A, Anderson, et al. et al. Impact of ICP instability and hypotension on outcome in patients with severe head trauma. J Neurosurg. 1991; 75(1, Suppl):S59–S66

[15] Scalea TM, Maltz S, Yelon J, Trooskin SZ, Duncan AO, Sclafani SJ. Resuscitation of multiple trauma and head injury: role of crystalloid fluids and inotropes. Crit Care Med. 1994; 22(10):1610–1615

[16] Härtl R, Ghajar J, Hochleuthner H, Mauritz W. Hypertonic/hyperoncotic saline reliably reduces ICP in severely head-injured patients with intracranial hypertension. Acta Neurochir Suppl (Wien). 1997; 70:126–129

[17] Wade CE, Grady JJ, Kramer GC, Younes RN, Gehlsen K, Holcroft JW. Individual patient cohort analysis of the efficacy of hypertonic saline/

dextran in patients with traumatic brain injury and hypotension. J Trauma. 1997; 42(5, Suppl):S61–S65

[18] Aibiki M, Maekawa S, Yokono S. Moderate hypothermia improves imbalances of thromboxane A2 and prostaglandin I2 production after traumatic brain injury in humans. Crit Care Med. 2000; 28(12):3902–3906

[19] Clifton GL, Allen S, Barrodale P, et al. A phase II study of moderate hypothermia in severe brain injury. J Neurotrauma. 1993; 10(3):263–271, discussion 273

[20] Jiang J, Yu M, Zhu C. Effect of long-term mild hypothermia therapy in patients with severe traumatic brain injury: 1-year follow-up review of 87 cases. J Neurosurg. 2000; 93(4):546–549

[21] Marion DW, Penrod LE, Kelsey SF, et al. Treatment of traumatic brain injury with moderate hypothermia. N Engl J Med. 1997; 336(8):540–546

[22] Qiu WS, Liu WG, Shen H, et al. Therapeutic effect of mild hypothermia on severe traumatic head injury. Chin J Traumatol. 2005; 8(1):27–32

[23] Zabramski JM, Whiting D, Darouiche RO, et al. Efficacy of antimicrobial-impregnated external ventricular drain catheters: a prospective, randomized, controlled trial. J Neurosurg. 2003; 98(4):725–730

[24] Knudson MM, Ikossi DG, Khaw L, Morabito D, Speetzen LS. Thromboembolism after trauma: an analysis of 1602 episodes from the American College of Surgeons National Trauma Data Bank. Ann Surg. 2004; 240(3):490–496, discussion 496–498

[25] Skillman JJ, Collins RE, Coe NP, et al. Prevention of deep vein thrombosis in neurosurgical patients: a controlled, randomized trial of external pneumatic compression boots. Surgery. 1978; 83(3):354–358

[26] Turpie AG, Hirsh J, Gent M, Julian D, Johnson J. Prevention of deep vein thrombosis in potential neurosurgical patients. A randomized trial comparing graduated compression stockings alone or graduated compression stockings plus intermittent pneumatic compression with control. Arch Intern Med. 1989; 149(3):679–681

[27] Kleindienst A, Harvey HB, Mater E, et al. Early antithrombotic prophylaxis with low molecular weight heparin in neurosurgery. Acta Neurochir (Wien). 2003; 145(12):1085–1090, discussion 1090–1091

[28] Gerlach R, Scheuer T, Beck J, Woszczyk A, Seifert V, Raabe A. Risk of postoperative hemorrhage after intracranial surgery after early nadroparin administration: results of a prospective study. Neurosurgery. 2003; 53(5):1028–1034, discussion 1034–1035

[29] Narayan RK, Kishore PR, Becker DP, et al. Intracranial pressure: to monitor or not to monitor? A review of our experience with severe head injury. J Neurosurg. 1982; 56(5):650–659

[30] Eisenberg HM, Gary HE, Jr, Aldrich EF, et al. Initial CT findings in 753 patients with severe head injury. A report from the NIH Traumatic Coma Data Bank. J Neurosurg. 1990; 73(5):688–698

[31] Cremer OL, van Dijk GW, van Wensen E, et al. Effect of intracranial pressure monitoring and targeted intensive care on functional outcome after severe head injury. Crit Care Med. 2005; 33(10):2207–2213

[32] Lane PL, Skoretz TG, Doig G, Girotti MJ. Intracranial pressure monitoring and outcomes after traumatic brain injury. Can J Surg. 2000; 43(6):442–448

[33] Chesnut RM, Temkin N, Carney N, et al; Global Neurotrauma Research Group. A trial of intracranial-pressure monitoring in traumatic brain injury. N Engl J Med. 2012; 367(26):2471–2481

[34] Sahuquillo J, Biestro A. Is intracranial pressure monitoring still required in the management of severe traumatic brain injury? Ethical and methodological considerations on conducting clinical research in poor and low-income countries. Surg Neurol Int. 2014; 5:86

[35] Chesnut RM, Temkin N, Dikmen S, et al. Ethical and methodological considerations on conducting clinical research in poor and low-income countries: viewpoint of the authors of the BEST TRIP ICP randomized trial in Latin America. Surg Neurol Int. 2015; 6:116

[36] Chesnut RM, Bleck TP, Citerio G, et al. A consensus-based interpretation of the Benchmark Evidence From South American Trials: Treatment of Intracranial Pressure Trial. J Neurotrauma. 2015; 32(22):1722–1724

[37] Chambers IR, Mendelow AD, Sinar EJ, Modha P. A clinical evaluation of the Camino subdural screw and ventricular monitoring kits. Neurosurgery. 1990; 26(3):421–423

[38] Holloway KL, Barnes T, Choi S, et al. Ventriculostomy infections: the effect of monitoring duration and catheter exchange in 584 patients. J Neurosurg. 1996; 85(3):419–424

[39] Gambardella G, Zaccone C, Cardia E, Tomasello F. Intracranial pressure monitoring in children: comparison of external ventricular device with the fiberoptic system. Childs Nerv Syst. 1993; 9(8):470–473

[40] Smith RW, Alksne JF. Infections complicating the use of external ventriculostomy. J Neurosurg. 1976; 44(5):567–570

[41] McGraw CP. A cerebral perfusion pressure greater than 80 mm Hg is more beneficial. In: Hoff JT, Betz AL, eds. Intracranial Pressure VII. Berlin: Springer-Verlag; 1989:839–841

[42] Contant CF, Valadka AB, Gopinath SP, Hannay HJ, Robertson CS. Adult respiratory distress syndrome: a complication of induced hypertension after severe head injury. J Neurosurg. 2001; 95(4):560–568

[43] Cormio M, Valadka AB, Robertson CS. Elevated jugular venous oxygen saturation after severe head injury. J Neurosurg. 1999; 90(1):9–15

[44] Robertson C. Desaturation episodes after severe head injury: influence on outcome. Acta Neurochir Suppl (Wien). 1993; 59:98–101

[45] Robertson CS, Gopinath SP, Goodman JC, Contant CF, Valadka AB, Narayan RK. SjvO2 monitoring in head-injured patients. J Neurotrauma. 1995; 12(5):891–896

[46] Valadka AB, Gopinath SP, Contant CF, Uzura M, Robertson CS. Relationship of brain tissue PO2 to outcome after severe head injury. Crit Care Med. 1998; 26(9):1576–1581

[47] van den Brink WA, van Santbrink H, Steyerberg EW, et al. Brain oxygen tension in severe head injury. Neurosurgery. 2000; 46(4):868–876, discussion 876–878

[48] Marshall LF, Smith RW, Shapiro HM. The outcome with aggressive treatment in severe head injuries. Part I: the significance of intracranial pressure monitoring. J Neurosurg. 1979; 50(1):20–25

[49] Eisenberg HM, Frankowski RF, Contant CF, Marshall LF, Walker MD. High-dose barbiturate control of elevated intracranial pressure in patients with severe head injury. J Neurosurg. 1988; 69(1):15–23

[50] Roberts I, Sydenham E. Barbiturates for acute traumatic brain injury. Cochrane Database Syst Rev. 2012; 12:CD000033

[51] Kelly DF, Goodale DB, Williams J, et al. Propofol in the treatment of moderate and severe head injury: a randomized, prospective double-blinded pilot trial. J Neurosurg. 1999; 90(6):1042–1052

[52] Rapp RP, Young B, Twyman D, et al. The favorable effect of early parenteral feeding on survival in head-injured patients. J Neurosurg. 1983; 58(6):906–912

[53] Lam AM, Winn HR, Cullen BF, Sundling N. Hyperglycemia and neurological outcome in patients with head injury. J Neurosurg. 1991; 75(4):545–551

[54] Young B, Ott L, Dempsey R, Haack D, Tibbs P. Relationship between admission hyperglycemia and neurologic outcome of severely brain-injured patients. Ann Surg. 1989; 210(4):466–472, discussion 472–473

[55] Suchner U, Senftleben U, Eckart T, et al. Enteral versus parenteral nutrition: effects on gastrointestinal function and metabolism. Nutrition. 1996; 12(1):13–22

[56] Young B, Ott L, Kasarskis E, et al. Zinc supplementation is associated with improved neurologic recovery rate and visceral protein levels of patients with severe closed head injury. J Neurotrauma. 1996; 13(1):25–34

[57] Temkin NR, Dikmen SS, Wilensky AJ, Keihm J, Chabal S, Winn HR. A randomized, double-blind study of phenytoin for the prevention of post-traumatic seizures. N Engl J Med. 1990; 323(8):497–502

[58] Wohns RN, Wyler AR. Prophylactic phenytoin in severe head injuries. J Neurosurg. 1979; 51(4):507–509

[59] Young B, Rapp R, Brooks WH, Madauss W, Norton JA. Posttraumatic epilepsy prophylaxis. Epilepsia. 1979; 20(6):671–681

[60] Temkin NR, Dikmen SS, Anderson GD, et al. Valproate therapy for prevention of posttraumatic seizures: a randomized trial. J Neurosurg. 1999; 91(4):593–600

[61] Miller JD, Becker DP, Ward JD, Sullivan HG, Adams WE, Rosner MJ. Significance of intracranial hypertension in severe head injury. J Neurosurg. 1977; 47(4):503–516

[62] Obrist WD, Langfitt TW, Jaggi JL, Cruz J, Gennarelli TA. Cerebral blood flow and metabolism in comatose patients with acute head injury. Relationship to intracranial hypertension. J Neurosurg. 1984; 61(2):241–253

[63] Imberti R, Bellinzona G, Langer M. Cerebral tissue PO2 and SjvO2 changes during moderate hyperventilation in patients with severe traumatic brain injury. J Neurosurg. 2002; 96(1):97–102

[64] Oertel M, Kelly DF, Lee JH, et al. Efficacy of hyperventilation, blood pressure elevation, and metabolic suppression therapy in controlling intracranial pressure after head injury. J Neurosurg. 2002; 97(5):1045–1053

[65] Sheinberg M, Kanter MJ, Robertson CS, Contant CF, Narayan RK, Grossman RG. Continuous monitoring of jugular venous oxygen saturation in head-injured patients. J Neurosurg. 1992; 76(2):212–217

[66] Muizelaar JP, Marmarou A, Ward JD, et al. Adverse effects of prolonged hyperventilation in patients with severe head injury: a randomized clinical trial. J Neurosurg. 1991; 75(5):731–739

[67] French LA, Galicich JH. The use of steroids for control of cerebral edema. Clin Neurosurg. 1964; 10:212–223

[68] Braakman R, Schouten HJ, Blaauw-van Dishoeck M, Minderhoud JM. Megadose steroids in severe head injury. Results of a prospective double-blind clinical trial. J Neurosurg. 1983; 58(3):326–330

[69] Cooper PR, Moody S, Clark WK, et al. Dexamethasone and severe head injury. A prospective double-blind study. J Neurosurg. 1979; 51(3):307–316

[70] Alderson P, Roberts I. Corticosteroids in acute traumatic brain injury: systematic review of randomised controlled trials. BMJ. 1997; 314(7098):1855–1859

[71] Roberts I, Yates D, Sandercock P, et al; CRASH trial collaborators. Effect of intravenous corticosteroids on death within 14 days in 10008 adults with clinically significant head injury (MRC CRASH trial): randomised placebo-controlled trial. Lancet. 2004; 364(9442):1321–1328

[72] Cordobés F, Lobato RD, Rivas JJ, et al. Observations on 82 patients with extradural hematoma. Comparison of results before and after the advent of computerized tomography. J Neurosurg. 1981; 54(2):179–186

[73] Gupta SK, Tandon SC, Mohanty S, Asthana S, Sharma S. Bilateral traumatic extradural haematomas: report of 12 cases with a review of the literature. Clin Neurol Neurosurg. 1992; 94(2):127–131

[74] Schutzman SA, Barnes PD, Mantello M, Scott RM. Epidural hematomas in children. Ann Emerg Med. 1993; 22(3):535–541

[75] Cucciniello B, Martellotta N, Nigro D, Citro E. Conservative management of extradural haematomas. Acta Neurochir (Wien). 1993; 120(1–2):47–52

[76] Haselsberger K, Pucher R, Auer LM. Prognosis after acute subdural or epidural haemorrhage. Acta Neurochir (Wien). 1988; 90(3–4):111–116

[77] Gennarelli TA, Spielman GM, Langfitt TW, et al. Influence of the type of intracranial lesion on outcome from severe head injury. J Neurosurg. 1982; 56(1):26–32

[78] Cohen JE, Montero A, Israel ZH. Prognosis and clinical relevance of anisocoria-craniotomy latency for epidural hematoma in comatose patients. J Trauma. 1996; 41(1):120–122

[79] Lee EJ, Hung YC, Wang LC, Chung KC, Chen HH. Factors influencing the functional outcome of patients with acute epidural hematomas: analysis of 200 patients undergoing surgery. J Trauma. 1998; 45(5):946–952

[80] Bullock R, Smith RM, van Dellen JR. Nonoperative management of extradural hematoma. Neurosurgery. 1985; 16(5):602–606

[81] Mathew P, Oluoch-Olunya DL, Condon BR, Bullock R. Acute subdural haematoma in the conscious patient: outcome with initial non-operative management. Acta Neurochir (Wien). 1993; 121(3–4):100–108

[82] Wilberger JE, Jr, Harris M, Diamond DL. Acute subdural hematoma: morbidity and mortality related to timing of operative intervention. J Trauma. 1990; 30(6):733–736

[83] Hatashita S, Koga N, Hosaka Y, Takagi S. Acute subdural hematoma: severity of injury, surgical intervention, and mortality. Neurol Med Chir (Tokyo). 1993; 33(1):13–18

[84] Seelig JM, Becker DP, Miller JD, Greenberg RP, Ward JD, Choi SC. Traumatic acute subdural hematoma: major mortality reduction in comatose patients treated within four hours. N Engl J Med. 1981; 304(25):1511–1518

[85] Bullock R, Golek J, Blake G. Traumatic intracerebral hematoma—which patients should undergo surgical evacuation? CT scan features and ICP monitoring as a basis for decision making. Surg Neurol. 1989; 32(3):181–187

[86] Yamaki T, Hirakawa K, Ueguchi T, Tenjin H, Kuboyama T, Nakagawa Y. Chronological evaluation of acute traumatic intracerebral haematoma. Acta Neurochir (Wien). 1990; 103(3–4):112–115

[87] Tseng SH. Delayed traumatic intracerebral hemorrhage: a study of prognostic factors. J Formos Med Assoc. 1992; 91(6):585–589

[88] Wong CW. The CT criteria for conservative treatment—but under close clinical observation—of posterior fossa epidural haematomas. Acta Neurochir (Wien). 1994; 126(2–4):124–127

[89] Jennett B, Miller JD. Infection after depressed fracture of skull. Implications for management of nonmissile injuries. J Neurosurg. 1972; 36(3):333–339

[90] Wylen EL, Willis BK, Nanda A. Infection rate with replacement of bone fragment in compound depressed skull fractures. Surg Neurol. 1999; 51(4):452–457

[91] Jennett B. Early traumatic epilepsy. Incidence and significance after nonmissile injuries. Arch Neurol. 1974; 30(5):394–398

[92] Barzilay Z, Augarten A, Sagy M, Shahar E, Yahav Y, Boichis H. Variables affecting outcome from severe brain injury in children. Intensive Care Med. 1988; 14(4):417–421

[93] Cruz J, Nakayama P, Imamura JH, Rosenfeld KG, de Souza HS, Giorgetti GV. Cerebral extraction of oxygen and intracranial hypertension in severe, acute, pediatric brain trauma: preliminary novel management strategies. Neurosurgery. 2002; 50(4):774–779, discussion 779–780

[94] Pfenninger J, Santi A. Severe traumatic brain injury in children—are the results improving? Swiss Med Wkly. 2002; 132(9–10):116–120

[95] White JR, Farukhi Z, Bull C, et al. Predictors of outcome in severely head-injured children. Crit Care Med. 2001; 29(3):534–540

[96] Wahlström MR, Olivecrona M, Koskinen LO, Rydenhag B, Naredi S. Severe traumatic brain injury in pediatric patients: treatment and outcome using an intracranial pressure targeted therapy—the Lund concept. Intensive Care Med. 2005; 31(6):832–839

[97] Bruce DA, Raphaely RC, Goldberg AI, et al. Pathophysiology, treatment and outcome following severe head injury in children. Childs Brain. 1979; 5(3):174–191

[98] Jagannathan J, Okonkwo DO, Yeoh HK, et al. Long-term outcomes and prognostic factors in pediatric patients with severe traumatic brain injury and elevated intracranial pressure. J Neurosurg Pediatr. 2008; 2(4):240–249

[99] Chambers IR, Treadwell L, Mendelow AD. Determination of threshold levels of cerebral perfusion pressure and intracranial pressure in severe head injury by using receiver-operating characteristic curves: an observational study in 291 patients. J Neurosurg. 2001; 94(3):412–416

[100] Downard C, Hulka F, Mullins RJ, et al. Relationship of cerebral perfusion pressure and survival in pediatric brain-injured patients. J Trauma. 2000; 49(4):654–658, discussion 658–659

[101] Figg RE, Stouffer CW, Vander Kolk WE, Connors RH. Clinical efficacy of serial computed tomographic scanning in pediatric severe traumatic brain injury. Pediatr Surg Int. 2006; 22(3):215–218

[102] Baldwin HZ, Rekate HL. Preliminary experience with controlled external lumbar drainage in diffuse pediatric head injury. Pediatr Neurosurg. 1991–1992; 17(3):115–120

[103] Levy DI, Rekate HL, Cherny WB, Manwaring K, Moss SD, Baldwin HZ. Controlled lumbar drainage in pediatric head injury. J Neurosurg. 1995; 83(3):453–460

[104] McManus ML, Soriano SG. Rebound swelling of astroglial cells exposed to hypertonic mannitol. Anesthesiology. 1998; 88(6):1586–1591

[105] Arjamaa O, Karlqvist K, Kanervo A, Vainionpää V, Vuolteenaho O, Leppäluoto J. Plasma ANP during hypertonic NaCl infusion in man. Acta Physiol Scand. 1992; 144(2):113–119

[106] Shapiro K, Marmarou A. Clinical applications of the pressure-volume index in treatment of pediatric head injuries. J Neurosurg. 1982; 56(6):819–825

[107] Pittman T, Bucholz R, Williams D. Efficacy of barbiturates in the treatment of resistant intracranial hypertension in severely head-injured children. Pediatr Neurosci. 1989; 15(1):13–17

[108] Kasoff SS, Lansen TA, Holder D, Filippo JS. Aggressive physiologic monitoring of pediatric head trauma patients with elevated intracranial pressure. Pediatr Neurosci. 1988; 14(5):241–249

[109] Bramwell KJ, Haizlip J, Pribble C, VanDerHeyden TC, Witte M. The effect of etomidate on intracranial pressure and systemic blood pressure in pediatric patients with severe traumatic brain injury. Pediatr Emerg Care. 2006; 22(2):90–93

[110] de Bray JM, Granry JC, Monrigal JP, Leftheriotis G, Saumet JL. Effects of thiopental on middle cerebral artery blood velocities: a transcranial Doppler study in children. Childs Nerv Syst. 1993; 9(4):220–223

[111] Yablon SA. Posttraumatic seizures. Arch Phys Med Rehabil. 1993; 74(9):983–1001

[112] Young B, Rapp RP, Norton JA, Haack D, Walsh JW. Failure of prophylactically administered phenytoin to prevent post-traumatic seizures in children. Childs Brain. 1983; 10(3):185–192

[113] Raimondi AJ, Hirschauer J. Head injury in the infant and toddler. Coma scoring and outcome scale. Childs Brain. 1984; 11(1):12–35

[114] Lewis RJ, Yee L, Inkelis SH, Gilmore D. Clinical predictors of post-traumatic seizures in children with head trauma. Ann Emerg Med. 1993; 22(7):1114–1118

[115] Polin RS, Shaffrey ME, Bogaev CA, et al. Decompressive bifrontal craniectomy in the treatment of severe refractory posttraumatic cerebral edema. Neurosurgery. 1997; 41(1):84–92, discussion 92–94

[116] Cho DY, Wang YC, Chi CS. Decompressive craniotomy for acute shaken/impact baby syndrome. Pediatr Neurosurg. 1995; 23(4):192–198

20 Special Considerations of Antiplatelet Therapy, Anticoagulation, and The Need For Reversal In Neurosurgical Emergencies

Drew A. Spencer, Paul D. Ackerman, Omer Q. Iqbal, and Christopher M. Loftus

Abstract

Neurosurgical emergencies are a variety of pathologic conditions that pose an imminent risk to the patient's life and functional capacity. These situations can be exacerbated when patients are on chronic antiplatelet or anticoagulant therapy prior to presentation, as these therapies have the potential to accentuate hemorrhagic or compressive pathology. Given the expanding indications for therapy and an aging population, there has been an imperative to develop new anticoagulant agents that offer more convenient therapy for providers and patients alike. Reversal strategies, however, have so far lagged behind this effort. The authors believe that operating neurosurgeons must have at least sophisticated knowledge of both antiplatelet or anticoagulant agents and the available measures to reverse therapy prior to emergent surgical intervention. Herein we review the available therapeutic agents, reversal agents, and the current literature regarding their management when emergent surgical intervention is required.

Keywords: anticoagulation, antiplatelet, coagulopathy, craniotomy, emergency, laminectomy, spinal fusion

20.1 Introduction

Neurosurgical emergencies require surgeons to expeditiously resolve a direct risk to the central nervous system (CNS) while considering the confounding factors that can make surgical intervention an additive insult. Two populations in particular are more susceptible in these scenarios: elderly patients and those on antiplatelet or anticoagulant medications are at a unique disadvantage when faced with a threat to their neurologic function. Elderly patients are at an age-specific increased risk of all trauma, with traumatic brain injury (TBI) being a primary concern.[1,2] This age group therefore accounts for a disproportionate number of TBI-related mortalities.[1,3] Patients on antiplatelet (AP) and/or anticoagulant (AC) medication are also a high-risk group, with quantified evidence of a higher morbidity and mortality.[1,3,4,5] These two groups often overlap, owing to the growing elderly population and their higher likelihood of comorbidities dictating therapy. The indications for AP and AC continue to expand and now include multiple systems (cerebrovascular, cardiovascular, peripheral vascular) and pathologic conditions (atrial fibrillation, clotting disorders).

The cohort of patients on antiplatelet (30%), anticoagulant (3%), or both medications continues to expand and become a more routine scenario encountered by neurosurgeons.[6,7,8,9] The real management conundrum is the paucity of high-level evidence guiding the management of these patients. Randomized, controlled trials would likely be dangerous and would expose a subgroup of patients to undue risk. In spite of this, case-series and other smaller studies have provided general guidelines that have proven safe and efficacious. Using these data, combined with a keen understanding of the available therapeutic and reversal agents, these patients can be safely treated in real time.

20.2 Antiplatelet

There are numerous antiplatelet agents. The targets of these agents include platelet activation and aggregation, which can be targeted alone or in combination to maximize therapeutic effect. There are three main classes of antiplatelet agents in clinical use at present. The first and most well-established class are the cyclooxygenase-1 (COX-1) inhibitors. These medications, including aspirin and others, irreversibly inhibit COX-1 and prevent thromboxane production from arachidonic acid. This is an early step in platelet activation, aggregation, and degranulation, and its inhibition severely impairs its function. Clopidogrel is the most known and widely used medication among those that inhibit the $P2Y_{12}$ or adenosine diphosphate (ADP) receptors on the platelet surface. This receptor, when activated, binds fibrin and participates in platelet cross-linking to form a preliminary clot soon after bleeding begins. The final class includes medications such as abciximab, eptifibatide, and tirofiban, which inhibit the glycoprotein IIb/IIIa (GPIIb/IIIa) receptor. These agents prevent platelet aggregation by blocking surface receptor interaction with von Willebrand factor (vWF) and fibrinogen.

The common thread among all antiplatelet classes is their influence on early clot formation that begins immediately after an injury, as platelets are the initial reactive agent in the clotting cascade to encounter the damage. This prolongs bleeding not only by disrupting the framework for a clot but also by disrupting platelet interaction with factors such as vWF and fibrinogen, which serve as the catalysts for the remaining clotting cascade. In some patients, therefore, simply reversing the platelet deficiency is not adequate treatment, and this will be addressed in the later section on reversal strategies.

20.3 Anticoagulation

Anticoagulant medications are also used with increasing frequency as the population continues to age.[6,7,8] The number of available medications has increased dramatically in recent years congruent with their demand in clinical practice. Agents exist that are best suited for either acute, inpatient care or long-term outpatient therapy, or in some cases both. All medications used target crucial catalytic points—such as thrombin and activated factor X—in the coagulation cascade that have a measurable impact on the ability of the blood to clot.

Unfractionated heparin (UFH) and the low-molecular-weight heparins (LMWHs) are medications used in the acute care setting and given by either subcutaneous or intravenous administration. Their primary indications are the prevention of acute thrombi and limiting the propagation of recently diagnosed intravascular clots. UFH is most useful when intravenous therapy is required. LMWH is effective in prevention and also as a bridging agent to outpatient therapy when indicated. Heparin binds to and catalyzes the activity of anti–thrombin III, increasing its ability to inactivate thrombin, factor X, and others by one thousand fold. LMWH is more specifically targeted to factor X, with lesser effects on thrombin (factor II). LMWH has a more predictable steady state and clinical effect, obviating the need for the frequent laboratory monitoring required for heparin use. Heparin-induced thrombocytopenia (HIT) is a risk with any heparin-based therapy, requiring at least intermittent monitoring of platelet levels and coagulation parameters. Newer agents have been introduced in the LMWH class relatively recently, the most widely used of which is fondaparinux. Fondaparinux is a pentasaccharide that performs similarly to UFH in activating anti–thrombin III, inhibiting activated factor X, and preventing venous thromboembolism (VTE).

Warfarin is the oldest and most widely used anticoagulant medication, introduced in 1954. Warfarin is an inhibitor of hepatic carboxylation of coagulation factors II, VII, IX, and X. Warfarin's efficacy is rarely questioned, although it has never been the easiest medication to use for patients or physicians. The international normalized ratio (INR) must be monitored frequently even in patients on the medication for chronic therapy with a well-established dosing pattern. Simple dietary variations that affect vitamin K intake or the activity of liver enzymes can cause wide variations in INR as well. Warfarin has a long half-life that must be carefully considered in dosing changes and when therapy must be interrupted for any reason.

The limitations of warfarin prompted the development of new, more convenient medications, a class referred to as the novel or target-specific oral anticoagulants (NOACs, TSOACs). This class includes agents with a more specific action than that of warfarin, directly inhibiting either activated factor X (Xa) (rivaroxaban, apixaban, and edoxaban) or thrombin (dabigatran). These agents offer several benefits over warfarin, most importantly a short half-life that begets their quick onset of action, and a reliable clinical effect that precludes the need for frequent laboratory monitoring.[10] Patient safety is improved when using NOACs versus warfarin as well. The literature suggests a lower risk of hemorrhage in patients on NOACs (compared with warfarin), with a 2 to 3% risk of major hemorrhage per year and a 0.2% risk of intracranial hemorrhage.[9,11,12] The short half-life of these medications is also advantageous in trauma, surgery, or other situations requiring a quick return to baseline coagulation parameters. The problem, at present, for surgeons encountering NOAC patients is that there is no specific antidote. This creates a vexing clinical scenario in trauma and other hemorrhagic conditions, although the experience to date is providing a basic framework for at least nonspecific reversal strategies and the promise of imminent direct reversal agents (idarucizumab, the agent to reverse dabigatran, was actually approved by the Food and Drug Administration [FDA] as this book was being prepared) for the NOACs.

20.4 Reversal of Antiplatelet and Anticoagulant Medications for Neurosurgical Emergencies

The medical necessity of pharmacologic antiplatelet and anticoagulation measures has led to much investigation of their effective reversal when emergency surgery is indicated. Publications on this topic continue to increase and provide a template for

the safe management of this difficult patient base. Here we will review the currently approved agents and protocols for the efficient reversal of coagulopathy for emergent neurosurgical intervention.

The reversal of antiplatelet treatment is relatively simple and largely very effective.[13] The obvious indications for reversal are any intracranial or spinal hemorrhages meeting surgical criteria. A more ambiguous indication exists in hemorrhages not requiring surgical management, with the growing body of evidence advocating for reversal in most, if not all, of these situations.[3,14, 15,16,17] The transfusion of platelets is the only proven method for correcting the almost exclusively irreversible platelet dysfunction induced by antiplatelet agents. This is a temporary measure in the overall management, and patients may require continued transfusion every 12 hours for 48 hours, when the physiologic turnover has had ample time to replete the functioning native platelet pool.[15,18] In extreme cases, the only approved adjunct is the administration of 1-desamino-8-D-arginine vasopressin (DDAVP). The administration of 0.3 µg/kg of DDAVP with platelets enhances platelet function via an increase in vWF and a potential activating impact on other procoagulant factors.[19,20]

The reversal of anticoagulant agents depends on not only the agent used but also the nature of the emergency and, perhaps most importantly, the medical condition of the patient. In choosing the correct agent, one must consider not only the mechanism of action of the medication but also the ability of the patient to tolerate large fluid volumes (e.g., congestive heart failure [CHF]) or the risk of thrombosis (mechanical valves, carotid disease). Warfarin is still the most frequently used anticoagulant medication and, as such, has the most literature data on reversal. Warfarin reversal is traditionally addressed by administration of vitamin K and fresh frozen plasma [FFP], which can require significant time and repeat doses to correct the coagulopathy to a safe threshold for surgical intervention. The only known reversal agent for UFH is protamine sulfate. Protamine is also effective, to a lesser degree, for the reversal of enoxaparin. The role of FFP is not clearly established, but it is frequently used as an adjunct.[18] Acute reversal strategies for NOACs are changing quickly. As mentioned, these compelling clinical agents were first released without a specific antidote. The direct thrombin inhibitor (DTI) anticoagulant dabigatran is now reversed by idarucizumab. The currently available indirect reversal options for the factor Xa inhibitors include FFP, activated factor VII, prothrombin complex concentrate, and factor eight inhibitor bypass activity (FEIBA). Obviously there is great interest in agents for direct reversal of the Xa inhibitors as well, and we anticipate that these agents, described elsewhere in this text, will soon be commercially available to surgeons. Preliminary trials of one such agent, andexanet alfa (AndexXa; Portola Pharmaceuticals, South San Francisco, CA), for the reversal of the Xa NOACs (rivaroxaban, apixaban, edoxaban) have started.[21,22]

There are indirect strategies for reversal of anticoagulant effects, including those of the NOACs. FFP has been in clinical use for nearly 40 years and is very familiar to most clinicians. FFP replenishes clotting factors II, V, VII, IX, X, and XI. It is more effective in replacing these factors and overcoming the effects of warfarin and factor X inhibitors than in bleeding due to intrinsic factor (factor VIII) deficiencies.[23] An infrequent complication is that individual factors also have different sensitivities, or minimum levels present for effective clotting,[7,18] which can require excessive transfusion volumes to definitively reverse the coagulopathy. This complicates patient management in those with cardiac comorbidities or multisystem injury after trauma, and of course patients with elevated ICP. FFP will continue to be useful in the emergent reversal of coagulopathy, both alone and as complementary therapy to the newer agents that have been introduced recently.

Relatively new agents are now available for the near-immediate correction of coagulopathy via repletion of activated factors at crucial checkpoints in the clotting cascade. The primary advantages of these agents are improved times to correction and flexibility in formulating an appropriate regimen for specific patients. The new agents offer the added benefit of a synergistic effect with traditional FFP, which replenishes factors to be consumed by active coagulation.[7] Activated factor VII serves as the catalyst necessary to activate factors V and X, with resultant completion of the clotting cascade. Activated factor VII has a short onset of action and requires concurrent administration of FFP.[7,18,24] Prothrombin complex concentrate (PCC) is a targeted reversal agent composed mainly of concentrated factors II, IX, and X with some activated factor VII as well.[7,18,24] Standard PCC has a variety of urgent and emergent applications, whereas derivatives with high concentrations of activated factor VII (Kcentra; CSL Behring, King of Prussia, PA) are most useful in situations where emergent intervention is indicated.[9,25] Clinical studies have shown these agents to reverse coagulopathy greater than 4 times as fast as FFP (and with a much lower volume load), although the appropriate intervals for laboratory monitoring and duration of their effect have not yet been established. FEIBA is the other relatively novel agent, and it consists of factors II, IX, X (mainly nonactivated), and VIIa (mainly activated) in addition to 1 to 6 units of FVIII coagulation antigen (FVIIIC:Ag) per milliliter. These agents have the advantage of providing concentrated factors, in amounts sufficient to reestablish normal factor function in the clotting cascade. Activated factor VII, Kcentra, PCC, and FEIBA are invaluable tools in the management of neurosurgical emergencies in this patient population, and their utility only stands to increase as we learn more about their clinical characteristics. Concomitant administration of FFP with these agents is increasingly recommended to replenish all clotting factors and avoid a consumptive complication or limitation in reversal.[7] All patients undergoing anticoagulant reversal have a clinically significant increase in their risk of thrombosis in the postoperative period as well.[7] Therefore, each patient's clinical scenario, including their volume status, must be considered carefully to derive the ideal reversal strategy.

high-level evidence exists, the total body of work provides a safe and effective framework. For antiplatelet agents, the available data suggest that postoperative day 5 is the soonest these medications can be started.[26] In high-risk patients, however, others have suggested that antiplatelet agents can be continued up to and through surgery, with a low rate of hemorrhagic complications.[27,28] In trauma patients, no clear recommendation can be made based on current literature, and at the authors' institution, antiplatelet agents are routinely held until outpatient follow-up.

Reinstitution of anticoagulant therapy is planned for patients in two different clinical groups: those able to tolerate a perioperative therapeutic holiday and those requiring a bridge. For patients not requiring a bridge, therapy is restarted at the discretion of the treating surgeon. If it must be resumed on an inpatient basis, warfarin can be started as early as 24 hours postoperatively with either in- or outpatient INR monitoring. In less urgent cases, the prudent option is to delay reinitiation of therapy until outpatient surgical follow-up to minimize bleeding risk. When a patient requires bridging, many have published their experiences culminating in a safe and reliable result.[29,30] In low-risk patients, current recommendations are to restart warfarin 24 hours after the operation with a UFH or LMWH bridge. The advantage of LMWH is the option of outpatient use without a need for laboratory monitoring, allowing for shorter hospital stays. In patients considered to be at high risk of hemorrhage, which likely involves most neurosurgical patients, current practice is to delay warfarin restart until 48 to 72 hours postoperatively, with an appropriate bridge beginning as soon as possible (~ 6 hours) after surgery.

Although appropriate timing of therapy is still open to provider interpretation, clinical experience is more robust regarding how to dose anticoagulants.[29,30,31,32] In the majority of cases, either the preoperative dose or a gradually escalating warfarin dose has been used until achieving a therapeutic INR. A recent study advocates an initial dose double the patient's maintenance dose, finding that more patients achieved a therapeutic INR at day 5 than those receiving their maintenance dose (50% vs. 13%).[31] No increase in adverse events was noted in response to the rapid increase in INR. When using the NOACs, recent evidence supports initiation of the preoperative dose 24 to 72 hours after surgery.[10] In extreme cases involving patients in both bridge and nonbridge situations, anticoagulation can be held for 1 to 4 weeks postoperatively, provided that the physician and the patient have an open understanding of the inherent thrombotic risk.

20.5 Resumption of Antiplatelet and Anticoagulant Medications after Definitive Treatment

After definitive treatment of the emergent pathology, the patient's greatest risk transitions to the pathology that originally mandated antiplatelet or anticoagulant therapy. Neurosurgeons must make shrewd decisions when restarting these therapies to avoid complications and avoidable returns to the operating room. Fortunately, this decision is now guided by a growing literature documenting other surgeons' experience. Although no

20.6 Conclusion

Patients presenting with a neurosurgical emergency are a vulnerable population to be treated with prudent and efficient judgment. When these patients are also on chronic antiplatelet or anticoagulant therapy, the situation can be precarious. Neurosurgeons treating these conditions must be cognizant of the pharmacologic effect of the various agents used for these purposes, as well as how to safely reverse and reinitiate them. A keen understanding of this dynamic balance will enable shrewd decision-making and a continued focus on the best possible outcome for patients.

References

[1] Grandhi R, Harrison G, Voronovich Z, et al. Preinjury warfarin, but not antiplatelet medications, increases mortality in elderly traumatic brain injury patients. J Trauma Acute Care Surg. 2015; 78(3):614–621

[2] Peck KA, Calvo RY, Schechter MS, et al. The impact of preinjury anticoagulants and prescription antiplatelet agents on outcomes in older patients with traumatic brain injury. J Trauma Acute Care Surg. 2014; 76(2):431–436

[3] Cull JD, Sakai LM, Sabir I, et al. Outcomes in traumatic brain injury for patients presenting on antiplatelet therapy. Am Surg. 2015; 81(2):128–132

[4] Pakraftar S, Atencio D, English J, Corcos A, Altschuler EM, Stahlfeld K. Dabigatran etixilate and traumatic brain injury: evolving anticoagulants require evolving care plans. World J Clin Cases. 2014; 2(8):362–366

[5] Moussouttas M. Challenges and controversies in the medical management of primary and antithrombotic-related intracerebral hemorrhage. Ther Adv Neurol Disord. 2012; 5(1):43–56

[6] Goy J, Crowther M. Approaches to diagnosing and managing anticoagulant-related bleeding. Semin Thromb Hemost. 2012; 38(7):702–710

[7] McCoy CC, Lawson JH, Shapiro ML. Management of anticoagulation agents in trauma patients. Clin Lab Med. 2014; 34(3):563–574

[8] Labuz-Roszak B, Pierzchala K, Skrzypek M, Swiech M, Machowska-Majchrzak A. Oral anticoagulant and antiplatelet drugs used in prevention of cardiovascular events in elderly people in Poland. BMC Cardiovasc Disord. 2012; 12:98

[9] Suryanarayan D, Schulman S. Potential antidotes for reversal of old and new oral anticoagulants. Thromb Res. 2014; 133(Suppl 2):S158–S166

[10] Mavrakanas TA, Samer C, Fontana P, Perrier A. Direct oral anticoagulants: efficacy and safety in patient subgroups. Swiss Med Wkly. 2015; 145:w14081

[11] Fox BD, Kahn SR, Langleben D, Eisenberg MJ, Shimony A. Efficacy and safety of novel oral anticoagulants for treatment of acute venous thromboembolism: direct and adjusted indirect meta-analysis of randomised controlled trials. BMJ. 2012; 345:e7498

[12] Chatterjee S, Sardar P, Biondi-Zoccai G, Kumbhani DJ. New oral anticoagulants and the risk of intracranial hemorrhage: traditional and Bayesian meta-analysis and mixed treatment comparison of randomized trials of new oral anticoagulants in atrial fibrillation. JAMA Neurol. 2013; 70(12):1486–1490

[13] Thiele T, Sümnig A, Hron G, et al. Platelet transfusion for reversal of dual antiplatelet therapy in patients requiring urgent surgery: a pilot study. J Thromb Haemost. 2012; 10(5):968–971

[14] Gordon JL, Fabian TC, Lee MD, Dugdale M. Anticoagulant and antiplatelet medications encountered in emergency surgery patients: a review of reversal strategies. J Trauma Acute Care Surg. 2013; 75(3):475–486

[15] Campbell PG, Sen A, Yadla S, Jabbour P, Jallo J. Emergency reversal of antiplatelet agents in patients presenting with an intracranial hemorrhage: a clinical review. World Neurosurg. 2010; 74(2–3):279–285

[16] Campbell PG, Yadla S, Sen AN, Jallo J, Jabbour P. Emergency reversal of clopidogrel in the setting of spontaneous intracerebral hemorrhage. World Neurosurg. 2011; 76(1–2):100–104, discussion 59–60

[17] Washington CW, Schuerer DJ, Grubb RL, Jr. Platelet transfusion: an unnecessary risk for mild traumatic brain injury patients on antiplatelet therapy. J Trauma. 2011; 71(2):358–363

[18] Levi M, Eerenberg E, Kamphuisen PW. Bleeding risk and reversal strategies for old and new anticoagulants and antiplatelet agents. J Thromb Haemost. 2011; 9(9):1705–1712

[19] Sarode R. How do I transfuse platelets (PLTs) to reverse anti-PLT drug effect? Transfusion. 2012; 52(4):695–701, quiz 694

[20] Colucci G, Stutz M, Rochat S, et al. The effect of desmopressin on platelet function: a selective enhancement of procoagulant COAT platelets in patients with primary platelet function defects. Blood. 2014; 123(12):1905–1916

[21] Na SY, Mracsko E, van Ryn J, Veltkamp R. Idarucizumab improves outcome in murine brain hemorrhage related to dabigatran. Ann Neurol. 2015; 78(1):137–141

[22] Glund S, Moschetti V, Norris S, et al. A randomised study in healthy volunteers to investigate the safety, tolerability and pharmacokinetics of idarucizumab, a specific antidote to dabigatran. Thromb Haemost. 2015; 113(5):943–951

[23] Agus N, Yilmaz N, Colak A, Liv F. Levels of factor VIII and factor IX in fresh-frozen plasma produced from whole blood stored at 4 °C overnight in Turkey. Blood Transfus. 2012; 10(2):191–193

[24] Medow JE, Dierks MR, Williams E, Zacko JC. The emergent reversal of coagulopathies encountered in neurosurgery and neurology: a technical note. Clin Med Res. 2015; 13(1):20–31

[25] Majeed A, Meijer K, Larrazabal R, et al. Mortality in vitamin K antagonist-related intracerebral bleeding treated with plasma or 4-factor prothrombin complex concentrate. Thromb Haemost. 2014; 111(2):233–239

[26] Carragee EJ, Golish SR, Scuderi GJ. A case of late epidural hematoma in a patient on clopidogrel therapy postoperatively: when is it safe to resume antiplatelet agents? Spine J. 2011; 11(1):e1–e4

[27] Rahman M, Donnangelo LL, Neal D, Mogali K, Decker M, Ahmed MM. Effects of perioperative acetyl salicylic acid on clinical outcomes in patients undergoing craniotomy for brain tumor. World Neurosurg. 2015; 84(1):41–47

[28] Ogawa Y, Tominaga T. Sellar and parasellar tumor removal without discontinuing antithrombotic therapy. J Neurosurg. 2015; 123(3):794–798

[29] Spyropoulos AC. Bridging therapy and oral anticoagulation: current and future prospects. Curr Opin Hematol. 2010; 17(5):444–449

[30] Ortel TL. Perioperative management of patients on chronic antithrombotic therapy. Hematology (Am Soc Hematol Educ Program). 2012; 2012:529–535

[31] Schulman S, Hwang HG, Eikelboom JW, Kearon C, Pai M, Delaney J. Loading dose vs. maintenance dose of warfarin for reinitiation after invasive procedures: a randomized trial. J Thromb Haemost. 2014; 12(8):1254–1259

[32] Yorkgitis BK, Ruggia-Check C, Dujon JE. Antiplatelet and anticoagulation medications and the surgical patient. Am J Surg. 2014; 207(1):95–101

21 Acute Intervention for Cervical, Thoracic, and Lumbar Spinal Disk Disease

Mazda K. Turel and Vincent C. Traynelis

Abstract

The natural history of spinal disk disease is often benign and self-limited. Most patients are managed conservatively, and the majority respond well to medical management alone. In contrast, less than 1% of patients with a herniated disk present with severe deficit or rapidly progressive neurologic deterioration. Although there is no consensus on the term "acute," most surgeons would agree on a time frame of 2 to 4 weeks of symptom duration. These patients may exhibit symptoms and signs that include marked radicular weakness, myelopathy, and bowel or bladder dysfunction. Inappropriate or delayed treatment of these individuals may result in increased morbidity or persistent neurologic deficit. This chapter reviews the clinicoradiologic presentation of acute cervical, thoracic, and lumbar disk disease. We also discuss the recommendations made on the optimal timing of management as well as the role of acute surgical intervention in patients with severe or progressive neurologic symptoms secondary to spinal disk disease. Various open and minimally invasive and endoscopic surgical approaches available in the modern era are alluded to. Outcomes and prognosis are also described, giving the reader a holistic paradigm to guide clinical practice when faced with a similar scenario.

Keywords: acute, cauda equina, cervical, disk disease, lumbar, thoracic

21.1 Introduction

Disk herniation usually occurs in patients with mild to moderate degenerative changes. These degenerative processes predispose the intervertebral disk to the formation of anulus fibrosus fissures, and increased intradiskal pressure can result in herniation of the nucleus pulposus through these fissures.[1] Understanding the collagen and ultrastructural substrate of degenerative changes in the human disk is an essential step in planning restorative therapies.[2] Current research also stresses upon the role of microRNAs, cytokines, enzymes, growth factors, and proapoptotic proteins in symptomatic disk disease.[3,4] Extreme axial loading with rotation may produce acute herniations in relatively normal intervertebral disks in the spine.

21.2 Clinical Evaluation

The initial evaluation of patients includes a careful history, which often assists in distinguishing between vascular, infectious, neoplastic, and traumatic causes of acute neurologic deterioration. This provides a functional baseline for subsequent examinations. The inclusion of the Nurick grade, modified Japanese Orthopedic Association score (mJOA), Oswestry Disability Index (ODI), and Neck Disability Index (NDI) provides an objective assessment of the severity of the condition and is helpful in estimating outcome.[5,6,7,8]

21.3 Radiographic Evaluation

Plain radiographs evaluate alignment, stability, bony anatomy, and degenerative disk disease but are inadequate for detecting an acute disk prolapse and have been reported as "normal" in 20 to 50% of acute herniations. Approximately one third of patients with disk herniations will have disk space narrowing evident on plain films; however, this is a common radiographic finding, especially in individuals over the age of 50 years.[9]

Computed tomography (CT) provides optimal visualization of bony detail and has a high sensitivity in detecting fractures, which may be associated with a disk herniation in patients with a history of trauma.[10] CT can also help distinguish neural compression due to soft-tissue versus bony anatomy. The addition of myelography to CT provides an excellent adjunctive study to further delineate specific anatomy, such as the lateral recess, or to reconcile against a magnetic resonance imaging (MRI) study in which the etiology of clinical symptoms is not demonstrated. It should be noted that myelography is usually nondiagnostic in cases of far-lateral disk herniation in which nerve root compression is distal to the dural nerve sheath, although the postmyelogram CT can be quite useful in this particular situation.

MRI is the most widely used imaging modality for detection of an acute disk herniation. MRI allows direct visualization of neural structures and provides the greatest soft-tissue detail. Although multiplanar unenhanced T1- and T2-weighted images are sufficient to diagnose disk herniation, contusions, syrinx, infarction, hematoma, and demyelinating spinal cord diseases, the addition of gadolinium-enhanced sequences assist in differentiating neurologic deterioration due infection and tumor. The use of diffusion tensor imaging and tractography is beginning to find relevance in the evaluation of herniated disk disease, but the clinical research is still in its infancy.[11] Because herniated disks can be found in about 20% of asymptomatic individuals between the ages of 20 and 40, MRI findings must be strictly corelated with the clinical presentation. Neurologic examination remains the cornerstone of decision-making despite the availability of advanced imaging, which is invaluable in confirming diagnosis and identifying treatment that has the best chance of clinical success.

21.4 Indications for Acute Surgical Intervention

The timing of surgical intervention for symptomatic disk disease is somewhat controversial. Emergent surgical intervention should be reserved for those patients with severe or rapidly progressive motor radiculopathy, myelopathy, or bowel or bladder dysfunction. In contrast, patients without evidence of spinal instability who present with pain, sensory disturbances, and mild or fixed motor deficits or those exhibiting neurologic improvement should not be considered for emergent surgical decompression. Instead, these patients should be treated with

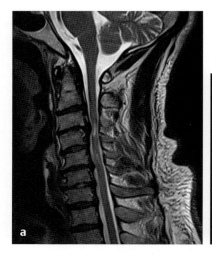
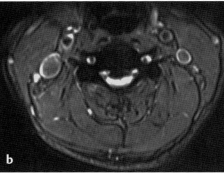

Fig. 21.1 T2-weighted (**a**) sagittal and (**b**) axial images of a 54-year-old man who presented with acute quadriparesis over 2 weeks showing a large central C3–C4 disk prolapse with signal changes within the cord. We did a C3–C4 anterior cervical diskectomy and fusion, following which he had a remarkable recovery.

conservative and supportive medical management. If they fail these treatment modalities, then elective surgical intervention should be considered.

21.5 Cervical Spine

Acute cervical radiculopathy usually results from lateral or posterolateral disk herniations. Early degenerative changes may produce mild foraminal narrowing secondary to osteophyte formation or facet hypertrophy. These changes can tether or stretch the nerve root so that even relatively small disk herniations may result in profound neurologic deficits. The exact pathophysiology of radiculopathy remains unclear; however, it appears that compression, ischemia of the nerve root, and inflammatory mediators are all part of the process. The most commonly affected levels in decreasing order of frequency are C5–C6, C6–C7, and C4–C5.[12]

Myelopathy secondary to acute disk herniation is probably the result of both spinal cord compression and vascular compromise, although sudden extrusion of the intervertebral disk may produce neurologic deterioration secondary to direct spinal cord pressure or contusion or both. In the absence of trauma, the acute onset of neurologic deficit is usually due to vascular compromise. Long transverse perforating arteries arising from the anterior spinal artery supply the ventral gray matter as well as the lateral funiculi of the spinal cord. Compression of the cord in a ventrodorsal direction compromises these transverse arteries and results in ischemia of the anterior gray matter and lateral white matter tracts. This ischemia produces lower motor neuron signs at the level of compression from anterior horn cell involvement, and upper motor neuron findings caudal to the disk herniation secondary to lateral corticospinal tract dysfunction.

21.5.1 Clinical Presentation

There is a slight male predominance, and the peak age is in the fourth and fifth decades. The risk of developing symptomatic cervical disk disease increases with congenital or degenerative narrowing of the spinal canal. Although pain and sensory

abnormalities are the most common complaints of acute cervical disk herniations, about 60% of patients will exhibit weakness and hyporeflexia by the time of evaluation.[12] A history of physical exertion or trauma precedes the onset of symptoms in only about 15% of cases.[13] Patients with symptomatic cervical spondylosis may present with radiculopathy, myelopathy, or both. Compression of the cervical spinal cord by central and centrolateral disk herniations may result in quadriparesis, painless sensory disturbances, and hyperreflexia (▶ Fig. 21.1). Acute nontraumatic rapidly progressive myelopathy in the context of cervical disk herniation (with or without comorbid ossification of the posterior longitudinal ligament) is rarely encountered clinically.[14] The population of patients with cervical disk herniation and rapidly progressive myelopathy are heterogeneous with respect to age, sex, relative acuity of onset, rapidity of quadraparesis onset, and spinal level of disk herniation. Both the onset and resolution of neurologic dysfunction are variable.[15,16,17,18,19,20,21,22]

21.5.2 Cervical Trauma

Patients with evidence of cervical trauma deserve special consideration, especially those with unilateral or bilateral facet dislocations. Facet dislocations with a concomitant traumatic disk herniation can produce cervical cord compression at the level of facet dislocation[23]; however, determining the significance of the disk herniation remains more difficult. Although neurologic injuries are commonly seen in patients sustaining bilateral facet dislocations, patients with unilateral facet dislocation may demonstrate evidence of an isolated nerve root injury. Some authors recommend rapid alignment of the spine through closed traction, followed by surgical stabilization, as it provides quick decompression of the cord and a better chance of neurologic recovery in awake patients in whom serial examinations are possible.[24] An alternative approach was advocated by Eismont et al[25] who recommend doing a prereduction MRI before attempting any signification reduction by traction to rule out the presence of a traumatic disk herniation. This is to avoid the rare neurologic deterioration that occurs after closed reduction, particularly if it's under anesthesia. The treatment of bilateral locked facets in the presence of a large anterior traumatic disk herniation warrants a ventral decompression, followed by an attempt to reduce the dislocation with or without posterior open reduction. The safety and efficacy of each approach for traumatic facet dislocation continue to generate debate.[26] According to evidence-based guidelines, several large clinical series have failed to establish a relationship between the presence of a prereduction herniated disk and the development of neurologic deterioration with attempted closed traction reduction in awake patients.[27] Current guidelines continue to recommend early closed reduction.[28] MRI does, however, have a proven role in two specific subsets of patients: patients with cervical spine fracture/dislocations who cannot be examined during attempted closed reduction and those who require an open reduction.

21.5.3 Surgical Approaches

Multiple surgical approaches to the cervical spinal canal or neural foramina are possible for the removal of an acute herniated disk. Each approach has its indications, advantages, and disadvantages.

Posterior

The dorsal approach makes use of a midline incision and subperiosteal dissection. With this approach, a hemilaminotomy and medial facetectomy are required to obtain adequate exposure of the lateral disk space and lateral recess of the spinal canal. Less surgical effort is required in exposing multiple levels, and fusion is rarely required. The risk of postoperative instability is minimal if less than one third of the facet joint is resected. The posterior approach lends itself well to the current trend toward more minimally invasive approaches, with the procedure being performed through an access tube or port.[29] Central disk herniations however, should be approached ventrally. Central disk herniations approached posteriorly require extensive bone and facet joint removal for adequate ventral exposure, which increases the risk of postoperative instability. This factor, combined with the potential need for spinal cord manipulation, makes this an unfavorable option, particularly with the ease of ventral approaches.

Lateral

Although rarely used today, lateral approaches should be included for a historical perspective, and the anterior lateral approach may be an alternative to posterior facetectomy or anterior diskectomy in highly selected patients.[30] The skin incision follows the anterior border of the sternocleidomastoid, and soft-tissue dissection is continued until the transverse processes are identified. This approach requires skeletonizing the vertebral artery and retracting it laterally to gain access to the neural foramen. The advantages include direct visualization of the nerve root as it exits the foramen and preservation of the posterior apophyseal joints as well as the supporting ligaments. The disadvantages include the risk of injury to the vertebral artery and sympathetic chain and limited access to the contralateral neural foramen.

Anterior

Anterior cervical diskectomy and fusion (ACDF) has been described by Cloward Robinson and Smith over 50 years ago.[31,32] This allows access to the entire anterior spinal canal and both neural foramina at each vertebral level. Most patients are fused after an anterior decompression, and in the United States, almost all patients are also plated. Cervical disk arthroplasty seems to be a promising nonfusion alternative, especially in cases of soft disk herniation, which are often acute.[33]

21.5.4 Prognosis

Postoperative neurologic outcome is related to the type, duration, acuteness, and severity of the preoperative deficit. Data from prospective observational studies indicate that 2 years after surgery for cervical radiculopathy caused by soft cervical disk herniation (without myelopathy), 75% of patients have substantial pain relief from radicular symptoms.[34] Radicular symptoms are more likely to improve with surgical decompression compared with myelopathy; however, several small reports note significant improvement in myelopathic patients if surgery is performed early.[14] Overall quality of life as assessed by the Short-Form 36 inventory and ODI also shows significant improvement.[35] Patients with deficits from acute disk herniations have a more favorable surgical outcome compared with those with deficits from spondylotic disease. Patients who present with severe or long-standing symptoms and signs have a poorer functional outcome than those with only a short clinical history and minor neurologic deficits.

21.6 Thoracic Spine

Acute disk herniations in the thoracic spine are very uncommon compared with those in the cervical or lumbar region. Compression of the thoracic spinal cord and/or nerve roots, resulting in myelopathy or radiculopathy, is rare, occurring in an estimated 1 in 1 million people.[36] Thoracic diskectomy procedures constitute between 0.15 and 4% of all disk surgeries.[37,38] There is a slight male predominance, and most patients are affected in the fourth through sixth decades.[36,37,38] Disk herniations have been reported at every level in the thoracic spine; however, 70 to 80% occur below T8.[38] T11–T12 is the most common level, and this increased frequency is thought to be secondary to greater mobility at these lower levels.[39] Multiple thoracic disk herniations are uncommon. Herniations occur most often in the midline (> 70%), followed by centrolateral and lateral prolapses (▶ Fig. 21.2) Associated risk factors for acute disk herniations include lifting or bending, trauma, and Scheuermann's disease.

21.6.1 Clinical Presentation

The signs and symptoms of an acute thoracic herniated disk can be divided into radicular or myelopathic presentation. A laterally displaced herniated disk is more likely to produce radicular symptoms. Band-like pain and sensory abnormalities involving the thorax and abdomen are the most common presentations. These symptoms are frequently misdiagnosed as

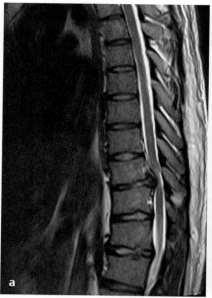
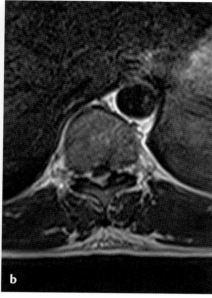

Fig. 21.2 T2-weighted (a) sagittal and (b) axial images of a 24-year-old man who presented with acute progressive spastic paraparesis and magnetic resonance imaging showing a T9–T10 central disk prolapse. We did T9–T10 diskectomy through transpedicular approach. Postoperatively, his spasticity in both the lower limbs had improved significantly.

pleuritis, angina, or cholecystitis. Radicular motor deficits involving the T1 nerve root may result in interosseous wasting and hand weakness. Central or centrolateral disk herniations may produce myelopathy secondary to spinal cord compression and ischemia.[40] The cross-sectional area of the thoracic spinal cord occupies a relatively larger portion of the spinal canal compared with the cervical region; consequently, a small disk herniation can produce a disproportionately significant canal compromise with a resultant myelopathy. Some of the pathophysiology of acute thoracic spinal cord dysfunction is related to vascular compromise resulting from anterior spinal artery territory ischemia.[41]

Central disk herniations present with leg weakness as the initial symptom in 20 to 30% of patients, and more than 50% of patients will have a frank myelopathy at the time of clinical evaluation. Bladder and bowel dysfunction occur in 30 to 70% of patients.[36,37,38,39] The natural history of symptomatic herniated thoracic disks is usually one of progressive neurologic deterioration, usually over several years. Acute presentations are very rare.

Conus medullaris compression secondary to T11–T12 or T12–L1 disk herniations presents primarily with sensory deficits that are usually in a saddle-like distribution and motor deficits that are more symmetrical than deficits produced by cauda equina compression. Sacral sparing of pain and temperature is present inconsistently and bladder and bowel sphincter dysfunction occur earlier in conus medullaris compression compared with disk herniations involving the upper thoracic spine or cauda equina.

21.6.2 Surgical Approaches

The natural history of symptomatic thoracic disk disease presenting with myelopathy is one of progressive deterioration; therefore, surgical intervention should be performed expeditiously. Emergent surgical intervention should be performed in patients with rapid progression or an acute sudden onset of severe neurologic deficits. Thoracic disk herniations can be decompressed through posterolateral or anterior approaches.[42] The surgical decision-making process involves assessment of anatomical factors, including the bony anatomy, rib cage location, scapula location, and mediastinal contents, including the lung and diaphragm. The extent of calcification and the laterality of the disk herniation are important in directing the operative approach. The most important goal when choosing a surgical approach is to minimize manipulation of an already compromised thoracic spinal cord.

Determination of Correct Level

Diskectomy at the wrong level is not an infrequent problem in the thoracic spine.[39] Vertebral counting is often hindered by differences in individual regional anatomy, the amount of subcutaneous fat, obliquity of the spinous process, and poor visibility, especially in the high thoracic levels. Several preoperative marking strategies have been used, but errors still do occur, albeit in small numbers. Radiographic skin markers, percutaneous injection of methylene blue dye, placement of radiopaque markers at the periosteum of the pedicle, flexible hook-wire markers inserted into the soft tissues under CT guidance, and percutaneous placement of a K-wire into a "fixed point" such as the pedicle of interest under image guidance have all been described to minimize these errors.[43,44,45] With the widespread use of navigation, these techniques, some of which are invasive, may not be necessary.

Posterior

Historically, thoracic diskectomies were performed through a midline posterior approach in conjunction with extensive laminotomies or laminectomies to decompress the spinal cord. Retraction of the spinal cord is often necessary for adequate ventral exposure. Such retraction is responsible for up to 50% increase in incidence of neurologic deficits postoperatively and is directly attributable to the decline in this approach's popularity.[46]

Several modifications of the posterior approach have been developed to improve ventral exposure, including medial facetectomy, division of the dentate ligaments, and rhizotomy of the spinal nerves; however, such maneuvers have not altered the unacceptably high incidence of postoperative deficits.[47] In the current era, open direct midline approaches have no role in the treatment of herniated thoracic disks. However, with the advent of the endoscope in spine surgery, this approach is being revisited.[48,49]

Transpedicular

Posterolateral decompression by the transpedicular approach, originally described by Patterson and Arbit in 1978, provides better ventral exposure of centrolateral or lateral disk herniations.[50] Transpedicular diskectomies are performed through a midline incision; however, the subperiosteal dissection is continued laterally until the entire facet is exposed. Bony resection is kept to a minimum, with only a single facet joint and the superior aspect of the inferior pedicle being removed to gain access to the disk space. The transpedicular approach is less invasive and significantly decreases the amount of manipulation of the spinal cord required to access the intervertebral space. The surgery avoids problems associated with thoracotomy, rib resection, and extensive muscle dissection. Operating time and blood loss also appear to be less than with other surgeries. Bilateral laminectomies and dorsal fusion can also be performed after ventral decompression through the same skin incision without repositioning the patient. Although the transpedicular approach increases the risk of instability, this occurs uncommonly owing to the stabilizing effects of the bony thorax. This approach is sufficient for a soft lateral disk; however, a large central disk often requires extensive ventral decompression. Limited access across the midline ventral to the spinal cord makes the unilateral transpedicular approach less effective than anterior exposures for these large ventral lesions. A bilateral transpedicular exposure can provide midline access but requires a spinal reconstructive procedure.

Costotransversectomy

Hulme modified the costotransversectomy approach, which had previously been used for tuberculous spondylitis in Pott's disease of the spine, and applied it to herniated thoracic disks.[51] Approximately 6 cm of the adjacent rib is resected to gain access to the lateral aspect of the vertebral body and neural foramen. Costotransversectomy provides improved exposure of the ventral spinal canal with minimal resection of the facet joint compared with the transpedicular approach.[52] Similarly, dorsal fusion can be accomplished after ventral decompression, if required, without repositioning the patient.[53] The disadvantages of this procedure include extensive soft-tissue dissection and the risk of pneumothorax.

Lateral Extracavitary

Larson and colleagues introduced the lateral extracavitary approach as a derivative of the costotransversectomy.[54] Since it is an entirely extrapleural approach, it avoids the complications associated with the transthoracic approach and placement of a chest tube yet provides significant anterior paraspinal exposure. The approach entails resection of 6 to 8 cm of the dorsal rib. After the partial pediculectomies are performed to enlarge the intervertebral foramen, a posterior vertebral body trough is fashioned so that disk and osteophytes are elevated away from the dura, thus decompressing the thecal sac.[55] One major advantage of this procedure is the enhanced safety during the disk removal because of direct visualization of the dura mater before and during the decompression, which is facilitated by the removal of the pedicle as well as the ability to perform anterior interbody fusion and posterior spinal fusion through a single incision. It is a formidable operation with a potential for significant perioperative pain, a potential for a prolonged operating time, and considerable blood loss.

Anterolateral

The transthoracic approach, first described in 1958 by Crafoord et al, provides the greatest exposure to the anterior thoracic spine for ventral decompression as compared with any other procedure.[56] A lateral thoracotomy and trans- or extrapleural dissection provide access to the anterolateral aspect of the vertebral bodies. Additional exposure, if needed, is attained with a one- or two-level rib resection. Ventral decompression can be performed across the midline of the vertebral body with direct visualization of the anterior thecal sac. The risk of instability after diskectomy using this technique is less than with posterolateral approaches. The disadvantages include increased risk of pulmonary complications, subarachnoid–pleural fistula, and injuries of the great vessels, heart, liver, or diaphragm. Pulmonary disease is a relative contraindication to this approach.

Minimally Invasive Lateral Transthoracic Retro/Transpleural Approach Diskectomy

Recently, the mini–open anterolateral approach using a tubular retractor has been introduced to represent a middle-ground alternative between endoscopic and open-approach procedures for the treatment of thoracic disks. The procedure enters the thoracic cavity in the space between the ribs and uses direct visualization, generating an adequate working field for the disk space.[57] If the procedure is performed using a retropleural approach, it does not require single-lung intubation or a chest tube.

Thoracoscopic

Anterior approaches to the thoracic spine have also benefited from the advent of minimally invasive technologies. Thoracoscopic discectomy provides acceptable surgical results and has several distinct advantages, including reduced postoperative pain, morbidity, hospital stay, and recovery time, along with improved cosmetic results. The major disadvantage is a steep learning curve. Complications included dural tear, transient atelectasis, pleural effusions, and a hemothorax.[58] The technical

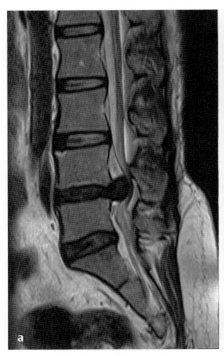
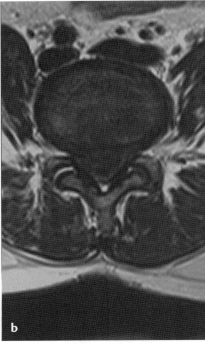

Fig. 21.3 T2-weighted (a) sagittal and (b) axial images of a 34-year-old woman who presented with an acute cauda equine syndrome and magnetic resonance imaging showing a large central L4–L5 disk prolapse with bilateral L5 nerve root compression. After an L4–L5 diskectomy, she made a complete recovery.

feasibility of the thoracoscopic approach has been sufficiently established and is ideally suited for the ventral thoracic disk herniation.

21.6.3 Prognosis

Long-term functional outcome after decompression appears to be related to the nature, rate of progression, severity, and duration of symptoms. There also appears to be a correlation between neurologic outcome with the timing of surgery and the operative approach selected. Neurologic outcome is variable in patients presenting with radicular complaints only. This is especially true for decompression of acute thoracic disk herniations presenting with pain. In their series of eight patients with an acute myelopathy due to thoracic disk herniation, Cornips at al[59] show that remarkable recovery is possible not only in myelopathy but also sphincter recovery even with profound neurologic deficit and a delay of several days, provided that the spinal cord is adequately decompressed. The greatest neurologic recovery commonly occurs within 6 weeks, but some patients may continue to improve for up to 2 years. Surgical excision of thoracic disk herniations via posterolateral and anterior approaches is reported to improve neurologic function in 75 to 100% of cases in the modern era.[39,48,55,57,58,59] Hence, however severe the presentation, every single patient with acute myelopathy due to thoracic disk herniation should be recommended surgical treatment.

21.7 Lumbar Spine

Lumbar discectomies account for approximately two thirds of all disk surgeries. Acute disk herniations occur more frequently in the fourth and fifth decades, which is significantly earlier than the peak age for symptomatic degenerative spinal disease.

Males account for 60% of acute lumbar disk herniations and are affected at a younger age than females.[60] Eighty percent of acute disk disease occurs at the L4–L5 and L5–S1 intervertebral disk spaces. This is most likely related to the lordotic curve, flexibility of the lumbar spine, and facet orientation. Clinical, radiographic, and biomechanical studies have shown an increased frequency of intervertebral disk disease with obliquely oriented facets.[61] Disk herniations occur most commonly through the posterolateral aspect of the anulus fibrosus where the anulus is relatively thin. In addition, the posterior longitudinal ligament is less adherent and provides less support to the anulus compared with the anterior longitudinal ligament (▶ Fig. 21.3).

21.7.1 Clinical Presentation

Large median or paramedian disk herniations producing a cauda equina syndrome account for 2 to 4% of operative lumbar disk herniations.[62,63] The symptoms and signs of cauda equina compression include asymmetrical sensory disturbances, pain, and weakness of the lower extremities. Symptoms may occur suddenly; however, most patients have a previous history of back pain or radiculopathy. Back and perianal pain often predominates, and radicular symptoms may be minimal. Sudden onset of cauda equina syndrome is associated with sphincter disturbances in greater than 50% of cases.[63] Urinary retention is likely to be painless secondary to deafferentation of the bladder. There is a strong association between intradural disk rupture and cauda equina syndrome as well.[64]

21.7.2 Surgical Approaches

Various nonoperative measures such as epidural and facetal injections, spinal manipulation, traction, ozone, and other pharmacotherapies have been tried with varying degrees of success for acute radiculopathy due to a herniated lumbar disk.[65,66] In a meta-analysis of randomized controlled trials, a short course of oral steroids, compared with placebo, resulted in modestly improved function and no improvement in pain.[67] Nearly universally accepted indications for early surgery include significant motor deficit, unmanageable refractory pain persisting for more than 6 to 12 weeks, and of course cauda equina syndrome.[68] Although controversy still persists regarding the timing of surgery for cauda equine syndrome, most surgeons recommend performing a surgical decompression with 24 hours.[69]

Posterior/Midline

Large median disk herniations may require bilateral exposure to decompress the cauda equina. Generous bilateral hemilaminectomies or laminectomies may be necessary to achieve adequate exposure without excessive retraction of the nerve roots or thecal sac. Posterolateral herniations are also approached by midline posterior procedures; however, a partial medial facetectomy is often required. Far-lateral disk herniations may be accessed via an extensive or even complete facetectomy, but this approach is associated with a relative increase in the risk of postoperative instability. Unilateral total facetectomy is associated with progressive instability in about 5% of cases.[70]

Paramedian

Paramedian approaches are used primarily for minimally invasive procedures and for decompression of far-lateral disk herniations, which account for less than 10% of all lumbar disk herniations.[71] Paramedian incisions with muscle splitting or midline incisions with lateral dissection are used to approach the lateral aspect of the facet. The advantages of these procedures include better exposure of lateral disk herniations, preservation of the facet joint and capsule, potentially reduced pain and discomfort, and early postoperative mobilization.

Anterior/Anterolateral

Transabdominal or retroperitoneal approaches to the anterior spine are rarely indicated in emergent surgical intervention for acute lumbar disk disease. These approaches are more commonly used for neoplasms or when and anterior interbody fusion is required. Anterior or anterolateral approaches provide adequate exposure to the ventral aspect of the spinal canal, and decompression may be performed with direct visualization of the anterior thecal sac. These approaches require repositioning of the patient and a separate skin incision if posterior stabilization is needed.

Minimally Invasive Lumbar Diskectomy

The modern era began with a combination of the traditional microsurgical disk removal with endoscopic viewing assistance, for which the term *microendoscopic diskectomy* (MED) was coined.[72] The technique is essentially the same as the open operation, but it is performed with a surgical endoscope or, more commonly today, an operative microscope. We prefer the microscope with its stereoscopic vision rather than the two-dimensional images of the endoscope. The fundamental objective is to reduce the scope and size of the incision and the resultant tissue disruption, thereby reducing hospital stay and postoperative recovery. On average, the mean hospital stay is 9.5 hours, making same-day discharge a reality. Conceptually, operative access is achieved through a paramedian muscle-splitting approach and then dilatation through a series of progressively larger tubes that eventually creates a working port of about 22 to 26 mm in width from which to perform the surgical procedure. This working port concept changed the operation substantially, and subperiosteal muscle dissection was replaced with an efficient muscle-splitting approach. Once surface landmarks are reconciled with the fluoroscopic image, the surgery proceeds in the traditional fashion: laminotomy, medial facetectomy, foraminotomy, ligamentum flavum removal, nerve root/thecal sac retraction, and disk incision and removal. Closure involves reapproximating the fascia and closing the small stab skin incision. It has been the authors' experience that this approach is actually easier in very obese patients because the muscle-splitting dilatation is technically easier than a deep subperiosteal dissection and the attendant retraction of a substantial muscle mass. Although minimally invasive discectomies are growing in popularity and have high reported success rates, it is important to acknowledge that a meta-analysis of prospective, randomized trials has not demonstrated them to be superior to the traditional open microsurgical diskectomy.[73]

21.7.3 Prognosis

Prognostic indicators of functional outcome after surgical intervention include preoperative neurologic status, acuteness and duration of symptoms, and bladder dysfunction. In general, patients with the rapid onset of symptoms and signs are less likely to have complete recovery of function postoperatively compared with those with slowly progressive deterioration[68,70,73]; however, functional outcome is also decreased in patients with prolonged duration of symptoms and surgical delay. Motor weakness is more likely to improve after surgical intervention as compared with bladder, bowel, or sensory disturbances.[69] Sensory deficits are least likely to resolve. Patients with more extensive weakness or sphincter involvement have relatively worse functional recovery.

21.8 Conclusion

Acute disk herniations resulting in severe or progressive neurologic deficits that require emergent decompression occur infrequently. Acute herniations tend to produce more severe neurologic dysfunction than spondylotic disease of the spine. Acute disk herniations secondary to trauma, bending, or lifting are reported infrequently in most series. Initial evaluation should include a detailed neurologic examination and prompt high-resolution MRI. Indications for urgent surgical intervention include acute severe or rapidly progressive neurologic deterioration, myelopathy, and bowel or bladder dysfunction.

The surgical approaches are based on clinical presentation, level and location of the disk herniation, and the need for postdecompression stabilization. Prognostic indicators of functional neurologic recovery include type, severity, and duration of symptoms. There is no consensus regarding optimal timing of decompression; however, it appears that early surgical intervention is associated with a better prognosis compared with delayed surgical treatment.

References

[1] Harris RI, Macnab I. Structural changes in the lumbar intervertebral discs; their relationship to low back pain and sciatica. J Bone Joint Surg Br. 1954; 36-B(2):304–322

[2] Fontes RB de V, Baptista JS, Rabbani SR, Traynelis VC, Liberti EA. Structural and ultrastructural analysis of the cervical discs of young and elderly humans. PLoS ONE. 2015; 10(10):e0139283

[3] Dagistan Y, Cukur S, Dagistan E, Gezici AR. Importance of IL-6, MMP-1, IGF-1, and BAX levels in lumbar herniated disks and posterior longitudinal ligament in patients with sciatic pain. World Neurosurg. 2015; 84(6):1739–1746

[4] Wang C, Wang W-J, Yan Y-G, et al. MicroRNAs: new players in intervertebral disc degeneration. Clin Chim Acta. 2015; 450(X):333–341

[5] Nurick S. The pathogenesis of the spinal cord disorder associated with cervical spondylosis. Brain. 1972; 95(1):87–100

[6] Revanappa KK, Rajshekhar V. Comparison of Nurick grading system and modified Japanese Orthopaedic Association scoring system in evaluation of patients with cervical spondylotic myelopathy. Eur Spine J. 2011; 20(9):1545–1551

[7] Fairbank JCT. Why are there different versions of the Oswestry Disability Index? J Neurosurg Spine. 2014; 20(1):83–86

[8] Vernon H. The Neck Disability Index: state-of-the-art, 1991–2008. J Manipulative Physiol Ther. 2008; 31(7):491–502

[9] Frymoyer J (ed). The adult spine: Principles and practice (2nd edition). Lippincott-Raven; 1997.

[10] Nuñez DB, Jr, Zuluaga A, Fuentes-Bernardo DA, Rivas LA, Becerra JL. Cervical spine trauma: how much more do we learn by routinely using helical CT? Radiographics. 1996; 16(6):1307–1318, discussion 1318–1321

[11] Oikawa Y, Eguchi Y, Inoue G, et al. Diffusion tensor imaging of lumbar spinal nerve in subjects with degenerative lumbar disorders. Magn Reson Imaging. 2015; 33(8):956–961

[12] Lunsford LD, Bissonette DJ, Jannetta PJ, Sheptak PE, Zorub DS. Anterior surgery for cervical disc disease. Part 1: treatment of lateral cervical disc herniation in 253 cases. J Neurosurg. 1980; 53(1):1–11

[13] Radhakrishnan K, Litchy WJ, O'Fallon WM, Kurland LT. Epidemiology of cervical radiculopathy. A population-based study from Rochester, Minnesota, 1976 through 1990. Brain. 1994; 117(Pt 2):325–335

[14] Westwick HJ, Goldstein CL, Shamji MF. Acute spontaneous cervical disc herniation causing rapidly progressive myelopathy in a patient with comorbid ossified posterior longitudinal ligament: case report and literature review. Surg Neurol Int. 2014; 5(Suppl 7):S368–S372

[15] Goh HK, Li YH. Non-traumatic acute paraplegia caused by cervical disc herniation in a patient with sleep apnoea. Singapore Med J. 2004; 45(5):235–238

[16] Liu C, Huang Y, Cai H-X, Fan S-W. Nontraumatic acute paraplegia associated with cervical disk herniation. J Spinal Cord Med. 2010; 33(4):420–424

[17] Suzuki T, Abe E, Murai H, Kobayashi T. Nontraumatic acute complete paraplegia resulting from cervical disc herniation: a case report. Spine. 2003; 28(6):E125–E128

[18] Ueyama T, Tamaki N, Kondoh T, Miyamoto H, Akiyama H, Nagashima T. Non-traumatic acute paraplegia associated with cervical disc herniation: a case report. Surg Neurol. 1999; 52(2):204–206, discussion 206–207

[19] Cheong HS, Hong BY, Ko Y-A, Lim SH, Kim JS. Spinal cord injury incurred by neck massage. Ann Rehabil Med. 2012; 36(5):708–712

[20] Eisenberg RA, Bremer AM, Northup HM. Intradural herniated cervical disk: a case report and review of the literature. AJNR Am J Neuroradiol. 1986; 7(3):492–494

[21] Hsieh J-H, Wu C-T, Lee S-T. Cervical intradural disc herniation after spinal manipulation therapy in a patient with ossification of posterior longitudinal ligament: a case report and review of the literature. Spine. 2010; 35(5):E149–E151

[22] Lourie H, Shende MC, Stewart DH, Jr. The syndrome of central cervical soft disk herniation. JAMA. 1973; 226(3):302–305

[23] Doran SE, Papadopoulos SM, Ducker TB, Lillehei KO. Magnetic resonance imaging documentation of coexistent traumatic locked facets of the cervical spine and disc herniation. J Neurosurg. 1993; 79(3):341–345

[24] Cotler JM, Herbison GJ, Nasuti JF, Ditunno JF, Jr, An H, Wolff BE. Closed reduction of traumatic cervical spine dislocation using traction weights up to 140 pounds. Spine. 1993; 18(3):386–390

[25] Eismont FJ, Arena MJ, Green BA. Extrusion of an intervertebral disc associated with traumatic subluxation or dislocation of cervical facets. Case report. J Bone Joint Surg Am. 1991; 73(10):1555–1560

[26] Lee JY, Nassr A, Eck JC, Vaccaro AR. Controversies in the treatment of cervical spine dislocations. Spine J. 2009; 9(5):418–423

[27] Hadley MN, Walters BC, Grabb PA, et al. Guidelines for the management of acute cervical spine and spinal cord injuries. Clin Neurosurg. 2002; 49:407–498

[28] Walters BC, Hadley MN, Hurlbert RJ, et al; American Association of Neurological Surgeons. Congress of Neurological Surgeons. Guidelines for the management of acute cervical spine and spinal cord injuries: 2013 update. Neurosurgery. 2013; 60(Suppl 1):82–91

[29] Branch BC, Hilton DL, Jr, Watts C. Minimally invasive tubular access for posterior cervical foraminotomy. Surg Neurol Int. 2015; 6:81

[30] Verbiest H. The lateral approach to the cervical spine. Clin Neurosurg. 1973; 20:295–305

[31] Cloward RB. The anterior approach for removal of ruptured cervical disks. J Neurosurg. 1958; 15(6):602–617

[32] Robinson RA, Smith GW. Anterolateral cervical disc removal and interbody fusion for cervical disc syndrome. Bull Johns Hopkins Hosp. 1955; 96:223–224

[33] Burkus JK, Traynelis VC, Haid RW, Jr, Mummaneni PV. Clinical and radiographic analysis of an artificial cervical disc: 7-year follow-up from the Prestige prospective randomized controlled clinical trial. J Neurosurg Spine. 2014; 21(4):516–528

[34] Hacker RJ, Cauthen JC, Gilbert TJ, Griffith SL. A prospective randomized multicenter clinical evaluation of an anterior cervical fusion cage. Spine. 2000; 25(20):2646–2654, discussion 2655

[35] Röllinghoff M, Zarghooni K, Hackenberg L, Zeh A, Radetzki F, Delank KS. Quality of life and radiological outcome after cervical cage fusion and cervical disc arthroplasty. Acta Orthop Belg. 2012; 78(3):369–375

[36] Carson J, Gumpert J, Jefferson A. Diagnosis and treatment of thoracic intervertebral disc protrusions. J Neurol Neurosurg Psychiatry. 1971; 34(1):68–77

[37] Stillerman CB, Chen TC, Couldwell WT, Zhang W, Weiss MH. Experience in the surgical management of 82 symptomatic herniated thoracic discs and review of the literature. J Neurosurg. 1998; 88(4):623–633

[38] Arce CA, Dohrmann GJ. Herniated thoracic disks. Neurol Clin. 1985; 3(2):383–392

[39] Vanichkachorn JS, Vaccaro AR. Thoracic disk disease: diagnosis and treatment. J Am Acad Orthop Surg. 2000; 8(3):159–169

[40] Yano S, Hida K, Seki T, Iwasaki Y, Akino M, Saitou H. [A case of thoracic disc herniation with sudden onset paraplegia on toilet straining: case report] No Shinkei Geka. 2003; 31(12):1297–1301

[41] Reynolds JM, Belvadi YS, Kane AG, Poulopoulos M. Thoracic disc herniation leads to anterior spinal artery syndrome demonstrated by diffusion-weighted magnetic resonance imaging (DWI): a case report and literature review. Spine J. 2014; 14(6):e17–e22

[42] Yoshihara H. Surgical treatment for thoracic disc herniation: an update. Spine. 2014; 39(6):E406–E412

[43] Paolini S, Ciappetta P, Missori P, Raco A, Delfini R. Spinous process marking: a reliable method for preoperative surface localization of intradural lesions of the high thoracic spine. Br J Neurosurg. 2005; 19(1):74–76

[44] Binning MJ, Schmidt MH. Percutaneous placement of radiopaque markers at the pedicle of interest for preoperative localization of thoracic spine level. Spine. 2010; 35(19):1821–1825

[45] Hsu W, Sciubba DM, Sasson AD, et al. Intraoperative localization of thoracic spine level with preoperative percutaneous placement of intravertebral polymethylmethacrylate. J Spinal Disord Tech. 2008; 21(1):72–75

[46] Logue V. Thoracic intervertebral disc prolapse with spinal cord compression. J Neurol Neurosurg Psychiatry. 1952; 15(4):227–241

[47] Ravichandran G, Frankel HL. Paraplegia due to intervertebral disc lesions: a review of 57 operated cases. Paraplegia. 1981; 19(3):133–139

[48] Choi KY, Eun SS, Lee SH, Lee HY. Percutaneous endoscopic thoracic discectomy; transforaminal approach. Minim Invasive Neurosurg. 2010; 53(1):25–28

[49] Smith JS, Eichholz KM, Shafizadeh S, Ogden AT, O'Toole JE, Fessler RG. Minimally invasive thoracic microendoscopic diskectomy: surgical technique and case series. World Neurosurg. 2013; 80(3–4):421–427

[50] Patterson RH, Jr, Arbit E. A surgical approach through the pedicle to protruded thoracic discs. J Neurosurg. 1978; 48(5):768–772

[51] Hulme A. The surgical approach to thoracic intervertebral disc protrusions. J Neurol Neurosurg Psychiatry. 1960; 23:133–137

[52] Kshettry VR, Healy AT, Jones NG, Mroz TE, Benzel EC. A quantitative analysis of posterolateral approaches to the ventral thoracic spinal canal. Spine J. 2015; 15(10):2228–2238

[53] Sagan LM, Madany L, Lickendorf M. [Costotransversectomy and interbody fusion for treatment of thoracic dyscopathy] Ann Acad Med Stetin. 2007; 53(1):23–26

[54] Larson SJ, Holst RA, Hemmy DC, Sances A, Jr. Lateral extracavitary approach to traumatic lesions of the thoracic and lumbar spine. J Neurosurg. 1976; 45(6):628–637

[55] Maiman DJ, Larson SJ, Luck E, El-Ghatit A. Lateral extracavitary approach to the spine for thoracic disc herniation: report of 23 cases. Neurosurgery. 1984; 14(2):178–182

[56] Crafoord C, Hiertonn T, Lindblom K, Olsson SE. Spinal cord compression caused by a protruded thoracic disc; report of a case treated with antero-lateral fenestration of the disc. Acta Orthop Scand. 1958; 28(2):103–107

[57] Kasliwal MK, Deutsch H. Minimally invasive retropleural approach for central thoracic disc herniation. Minim Invasive Neurosurg. 2011; 54(4):167–171

[58] Han PP, Kenny K, Dickman CA. Thoracoscopic approaches to the thoracic spine: experience with 241 surgical procedures. Neurosurgery. 2002; 51(5, Suppl):S88–S95

[59] Cornips EMJ, Janssen MLF, Beuls EAM. Thoracic disc herniation and acute myelopathy: clinical presentation, neuroimaging findings, surgical considerations, and outcome. J Neurosurg Spine. 2011; 14(4):520–528

[60] Friberg S, Hirsch C. Anatomical and clinical studies on lumbar disc degeneration. Acta Orthop Scand. 1949; 19(2):222–242, illust

[61] Farfan HF, Sullivan JD. The relation of facet orientation to intervertebral disc failure. Can J Surg. 1967; 10(2):179–185

[62] Raaf J. Removal of protruded lumbar intervertebral discs. J Neurosurg. 1970; 32(5):604–611

[63] Gleave JR, MacFarlane R. Prognosis for recovery of bladder function following lumbar central disc prolapse. Br J Neurosurg. 1990; 4(3):205–209

[64] Dinning TA, Schaeffer HR. Discogenic compression of the cauda equina: a surgical emergency. Aust N Z J Surg. 1993; 63(12):927–934

[65] Spijker-Huiges A, Vermeulen K, Winters JC, van Wijhe M, van der Meer K. Costs and cost-effectiveness of epidural steroids for acute lumbosacral radicular syndrome in general practice: an economic evaluation alongside a pragmatic randomized control trial. Spine. 2014; 39(24):2007–2012

[66] Melchionda D, Milillo P, Manente G, Stoppino L, Macarini L. Treatment of radiculopathies: a study of efficacy and tollerability of paravertebral oxygen-ozone injections compared with pharmacological anti-inflammatory treatment. J Biol Regul Homeost Agents. 2012; 26(3):467–474

[67] Goldberg H, Firtch W, Tyburski M, et al. Oral steroids for acute radiculopathy due to a herniated lumbar disk: a randomized clinical trial. JAMA. 2015; 313(19):1915–1923

[68] Baldwin NG. Lumbar disc disease: the natural history. Neurosurg Focus. 2002; 13(2):E2

[69] Srikandarajah N, Boissaud-Cooke MA, Clark S, Wilby MJ. Does early surgical decompression in cauda equina syndrome improve bladder outcome? Spine. 2015; 40(8):580–583

[70] Garrido E, Connaughton PN. Unilateral facetectomy approach for lateral lumbar disc herniation. J Neurosurg. 1991; 74(5):754–756

[71] Pirris SM, Dhall S, Mummaneni PV, Kanter AS. Minimally invasive approach to extraforaminal disc herniations at the lumbosacral junction using an operating microscope: case series and review of the literature. Neurosurg Focus. 2008; 25(2):E10

[72] Maroon JC. Current concepts in minimally invasive discectomy. Neurosurgery. 2002; 51(5, Suppl):S137–S145

[73] Rasouli MR, Rahimi-Movaghar V, Shokraneh F, Moradi-Lakeh M, Chou R. Minimally invasive discectomy versus microdiscectomy/open discectomy for symptomatic lumbar disc herniation. Cochrane Database Syst Rev. 2014(9):CD010328

22 Is Cervical Stenosis An Emergency?

Daipayan Guha, Allan R. Martin, and Michael G. Fehlings

Abstract

Cervical spinal canal stenosis may lead to chronic progressive myelopathy from static and/or dynamic cord compression. However, in certain patients, cervical stenosis can result in rapid deterioration or may predispose healthy individuals to acute spinal cord injury following relatively mild trauma. The evaluation of patients with suspected cervical stenosis includes the radiographic determination of osseous and soft-tissue canal encroachment, with multiple grading systems with poor predictive value for the likelihood of future neurologic deterioration. Although the overall likelihood of catastrophic injury in patients with preexisting cervical stenosis appears minimal, in this chapter three clinical scenarios in which acute surgical intervention should be considered more carefully are reviewed. In patients with rapidly progressive degenerative cervical myelopathy, although the precise timing of surgical decompression has not yet been studied explicitly, postoperative functional outcomes are highly dependent on baseline status; hence, surgical decompression within days of clinical presentation may be appropriate. In cases of acute traumatic central cord syndrome, patients should be monitored closely and early surgical decompression considered within 1 to 3 days for patients with persistent deficits and ongoing radiographic compression. In patients with cervical cord neurapraxia, a condition most commonly seen in athletes, neurologic status should be carefully monitored for improvement over the first 1 to 3 days following injury, to distinguish this diagnosis from other injuries that require urgent surgical intervention.

Keywords: central cord syndrome, cervical neurapraxia, cervical stenosis, myelopathy, surgical decompression, surgical timing

22.1 Introduction

Stenosis of the cervical spinal canal may lead to progressive myelopathy due to static and/or dynamic cord compression, which is most commonly observed as a chronic process occurring over months to years.[1] However, in a subset of patients, cervical stenosis can cause rapidly progressive deterioration.[2] Furthermore, stenosis of the cervical canal may predispose individuals to acute spinal cord injury (SCI) following a traumatic insult, which may occur with a relatively innocuous mechanism.[3]

In cadaveric studies, the incidence of osseous cervical stenosis has been estimated to be 4.9% of the adult North American population, rising to 6.8% in those over 50 and 9% in those over 70 years of age.[4] The true prevalence of cervical stenosis is likely higher when soft-tissue canal encroachment is accounted for, particularly among susceptible Asian populations. In a Japanese population-based cohort of 977 subjects, 24.4% showed cervical cord compression on magnetic resonance imaging (MRI), the vast majority of which were clinically asymptomatic.[5] Degenerative disorders are by far the commonest etiology of cervical stenosis, including soft-tissue encroachment from protruding or herniated disks, buckling, hypertrophy and/or ossification of the intervertebral ligaments, bony remodeling (spondylosis) and osteophyte formation, and joint hypermobility and listhesis.[1]

Although some have advocated for prophylactic surgical decompression to prevent acute or progressive tetraparesis,[6] the likelihood of catastrophic injury in patients with preexisting cervical stenosis appears to be minimal.[7,8] The aim of this chapter is to review the management of clinical syndromes, in patients with preexisting congenital or degenerative cervical stenosis, in which acute surgical intervention may be warranted.

22.2 Initial Evaluation

A complete history and thorough neurologic evaluation should be performed in all patients presenting with clinical symptoms of cervical cord or nerve root dysfunction, and it may assist in distinguishing vascular, neoplastic, infectious, inflammatory, or traumatic etiologies of acute deterioration. The clinical examination may also guide the choice of subsequent radiographic studies. Degenerative cervical myelopathy (DCM) typically presents with one or more of the following symptoms, which constitute the modified Japanese Orthopedic Association (mJOA) score: hand dyscoordination, gait dysfunction, hand numbness and paresthesias, and bowel/bladder dysfunction. Patients may also show axial neck pain, Lhermitte's phenomenon, upper and lower extremity hyperreflexia, weakness and muscle atrophy, fasciculations, and neuropathic pain. However, the clinical presentation of DCM is highly variable, and there is no single symptom or sign that is reliably present.[1,5]

22.3 Radiographic Evaluation

In the current era, patients with any symptoms or signs consistent with cervical myelopathy should be investigated with MRI, barring any contraindications, to evaluate for cervical spinal cord compression. Radiographic work-up may also include anteroposterior (AP) and lateral X-rays of the cervical spine, with selected patients benefiting from dynamic lateral flexion–extension views to assess bony instability. Computed tomography (CT) may also be beneficial to visualize bony anatomy and identify ossification of ligamentous structures. In patients who cannot undergo MRI, CT myelography is an acceptable alternative for identifying and visualizing spinal cord compression.

Cervical stenosis historically has been defined on plain radiographs by the segmental sagittal canal diameter, measured from the midposterior vertebral body to the most anterior point on the corresponding spinolaminar line (▶Fig. 22.1).[9] Sagittal diameters of less than 14 mm are considered stenotic. To minimize interrater variability and to account for differences in X-ray magnification, Torg and Pavlov and colleagues subsequently defined an eponymous ratio of the sagittal canal diameter to vertebral body diameter (▶Fig. 22.1).[10] Numerous cutoffs for Torg–Pavlov ratios have been described, with a ratio < 0.8 portending increased risk of cervical cord neurapraxia (CCN) in

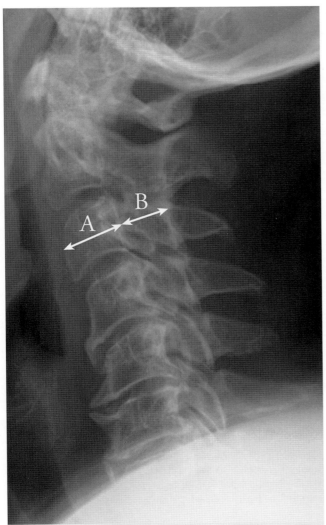

Fig. 22.1 Lateral cervical spine X-ray. Vertebral body width shown by arrow A. Segmental sagittal canal diameter shown by arrow B. Torg–Pavlov ratio is defined as B/A.

normal; grade 1, obliteration of the anterior or posterior CSF space by greater than 50%; grade 2, cord compression or displacement; and grade 3, cord compression or displacement with intramedullary T2 hyperintensity.[18] Torg et al have also defined a "functional reserve" of the cervical cord on MRI, the ratio of the sagittal AP cord diameter to the spinal canal diameter at the adjacent disk level (▶ Fig. 22.2).[19]

22.4 Indications for Acute Surgical Intervention

The timing of surgical intervention for patients with cervical stenosis is controversial. Patients with rapidly progressive myelopathy or persistent neurologic deficits following an acute traumatic incident, with radiographic evidence of ongoing cord compression, warrant consideration for emergent surgical decompression. In contrast, neurologically intact patients or those with improving deficits and without frank spinal instability, even in the presence of radiographic cord compression, are not necessarily appropriate for urgent surgery. We review here three clinical syndromes, in the setting of existing cervical stenosis, in which emergent decompression merits consideration: rapidly progressive DCM, acute cervical spinal cord injury (SCI) with tetraparesis, a subset of which includes acute traumatic central cord syndrome (tCCS), and cervical cord neurapraxia (CCN).

22.4.1 Degenerative Cervical Myelopathy

Nontraumatic degenerative etiologies of cervical myelopathy constitute the commonest cause of spinal cord impairment in the elderly.[20] DCM encompasses the pathologies of degenerative disk disease (DDD), cervical spondylotic myelopathy (CSM), ossification of the posterior longitudinal ligament (OPLL), and ossification of the ligamentum flavum (OLF).

The prevalence of DCM has been estimated at up to 605 per million in North America, increasing with age and more common in males.[21] Population estimates of OPLL in isolation are between 1.5 and 4.3%, depending on the population studied.[22] In cross-sectional studies, OLF has been found in 3.8% of Asian populations, predominantly in the lower thoracic spine.[23] OLF as the sole lesion underlying cervical myelopathy has been described rarely in case reports.[24]

Pathophysiology

Neurologic impairment in DCM may result from static cord compression, altered cord tension from global cervical malalignment, and repetitive dynamic injury due to segmental hypermobility. Cord compression may result from protruding annulus fibrosus or herniated nucleus pulposus in DDD, with more severe spondylosis resulting in posterior osteophytosis as well as buckling and laxity of the canal ligaments associated with CSM. Osseous narrowing anterior or posterior to the cord is seen in OPLL and OLF, respectively (▶ Fig. 22.3). Multiple ischemic, inflammatory, and immune pathways have been implicated in the subsequent responses to chronic cord compression.[21]

the original study[10] and < 0.7 associated with increased risk of acute spinal cord injury (SCI) following minor trauma.[11] Plain radiographs remain imperfect, however, with Torg–Pavlov ratios corresponding poorly to the true canal diameter measured on CT[12] and varying significantly with age, gender, and ethnicity.[13] Unsurprisingly, the predictive value of the Torg–Pavlov ratio for neurologic deterioration in patients with preexisting stenosis is questionable.[14,15,16]

Although CT imaging provides accurate measurements of the bony canal diameter, the resolution of MRI in assessing soft-tissue canal encroachment, as well as the true space available for the cord, is unparalleled. Multiple grading systems for the assessment of cervical stenosis on MRI have been proposed. Muhle et al developed a 4-point scale, with grade 0 defined as normal, grade 1, partial obliteration of the anterior or posterior cerebrospinal fluid (CSF) space; grade 2, complete obliteration of the CSF space; and grade 3, compression or displacement of the cord.[17] This was subsequently modified by Kang et al to improve predictive performance, such that grade 0 indicates

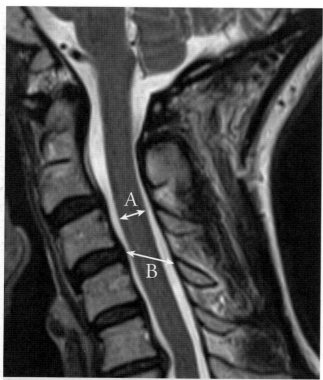

Fig. 22.2 Midsagittal cervical spine T2-weighted MRI. Spinal cord diameter shown by arrow A. Adjacent disk-level canal diameter shown by arrow B. "Space available for cord" (SAC) is defined as (B − A). "Functional reserve" is defined as A/B.

Natural History

The vast majority of patients with cervical stenosis do not develop clinical myelopathy. In one of the largest studies to date of a predominantly elderly population, 24% showed radiographic cervical cord compression, with no association between cord compression and the development of myelopathic signs.[5] Among patients with asymptomatic cervical cord compression of any etiology identified on MRI, a ystematic review has identified the risk of developing clinical myelopathy at 8% at 1 year, and 23% at a median of 44 months.[25] Age, gender, Torg–Pavlov ratios, and the mechanism of cervical cord compression are all not associated with the development of clinical myelopathy in asymptomatic patients.[25,26] Of patients who do develop clinical myelopathy, it is estimated that 20 to 60% will deteriorate neurologically over 2 years without surgical intervention.[1,26]

Classically, the time course of neurologic deterioration in patients with clinical myelopathy has been described as stepwise in 75%, and slowly progressive over years in 20%.[27] For these patients, surgical decompression if indicated is performed on an elective basis. Much less common, constituting the remaining 5%, are scenarios involving the acute development of myelopathy or rapidly progressive myelopathy, which merit consideration for urgent surgery within days of presentation. These patients may be categorized into three groups:

1. Group I: rapidly progressive myelopathy, without antecedent trauma.
2. Group II: new myelopathy following minor trauma in a patient with preexisting stenosis.
3. Group III: rapid exacerbation of existing myelopathy, following minor trauma in a patient with preexisting stenosis.

Among patients with symptomatic myelopathy, 5 to 18% may be classified as group I.[2,27] In a retrospective review of an Asian population, up to 28% of patients presenting with cervical

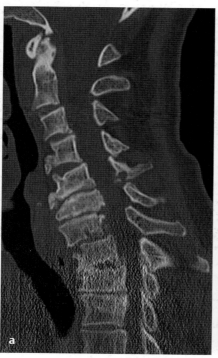
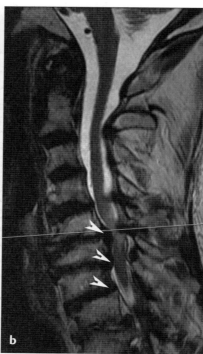

Fig. 22.3 Midsagittal cervical spine **(a)** computed tomography and **(b)** T2-weighted magnetic resonance imaging, demonstrating cervical spondylotic myelopathy and evidence of degenerative disk disease, most significantly at C5–C6, C6–C7, and C7–T1 (arrowheads). Cord compression with intramedullary T2 signal change is also demonstrated.

myelopathy were categorized in group II and 20% in group III.[28] Although the precise timing of surgical decompression in patients with rapidly progressive myelopathy has not been studied explicitly, it is well known that baseline neurologic and functional status portend postoperative functional outcome.[29] Early surgical decompression, within days of clinical presentation, is therefore reasonable for appropriate surgical candidates. Markers predicting rapidly progressive symptomatology have yet to be identified; however, some studies have reported associations between a fibroadipose–vascular epidural membrane at the most focal segment of compression, seen intraoperatively, and the development of rapidly progressive myelopathy.[2,30]

22.4.2 Acute Traumatic Central Cord Syndrome

Acute traumatic central cord syndrome (tCCS) was first described by Schneider in 1954 as an incomplete SCI, characterized by weakness predominantly in the upper extremities, bladder dysfunction typically with urinary retention, and various patterns of sensory deficit below the level of injury.[31] tCCS is the commonest type of incomplete SCI, representing approximately 16 to 25% of all SCI and increasing as the population ages.[32]

tCCS is seen most commonly following motor vehicle accidents, falls, and diving accidents, resulting in hyperextension or, less frequently, hyperflexion injuries. Three distinct groups of patients have been described: younger patients (< 50 years of age) with severe traumatic fracture/dislocation and cord compression, older patients (> 50 years of age) with hyperextension injury without fracture in the context of a stenotic cervical spine, and younger patients sustaining a low-velocity injury resulting in acute central disk herniation without bony injury.[33,34,35,36] Among patients with tCCS, cervical stenosis of various etiologies is seen in 50 to 65% of patients (▶ Fig. 22.4).[36,37] A greater degree of stenosis may be correlated with poorer neurologic recovery, independent of surgical intervention.[38]

Pathophysiology

Following hyperextension injury in spondylotic canals, inward buckling of the ligamentum flavum is presumed to compress the spinal cord against disk–osteophyte complexes anteriorly. Microvascular ischemia results in selective damage to the most medial white matter tracts located within the lateral funiculi, consistent with the anatomical location of the lateral corticospinal and rubrospinal tracts. These tracts have been shown evolutionarily to be progressively important for upper extremity and hand function, supporting the clinical findings of predominantly upper extremity weakness.[34]

Natural History

Some degree of neurologic recovery is made in more than 75% of patients with tCCS with conservative management. Age appears to be the strongest predictor of prognosis; patients younger than 50 years of age regain independent ambulation in almost all cases, dropping to less than 40% of those older

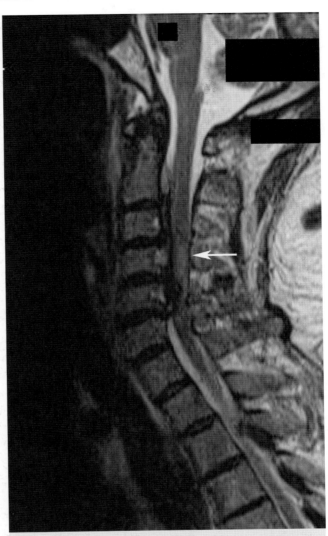

Fig. 22.4 Midsagittal cervical spine T2-weighted magnetic resonance imaging, in a patient with acute traumatic central cord syndrome. Cervical stenosis with intramedullary T2 signal change (arrow) is demonstrated, secondary to ossification of the posterior longitudinal ligament and mild cervical spondylosis.

than 70 years.[39] Neurologic function tends to return first in the lower extremities, followed by the bladder and proximal upper extremities. Recovery of hand function is often limited and is the primary cause of long-term functional impairment in tCCS patients.[40]

Treatment Options

Following Schneider's initial observations of spontaneous neurologic recovery in six patients with tCCS, multiple series with short-term follow-up have echoed the potential for recovery without surgical intervention.[39,40,41] However, in series following patients several years post injury, up to 25% of patients had eventual plateau and subsequent decline in neurologic function due to persistent cord compression.[42] Surgical decompression for patients with nonimproving deficits and evidence of radiographic cord compression was therefore revisited, and it was shown in multiple studies to allow faster and more complete neurologic recovery while minimizing immobility-related complications and hospital length of stay (LOS).[43,44,45]

The optimal timing of surgical decompression in tCCS remains uncertain. Although the initial surgical series for tCCS demonstrated improved neurologic recovery even when delayed by several months, after failure of conservative therapy, there has been a growing body of evidence in favor of surgery in the subacute period post injury.[43,44] In a retrospective review of 114 patients, Chen et al demonstrated improved motor and sensory recovery with surgical decompression, particularly in younger patients, with more rapid motor improvement in patients operated on within 1 to 2 weeks of injury.[46] In 23 surgical patients, Yamazaki et al demonstrated improved motor recovery and postoperative JOA scores at 44-month follow-up, for patients operated on within versus later than 2 weeks.[38] Other studies have demonstrated improved motor outcomes with surgery within 24 hours, specifically in patients with acute fracture/dislocations or disk herniations,[47] or in those with profound initial neurologic deficits (American Spinal Injury Association [ASIA] grade C or worse) and persistent cord compression.[32] In a prospective cohort study of cervical SCI, surgical decompression within 24 hours was shown to significantly improve the odds of a 2-grade improvement in ASIA Impairment Scale (AIS) at 6-month follow-up; however, this study was not limited to tCCS, and roughly one third of the patients had complete SCI.[48] In contrast, one retrospective study of 49 surgical patients, with almost 5-year follow-up, found no difference in AIS score between patients undergoing decompression before or after 4 days.[49] Similarly, Kepler et al found no effect of surgical intervention within 24 hours on motor recovery and intensive care unit (ICU) or overall LOS, in patients with bony injury or with hyperextension in the context of a spondylotic canal.[50]

The current evidence for the timing of surgery for tCCS is best summarized in a systematic review by Anderson et al.[51] Early surgical decompression, within 2 weeks of injury, is likely beneficial for long-term neurologic and functional outcomes, particularly in patients with ongoing radiographic cord compression and persistent or nonimproving motor deficits after a few days. However, in patients with fracture–dislocations or frank instability, surgery within 72 hours rather than 2 weeks may be considered to promote early mobilization and minimize confinement-related complications. Patients undergoing surgical decompression in delayed fashion, after 2 weeks, retain the potential for long-term neurologic improvement; however, this may occur more slowly and incompletely than if surgery is performed early.[52]

22.4.3 Cervical Cord Neurapraxia

CCN is defined as a transient cervical neurologic deficit following a traumatic insult.[10] It has been best described in athletes, particularly football and professional soccer players, with an incidence of 1.3 to 6 per 10,000.[53] Reports of non–sports-related CCN have also been described.[54]

Up to 86% of cases are associated with cervical stenosis on the basis of a Torg–Pavlov ratio of less than 0.8.[19] However, multiple subsequent studies have demonstrated that the Torg–Pavlov ratio has high sensitivity but poor positive predictive value for

the future development of CCN in asymptomatic athletes.[15] MRI measurements of "functional reserve," and the similar "space available for cord" (SAC), i.e., the sagittal cord diameter subtracted from the disk-level canal diameter, have shown better predictive value: a SAC of less than 5 mm has 80% sensitivity and a negative predictive value of 0.23 for the future risk of developing CCN.[55]

Pathophysiology

CCN typically results from an acute hyperextension injury on the background of a stenotic cervical canal, resulting in temporary derangement of axonal permeability.[56] Rapid axonal stretch leads to altered ion currents and prolonged depolarization, as well as microvascular constriction and vasospasm.

Natural History

By definition, neurologic impairment in CCN is transient, with eventual complete resolution of all motor and sensory deficits. Patients may be classified according to their duration of neurologic symptoms: grade I, less than 15 minutes; grade II, 15 minutes to 24 hours; grade III, more than 24 hours.[19] Patients may also be classified on the basis of anatomical pattern of deficits: affecting all four extremities, the upper extremities only, the lower extremities only, or a hemibody distribution.[19]

Recurrence of CCN is seen in up to 56% of patients and may be career-ending for some athletes.[19] Lower Torg–Pavlov ratios and disk-level canal diameters appear to predispose individuals to an increased risk of recurrence; however, there does not appear to be any significantly increased risk of permanent catastrophic SCI if the CSF space around the cord is preserved.[7]

Treatment Options

Surgical decompression for CCN has been reserved for patients with ongoing focal compressive pathology at the neurologically injured level.[19,57] If indicated, surgery is typically performed on an elective basis, prior to return to contact activities for athletes. The clinical history and physical examination therefore become paramount in differentiating patients with tCCS from grade III CCN. Particularly in younger patients with cervical stenosis and neurologic deficits following a traumatic hyperextension insult, without bony or ligamentous injury, it may be wise to delay surgical treatment until at least 24 hours have passed, in order to allow time for the spontaneous resolution of symptoms, except in cases where the neurologic injury is severe or imaging reveals a dramatic degree of spinal cord compression.

22.5 Conclusion

Spondylotic cervical stenosis is seen commonly in the elderly population, but it becomes symptomatic infrequently. Prophylactic surgical decompression in asymptomatic patients with canal stenosis is not recommended. Most symptomatic presentations occur with insidious onset, typically with myelopathy or radiculopathy, and elective surgery is an appropriate treatment option. However, acute neurologic deterioration can occur in the setting of canal stenosis with or without antecedent trauma. Patients with rapidly progressive myelopathy should be considered for urgent surgical decompression within days of presentation. Acute traumatic central cord syndrome should be monitored closely, and early surgical decompression should be considered within 1 to 3 days for patients with persistent non-improving neurologic deficits and ongoing radiographic compression. Cases of suspected cervical cord neurapraxia, most commonly seen in athletes with axial loading or hyperextension injuries, should be carefully assessed over the first 1 to 3 days following injury to distinguish this diagnosis from other injuries that could merit urgent surgical intervention.

References

[1] Karadimas SK, Erwin WM, Ely CG, Dettori JR, Fehlings MG. Pathophysiology and natural history of cervical spondylotic myelopathy. Spine. 2013; 38(22, Suppl 1):S21–S36

[2] Morishita Y, Matsushita A, Maeda T, Ueta T, Naito M, Shiba K. Rapid progressive clinical deterioration of cervical spondylotic myelopathy. Spinal . 2015; 53(5):408–412

[3] Kang JD, Figgie MP, Bohlman HH. Sagittal measurements of the cervical spine in subaxial fractures and dislocations. An analysis of two hundred and eighty-eight patients with and without neurological deficits. J Bone Joint Surg Am. 1994; 76(11):1617–1628

[4] Lee MJ, Cassinelli EH, Riew KD. Prevalence of cervical spine stenosis. Anatomic study in cadavers. J Bone Joint Surg Am. 2007; 89(2):376–380

[5] Nagata K, Yoshimura N, Muraki S, et al. Prevalence of cervical cord compression and its association with physical performance in a population-based cohort in Japan: the Wakayama Spine Study. Spine. 2012; 37(22):1892–1898

[6] Boden SD, Dodge LD, Bohlman HH, Rechtine GR. Rheumatoid arthritis of the cervical spine. A long-term analysis with predictors of paralysis and recovery. J Bone Joint Surg Am. 1993; 75(9):1282–1297

[7] Bailes JE. Experience with cervical stenosis and temporary paralysis in athletes. J Neurosurg Spine. 2005; 2(1):11–16

[8] Bednarik J, Kadanka Z, Dusek L, et al. Presymptomatic spondylotic cervical cord compression. Spine. 2004; 29(20):2260–2269

[9] Edwards WC, LaRocca H. The developmental segmental sagittal diameter of the cervical spinal canal in patients with cervical spondylosis. Spine. 1983; 8(1):20–27

[10] Torg JS, Pavlov H, Genuario SE, et al. Neurapraxia of the cervical spinal cord with transient quadriplegia. J Bone Joint Surg Am. 1986; 68(9):1354–1370

[11] Aebli N, Wicki AG, Rüegg TB, Petrou N, Eisenlohr H, Krebs J. The Torg-Pavlov ratio for the prediction of acute spinal cord injury after a minor trauma to the cervical spine. Spine J. 2013; 13(6):605–612

[12] Blackley HR, Plank LD, Robertson PA. Determining the sagittal dimensions of the canal of the cervical spine. The reliability of ratios of anatomical measurements. J Bone Joint Surg Br. 1999; 81(1):110–112

[13] Lim J-K, Wong H-K. Variation of the cervical spinal Torg ratio with gender and ethnicity. Spine J. 2004; 4(4):396–401

[14] Chen IH, Liao KK, Shen WY. Measurement of cervical canal sagittal diameter in Chinese males with cervical spondylotic myelopathy. Zhonghua Yi Xue Za Zhi (Taipei). 1994; 54(2):105–110

[15] Herzog RJ, Wiens JJ, Dillingham MF, Sontag MJ. Normal cervical spine morphometry and cervical spinal stenosis in asymptomatic professional football players. Plain film radiography, multiplanar computed tomography, and magnetic resonance imaging. Spine. 1991; 16(6, Suppl):S178–S186

[16] Yue WM, Tan SB, Tan MH, Koh DC, Tan CT. The Torg–Pavlov ratio in cervical spondylotic myelopathy: a comparative study between patients with cervical spondylotic myelopathy and a nonspondylotic, nonmyelopathic population. Spine. 2001; 26(16):1760–1764

[17] Muhle C, Metzner J, Weinert D, et al. Classification system based on kinematic MR imaging in cervical spondylitic myelopathy. AJNR Am J Neuroradiol. 1998; 19(9):1763–1771

[18] Kang Y, Lee JW, Koh YH, et al. New MRI grading system for the cervical canal stenosis. AJR Am J Roentgenol. 2011; 197(1):W134–40

[19] Torg JS, Corcoran TA, Thibault LE, et al. Cervical cord neurapraxia: classification, pathomechanics, morbidity, and management guidelines. J Neurosurg. 1997; 87(6):843–850

[20] Kalsi-Ryan S, Karadimas SK, Fehlings MG. Cervical spondylotic myelopathy: the clinical phenomenon and the current pathobiology of an increasingly prevalent and devastating disorder. Neuroscientist. 2013; 19(4):409–421

[21] Nouri A, Tetreault L, Singh A, Karadimas SK, Fehlings MG. Degenerative cervical myelopathy: epidemiology, genetics, and pathogenesis. Spine. 2015; 40(12):E675–E693

[22] Matsunaga S, Sakou T. OPLL: ossification of the posterior longitudinal ligament. In: Yonenobu K, Nakamura K, Toyama Y, eds. Tokyo: Springer Japan; 2006:11–17

[23] Guo JJ, Luk KDK, Karppinen J, Yang H, Cheung KMC. Prevalence, distribution, and morphology of ossification of the ligamentum flavum: a population study of one thousand seven hundred thirty-six magnetic resonance imaging scans. Spine. 2010; 35(1):51–56

[24] Kotani Y, Takahata M, Abumi K, Ito M, Sudo H, Minami A. Cervical myelopathy resulting from combined ossification of the ligamentum flavum and posterior longitudinal ligament: report of two cases and literature review. Spine J. 2013; 13(1):e1–e6

[25] Wilson JR, Barry S, Fischer DJ, et al. Frequency, timing, and predictors of neurological dysfunction in the nonmyelopathic patient with cervical spinal cord compression, canal stenosis, and/or ossification of the posterior longitudinal ligament. Spine. 2013; 38(22, Suppl 1):S37–S54

[26] Oshima Y, Seichi A, Takeshita K, et al. Natural course and prognostic factors in patients with mild cervical spondylotic myelopathy with increased signal intensity on T2-weighted magnetic resonance imaging. Spine. 2012; 37(22):1909–1913

[27] Lees F, Turner JW. Natural history and prognosis of cervical spondylosis. BMJ. 1963; 2(5373):1607–1610

[28] Yoo D-S, Lee S-B, Huh P-W, Kang S-G, Cho K-S. Spinal cord injury in cervical spinal stenosis by minor trauma. World Neurosurg. 2010; 73(1):50–52, discussion e4

[29] Tetreault L, Kopjar B, Côté P, Arnold P, Fehlings MG. A clinical prediction rule for functional outcomes in patients undergoing surgery for degenerative cervical myelopathy: analysis of an international prospective multicenter data set of 757 subjects. J Bone Joint Surg Am. 2015; 97(24):2038–2046

[30] Miyauchi A, Sumida T, Manabe H, et al. Morphological features and clinical significance of epidural membrane in the cervical spine. Spine. 2012; 37(19):E1182–E1188

[31] Schneider RC, Cherry G, Pantek H. The syndrome of acute central cervical spinal cord injury; with special reference to the mechanisms involved in hyperextension injuries of cervical spine. J Neurosurg. 1954; 11(6):546–577

[32] Lenehan B, Fisher CG, Vaccaro A, Fehlings M, Aarabi B, Dvorak MF. The urgency of surgical decompression in acute central cord injuries with spondylosis and without instability. Spine. 2010; 35(21, Suppl):S180–S186

[33] Dai L, Jia L. Central cord injury complicating acute cervical disc herniation in trauma. Spine. 2000; 25(3):331–335, discussion 336

[34] Harrop JS, Sharan A, Ratliff J. Central cord injury: pathophysiology, management, and outcomes. Spine J. 2006; 6(6, Suppl):198S–206S

[35] Hayes KC, Askes HK, Kakulas BA. Retropulsion of intervertebral discs associated with traumatic hyperextension of the cervical spine and absence of vertebral fracture: an uncommon mechanism of spinal cord injury. Spinal Cord. 2002; 40(10):544–547

[36] Ishida Y, Tominaga T. Predictors of neurologic recovery in acute central cervical cord injury with only upper extremity impairment. Spine. 2002; 27(15):1652–1658, discussion 1658

[37] Song J, Mizuno J, Nakagawa H, Inoue T. Surgery for acute subaxial traumatic central cord syndrome without fracture or dislocation. J Clin Neurosci. 2005; 12(4):438–443

[38] Yamazaki T, Yanaka K, Fujita K, Kamezaki T, Uemura K, Nose T. Traumatic central cord syndrome: analysis of factors affecting the outcome. Surg Neurol. 2005; 63(2):95–99, discussion 99–100

[39] Newey ML, Sen PK, Fraser RD. The long-term outcome after central cord syndrome: a study of the natural history. J Bone Joint Surg Br. 2000; 82(6):851–855

[40] Roth EJ, Lawler MH, Yarkony GM. Traumatic central cord syndrome: clinical features and functional outcomes. Arch Phys Med Rehabil. 1990; 71(1):18–23

[41] Penrod LE, Hegde SK, Ditunno JF, Jr. Age effect on prognosis for functional recovery in acute, traumatic central cord syndrome. Arch Phys Med Rehabil. 1990; 71(12):963–968

[42] Bosch A, Stauffer ES, Nickel VL. Incomplete traumatic quadriplegia. A ten-year review. JAMA. 1971; 216(3):473–478

[43] Bose B, Northrup BE, Osterholm JL, Cotler JM, DiTunno JF. Reanalysis of central cervical cord injury management. Neurosurgery. 1984; 15(3):367–372

[44] Brodkey JS, Miller CF, Jr, Harmody RM. The syndrome of acute central cervical spinal cord injury revisited. Surg Neurol. 1980; 14(4):251–257

[45] Chen TY, Dickman CA, Eleraky M, Sonntag VK. The role of decompression for acute incomplete cervical spinal cord injury in cervical spondylosis. Spine. 1998; 23(22):2398–2403

[46] Chen TY, Lee ST, Lui TN, et al. Efficacy of surgical treatment in traumatic central cord syndrome. Surg Neurol. 1997; 48(5):435–440, discussion 441

[47] Guest J, Eleraky MA, Apostolides PJ, Dickman CA, Sonntag VK. Traumatic central cord syndrome: results of surgical management. J Neurosurg. 2002; 97(1, Suppl):25–32

[48] Fehlings MG, Vaccaro A, Wilson JR, et al. Early versus delayed decompression for traumatic cervical spinal cord injury: results of the Surgical Timing in Acute Spinal Cord Injury Study (STASCIS). PLoS ONE. 2012; 7(2):e32037

[49] Chen L, Yang H, Yang T, Xu Y, Bao Z, Tang T. Effectiveness of surgical treatment for traumatic central cord syndrome. J Neurosurg Spine. 2009; 10(1):3–8

[50] Kepler CK, Kong C, Schroeder GD, et al. Early outcome and predictors of early outcome in patients treated surgically for central cord syndrome. J Neurosurg Spine. 2015; 23(4):490–494

[51] Anderson KK, Tetreault L, Shamji MF, et al. Optimal timing of surgical decompression for acute traumatic central cord syndrome: a systematic review of the literature. Neurosurgery. 2015; 77(Suppl 4):S15–S32

[52] Park MS, Moon S-H, Lee H-M, et al. Delayed surgical intervention in central cord syndrome with cervical stenosis. Global Spine J. 2015; 5(1):69–72

[53] Clark AJ, Auguste KI, Sun PP. Cervical spinal stenosis and sports-related cervical cord neurapraxia. Neurosurg Focus. 2011; 31(5):E7

[54] Andrews FJ. Transient cervical neurapraxia associated with cervical spine stenosis. Emerg Med J. 2002; 19(2):172–173

[55] Presciutti SM, DeLuca P, Marchetto P, Wilsey JT, Shaffrey C, Vaccaro AR. Mean subaxial space available for the cord index as a novel method of measuring cervical spine geometry to predict the chronic stinger syndrome in American football players. J Neurosurg Spine. 2009; 11(3):264–271

[56] Torg JS, Thibault L, Sennett B, Pavlov H. The Nicolas Andry Award. The pathomechanics and pathophysiology of cervical spinal cord injury. Clin Orthop Relat Res. 1995(321):259–269

[57] Maroon JC, El-Kadi H, Abla AA, et al. Cervical neurapraxia in elite athletes: evaluation and surgical treatment. Report of five cases. J Neurosurg Spine. 2007; 6(4):356–363

23 The Intensive Care Management of Spine– and Spinal Cord–Injured Patients

Christopher D. Baggott, Joshua E. Medow, and Daniel K. Resnick

Abstract

In North America, acute spinal cord injury affects between 12,000 and 14,000 people per year, and 200,000 people have suffered a significant spinal cord injury. The average age of injury is 34, and men are 4 times more often affected than women. Many of these patients have other life-threatening injuries to the limbs, abdomen, thorax, and head and the vascular structures contained therein. Management of patients with spinal trauma requires trained prehospital personnel, well-established triage and resuscitation protocols, multidisciplinary medical/surgical acute management, and appropriate rehabilitation care providers. The purpose of this chapter is to review the medical management of these patients from prehospital care through transition to rehabilitation services. Management of the unique pulmonary, hemodynamic, thromboembolic, and nutritional needs of this patient population are described.

Keywords: critical care, induced hypertension, spinal cord injury, thromboembolism

23.1 Introduction

In North America, acute spinal cord injury affects between 12,000 and 14,000 people per year,[1] and 200,000 people have suffered a significant spinal cord injury.[1,2] The average age of injury is 34, and men are 4 times more often affected than women. Approximately 3 to 25% of spinal cord injuries occur after the initial traumatic insult.[3,4,5,6,7,8] Many of these patients have other life-threatening injuries to the limbs, abdomen, thorax, and head and the vascular structures contained therein. Management of patients with spinal trauma requires trained prehospital personnel, well-established triage and resuscitation protocols, multidisciplinary medical/surgical acute management, and appropriate rehabilitation care providers.

23.2 Prehospital Management

Early management of spine injuries begins with immobilization in the field. Although there is not a valid, reliable, sensitive prehospital triage protocol for which patients require immobilization, patients with head/neck injuries or mechanisms of injury with the potential to cause cervical spine injury should be immobilized. Patients who are neurologically intact, awake, alert, and not intoxicated and who do not have neck pain/tenderness, do not have neurologic abnormality, and do not have distracting injury do not require immobilization.[9] Additionally, application of spinal immobilization does have reported morbidity. Immobilization can delay resuscitation, which has been shown to cause increased morbidity and mortality in penetrating trauma patients.[10] Immobilization-related neurologic decline in ankylosing spondylitis has been reported as well.[11] Development of appropriate inclusion/exclusion criteria for complete spinal immobilization is necessary to limit both secondary neurologic injury and immobilization-related morbidity. Discontinuation of spine immobilization should be done promptly once the spine is cleared of potential injury.

23.3 Clearance of the Spine

Ruling out a significant spinal injury is important, to allow the discontinuation of unnecessary immobilization and to facilitate resuscitation, nursing care, and patient mobilization.

In asymptomatic, alert patients without a distracting injury, who have not received pain/sedative medications, and who do not have spine pain or tenderness, functional range of motion examination is appropriate. If the range of motion is not limited, and there is no pain, cervical immobilization can be discontinued without spine imaging. In awake patients with neck pain or tenderness, computed tomography (CT) is recommended for initial imaging.[12,13] Anteroposterior (AP), lateral, and odontoid X-rays can be used where CT is not available, but suspicious or nonvisible areas require supplemental CT. The craniocervical junction as well as the cervicothoracic junction must be clearly imaged to radiographically clear the cervical spine. In the setting of normal imaging, the awake patient with neck pain/tenderness can be maintained in cervical immobilization until asymptomatic; alternatively, cervical immobilization can be discontinued after either a normal magnetic resonance imaging (MRI) within 48 hours of the injury or normal dynamic flexion/extension X-rays.[13]

The vast majority of patients who present to the intensive care unit (ICU) have multiple injuries and may have an altered level of consciousness. In obtunded patients or patients with an unreliable examination, CT of the cervical spine is the initial imaging modality of choice.[13] If a high-quality CT of the cervical spine is negative for injury, MRI within 48 hours of injury likely is adequate to evaluate for cervical ligamentous or neurologic injury.[13,14] With a normal MRI in this scenario, discontinuation of cervical immobilization is reasonable. Rigid cervical immobilization should be maintained until the cervical spine is cleared.

Anteroposterior and lateral radiographs are required for the clearance of the thoracic and lumbar spine.[13] These films must show views of all vertebrae so that deformity, malalignment, or fracture can be ruled out. In the thoracic and lumbar spine, entirely normal radiographs preclude the need for any further work-up. Patients should be removed from the hard, immobilization backboard as soon as possible to prevent skin breakdown.

If there is any question as to the presence or absence of a fracture, CT may be used as a definitive means to rule out bony injury. Fractures of the spinous and transverse processes are often inconsequential and usually do not require further work-up unless the patient is symptomatic. Isolated ligamentous injury without bony injury or malalignment of the spine is rare but can occur. In the presence of persistent pain, or if there is any relevant neurologic deficit, MRI should be employed to rule out a ligamentous injury or epidural hematoma.

Unlike with thoracic and lumbar spine injuries, ligamentous injury is not uncommon in the cervical spine. In patients who are alert and oriented and not receiving pain medications, clinical clearance can be obtained by having the patient move the neck in all orthogonal planes. If pain is present, then this method of cervical spine clearance will be inadequate. Within 48 hours of the injury, an MRI of the cervical spine can be performed to assess for soft-tissue edema, which is a predictor of ligamentous injury.[14] A negative MRI study is predictive of a lack of injury given the sensitivity of MRI. A positive finding is not necessarily indicative of injury, however, because the MRI is not particularly specific. Dynamic flexion/extension X-rays may be helpful in deciding whether cervical immobilization should be discontinued when there has been a positive MRI.

23.4 Immobilization and Reduction

Patients with evidence of a fracture dislocation of the spine should remain in an immobilizing device until reduction and stabilization can be safely performed. Depending on the level and the type of injury, certain external orthotic devices may be indicated, whereas other injuries may require surgical intervention.

23.4.1 Choice of Immobilization Device

A hard cervical collar provides some stability for many fractures or minor ligamentous injuries from the occiput to T1 but generally has its greatest effect from the occiput to C3.[15] A cervicothoracic orthotic (CTO) provides additional stability from the occiput to about T3.[15] A properly placed halo device will provide more stability than a CTO at the same levels (occiput to T3).[15] The Lerman Minerva orthotic device (Trulife, Inc., Poulsbo, WA) provides stability at the cervicothoracic junction from about C2 to T3, but support above C2 is significantly less.[16] The thoracolumbar spine orthotic (TLSO) provides support from T9 to S1 but poorly controls lower lumbar levels and the lumbosacral junction.[16] Additional stability from T2 to T8 can be obtained if a chin extender is added to the TLSO construct. A Jewett brace (Florida Brace Corporation, Winter Park, FL) can be employed for injuries located at the thoracolumbar junction spanning from T8 to L2 and is generally ineffective for two- or three-column injuries.[16] Thus, there are several bracing options available to patients with damage to the structural components of the spine. The correct brace is determined by the level and biomechanical characteristics of the injury.

23.4.2 Complications of Immobilization Devices

Orthotic devices are not entirely benign, and their use has been associated with a variety of complications. Some complications are more common in patients with spinal cord injuries and in patients who need to wear a brace for a relatively long period of time.

Pressure Ulcers

Decubitus ulcers are found under cervical collars in 44% of patients within 6 days of placement of the orthotic device.[17] The consequences of these ulcers can be significant and may involve osteomyelitis, significant scarring, nerve compression and dysfunction, local infection, and sepsis. Thus, it is extremely important to ensure a properly fitted orthotic device, especially if the patient needs to wear the device long term. It is imperative to check for decubitus ulcers regularly and to treat them early. It is also important to remove the orthotic device as soon as possible to help prevent decubitus ulcers from occurring without sacrificing the safety of needed immobilization.

Spine immobilization also increases the risk of pressure ulcers in other parts of the body when the patient is not turned frequently enough, and it can occur in as little as 2 hours.[18] The length of time on a hard backboard has also been associated with the development of pressure sores. The best ways to prevent the development of decubitus ulcers include turning the patient frequently, applying a properly fitted orthotic device, and keeping the skin clean and dry.[19,20]

Intracranial Hypertension and Cervical Collars

Stiff cervical collars can result in marked elevation of intracranial pressure, with a mean increase of 4.5 mm Hg associated with cervical collar application.[21] This is most likely due to venous congestion caused by compression of the jugular veins.

Pulmonary Issues

Appropriately applied orthotic devices can significantly impact respiratory parameters in normal human subjects and may also increase the risk of aspiration.[22] The effects are consistent with restrictive lung disease on pulmonary function tests. The implication is that orthotic devices can complicate potentially impaired respiratory function in patients with acute spinal cord injury.

23.4.3 Closed Reduction of Cervical Dislocation Injuries

Closed reduction of cervical spine facet dislocation injuries is safe in the awake patient without upper cervical spine injury.[23] Early closed reduction is advisable when possible for prompt decompression of the spinal cord when there is a deformity causing ongoing neurologic compression. Because tongs are often used in the reduction, care must be taken to ensure that there is no fracture of the cranium that could result in an adverse outcome from pin placement. An MRI is not necessary to rule out an acute herniated disk prior to awake closed reduction but is frequently obtained in patients who are not completely awake, patients who fail attempted closed reduction, or patients who are treated with open reduction while anesthetized. Thirty percent to 50% of patients with a fracture subluxation will be found to have a traumatic herniated disk. The importance of this finding is unclear.[23] During closed reduction, muscle relaxants may be used to prevent splinting of the neck muscles, and mild sedation is often indicated for relief of anxiety. Tongs are placed just above the pinna of the ear using local anesthetic. Slight variation in placement of the tongs may be used to promote upper cervical flexion or extension to some extent. As a rule of thumb, weight is added in 5- to 10-pound increments up to approximately 10 pounds per level.[24] Thus, if C6 is subluxed on C7, then 60 pounds of traction may be safely applied. Some authors advocate the use of more weight, however, and there is some variance in technique from center to center. X-ray or fluoroscopic imaging is obtained after each change in weight. Once the deformity is reduced, the weight should be reduced to prevent overdistraction; however, the patient should be maintained in traction or in a brace until definitive stabilization can be achieved. The onset of neurologic symptoms, the inability of the patient to tolerate the procedure, and the presence of overdistraction on imaging are all indications that the attempted reduction has failed. In these instances, the weight should be removed, the spine immobilized, and further study performed to determine the reason for failure. MRI is often indicated in patients who fail closed reduction because they will usually require open reduction.

23.5 Acute Medical Management

As with any trauma patient, assessment should begin with airway, breathing, and cardiovascular status and should include in-line stabilization of the entire spine until it can be clinically and/or radiographically cleared. The assessment should continue with a scaled score of function that reflects the level of injury. The Guidelines for the Management of Acute Cervical Spine and Spinal Cord Injuries recommends validated clinical assessment tools to facilitate communication, prognostication, and research.[12] The American Spinal Injury Association (ASIA) score is the recommended tool to evaluate motor and sensory function.[12] The Spinal Cord Independence Measure (SCIM III) is recommended by the guidelines as the preferred functional outcome assessment tool.[12] The assessment of pain severity, along with physical and emotional functioning affected by pain, using the International Spinal Cord Injury Basic Pain Data Set (ISCIB-PDS) is recommended.[12]

It is recommended that acute spinal cord injuries be managed in the ICU setting, especially in upper cervical lesions.[25] Monitoring should include blood pressure and pulse, respiratory status, and neurologic function. Additional management of patients with acute spinal cord injuries is often difficult and not necessarily supported by clear evidence as to method or duration of treatment. Consequently, it is often difficult for caregivers to address the multiple medical issues that present in this patient population.

23.5.1 Steroids

In the updated Guidelines for the Management of Acute Cervical Spine and Spinal Cord Injuries, methylprednisolone is specifically not recommended in the treatment of acute spinal cord injury.[26]

The National Acute Spinal Cord Injury Study (NASCIS I) reported no significant change in motor or sensory function with steroid treatment.[27] However, animal studies suggested that the doses of methylprednisolone used in NASCIS I were too low to demonstrate a significant improvement in outcome.[28,29,30,31,32] This prompted NASCIS II.[29] In this study, methylprednisolone was administered at higher doses. Improved neurologic outcome was reported with this protocol when it was started within 8 hours of the injury. However, this conclusion was drawn after over half of the randomized patients were excluded post hoc because they were treated outside an arbitrarily defined therapeutic window of 8 hours post injury.[33] Although clinical practice was widely influenced by the NASCIS II results, the conclusion of clinical benefit derived from post hoc analysis of the randomized, controlled, double-blind data set is methodologically flawed. Analysis of the entire NASCIS II data set is class I medical evidence that demonstrates a trend toward more serious complications, whereas the widely syndicated reported benefit is class III medical evidence at best.[26] NASCIS III, which compared various steroid dosing protocols without placebo control, demonstrated a higher risk of complications with higher doses of steroids.[26]

Although there has been extensive investment in the evaluation of steroids in the treatment of acute spinal cord injury because of scattered reports of minor improvements in motor or sensory function on detailed clinical examination, there has never been any significant functional or behavioral improvement demonstrated as a result of steroid administration. This in combination with the clear harmful effect of steroid administration has led to the recommendation that steroid administration after acute spinal cord injury should not be considered. The Guidelines for the Management of Acute Cervical Spine and Spinal Cord Injuries adds to the statement that steroids are not recommended by stating the following: "Clinicians considering MP [methylprednisolone] therapy should bear in mind that the drug is not FDA approved for this application … Class I, II, and III evidence exists that high-dose steroids are associated with harmful side effects including death."[26]

23.5.2 Blood Pressure Management

Maintenance of mean arterial blood pressure (MAP) of 85 to 90 mm Hg is advisable for 5 days after spinal cord injury. Spinal cord blood flow may be compromised following injury because of multiple factors. Often there is a combination of systemic hypotension and local vascular changes that include direct injury and focal vasospasm.[28,34,35,36,37,38,39,40] Spinal cord injury itself may cause decreased blood pressure because of neurogenic shock resulting from the loss of normal sympathetic tone. Typical findings of neurogenic shock include bradycardia and rhythm disturbances, decreased systemic vascular resistance (SVR), which results in decreased MAP, and consequently decreased cardiac output.[7,28,34,38,39,40,41,42,43] It is the lack of sinoatrial and vasomotor innervation that results in decreased cardiac output. Once the ability to maintain perfusion is compromised because of an inability to autoregulate blood flow, spinal cord ischemia develops.[28,40,42] The first week after surgery is when most patients have cardiovascular instability.[41] Clinical outcomes may be improved by maintaining systolic blood pressure greater than 90 mm Hg and MAP greater than 85 mm Hg using a combination of pressors and fluid resuscitation.[25,42,44,45,46,47,48] Typically pressors, such as dopamine, that have both α and β agonist properties are employed. Other agents that independently cause ionotropic/chronotropic responses separate from vasoconstriction can be used to emphasize one response over another. For example, if the pulse is too fast, a more potent vasoconstrictor can be used. Norepinephrine (Levophed; Sanofi-Aventis, Bridgewater, NJ) has primarily α-agonist functions but does have some β activity as well. It causes profound vasoconstriction. Phenylephrine has pure vasoconstrictor properties but is not quite as potent as norepinephrine. Depending on the circumstances, these different medications can be used to maintain MAP. However, it is important to maintain an appropriate intravascular volume to perfuse the renal and splanchnic vascular beds because vasoconstriction occurs primarily here and in the limbs. If the vascular volume is low and the SVR is too high, end organs can become ischemic.[49]

23.5.3 Autonomic Dysreflexia

Autonomic dysreflexia occurs in 85% of patients with acute spinal cord injuries above T6.[50,51,52] Symptoms include substantial elevations in blood pressure, tachycardia or bradycardia, headaches, flushing, diaphoresis above the level of injury, and pupillary changes.[50,51,52] It is most common in the early period after spinal cord injury and is the consequence of significant reflex sympathetic discharge triggered by a noxious stimulus (i.e., bladder distension). Treatment can involve α and β blockade and perhaps other neuromodulating medications such as gabapentin.

23.5.4 Pulmonary Care

Several issues must be considered in the respiratory management of patients with acute spinal cord injuries. Many of these pertain to direct injury to the lungs sustained during the trauma, aspiration, pneumonias, pulmonary edema (often neurogenic), and adult respiratory distress syndrome (ARDS). Abnormal airway reactivity has been reported in patients with spinal cord injury as well.[53] Bronchospasm that develops as a consequence of the injury typically responds to bronchodilators. Many spinal cord injury patients have bronchial mucus hypersecretion as well. Patients with spinal cord injuries are also at increased risk of obstructive or mixed sleep apnea.[54,55] A significant concern in patients with spinal cord injuries is the denervation of the muscles of respiration because pulmonary dysfunction accounts for the largest cause of morbidity in spinal cord injured patients.[56] In one study, only 25% of patients who required chronic positive pressure ventilation survived for 1 year and only 60% of them were alive at 14 years.[57]

The anatomical location of the injury influences the physiology of respiration. During inspiration, the rib cage expands as a result of the contraction of the external intercostal muscles and the diaphragm. When the external intercostal muscles are paralyzed, the ribs may move inward during respiration rather than outward. This paradoxical motion decreases the development of negative inspiratory pressure and compromises ventilation.[58,59] The tone of the abdominal muscles is also important in providing the appropriate amount of intra-abdominal pressure. Intra-abdominal pressure provides apposition and tension on the diaphragm, allowing it to contract effectively. After a spinal cord injury, the abdominal muscle tone present in normal individuals is often lost.[60,61,62,63] Consequently, inhalation is often more difficult and less efficient. A change from the seated to the supine position generally results in a decrease in functional residual capacity (FRC) by 500 mL, whereas vital capacity (VC) increases. Over time, the neural input to the diaphragm may increase. This is known as operational length compensation (OLC).[64,65] When normal subjects are upright, abdominal pressure decreases, and this may be exaggerated in patients with spinal cord injuries. In this situation, OLC may be inadequate, resulting in the inability of the patient to ventilate adequately when upright.[66] In patients with abdominal muscle paralysis, the use of an abdominal binder may augment ventilation, whereas a rocking bed may help patients with marked diaphragm weakness.[62,67,68,69]

Patients with high cervical injuries have the highest incidence of respiratory complications, including recurrent pneumonias, atelectasis, and respiratory failure. They also recover more slowly and have the highest mortality rate compared with other spinal cord injured patients.[56,70,71] Quadriplegic patients have blunted responses to hypercapnia and small increases in respiratory drive.[72] Patients with injuries above C3 require diaphragmatic pacing or chronic ventilatory support.

Patients with injuries between C3 and C5 have variable impairment of diaphragmatic strength. Chronic ventilator dependence is most common among patients older than 50 with underlying lung disease. For many patients, however, mechanical ventilation is often necessary only in the acute phase and is usually not necessary long term.[73,74,75] Improvements tend to follow as spinal cord edema resolves, accessory ventilatory muscles are recruited, deconditioned muscles gain strength, and flaccidity gives way to spasticity.[73,74,75,76,77] These patients may utilize intermittent glossopharyngeal breathing (which is a combination of oral, pharyngeal, and laryngeal muscle movements to project a bolus of air past the glottis) to help with coughing, increasing VC for deeper breathing, and for raising the vocal volume.[78,79,80] Patients with diaphragmatic pacers can also demonstrate improvements in the fluidity of speech.

Patients with injuries between C5 and C8 have intact diaphragm innervation and can use accessory muscles in the neck and the clavicular portion of the pectoralis major muscles to inhale adequately. Exhalation is by passive recoil.[81,82] Thus, spinal cord injured patients may have increased residual volumes (RVs) because of an inability to exhale and may appear to have restrictive ventilatory defects during pulmonary function testing.[74,77,82,83,84,85] Patients with thoracic spinal cord injuries may still have ventilatory complications but not necessarily as a consequence of neurologic compromise. Many of these patients have other direct chest trauma, including pulmonary contusions, hemo-/pneumothorax, and so forth.[55,56] Furthermore, these patients may develop ARDS from direct injury, chemical pneumonitis from aspiration, and aspiration pneumonia.

All patients with central nervous system injuries are at some risk for the development of neurogenic pulmonary edema; however, it rarely occurs in complete spinal cord injuries above C7.[86,87,88,89] It is thought to be related to secretion of protein-rich fluid in the presence of vasogenic instability from aberrant sympathetic discharge. Primary management is supportive therapy until the problem clears. Cardiogenic pulmonary edema can also occur as a consequence of spinal cord-induced bradycardia.

Chest physiotherapy appears to decrease the risk of mucus retention, atelectasis, and pneumonia in patients with spinal cord injuries.[71,89] This strategy includes incentive spirometry, frequent changes of position/postural drainage of secretions, nasotracheal suctioning, and, in patients with a weak cough, manually assisted coughing using forceful abdominal thrusts if no precluding abdominal or spinal injury exists. In quadriplegics, surface stimulation of abdominal muscles with an electrical charge was shown to be as effective as abdominal cough assistance.[90] There are no data to support prophylactic use of bronchodilators or intermittent positive-pressure ventilation.[91,92]

Patients with severe high cervical cord injuries, or those with concomitant head or pulmonary injuries, may require prolonged mechanical ventilation. In these patients, tracheostomy should be considered early because of the risk of laryngeal damage resulting from chronic endotracheal intubation.

23.5.5 Deep Venous Thrombosis and Venous Thromboembolism

The incidence of deep venous thrombosis (DVT) in chronic spine injured patients within 1 year has been reported at 2.1% and 0.5 to 1.0% per year thereafter.[93] The concern of DVT is progressive loss of circulation in the limb with concomitant pain and ischemia, chronic limb swelling, and venous thromboembolism (VTE). The incidence of thromboembolic events in patients with spinal cord injuries ranges from 7 to 100%,[94,95,96,97,98,99,100,101,102,103,104,105] and morbidity and mortality are quite high in the acute injury setting.[106,107] Most pulmonary emboli (PE) occur in the first 2 to 3 months after injury,[101,108,109,110] and patients with acute spinal cord injuries have a 500-fold increase in mortality from a PE compared with age- and sex-matched noninjured patients.[107] This risk decreases to a 20-fold mortality rate between spinal cord injury patients who are 6 months out from their injury and their noninjured counterparts.[107] The diagnosis of DVT may be made with a variety of tests. After careful consideration of these different modalities, the Consortium of Spinal Cord Medicine has recommended the use of Doppler ultrasound to diagnose DVT.[106] Modalities including Doppler ultrasound, impedance plethysmography, venography, and fibrinogen and D-dimer levels have been used to detect DVT.[94,95,96,97,98,99,101,102,103,108,109,110] The gold standard is venography, but because of its expense and the invasive nature of the test, it is often impractical to use.[60] Venography also carries a 10% risk of phlebitis and allergic reaction to the contrast.[93] Pulmonary embolism has been known to occur in patients with negative venograms.[96,108] Doppler ultrasound and impedance plethysmography are 80 to 100% accurate for the diagnosis of DVT compared with venography.[111] Doppler ultrasound is less sensitive for DVTs below the knee than it is above the knee because of the smaller size of distal veins. D-dimer and fibrinogen tests are very sensitive but are often unspecific, meaning that they will not miss a DVT, but when positive, the chance that a DVT is present might not be very high.[112,113] Routine surveillance for DVT is not necessary, but a high index of suspicion in spinal cord injury patients is appropriate.

Venous thromboembolism can be a devastating adverse event after spinal cord injury. Signs and symptoms of pulmonary embolism include tachycardia, hypotension/shock, myocardial infarct, tachypnea/dyspnea, apprehension, diaphoresis, fever, chest pain, cyanosis, cough/hemoptysis, and complete cardiovascular collapse with sudden death.[114,115] Diagnostic findings can include platelike atelectasis on chest X-ray, right ventricular axis shift on electrocardiogram (ECG), and supraventricular tachycardia.[116] With severe pulmonary embolism, ST segment changes and T-wave inversion may be present as well.[116] Although hypoxemia and a large A–a gradient on blood gas analysis is classically reported with PE, partial arterial pressure of oxygen (PaO_2), and O_2 saturation values are very inconsistent and should not be used to rule out PE.[117,118,119,120]

Death from PE is unlikely in patients without evidence of shock.[116] These patients should begin full-dose anticoagulation with heparin, if possible, and a confirmatory diagnostic study should be obtained.[116] In this patient population ventilation–perfusion (V/Q) scans, MRI, helical CT angiography, and the gold standard percutaneous venous angiogram are all viable options.[121,122,123]

Patients with shock due to PE are far more likely to die within the first hour, making rapid diagnosis extremely important.[116] CT and V/Q scans may not be plausible because of the time delay incurred in obtaining a confirmatory study. Percutaneous angiography may be reasonable if the intention is to treat the PE with catheter embolectomy, mechanical clot disruption, or selective tissue plasminogen activator (tPA) injection.[116] Oftentimes it is beneficial to obtain a bedside echocardiogram because it can be mobilized to the patient in the ICU rather than moving an unstable patient to an imaging department where ICU staff, equipment, and medical therapies are in short supply.

Echocardiography (transthoracic or transesophageal) is useful in the recognition and differentiation of PE and the patient's response to therapy.[124,125] Echocardiography can detect emboli in transit and may provide alternative diagnoses for the cause of shock, including aortic dissection, myocardial dysfunction/infarction, pericardial disease, hypovolemia, and valvular insufficiency.[126,127] Echocardiographic findings of PE include right ventricle pressure overload, enlarged right to left ventricle ratio, paradoxical septal motion, pulmonary artery dilatation, and tricuspid regurgitation.[124,125,127,128] It appears that an embolism that causes 30% or greater pulmonary artery (PA) occlusion is required to produce right ventricle dilatation and hemodynamic instability.[129,130,131] Smaller, hemodynamically insignificant emboli (those that cause < 20% PA occlusion) may not be detected with echocardiography.[132,133] Echocardiography is also not able to establish the severity of a superimposed event in patients with preexisting left ventricle dysfunction.[133]

V/Q scans have been used for the diagnosis of PE. The majority of patients with angiographically documented PE (59%) do not have a high probability V/Q scan.[134] Scan interpretations that are conclusively normal or read as high probability are rare, only 15% and 13%, respectively.[134] The remainder of scans are interpreted as intermediate (38%) or low (34%) probability.[8] In patients with chronic obstructive pulmonary disease (COPD), V/Q scans are even less diagnostic.[135] Part of this may be due to the difficulty in performing ventilation scans in critically ill patients.[136] Consequently V/Q scanning will often require an angiographic study to definitively confirm the diagnosis of PE.[137]

Angiography is recognized as the gold standard test to confirm PE but is invasive, expensive, and requires skilled staff to perform it.[110] It is not uniformly available and is associated with multiple complications,[137,138,139] particularly in critically ill patients[135] and in patients with pulmonary hypertension.[140] Although selective tPa delivery with a catheter is an accepted treatment modality, nonselective intravenous (IV) tPa with angiography has been shown to have an increased bleeding complication rate.[141]

Helical CT angiography is appealing as a diagnostic tool because it is readily available, noninvasive, can define alternative diagnoses,[142,143] and can detect right ventricle dilatation similarly to echocardiography.[144] When the findings of a helical CT are compared with those of a percutaneous angiogram for PE in the central arteries, helical CT was 94% sensitive, 94% specific, and had a 93% positive predictive value.[145,146,147,148,149,150] Specificities nearing 100% have been reported in cases of PE that were clinically important with right ventricle pressure overload.[148,150,151] Optimal scanning involves breath holding,[152] but recent technology allows for faster slice acquisition, making motion less of a problem. MRI has also been employed for the diagnosis of PE. MRI accurately visualizes the central vessels, can be used to interpret heart function, and can provide alternative diagnoses with comparable sensitivity and specificity to helical CT angiography.[153,154,155] It does not require iodine contrast, which can be nephrotoxic, and unlike CT can allow for MR venography during the same session.[153,156] However, setup time, the duration of the scan, isolation of the patient in the bore of the magnet away from health care workers, and implantable devices that may not be MRI compatible often preclude the use of MRI in patients with hemodynamically significant PE.

23.5.6 Venous Thromboembolism Prophylaxis and Treatment

VTE prophylaxis should be administered within 72 hours of injury to reduce the risk of DVT/VTE. Subcutaneous (SQ) unfractionated heparin, 5,000 units three times a day has been shown to substantially reduce DVT formation.[95,99,102,103,123,157,158,159,160,161,162] However, in patients with acute spinal cord injury, low-dose unfractionated heparin has been considered inadequate by some authors.[97,163] Attaining an activated partial thromboplastin time (aPTT) of 1.5 times normal has been suggested but does result in a higher bleeding complication rate compared with fixed dose SQ heparin. As compared with oral anticoagulation, low-dose heparin was shown to have better efficacy in preventing DVT.[160] The use of low-molecular-weight heparin (LMWH), otherwise known as fractionated heparin, has been studied as well and has had favorable results as compared with unfractionated heparin in both prevention of DVT and decreased bleeding complications.[98] Other reports have shown significant efficacy of LMWH against DVT and PE in patients with spinal cord injuries.[112,164] Because most pulmonary emboli occur within 2 to 3 months, prophylaxis with anticoagulation usually spans an 8- to 12-week period. Patients with other risk factors such as obesity, previous DVT or PE, and malignancy may stay on prophylactic anticoagulation therapy longer.[108] Patients who have useful motor function in the lower extremities may run shorter courses of anticoagulation because they are at less risk for developing a DVT.[100,106]

Inferior vena cava (IVC) filters have been used for patients who do not tolerate anticoagulation, as well for the prevention of massive PE. The filter device can prevent large thromboembolic events from occurring but does not necessarily prevent smaller thromboemboli from resulting in PE. They do not prevent upper extremity pulmonary emboli. IVC filters can also contribute to the formation or enlargement of DVTs because they cause resistance to flow. Complications of filter placement include distal migration, intraperitoneal erosion, and symptomatic IVC occlusion.[165,166,167] In a randomized trial that evaluated routine placement of vena cava filters as an adjunct to anticoagulant therapy in patients with proximal DVT, filters were shown to reduce the frequency of PE during the first 12 days but to almost double the long-term risk of recurrent DVT.[168] Hence, removal IVC filters may be appropriate for patients in whom the risk for PE is high but anticoagulation cannot be used. IVC filters should not be used as a routine prophylactic measure.

Other preventive measures include compression stockings and sequential compression devices, which have been shown to lower the risk of PE.[169] The use of rotating beds for 10 days in patients with acute spinal cord injuries has also demonstrated a decreased incidence of DVT by 80%.[170] We generally apply pneumatic compression devices immediately and start LMWH within 24 to 72 hours, depending upon other injuries and contraindications to anticoagulation. Treatment of a known DVT should include full anticoagulation with unfractionated or fractionated heparin followed by warfarin therapy, usually for more than 3 months and with a goal international normalized ratio (INR) of 2.5.[171] In patients who cannot undergo anticoagulation, an IVC filter should be considered.[171]

Patients with PE may maintain hemodynamic stability with an intense catecholamine surge.[116] This is necessary to maintain blood pressure to the heart and central nervous system. Mechanical ventilation during a hemodynamically significant PE may be necessary if refractory hypoxia and shock ensue. However, starting mechanical ventilation can often blunt the catecholamine surge and precipitate cardiovascular collapse.[116] This can be due in part to sedative/hypnotic medications that decrease consciousness and catecholamine release and can also be due to direct vasodilatation.[116] Furthermore, positive-pressure ventilation can cause a decrease in venous return to the right ventricle and can also increase pulmonary vascular resistance, resulting in further compromise of right ventricular function with a concomitant decrease in cardiac output and a drop in systemic blood pressure.[116] Accordingly, intubation should be undertaken judiciously while weighing its risks and benefits.[116] An awake fiberoptic intubation provides no loss of consciousness and permits direct visualization of the vocal cords, often with less stimulation than direct laryngoscopy. Etomidate should be used if sedation is necessary because it does not cause hypotension.[116]

Volume expansion with 1 to 2 L of crystalloid solution is the traditional treatment for hypotension in undifferentiated shock and is frequently helpful in driving cardiac output in patients with massive PE unless right ventricular failure is severe.[116] Pressors such as norepinephrine are instrumental in improving systemic blood pressure and blood flow to the heart, resulting in less cardiac ischemia.[172] Furthermore, norepinephrine has β_1 effects resulting in improved cardiac contractility and thus right ventricular function,[173,174] which is why it is indicated in patients suffering from severe shock.[175,176] Dobutamine and other pressors with strong b activity may cause hypotension from vasodilatation, and their use should be limited in PE.[116] Inhaled prostacyclin and nitric oxide have been reported to increase cardiac output, decrease pulmonary pressures, and improve gas exchange in cases of severe PE.[177,178] Placing the embolized lung in the dependent position can also improve oxygenation.[179]

Heparin should be started at full therapeutic doses until PE is excluded, provided that no contraindications to heparin therapy exist.[180] The efficacy of heparin is attributed to the impairment of clot propagation and the prevention of recurrent PE.[181] Heparin therapy should be aggressively pursued in patients with suspected PE because recurrent PE is reported to be the most common cause of death in hemodynamically stable patients.[182,183] Heparin boluses can be associated with hypotension as a consequence of histamine release and can be treated with histamine 1 and 2 receptor blockers to help prevent/treat hypotension.[184,185] Long-term treatment often requires warfarin therapy for more than 3 months and with a goal INR of 2.5.

Cardiac arrest will occur within 1 to 2 hours after the onset of clinical presentation in two thirds of fatal PE cases[182,186] and is almost uniformly due to pulseless electrical activity (PEA).[116] PEA is at least momentarily reversible in one third of cases.[116] The survival rate for patients presenting with cardiac arrest is reported at 35%.[187] Those patients who experience intermittent cardiac arrest have a lower mortality rate than those requiring continuous resuscitation.[188,189]

Cardiopulmonary resuscitation (CPR) not only promotes circulation by pumping the heart but can also mechanically disrupt the embolus, permitting improved flow through the pulmonary artery.[116] Thrombolysis is uniformly accepted as the treatment of choice in hemodynamically unstable PE[190,191,192] but is not without bleeding complications. Relative and absolute contraindications may prevent the use of this medication. Selective tPA delivery during angiography may help reduce the dose necessary to be effective and consequently may decrease risks of bleeding.

Catheter embolectomy or fragmentation is an option for patients not in cardiac arrest[193] where tPa is contraindicated. Open embolectomy is another treatment possibility, but it requires cardiopulmonary bypass and full anticoagulation with heparin. Cardiac arrest does not preclude open embolectomy; however, it requires general anesthesia, which can decrease cardiac output and precipitate cardiac arrest, complicating matters further for patients with hemodynamically significant PE.[194]

23.5.7 Vertebral Artery Injury

Vertebral artery injuries occur in up to 11% of nonpenetrating cervical spine injuries.[6] They are most often due to fractures through the foramen transversarium, facet fracture–dislocation, or vertebral subluxation,[195,196,197,198,199,200,201,202] all of which are readily seen with CT scans of the cervical spine.

After blunt cervical trauma, patients at particularly high risk for cerebrovascular injury are patients with complete spinal cord injury, fractures through the foramen transversarium, facet fracture–dislocation, or vertebral subluxation.[195,197,201] Many centers used the Modified Denver Screening Criteria to identify patients who should undergo cerebrovascular imaging; the sensitivity, specificity, positive predictive value, and negative predictive value of these criteria remain unknown.

Practically, the vascular imaging of choice is CT angiography. Although catheter-based diagnostic angiography may still have a role in confirming or refuting CTA findings, the diagnostic accuracy of a high-quality CTA for cervical vascular injury has been reported to be 99.3% in patients with blunt cervical trauma meeting the Modified Denver Screening Criteria.[203] The incidence of vascular injury identified by CTA in blunt trauma patients meeting the Modified Denver Screening Criteria was reported as 5.5%.[204]

Although there is a risk for vertebral artery injury after blunt cervical trauma, there is no established or evidence-based treatment. Antiplatelet agents, anticoagulation, endovascular treatment, and observation have all been proposed. Most patients remain asymptomatic after vertebral artery injury regardless of the treatment paradigm, calling into question the importance of screening patients for vascular injury at all.[195]

Aspirin is often the most appropriate treatment after considering the specific circumstance: the presence of stroke, the nature of the vascular injury, and the risk for hemorrhagic complications. There does not appear to be any difference in the outcome between antiplatelet treatment and anticoagulant treatment; however, it is reported that anticoagulation with IV heparin is associated with increased rate of complications (31%), including hemorrhagic complications (14%), in the literature.[195] The role of endovascular stent reconstruction is uncertain. Careful attention to all injuries sustained in a trauma and monitoring of neurologic status in patients with vertebral artery injuries can lead to favorable outcomes.

23.5.8 Nutrition

Patients with spinal cord injuries require nutritional support. Enteral feedings (EFs) should be started as soon as feasible, and it is recommended that enteral nutrition be administered within 72 hours. Total parenteral nutrition (TPN), if necessary, is generally not started before day 5 because of higher morbidity concerns related to electrolyte and fluid shifts.

Patients capable of safely taking nutrition orally should do so. If patients cannot tolerate oral intake, a nasogastric (NG) or orogastric (OG) tube should be placed to start EF early. NG and OG tubes provide the ability to evacuate the stomach to help reduce enteric distension and to measure residual secretions and feeds. Once the gastrointestinal (GI) tract is functioning satisfactorily, a Dobhoff tube can replace the NG tube. Because it is narrower, the Dobhoff tube is thought to induce less nasopharyngeal swelling and may perhaps decrease the incidence of sinusitis compared with the larger NG tubes. Gastrostomy tubes should be employed early for those patients who will definitely need long-term nutritional support.

Caloric intake should be 140% of the predicted basal energy expenditure (BEE) and 100% of the BEE in paralyzed individuals because of the elevated energy requirements within the first 2 weeks after injury. BEE can be calculated using the Harris–Benedict equation. Indirect calorimetry is probably the best way to assess nutritional requirements.[205] Fifteen percent of the total calories should come from protein.

Overfeeding can result in cholestasis and significantly elevated liver function tests (LFTs). Patients receiving nutritional support will often demonstrate mild elevations in LFTs. This should not prompt halting of nutritional supplementation, but it should be monitored closely.

23.6 Conclusion

Patients with acute spinal injuries encounter considerable obstacles during recovery. Recognizing the limitations of current therapies and the risks involved with their use is of the utmost importance. Careful attention to detail during the early phases of treatment can lead to lower morbidity and mortality rates. Some of the longer-term problems can potentially be avoided with good skin and wound care, appropriate use of orthotic devices, and careful anticoagulation. A multidisciplinary approach that treats the whole patient is necessary to improve quality of life and to facilitate functional recovery in this patient population.

References

[1] National Spinal Cord Injury Statistical Center (NSCISC). Spinal Cord Injury: Facts and Figures at a Glance. Birmingham, AL: University of Alabama Press; 1996

[2] Lasfargues JE, Custis D, Morrone F, Carswell J, Nguyen T. A model for estimating spinal cord injury prevalence in the United States. Paraplegia. 1995; 33(2):62–68

[3] Bohlman HH. Acute fractures and dislocations of the cervical spine. An analysis of three hundred hospitalized patients and review of the literature. J Bone Joint Surg Am. 1979; 61(8):1119–1142

[4] Burney RE, Waggoner R, Maynard FM. Stabilization of spinal injury for early transfer. J Trauma. 1989; 29(11):1497–1499

[5] Geisler WO, Wynne-Jones M, Jousse AT. Early management of the patient with trauma to the spinal cord. Med Serv J Can. 1966; 22(7):512–523

[6] Hachen HJ. Emergency transportation in the event of acute spinal cord lesion. Paraplegia. 1974; 12(1):33–37

[7] Prasad VS, Schwartz A, Bhutani R, Sharkey PW, Schwartz ML. Characteristics of injuries to the cervical spine and spinal cord in polytrauma patient population: experience from a regional trauma unit. Spinal Cord. 1999; 37(8):560–568

[8] Totten VY, Sugarman DB. Respiratory effects of spinal immobilization. Prehosp Emerg Care. 1999; 3(4):347–352

[9] Theodore N, Hadley MN, Aarabi B, et al. Prehospital cervical spinal immobilization after trauma. Neurosurgery. 2013; 72(Suppl 2):22–34

[10] Haut ER, Kalish BT, Efron DT, et al. Spine immobilization in penetrating trauma: more harm than good? J Trauma. 2010; 68(1):115–120, discussion 120–121

[11] Thumbikat P, Hariharan RP, Ravichandran G, McClelland MR, Mathew KM. Spinal cord injury in patients with ankylosing spondylitis: a 10-year review. Spine. 2007; 32(26):2989–2995

[12] Hadley MN, Walters BC, Aarabi B, et al. Clinical assessment following acute cervical spinal cord injury. Neurosurgery. 2013; 72(Suppl 2):40–53

[13] Ryken TC, Hadley MN, Walters BC, et al. Radiographic assessment. Neurosurgery. 2013; 72(Suppl 2):54–72

[14] Benzel EC, Hart BL, Ball PA, Baldwin NG, Orrison WW, Espinosa MC. Magnetic resonance imaging for the evaluation of patients with occult cervical spine injury. J Neurosurg. 1996; 85(5):824–829

[15] Johnson RM, Hart DL, Simmons EF, Ramsby GR, Southwick WO. Cervical orthoses. A study comparing their effectiveness in restricting cervical motion in normal subjects. J Bone Joint Surg Am. 1977; 59(3):332–339

[16] Woodard EJ, Kowalski RJ, Benzel EC. Orthoses: complication prevention and management. In: Benzel EC, ed. Spine Surgery Techniques, Complication Avoidance, and Management. Vol. 2. Philadelphia, PA: Elsevier Churchill Livingstone; 2005:1915–1934

[17] Davis JW, Phreaner DL, Hoyt DB, Mackersie RC. The etiology of missed cervical spine injuries. J Trauma. 1993; 34(3):342–346

[18] Linares HA, Mawson AR, Suarez E, Biundo JJ. Association between pressure sores and immobilization in the immediate post-injury period. Orthopedics. 1987; 10(4):571–573

[19] Black CA, Buderer NM, Blaylock B, Hogan BJ. Comparative study of risk factors for skin breakdown with cervical orthotic devices: Philadelphia and Aspen. J Trauma Nurs. 1998; 5(3):62–66

[20] Blaylock B. Solving the problem of pressure ulcers resulting from cervical collars. Ostomy Wound Manage. 1996; 42(4):26–28, 30, 32–33

[21] Davies G, Deakin C, Wilson A. The effect of a rigid collar on intracranial pressure. Injury. 1996; 27(9):647–649

[22] Bauer D, Kowalski R. Effect of spinal immobilization devices on pulmonary function in the healthy, nonsmoking man. Ann Emerg Med. 1988; 17(9):915–918

[23] Gelb DE, Hadley MN, Aarabi B, et al. Initial closed reduction of cervical spinal fracture-dislocation injuries. Neurosurgery. 2013; 72(Suppl 2):73–83

[24] Greenberg MS. Spine injuries: cranial-cervical traction. In: Greenberg MS, ed. Handbook of Neurosurgery. Vol. 2. Lakeland, FL: Greenberg Graphics; 1997:778

[25] Ryken TC, Hurlbert RJ, Hadley MN, et al. The acute cardiopulmonary management of patients with cervical spinal cord injuries. Neurosurgery. 2013; 72(Suppl 2):84–92

[26] Hurlbert RJ, Hadley MN, Walters BC, et al. Pharmacological therapy for acute spinal cord injury. Neurosurgery. 2013; 72(Suppl 2):93–105

[27] Bracken MB, Collins WF, Freeman DF, et al. Efficacy of methylprednisolone in acute spinal cord injury. JAMA. 1984; 251(1):45–52

[28] Amar AP, Levy ML. Pathogenesis and pharmacological strategies for mitigating secondary damage in acute spinal cord injury. Neurosurgery. 1999; 44(5):1027–1039, discussion 1039–1040

[29] Bracken MB, Shepard MJ, Collins WF, et al. A randomized, controlled trial of methylprednisolone or naloxone in the treatment of acute spinal-cord injury. Results of the Second National Acute Spinal Cord Injury Study. N Engl J Med. 1990; 322(20):1405–1411

[30] Ducker TB, Zeidman SM. Spinal cord injury. Role of steroid therapy. Spine. 1994; 19(20):2281–2287

[31] Young W, Bracken MB. The Second National Acute Spinal Cord Injury Study. J Neurotrauma. 1992; 9(Suppl 1):S397–S405

[32] Zeidman SM, Ling GS, Ducker TB, Ellenbogen RG. Clinical applications of pharmacologic therapies for spinal cord injury. J Spinal Disord. 1996; 9(5):367–380

[33] Bracken MB, Shepard MJ, Collins WF, Jr, et al. Methylprednisolone or naloxone treatment after acute spinal cord injury: 1-year follow-up data. Results of the second National Acute Spinal Cord Injury Study. J Neurosurg. 1992; 76(1):23–31

[34] Dolan EJ, Tator CH. The effect of blood transfusion, dopamine, and gamma hydroxybutyrate on posttraumatic ischemia of the spinal cord. J Neurosurg. 1982; 56(3):350–358

[35] Hall ED, Wolf DL. A pharmacological analysis of the pathophysiological mechanisms of posttraumatic spinal cord ischemia. J Neurosurg. 1986; 64(5):951–961

[36] Lehmann KG, Lane JG, Piepmeier JM, Batsford WP. Cardiovascular abnormalities accompanying acute spinal cord injury in humans: incidence, time course and severity. J Am Coll Cardiol. 1987; 10(1):46–52

[37] Sandler AN, Tator CH. Effect of acute spinal cord compression injury on regional spinal cord blood flow in primates. J Neurosurg. 1976; 45(6):660–676

[38] Sandler AN, Tator CH. Review of the effect of spinal cord trama on the vessels and blood flow in the spinal cord. J Neurosurg. 1976; 45(6):638–646

[39] Tator CH. Experimental and clinical studies of the pathophysiology and management of acute spinal cord injury. J Spinal Cord Med. 1996; 19(4):206–214

[40] Tator CH, Fehlings MG. Review of the secondary injury theory of acute spinal cord trauma with emphasis on vascular mechanisms. J Neurosurg. 1991; 75(1):15–26

[41] Piepmeier JM, Lehmann KB, Lane JG. Cardiovascular instability following acute cervical spinal cord trauma. Cent Nerv Syst Trauma. 1985; 2(3):153–160

[42] Levi L, Wolf A, Rigamonti D, Ragheb J, Mirvis S, Robinson WL. Anterior decompression in cervical spine trauma: does the timing of surgery affect the outcome? Neurosurgery. 1991; 29(2):216–222

[43] Lu K, Lee TC, Liang CL, Chen HJ. Delayed apnea in patients with mid- to lower cervical spinal cord injury. Spine. 2000; 25(11):1332–1338

[44] Levi L, Wolf A, Belzberg H. Hemodynamic parameters in patients with acute cervical cord trauma: description, intervention, and prediction of outcome. Neurosurgery. 1993; 33(6):1007–1016, discussion 1016–1017

[45] Tator CH, Rowed DW, Schwartz ML, et al. Management of acute spinal cord injuries. Can J Surg. 1984; 27(3):289–293, 296

[46] Vale FL, Burns J, Jackson AB, Hadley MN. Combined medical and surgical treatment after acute spinal cord injury: results of a prospective pilot study to assess the merits of aggressive medical resuscitation and blood pressure management. J Neurosurg. 1997; 87(2):239–246

[47] King BS, Gupta R, Narayan RK. The early assessment and intensive care unit management of patients with severe traumatic brain and spinal cord injuries. Surg Clin North Am. 2000; 80(3):855–870, viii–ix

[48] Wolf A, Levi L, Mirvis S, et al. Operative management of bilateral facet dislocation. J Neurosurg. 1991; 75(6):883–890

[49] Kumar A, Parrillo JE. Shock: classification, pathophysiology, and approach to management. In: Parrillo J, Dellinger R, eds. Critical Care Medicine Principles of Diagnosis and Management in the Adult. St. Louis, MO: Mosby; 2002:371–420

[50] Colachis SC, III. Autonomic hyperreflexia with spinal cord injury. J Am Paraplegia Soc. 1992; 15(3):171–186

[51] Lee BY, Karmakar MG, Herz BL, Sturgill RA. Autonomic dysreflexia revisited. J Spinal Cord Med. 1995; 18(2):75–87

[52] Mathias CJ, Frankel HL. Cardiovascular control in spinal man. Annu Rev Physiol. 1988; 50:577–592

[53] Dicpinigaitis PV, Spungen AM, Bauman WA, Absgarten A, Almenoff PL. Bronchial hyperresponsiveness after cervical spinal cord injury. Chest. 1994; 105(4):1073–1076

[54] McEvoy RD, Mykytyn I, Sajkov D, et al. Sleep apnoea in patients with quadriplegia. Thorax. 1995; 50(6):613–619

[55] Short DJ, Stradling JR, Williams SJ. Prevalence of sleep apnoea in patients over 40 years of age with spinal cord lesions. J Neurol Neurosurg Psychiatry. 1992; 55(11):1032–1036

[56] Fishburn MJ, Marino RJ, Ditunno JF, Jr. Atelectasis and pneumonia in acute spinal cord injury. Arch Phys Med Rehabil. 1990; 71(3):197–200

[57] DeVivo MJ, Ivie CS, III. Life expectancy of ventilator-dependent persons with spinal cord injuries. Chest. 1995; 108(1):226–232

[58] Ayas NT, Garshick E, Lieberman SL, Wien MF, Tun C, Brown R. Breathlessness in spinal cord injury depends on injury level. J Spinal Cord Med. 1999; 22(2):97–101

[59] Whiteneck GG, Charlifue SW, Frankel HL, et al. Mortality, morbidity, and psychosocial outcomes of persons spinal cord injured more than 20 years ago. Paraplegia. 1992; 30(9):617–630

[60] Estenne M, De Troyer A. The effects of tetraplegia on chest wall statics. Am Rev Respir Dis. 1986; 134(1):121–124

[61] Goldman JM, Rose LS, Morgan MD, Denison DM. Measurement of abdominal wall compliance in normal subjects and tetraplegic patients. Thorax. 1986; 41(7):513–518

[62] McCool FD, Pichurko BM, Slutsky AS, Sarkarati M, Rossier A, Brown R. Changes in lung volume and rib cage configuration with abdominal binding in quadriplegia. J Appl Physiol (1985). 1986; 60(4):1198–1202

[63] Urmey W, Loring S, Mead J, et al. Upper and lower rib cage deformation during breathing in quadriplegics. J Appl Physiol (1985). 1986; 60(2):618–622

[64] Banzett RB, Inbar GF, Brown R, Goldman M, Rossier A, Mead J. Diaphragm electrical activity during negative lower torso pressure in quadriplegic men. J Appl Physiol. 1981; 51(3):654–659

[65] McCool FD, Brown R, Mayewski RJ, Hyde RW. Effects of posture on stimulated ventilation in quadriplegia. Am Rev Respir Dis. 1988; 138(1):101–105

[66] Danon J, Druz WS, Goldberg NB, Sharp JT. Function of the isolated paced diaphragm and the cervical accessory muscles in C1 quadriplegics. Am Rev Respir Dis. 1979; 119(6):909–919

[67] Maloney FP. Pulmonary function in quadriplegia: effects of a corset. Arch Phys Med Rehabil. 1979; 60(6):261–265

[68] Miller HJ, Thomas E, Wilmot CB. Pneumobelt use among high quadriplegic population. Arch Phys Med Rehabil. 1988; 69(5):369–372

[69] Weingarden SI, Belen JG. Alternative approach to the respiratory management of the high cervical spinal cord injury patient. Int Disabil Stud. 1987; 9(3):132–133

[70] DeVivo MJ, Stover SL, Black KJ. Prognostic factors for 12-year survival after spinal cord injury. Arch Phys Med Rehabil. 1992; 73(2):156–162

[71] Jackson AB, Groomes TE. Incidence of respiratory complications following spinal cord injury. Arch Phys Med Rehabil. 1994; 75(3):270–275

[72] Manning HL, Brown R, Scharf SM, et al. Ventilatory and P0.1 response to hypercapnia in quadriplegia. Respir Physiol. 1992; 89(1):97–112

[73] Ledsome JR, Sharp JM. Pulmonary function in acute cervical cord injury. Am Rev Respir Dis. 1981; 124(1):41–44

[74] McMichan JC, Michel L, Westbrook PR. Pulmonary dysfunction following traumatic quadriplegia. Recognition, prevention, and treatment. JAMA. 1980; 243(6):528–531

[75] Wicks AB, Menter RR. Long-term outlook in quadriplegic patients with initial ventilator dependency. Chest. 1986; 90(3):406–410

[76] Axen K, Pineda H, Shunfenthal I, Haas F. Diaphragmatic function following cervical cord injury: neurally mediated improvement. Arch Phys Med Rehabil. 1985; 66(4):219–222

[77] Haas F, Axen K, Pineda H, Gandino D, Haas A. Temporal pulmonary function changes in cervical cord injury. Arch Phys Med Rehabil. 1985; 66(3):139–144

[78] Bach JR, Alba AS. Noninvasive options for ventilatory support of the traumatic high level quadriplegic patient. Chest. 1990; 98(3):613–619

[79] Bach JR, Alba AS, Bodofsky E, Curran FJ, Schultheiss M. Glossopharyngeal breathing and noninvasive aids in the management of post-polio respiratory insufficiency. Birth Defects Orig Artic Ser. 1987; 23(4):99–113

[80] Montero JC, Feldman DJ, Montero D. Effects of glossopharyngeal breathing on respiratory function after cervical cord transection. Arch Phys Med Rehabil. 1967; 48(12):650–653

[81] De Troyer A, Estenne M, Heilporn A. Mechanism of active expiration in tetraplegic subjects. N Engl J Med. 1986; 314(12):740–744

[82] Estenne M, Knoop C, Vanvaerenbergh J, Heilporn A, De Troyer A. The effect of pectoralis muscle training in tetraplegic subjects. Am Rev Respir Dis. 1989; 139(5):1218–1222

[83] Almenoff PL, Spungen AM, Lesser M, Bauman WA. Pulmonary function survey in spinal cord injury: influences of smoking and level and completeness of injury. Lung. 1995; 173(5):297–306

[84] Hemingway A, Bors E, Hobby RP. An investigation of the pulmonary function of paraplegics. J Clin Invest. 1958; 37(5):773–782

[85] McKinley AC, Auchincloss JH, Jr, Gilbert R, Nicholas JJ. Pulmonary function, ventilatory control, and respiratory complications in quadriplegic subjects. Am Rev Respir Dis. 1969; 100(4):526–532

[86] Brown BT, Carrion HM, Politano VA. Guanethidine sulfate in the prevention of autonomic hyperreflexia. J Urol. 1979; 122(1):55–57

[87] Kiker JD, Woodside JR, Jelinek GE. Neurogenic pulmonary edema associated with autonomic dysreflexia. J Urol. 1982; 128(5):1038–1039

[88] Poe RH, Reisman JL, Rodenhouse TG. Pulmonary edema in cervical spinal cord injury. J Trauma. 1978; 18(1):71–73

[89] Kirby NA, Barnerias MJ, Siebens AA. An evaluation of assisted cough in quadriparetic patients. Arch Phys Med Rehabil. 1966; 47(11):705–710

[90] Jaeger RJ, Turba RM, Yarkony GM, Roth EJ. Cough in spinal cord injured patients: comparison of three methods to produce cough. Arch Phys Med Rehabil. 1993; 74(12):1358–1361

[91] McCool FD, Mayewski RF, Shayne DS, Gibson CJ, Griggs RC, Hyde RW. Intermittent positive pressure breathing in patients with respiratory muscle weakness. Alterations in total respiratory system compliance. Chest. 1986; 90(4):546–552

[92] Stiller K, Simionato R, Rice K, Hall B. The effect of intermittent positive pressure breathing on lung volumes in acute quadriparesis. Paraplegia. 1992; 30(2):121–126

[93] McKinley WO, Jackson AB, Cardenas DD, DeVivo MJ. Long-term medical complications after traumatic spinal cord injury: a regional model systems analysis. Arch Phys Med Rehabil. 1999; 80(11):1402–1410

[94] Burns GA, Cohn SM, Frumento RJ, Degutis LC, Hammers L. Prospective ultrasound evaluation of venous thrombosis in high-risk trauma patients. J Trauma. 1993; 35(3):405–408

[95] Frisbie JH, Sasahara AA. Low dose heparin prophylaxis for deep venous thrombosis in acute spinal cord injury patients: a controlled study. Paraplegia. 1981; 19(6):343–346

[96] Geerts WH, Code KI, Jay RM, Chen E, Szalai JP. A prospective study of venous thromboembolism after major trauma. N Engl J Med. 1994; 331(24):1601–1606

[97] Green D, Lee MY, Ito VY, et al. Fixed- vs adjusted-dose heparin in the prophylaxis of thromboembolism in spinal cord injury. JAMA. 1988; 260(9):1255–1258

[98] Green D, Lee MY, Lim AC, et al. Prevention of thromboembolism after spinal cord injury using low-molecular-weight heparin. Ann Intern Med. 1990; 113(8):571–574

[99] Kulkarni JR, Burt AA, Tromans AT, Constable PD. Prophylactic low dose heparin anticoagulant therapy in patients with spinal cord injuries: a retrospective study. Paraplegia. 1992; 30(3):169–172

[100] Myllynen P, Kammonen M, Rokkanen P, Böstman O, Lalla M, Laasonen E. Deep venous thrombosis and pulmonary embolism in patients with acute spinal cord injury: a comparison with nonparalyzed patients immobilized due to spinal fractures. J Trauma. 1985; 25(6):541–543

[101] Perkash A, Prakash V, Perkash I. Experience with the management of thromboembolism in patients with spinal cord injury: part I. Incidence, diagnosis and role of some risk factors. Paraplegia. 1978; 16(3):322–331

[102] Powell M, Kirshblum S, O'Connor KC. Duplex ultrasound screening for deep vein thrombosis in spinal cord injured patients at rehabilitation admission. Arch Phys Med Rehabil. 1999; 80(9):1044–1046

[103] Watson N. Anti-coagulant therapy in the prevention of venous thrombosis and pulmonary embolism in the spinal cord injury. Paraplegia. 1978; 16(3):265–269

[104] Lamb GC, Tomski MA, Kaufman J, Maiman DJ. Is chronic spinal cord injury associated with increased risk of venous thromboembolism? J Am Paraplegia Soc. 1993; 16(3):153–156

[105] Tator CH, Duncan EG, Edmonds VE, Lapczak LI, Andrews DF. Comparison of surgical and conservative management in 208 patients with acute spinal cord injury. Can J Neurol Sci. 1987; 14(1):60–69

[106] Consortium for Spinal Cord Medicine. Prevention of thromboembolism in spinal cord injury. J Spinal Cord Med. 1997; 20(3):259–283

[107] DeVivo MJ, Kartus PL, Stover SL, Rutt RD, Fine PR. Cause of death for patients with spinal cord injuries. Arch Intern Med. 1989; 149(8):1761–1766

[108] El Masri WS, Silver JR. Prophylactic anticoagulant therapy in patients with spinal cord injury. Paraplegia. 1981; 19(6):334–342

[109] Naso F. Pulmonary embolism in acute spinal cord injury. Arch Phys Med Rehabil. 1974; 55(6):275–278

[110] Perkash A. Experience with the management of deep vein thrombosis in patients with spinal cord injury. Part II: a critical evaluation of the anticoagulant therapy. Paraplegia. 1980; 18(1):2–14

[111] Chu DA, Ahn JH, Ragnarsson KT, Helt J, Folcarelli P, Ramirez A. Deep venous thrombosis: diagnosis in spinal cord injured patients. Arch Phys Med Rehabil. 1985; 66(6):365–368

[112] Roussi J, Bentolila S, Boudaoud L, et al. Contribution of D-dimer determination in the exclusion of deep venous thrombosis in spinal cord injury patients. Spinal Cord. 1999; 37(8):548–552

[113] Todd JW, Frisbie JH, Rossier AB, et al. Deep venous thrombosis in acute spinal cord injury: a comparison of 125I fibrinogen leg scanning, impedance plethysmography and venography. Paraplegia. 1976; 14(1):50–57

[114] Bell WR, Simon TL, DeMets DL. The clinical features of submassive and massive pulmonary emboli. Am J Med. 1977; 62(3):355–360

[115] Stein PD, Willis PW, III, DeMets DL. History and physical examination in acute pulmonary embolism in patients without preexisting cardiac or pulmonary disease. Am J Cardiol. 1981; 47(2):218–223

[116] Wood KE. Major pulmonary embolism: review of a pathophysiologic approach to the golden hour of hemodynamically significant pulmonary embolism. Chest. 2002; 121(3):877–905

[117] Overton DT, Bocka JJ. The alveolar-arterial oxygen gradient in patients with documented pulmonary embolism. Arch Intern Med. 1988; 148(7):1617–1619

[118] Stein PD, Goldhaber SZ, Henry JW. Alveolar-arterial oxygen gradient in the assessment of acute pulmonary embolism. Chest. 1995; 107(1):139–143

[119] Stein PD, Goldhaber SZ, Henry JW, Miller AC. Arterial blood gas analysis in the assessment of suspected acute pulmonary embolism. Chest. 1996; 109(1):78–81

[120] Stein PD, Terrin ML, Hales CA, et al. Clinical, laboratory, roentgenographic, and electrocardiographic findings in patients with acute pulmonary embolism and no pre-existing cardiac or pulmonary disease. Chest. 1991; 100(3):598–603

[121] Lorut C, Ghossains M, Horellou MH, Achkar A, Fretault J, Laaban JP. A noninvasive diagnostic strategy including spiral computed tomography in patients with suspected pulmonary embolism. Am J Respir Crit Care Med. 2000; 162(4 Pt 1):1413–1418

[122] Stein PD, Hull RD, Saltzman HA, Pineo G. Strategy for diagnosis of patients with suspected acute pulmonary embolism. Chest. 1993; 103(5):1553–1559

[123] Wells PS, Ginsberg JS, Anderson DR, et al. Use of a clinical model for safe management of patients with suspected pulmonary embolism. Ann Intern Med. 1998; 129(12):997–1005

[124] Come PC. Echocardiographic evaluation of pulmonary embolism and its response to therapeutic interventions. Chest. 1992; 101(4, Suppl):151S–162S

[125] Torbicki A, Tramarin R, Morpurgo M. Role of echo/Doppler in the diagnosis of pulmonary embolism. Clin Cardiol. 1992; 15(11):805–810

[126] Cheriex EC, Sreeram N, Eussen YF, Pieters FA, Wellens HJ. Cross sectional Doppler echocardiography as the initial technique for the diagnosis of acute pulmonary embolism. Br Heart J. 1994; 72(1):52–57

[127] Kasper W, Meinertz T, Henkel B, et al. Echocardiographic findings in patients with proved pulmonary embolism. Am Heart J. 1986; 112(6):1284–1290

[128] Jardin F, Dubourg O, Bourdarias JP. Echocardiographic pattern of acute cor pulmonale. Chest. 1997; 111(1):209–217

[129] Kasper W, Geibel A, Tiede N, Hofmann T, Meinertz T, Just H. [Echocardiography in the diagnosis of lung embolism] [in German]. Herz. 1989; 14(2):82–101

[130] Ribeiro A, Juhlin-Dannfelt A, Brodin LA, Holmgren A, Jorfeldt L. Pulmonary embolism: relation between the degree of right ventricle overload and the extent of perfusion defects. Am Heart J. 1998; 135(5 Pt 1):868–874

[131] Wolfe MW, Lee RT, Feldstein ML, Parker JA, Come PC, Goldhaber SZ. Prognostic significance of right ventricular hypokinesis and perfusion lung scan defects in pulmonary embolism. Am Heart J. 1994; 127(5):1371–1375

[132] Kasper W, Geibel A, Tiede N, et al. Distinguishing between acute and subacute massive pulmonary embolism by conventional and Doppler echocardiography. Br Heart J. 1993; 70(4):352–356

[133] Vardan S, Mookherjee S, Smulyan HS, Obeid AI. Echocardiography in pulmonary embolism. Jpn Heart J. 1983; 24(1):67–78

[134] PIOPED Investigators. Value of the ventilation/perfusion scan in acute pulmonary embolism. Results of the prospective investigation of pulmonary embolism diagnosis (PIOPED). JAMA. 1990; 263(20):2753–2759

[135] Lesser BA, Leeper KV, Jr, Stein PD, et al. The diagnosis of acute pulmonary embolism in patients with chronic obstructive pulmonary disease. Chest. 1992; 102(1):17–22

[136] Davis LP, Fink-Bennett D. Nuclear medicine in the acutely ill patient—I. Crit Care Clin. 1994; 10(2):365–381

[137] Stein PD, Athanasoulis C, Alavi A, et al. Complications and validity of pulmonary angiography in acute pulmonary embolism. Circulation. 1992; 85(2):462–468

[138] Cooper TJ, Hayward MW, Hartog M. Survey on the use of pulmonary scintigraphy and angiography for suspected pulmonary thromboembolism in the UK. Clin Radiol. 1991; 43(4):243–245

[139] Mills SR, Jackson DC, Older RA, Heaston DK, Moore AV. The incidence, etiologies, and avoidance of complications of pulmonary angiography in a large series. Radiology. 1980; 136(2):295–299

[140] Zuckerman DA, Sterling KM, Oser RF. Safety of pulmonary angiography in the 1990s. J Vasc Interv Radiol. 1996; 7(2):199–205

[141] Stein PD, Hull RD, Raskob G. Risks for major bleeding from thrombolytic therapy in patients with acute pulmonary embolism. Consideration of noninvasive management. Ann Intern Med. 1994; 121(5):313–317

[142] Coche EE, Müller NL, Kim KI, Wiggs BR, Mayo JR. Acute pulmonary embolism: ancillary findings at spiral CT. Radiology. 1998; 207(3):753–758

[143] Cross JJ, Kemp PM, Walsh CG, Flower CD, Dixon AK. A randomized trial of spiral CT and ventilation perfusion scintigraphy for the diagnosis of pulmonary embolism. Clin Radiol. 1998; 53(3):177–182

[144] Reid JH, Murchison JT. Acute right ventricular dilatation: a new helical CT sign of massive pulmonary embolism. Clin Radiol. 1998; 53(9):694–698

[145] Blum AG, Delfau F, Grignon B, et al. Spiral-computed tomography versus pulmonary angiography in the diagnosis of acute massive pulmonary embolism. Am J Cardiol. 1994; 74(1):96–98

[146] Goodman LR, Curtin JJ, Mewissen MW, et al. Detection of pulmonary embolism in patients with unresolved clinical and scintigraphic diagnosis: helical CT versus angiography. AJR Am J Roentgenol. 1995; 164(6):1369–1374

[147] Remy-Jardin M, Remy J, Deschildre F, et al. Diagnosis of pulmonary embolism with spiral CT: comparison with pulmonary angiography and scintigraphy. Radiology. 1996; 200(3):699–706

[148] Remy-Jardin M, Remy J, Wattinne L, Giraud F. Central pulmonary thromboembolism: diagnosis with spiral volumetric CT with the single-breath-hold technique—comparison with pulmonary angiography. Radiology. 1992; 185(2):381–387

[149] Stein PD, Hull RD, Pineo GF. The role of newer diagnostic techniques in the diagnosis of pulmonary embolism. Curr Opin Pulm Med. 1999; 5(4):212–215

[150] Teigen CL, Maus TP, Sheedy PF, II, et al. Pulmonary embolism: diagnosis with contrast-enhanced electron-beam CT and comparison with pulmonary angiography. Radiology. 1995; 194(2):313–319

[151] Pruszczyk P, Torbicki A, Pacho R, et al. Noninvasive diagnosis of suspected severe pulmonary embolism: transesophageal echocardiography vs spiral CT. Chest. 1997; 112(3):722–728

[152] Kuzo RS, Goodman LR. CT evaluation of pulmonary embolism: technique and interpretation. AJR Am J Roentgenol. 1997; 169(4):959–965

[153] Erdman WA, Peshock RM, Redman HC, et al. Pulmonary embolism: comparison of MR images with radionuclide and angiographic studies. Radiology. 1994; 190(2):499–508

[154] Loubeyre P, Revel D, Douek P, et al. Dynamic contrast-enhanced MR angiography of pulmonary embolism: comparison with pulmonary angiography. AJR Am J Roentgenol. 1994; 162(5):1035–1039

[155] Meaney JF, Weg JG, Chenevert TL, Stafford-Johnson D, Hamilton BH, Prince MR. Diagnosis of pulmonary embolism with magnetic resonance angiography. N Engl J Med. 1997; 336(20):1422–1427

[156] Gefter WB, Hatabu H, Holland GA, Gupta KB, Henschke CI, Palevsky HI. Pulmonary thromboembolism: recent developments in diagnosis with CT and MR imaging. Radiology. 1995; 197(3):561–574

[157] Casas ER, Sánchez MP, Arias CR, Masip JP. Prophylaxis of venous thrombosis and pulmonary embolism in patients with acute traumatic spinal cord lesions. Paraplegia. 1977; 15(3):209–214

[158] Frisbie JH, Sharma GV. Pulmonary embolism manifesting as acute disturbances of behavior in patients with spinal cord injury. Paraplegia. 1994; 32(8):570–572

[159] Gündüz S, Oğur E, Möhür H, Somuncu I, Açjksöz E, Ustünsöz B. Deep vein thrombosis in spinal cord injured patients. Paraplegia. 1993; 31(9):606–610

[160] Hachen HJ. Anticoagulant therapy in patients with spinal cord injury. Paraplegia. 1974; 12(3):176–187

[161] Weingarden SI, Weingarden DS, Belen J. Fever and thromboembolic disease in acute spinal cord injury. Paraplegia. 1988; 26(1):35–42

[162] Chen D, Apple DF, Jr, Hudson LM, Bode R. Medical complications during acute rehabilitation following spinal cord injury—current experience of the Model Systems. Arch Phys Med Rehabil. 1999; 80(11):1397–1401

[163] Merli GJ, Herbison GJ, Ditunno JF, et al. Deep vein thrombosis: prophylaxis in acute spinal cord injured patients. Arch Phys Med Rehabil. 1988; 69(9):661–664

[164] Harris S, Chen D, Green D. Enoxaparin for thromboembolism prophylaxis in spinal injury: preliminary report on experience with 105 patients. Am J Phys Med Rehabil. 1996; 75(5):326–327

[165] Balshi JD, Cantelmo NL, Menzoian JO. Complications of caval interruption by Greenfield filter in quadriplegics. J Vasc Surg. 1989; 9(4):558–562

[166] Greenfield LJ. Does cervical spinal cord injury induce a higher incidence of complications after prophylactic Greenfield filter usage? J Vasc Interv Radiol. 1997; 8(4):719–720

[167] Kinney TB, Rose SC, Valji K, Oglevie SB, Roberts AC. Does cervical spinal cord injury induce a higher incidence of complications after prophylactic Greenfield inferior vena cava filter usage? J Vasc Interv Radiol. 1996; 7(6):907–915

[168] Decousus H, Leizorovicz A, Parent F, et al. A clinical trial of vena caval filters in the prevention of pulmonary embolism in patients with proximal deep-vein thrombosis. Prévention du Risque d'Embolie Pulmonaire par Interruption Cave Study Group. N Engl J Med. 1998; 338(7):409–415

[169] Winemiller MH, Stolp-Smith KA, Silverstein MD, Therneau TM. Prevention of venous thromboembolism in patients with spinal cord injury: effects of sequential pneumatic compression and heparin. J Spinal Cord Med. 1999; 22(3):182–191

[170] Becker DM, Gonzalez M, Gentili A, Eismont F, Green BA. Prevention of deep venous thrombosis in patients with acute spinal cord injuries: use of rotating treatment tables. Neurosurgery. 1987; 20(5):675–677

[171] López JA, Kearon C, Lee AY. Deep venous thrombosis. Hematology (Am Soc Hematol Educ Program). 2004:439–456

[172] Vlahakes GJ, Turley K, Hoffman JI. The pathophysiology of failure in acute right ventricular hypertension: hemodynamic and biochemical correlations. Circulation. 1981; 63(1):87–95

[173] Angle MR, Molloy DW, Penner B, Jones D, Prewitt RM. The cardiopulmonary and renal hemodynamic effects of norepinephrine in canine pulmonary embolism. Chest. 1989; 95(6):1333–1337

[174] Hirsch LJ, Rooney MW, Wat SS, Kleinmann B, Mathru M. Norepinephrine and phenylephrine effects on right ventricular function in experimental canine pulmonary embolism. Chest. 1991; 100(3):796–801

[175] Layish DT, Tapson VF. Pharmacologic hemodynamic support in massive pulmonary embolism. Chest. 1997; 111(1):218–224

[176] Prewitt RM. Hemodynamic management in pulmonary embolism and acute hypoxemic respiratory failure. Crit Care Med. 1990; 18(1 Pt 2):S61–S69

[177] Capellier G, Jacques T, Balvay P, Blasco G, Belle E, Barale F. Inhaled nitric oxide in patients with pulmonary embolism. Intensive Care Med. 1997; 23(10):1089–1092

[178] Webb SA, Stott S, van Heerden PV. The use of inhaled aerosolized prostacyclin (IAP) in the treatment of pulmonary hypertension secondary to pulmonary embolism. Intensive Care Med. 1996; 22(4):353–355

[179] Badr MS, Grossman JE. Positional changes in gas exchange after unilateral pulmonary embolism. Chest. 1990; 98(6):1514–1516

[180] Goldhaber SZ. Pulmonary embolism. N Engl J Med. 1998; 339(2):93–104

[181] Kearon C. Initial treatment of venous thromboembolism. Thromb Haemost. 1999; 82(2):887–891

[182] Dalen JE, Alpert JS. Natural history of pulmonary embolism. Prog Cardiovasc Dis. 1975; 17(4):259–270

[183] Goldhaber SZ, Haire WD, Feldstein ML, et al. Alteplase versus heparin in acute pulmonary embolism: randomised trial assessing right-ventricular function and pulmonary perfusion. Lancet. 1993; 341(8844):507–511

[184] Casthely PA, Yoganathan D, Karyanis B, et al. Histamine blockade and cardiovascular changes following heparin administration during cardiac surgery. J Cardiothorac Anesth. 1990; 4(6):711–714

[185] Kanbak M, Kahraman S, Celebioglu B, Akpolat N, Ercan S, Erdem K. Prophylactic administration of histamine 1 and/or histamine 2 receptor blockers in the prevention of heparin- and protamine-related haemodynamic effects. Anaesth Intensive Care. 1996; 24(5):559–563

[186] Soloff LA, Rodman T. Acute pulmonary embolism. II. Clinical. Am Heart J. 1967; 74(6):829–847

[187] Kasper W, Konstantinides S, Geibel A, et al. Management strategies and determinants of outcome in acute major pulmonary embolism: results of a multicenter registry. J Am Coll Cardiol. 1997; 30(5):1165–1171

[188] Schmid C, Zietlow S, Wagner TO, Laas J, Borst HG. Fulminant pulmonary embolism: symptoms, diagnostics, operative technique, and results. Ann Thorac Surg. 1991; 52(5):1102–1105, discussion 1105–1107

[189] Stulz P, Schläpfer R, Feer R, Habicht J, Grädel E. Decision making in the surgical treatment of massive pulmonary embolism. Eur J Cardiothorac Surg. 1994; 8(4):188–193

[190] Anderson DR, Levine MN. Thrombolytic therapy for the treatment of acute pulmonary embolism. CMAJ. 1992; 146(8):1317–1324

[191] Arcasoy SM, Kreit JW. Thrombolytic therapy of pulmonary embolism: a comprehensive review of current evidence. Chest. 1999; 115(6):1695–1707

[192] Dalen JE, Alpert JS, Hirsh J. Thrombolytic therapy for pulmonary embolism: is it effective? Is it safe? When is it indicated? Arch Intern Med. 1997; 157(22):2550–2556

[193] Elliott CG. Embolectomy, catheter extraction, or disruption of pulmonary emboli: editorial review. Curr Opin Pulm Med. 1995; 1(4):298–302

[194] Satter P. Pulmonary embolectomy with the aid of extracorporeal circulation. Thorac Cardiovasc Surg. 1982; 30(1):31–35

[195] Harrigan MR, Hadley MN, Dhall SS, et al. Management of vertebral artery injuries following non-penetrating cervical trauma. Neurosurgery. 2013; 72(Suppl 2):234–243

[196] Biffl WL, Moore EE, Elliott JP, et al. The devastating potential of blunt vertebral arterial injuries. Ann Surg. 2000; 231(5):672–681

[197] Friedman D, Flanders A, Thomas C, Millar W. Vertebral artery injury after acute cervical spine trauma: rate of occurrence as detected by MR angiography and assessment of clinical consequences. AJR Am J Roentgenol. 1995; 164(2):443–447, discussion 448–449

[198] Giacobetti FB, Vaccaro AR, Bos-Giacobetti MA, et al. Vertebral artery occlusion associated with cervical spine trauma. A prospective analysis. Spine. 1997; 22(2):188–192

[199] Louw JA, Mafoyane NA, Small B, Neser CP. Occlusion of the vertebral artery in cervical spine dislocations. J Bone Joint Surg Br. 1990; 72(4):679–681

[200] Weller SJ, Rossitch E, Jr, Malek AM. Detection of vertebral artery injury after cervical spine trauma using magnetic resonance angiography. J Trauma. 1999; 46(4):660–666

[201] Willis BK, Greiner F, Orrison WW, Benzel EC. The incidence of vertebral artery injury after midcervical spine fracture or subluxation. Neurosurgery. 1994; 34(3):435–441, discussion 441–442

[202] Woodring JH, Lee C, Duncan V. Transverse process fractures of the cervical vertebrae: are they insignificant? J Trauma. 1993; 34(6):797–802

[203] Eastman AL, Chason DP, Perez CL, McAnulty AL, Minei JP. Computed tomographic angiography for the diagnosis of blunt cervical vascular injury: is it ready for primetime? J Trauma. 2006; 60(5):925–929, discussion 929

[204] Berne JD, Reuland KS, Villarreal DH, McGovern TM, Rowe SA, Norwood SH. Sixteen-slice multi-detector computed tomographic angiography improves the accuracy of screening for blunt cerebrovascular injury. J Trauma. 2006; 60(6):1204–1209, discussion 1209–1210

[205] Young B, Ott L, Rapp R, Norton J. The patient with critical neurological disease. Crit Care Clin. 1987; 3(1):217–233

24 Biomechanical Considerations for Operative Interventions in Vertebral Column Fractures and Dislocations

Christopher E. Wolfla

Abstract

Spinal column fractures and dislocations are commonly seen in neurosurgical practice and are the source of a great deal of short- and intermediate-term morbidity and long-term disability. Rapid diagnosis and efficacious treatment are essential and are aided by knowledge of spine biomechanics. In this chapter, readers are introduced to basic principles regarding the diagnosis and treatment of cervical, thoracic, and lumbar injuries. Regardless of the spinal region, the goals of treatment are to prevent neurologic injury, reduce deformity, and stabilize the spine.

Keywords: biomechanics, diagnosis, fracture, spine, treatment

24.1 Epidemiology

Although the precise incidence of vertebral column fractures is not known, the National Inpatient Sample shows that in 2013 they were present in 277,335 hospital patient discharges and were the principal diagnosis in 110,730 discharges, with a mean hospital charge of over $70,000 per patient.[1] Spinal cord injuries (SCIs) occur in approximately 12,500 patients per year, and an estimated 240,000 to 337,000 individuals currently live with SCI. The most common neurologic category is incomplete tetraplegia (45%), followed by incomplete paraplegia (21%), complete paraplegia (20%), and complete tetraplegia (14%).[2]

Motor vehicle crashes (MVCs), particularly in the absence of occupant restraints, account for the majority of spine and spinal cord trauma. Less common causes are falls, acts of violence (most commonly gunshot wounds), and recreational sporting activities such as diving and contact sports. The average age at injury has steadily increased over time and is currently 42 years, likely reflecting the increase in the median age of the general population of the United States since the mid-1970s.[2] Among adults, vertebral column fractures and fracture dislocations are the most common injury types. Most often, the degree of associated neurologic injury correlates with the extent of vertebral column fracture and with associated dislocation or subluxation.[3,4] In both adults and children, the cervical spine is the most frequently injured region of the spinal column following high-velocity or blunt trauma and is estimated to be 2 to 4% of all trauma patients.[3,5] Accordingly, these injuries may be associated with neurologic impairment. Although lower cervical injuries are common in both adult and pediatric population, atlanto-occipital dislocation (AOD) is more prevalent in the pediatric age group.[3]

For all vertebral column injuries, initial management is focused on basic emergency and trauma management.[4,6,7] Acute clinical assessment and management of spinal cord–injured patients requires a skillful neurologic examination and knowledge of multisystem management issues (cardiac, hemodynamic, pulmonary, urogenital) specific to this patient population, with the preeminent objective of medical and neurologic stabilization and prevention of secondary injury. The primary focus of this chapter is to review the typical fractures or fracture dislocations that occur at a given vertebral column level and identify optimal nonsurgical or surgical treatment options.

24.2 General Consideration Regarding Timing of Surgical Treatment

Generally, the decision for surgical intervention in spinal column injury is based on numerous factors, including, but certainly not limited to, degree of spinal deformity, biomechanical stability, and neurologic status. Regardless of level, the principal management objectives are preservation of neurologic function, prevention of secondary injury, and provision of an optimal milieu for neurologic recovery.[8,9] Frequently, the injured patient will require reduction of deformity, decompression of neural elements, and stabilization to achieve these goals. Early, and often urgent, surgical treatment is preferred if biomechanical stability of the spine is severely compromised or if neurologic deficit is imminent or progressive. Yet, even the definitions of *early* and *delayed* remain controversial, and neurologic outcomes are equivalent irrespective of timing of surgical intervention.[8,9,10,11] Pulmonary failure and pneumonia are the leading causes of death in patients with spine trauma and SCI.[2,12] Recent studies, however, emphasize the non-neurologic benefits afforded by earlier surgical intervention when appropriate. Early surgical stabilization allows for more rapid mobilization and rehabilitation and has been shown to decrease complications such as pneumonia, decubitus ulcer formation, deep vein thrombosis, and urinary tract infections.[9,12]

24.3 Occipitocervical Junction Injuries

Stability of the atlanto-occipital junction relies primarily on the integrity of the ligamentous structures[1]: anterior and posterior atlanto-occipital membranes,[2] tectorial membrane,[3] cruciate ligament,[4] apical ligament of the dens, and[5] alar ligaments. The tectorial membrane and alar ligaments are the principal structures in maintaining atlanto-occipital stability, and disruption of these structures results in an unstable injury.

Traumatic AODs (▶ Fig. 24.1) are uncommon injuries caused by hyperflexion and distraction forces during high-energy blunt trauma.[4,5,13] Although often fatal, improvements in emergent patient management, transport, and early recognition have resulted in more survivors of AOD. Nearly 20% of survivors may show no initial focal neurologic deficit, leading to a low suspicion for

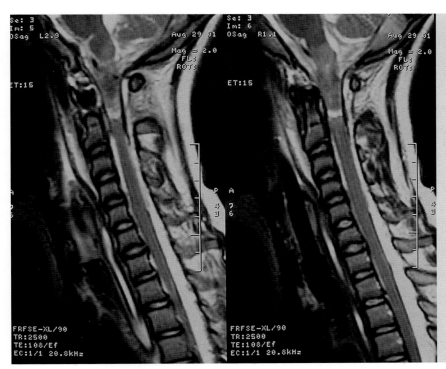

Fig. 24.1 Midsagittal T2-weighted magnetic resonance images show an atlanto-occipital dislocation. High signal intensity present in the ligamentous complex and spinal cord reflects severe injury to these structures.

diagnosis of AOD.[13,14] Consequently, 36% of patients with undiagnosed AOD experience neurologic deterioration from inadequate cervical immobilization.[13,14] In other cases where AOD is suspected, patients often have significant neurologic deficits that include lower cranial nerve neuropathies, unilateral or bilateral weakness, and quadriplegia resulting from compression or distortion of the lower cranial nerves, brainstem, or spinal cord.[4,13] Therefore, early identification and management of these injuries may limit progression of further neurologic impairment.[4,13,14,15]

Although several radiographic methods based on the relationship between the skull base and cervical spine have been well described to diagnose AOD from lateral cervical spine radiographs (▶Table 24.1), the basion–axial interval–basion dental interval is preferred.[13] Nevertheless, the diagnosis from plain radiographic film is often missed.[13] Because of this, additional imaging of the occipitocervical junction with reconstructive computed tomography (CT) or magnetic resonance

imaging (MRI) should be considered. This is particularly the case in pediatric patients, where the measurement of the condyle–C1 interval on CT is the recommended method.[13] Moreover, the presence of prevertebral soft-tissue swelling or an increase in the dens–basion distance on lateral cervical spine radiograph, or subarachnoid hemorrhage at the craniovertebral junction on CT, may provide diagnostic clues.[4,13,14]

AOD injuries have been classified into four types based on the ligamentous injury pattern, all of which are unstable (▶Table 24.2).[4,13] Initial treatment is immobilization of the cervical spine, preferably with a halo orthosis. Traction is not recommended and carries a 10% risk of neurologic injury.[13] Nonoperative management alone is inadequate and has been found to lead to persistent instability and worsening neurologic function.[4,15,16] Thus, definitive treatment for stabilization of AOD injuries is occipitocervical arthrodesis and rigid internal fixation, often accompanied by decompression and reduction to maximize neurologic recovery.[4,13,15]

Table 24.1 Radiographic criteria of atlanto-occipital dislocation

Method	Anatomical relationship
Wackenheim's clival line	Tangential line along posterior clivus to odontoid tip with no posterior or anterior displacement
Power's ratio (BC:OA)	Distance ratio between basion to C1 posterior arch (BC) and opisthion to anterior C1 arch ≤ 1
Wholey dens–basion technique	Distance from basion to dens ≤ 10 mm
Dublin's method	Distance from posterior mandible to anterior atlas ≤ 13 mm; or distance from posterior mandible to dens ≤ 20 mm
Harris BAI–BDI method[a]	Basion to posterior C2 line (basion–axial interval, BAI) with the caudal cortical line of the axis ≤ 12 mm ventrally or ≤ 4 mm dorsally; and basion to dens (basion–dens interval, BDI) distance ≤ 12 mm

[a]Most reliable means to diagnose atlanto-occipital dislocation.

Table 24.2 Classification of fractures of the upper cervical spine

Type	Description of disruption
Atlanto-occipital dislocations	
• I	Anterior ligament dislocation
• II	Longitudinal ligament dislocation
• III	Posterior ligament dislocation
• Other	Complex dislocation
Atlantoaxial ligamentous injuries	
• IA	Midportion of transverse ligament
• IB	Periosteal insertion with no bony fracture
• IIA	Disconnection with C1 lateral mass with comminuted fracture
• IIB	Disconnection with C1 lateral mass with avulsion fracture
Isolated C1 fractures	
• I	Posterior arch only, often bilateral
• II	Unilateral fracture with lateral mass involvement
• III	Burst-type fracture, involves three or more fractures through the anterior and posterior C1 ring; Jefferson's fracture
Odontoid fractures	
• I	Superior tip of the dens
• II	Base of dens at junction between dens and C2 vertebral body
• IIA	Type II with comminuted bone fracture at base of the dens with free bony fragments
• III	Fracture extension into vertebral body
Hangman's fractures	
• I	Isolated hairline fracture of the neural arch posterior to the vertebral body; < 3 mm subluxation of C2 on C3
• II	Disruption of the posterior longitudinal ligament and the disk space below C2; > 4 mm subluxation of C2 on C3 or > 11 degrees angulation
• IIA	Type II with less displacement but greater angulation
• III	Pars articularis fracture with bilateral facet dislocation at C2–C3
C2 body fractures	
• I	Vertical, coronal orientation
• II	Vertical, sagittal orientation
• III	Transverse, axial orientation
C1–C2 rotary subluxation	
• I	Rotary displacement without anterior shift
• II	Rotary displacement with anterior displacement 3–5 mm
• III	Rotary displacement with anterior displacement > 5 mm
• IV	Rotary displacement with posterior translation
Combined C1–C2 fractures	
• C1–type II odontoid	
• C1–miscellaneous axis	
• C1–type III odontoid	
• C1–hangman's type	

24.4 Atlantoaxial Ligamentous Injuries

Although not true fractures, isolated traumatic transverse atlantal ligament injuries are unstable, result from high-energy flexion forces to the cervical spine, and are often associated with significant upper cervical SCI.[17] Diagnosis may be made from lateral flexion cervical radiographs demonstrating a widened atlantodental interval, from CT imaging showing a C1 lateral mass avulsion fracture, or by direct visualization with MRI. Two categories of injury are disruption of the ligament alone (type I) and with avulsion of the tubercle connecting the ligament to the C1 lateral mass (type II) (▶Table 24.2). Although type II injuries may occasionally be successfully treated nonoperatively with rigid cervical immobilization, results are often unsatisfactory and C1–C2 fusion is the treatment of choice. Type I ligamentous injuries do not heal with external immobilization and require surgical stabilization. Surgical options include C1–C2 arthrodesis supplemented by posterior wiring, transarticular screws, and/or segmental screw fixation.[4,18]

24.5 Isolated C1 Fractures

Atlas fractures (▶Fig. 24.2) account for approximately 2 to 13% of acute cervical spine fractures and occur typically with axial load trauma, with or without lateral bending.[4,17,19] Any part of the C1 ring or lateral mass may be involved and fractures typically occur at multiple sites (▶Table 24.2). A Jefferson fracture is classically referred to as a four-point fracture (bilateral anterior and posterior ring) but more recently includes the more common two- or three-point fractures.[19] Neurologic deficit is rare and likely due to the larger spinal canal at this level and the tendency of the bone fragments to burst outward.[4] Assessment of C1 fractures for stability is dependent on the integrity of the transverse ligament, which may be evaluated by odontoid plain radiographs or direct visualization with high-resolution MRI. Generally, the transverse ligament is considered disrupted if the sum of displacement of the lateral masses of C1 over C2 is greater than 6.9 mm (rule of Spence) or the atlantodental interval is greater than 3 mm observed in the odontoid view radiograph.[20]

Treatment is based on the type of fracture and integrity of the transverse ligament. If, however, the transverse ligament is intact, treatment with external orthosis is recommended. In the presence of transverse ligament disruption, management may be with either an external orthosis or with operative treatment, although the latter is usually preferred.[19] Operative treatment may be considered for burst fractures with transverse atlantal ligamentous injury. Stabilization may be achieved by arthrodesis supplemented by posterior (or anterior) C1–C2 transarticular screws, C1 lateral mass–C2 pars/pedicle screws, or, more commonly, occipital–C1–C2 constructs. Wiring techniques are generally ineffective because they often fail to fixate the load-bearing lateral masses. The type of internal fixation performed may influence the requirement for postoperative immobilization.[19,20]

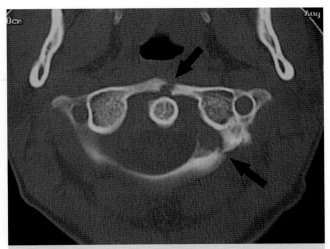

Fig. 24.2 Axial computed tomography image shows a two-point fracture through the anterior and posterior ring elements of C1 (black arrows).

24.6 C2 Fractures

Axis fractures represent nearly 20% of cervical fractures.[5,21] Classifiable fractures include odontoid fractures, hangman's fractures, and C2 body fractures.[4,22,23] Subtypes exist for each fracture classification based on the anatomical features and functional significance of the injury (▶Table 24.2). The unique anatomy and biomechanics of the C1–C2 complex provides weight-bearing support and axial rotation of the head on the spine.[17] Although atlantoaxial dislocation is one of the most common sites of fatal cervical spine injuries, the majority with isolated C2 fractures have minimal to no SCI.[21] Reconstructed CT imaging provides excellent radiographic evaluation of the bony injury. MRI provides important information regarding soft-tissue structures, particularly ligamentous structures, and is occasionally useful for judging the chronicity of C2 fractures.

24.7 Odontoid Fractures

Odontoid fractures result most often from a combination of compression and anterior or anterolateral shear. In younger patients, these fractures are usually due to high-energy trauma, such as MVCs, and from lower-energy injuries, such as falls from standing or sitting heights in the elderly.[21,24] The transverse atlantal ligament restricts the translational motion of C1 on C2 and anchors the odontoid process to the anterior arch of C1. Consequently, fractures of the odontoid process result in potential loss of restriction of translational movement.[17] Odontoid fractures are classified as either through the tip of the dens above the transverse ligament (type I), through its base (type II), through its base with comminution (type IIA), or through the base of the dens and extending into the C2 body (type III) (▶Table 24.2).[19,21,24] All odontoid fractures may be treated initially with external immobilization. Isolated type I and well-aligned type III fractures are considered stable and treated with nonoperative external immobilization, although the presence of a

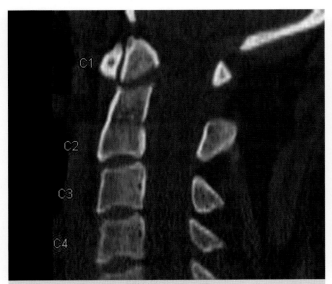

Fig. 24.3 C2 fracture through the odontoid (type II) is demonstrated on this reformatted midsagittal computed tomography image. Note minimal displacement of the odontoid and lack of comminuted bone fragments at the fracture site

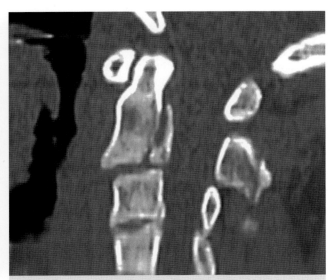

Fig. 24.4 Reformatted midsagittal computed tomography image of a coronally oriented (type I) C2 vertebral body fracture.

type I fracture is associated with AOD.[20,21] Poorly aligned type III fractures (≥ 5 mm displacement) should be given strong consideration for surgical treatment.[22]

Type II fractures are the most common odontoid fracture (▶ Fig. 24.3), they are considered unstable, and their treatment is controversial.[21,22,24] Nonoperative immobilization and reduction may be employed; however, this treatment is associated with high rates of nonunion. Subsequently, type II or IIA odontoid fractures should be considered for surgical fixation if any of the following factors are present[1]: dens displacement ≥ 5 mm[2], loss of fracture reduction with external immobilization,[3] comminution of the fracture,[4] and patient age ≥ 50 years.[22] Disruption of the transverse atlantal ligament, patient age, and medical comorbidities should also be considered when deciding on external versus surgical treatment. If the transverse ligament is ruptured (10% of odontoid fractures), early surgical stabilization to avoid delayed instability and nonunion is recommended. Operative management options are varied and include posterior C1–C2 wiring and bone grafting with or without transarticular screw fixation, C1–C2 wiring and bone grafting with posterior instrumentation of the lateral masses of C1 and C2, and, if the transverse ligament is intact, odontoid screw fixation.[21,24]

24.8 Hangman's Fractures

Traumatic spondylolisthesis of the axis (hangman's fracture) is characterized by bilateral fractures through the pars interarticularis of C2. Rather than the distraction and hyperextension mechanism associated with judicial hanging, the more common mechanism for this injury is hyperextension, axial loading, and possibly rebound flexion, or a combination of these forces associated with MVCs.[4,17,22,25] Neurologic deficit is uncommon or minimal and frequently resolves.[23,25] The three major types are those with < 3 mm of subluxation of C2 on C3 (type I); disruption of the C2–C3 disk and posterior longitudinal ligament

with resultant subluxation ≥ 4 mm C2 on C3 or angulation > 11 degrees (type II); similar to type II but less displacement with greater angulation (type IIA); and bilateral C2–C3 facet disruption with C2 bipedicle fracture (type III) (▶ Table 24.2).[4,22] Type I fractures are considered biomechanically stable fractures and may be treated with rigid cervical immobilization for 12 weeks.[23,25] Type II, IIA, and III fractures are considered biomechanically unstable and surgical treatment is recommended, particularly those that are ineffectively immobilized by a halo.[4,22,25] Surgical options depend upon the fracture anatomy but may include anterior C2–C3 interbody fusion and instrumentation as well as posterior C1–C3 fusion and instrumentation procedures.

24.9 C2 Body Fractures

C2 body fractures can be defined as fractures anterior to the pars articularis and inferior to the base of the dens and are categorized on the basis of the orientation of their fracture line as coronal, sagittal, or transverse (▶ Fig. 24.4).[23,26] The latter is considered identical to a type III odontoid fracture and should be managed accordingly. Evaluation with CT or MR angiography of the foramen transversarium can be considered to assess possible injury to the vertebral artery. Stability of these fractures is dependent on alignment, degree of displacement, and fracture location. Nonetheless, most fractures are successfully managed with external cervical immobilization, with surgical intervention reserved for fractures that are difficult to reduce, highly unstable, or in patients prone to nonunion.[4,22,23,25]

24.10 Combined Atlas–Axis Fractures

Combined atlas–axis fractures are infrequent, possibly because of the magnitude of force thought to be associated with these fractures and resultant increased mortality rate.[5,14] These fractures are usually unstable and are categorized into four subtypes (▶Table 24.2). Treatment options are based primarily on the specific characteristics of the axis fracture. As with isolated C1 or C2 fractures, external immobilization is recommended for most combined fractures except for C1–type II odontoid fractures with an atlantodens interval ≥ 5 mm or C1–hangman's type with C2–C3 angulation ≥ 11 degrees, for which surgical stabilization and fusion are recommended.[3,4,27]

24.11 C1–C2 Rotatory Subluxation

Acute C1–C2 rotary subluxation injuries are most common in the pediatric population, and four subtypes have been identified (▶Table 24.2).[3,4,5,28] Type I is most common; however, types II and III are both associated with transverse atlantal ligament disruption.[3,4,29] Odontoid view radiographs may show asymmetry of the C1 and C2 lateral masses; however, CT imaging better demonstrates rotary subluxation, and MRI permits optimal evaluation of ligament integrity. Treatment is primarily nonoperative, with external reduction by craniocervical traction followed by immobilization.[29] Irreducible or recurrent subluxations, transverse ligamentous injuries, or delayed instability should be managed surgically with a posterior stabilization procedure.[28,29]

24.12 Subaxial (C3–C7) Cervical Column Injuries

Subaxial cervical vertebral injuries are common, generally result from blunt traumatic injury to the cervical spine, and are often associated with devastating neurologic sequelae from associated cervical cord injury.[5] The work-up for these injuries generally includes CT to define the bony extent of the injury and MRI to evaluate the disks, ligaments, and neurologic structures.

Although many classification systems have been developed for these injuries, the use of the Subaxial Injury Classification (SLIC) or Cervical Spine Injury Severity Score (CSISS) is currently recommended. Both have the advantage of excellent reliability and intraclass correlation. The SLIC, however, includes morphological, ligamentous, and neurologic information and thus may be more useful in the clinical situation.

The SLIC divides subaxial injuries into four morphological categories: Normal, compression/burst, distraction, and translation/rotation. Translation/rotation injuries include bilateral and unilateral facet dislocations. Ligamentous categories include normal, indeterminate with MRI signal change only, and disrupted. Finally, neurologic categories take into account complete/incomplete spinal cord injuries, root injuries, and ongoing spinal cord compression. Each of these findings is assigned a point value and the sum determines the "threshold for surgical intervention" (▶Table 24.3). Injuries with a score of 1 to 3 are generally treated nonoperatively, whereas injuries with a score of 5 or higher are generally treated surgically. There is currently equipoise regarding the treatment of injuries with a score of 4.[30, 31,32]

The initial treatment of subaxial cervical spine injuries is immobilization with a rigid cervical collar and supportive blocks. Sandbags and tape are inadequate.[33] Subsequent treatment goals include decompression of the spinal cord and nerve roots,

Table 24.3 Subaxial injury classification and severity scale[30,31,32]

Subaxial injury classification	Points
Morphology	
• No abnormality	0
• Compression	1
• Burst	+1 = 2
• Distraction (facet perch, hyperextension)	3
• Rotation/translation (facet dislocation, unstable tear-drop, or advanced	4
• flexion compression injury)	
Discoligamentous complex (DLC)	
• Intact	0
• Indeterminate (isolated intraspinous widening, MRI signal change only)	1
• Disrupted (widening of disc space, facet perch or dislocation)	2
Neurologic status	
• Intact	0
• Root injury	1
• Complete cord injury	2
• Incomplete cord injury	3
• Continuous cord compression in setting of neurologic deficit (NeuroModifier)	+1 = 1

Abbreviation: MRI, magnetic resonance imaging.

as well as restoration of spinal stability. When surgical treatment is indicated, such treatment should be tailored to the patient's pattern of injury to accomplish these goals. At present, there is no compelling evidence that an anterior, posterior, or combined approach is superior in patients not requiring a specific approach for decompression.[34] There is a growing body of evidence that decompression prior to 24 hours after spinal cord injury results in improved outcomes.[35] Ankylosing spondylitis patients, however, represent an exception. Patients with this condition should undergo an aggressive work-up for even minor injuries. If an operative fracture is found, long segment posterior stabilization is recommended, as anterior stabilization is associated with an unacceptably high rate of failure.[34]

24.13 Thoracic and Thoracolumbar Column Injuries

The biomechanics of the thoracic spine are unique because of its relatively rigid kyphotic posture and articulation with the rib cage, which provide stability and resistance to compressive, bending, and axial rotation forces.[4,11,17,36] Distal to the rib cage, the thoracolumbar region is more vulnerable and more commonly injured.[4,17] Additionally, stability is maintained by the anterior longitudinal ligament, anulus fibrosus, and posterior longitudinal ligament rather than the facet capsules as in the cervical and lumbar spine.[36] Injury to the thoracic spine may be associated with varying degrees of paraplegia because the spinal canal is narrow and occupied mostly by the spinal cord.

Table 24.4 Classification of fractures of the thoracic, thoracolumbar, and lumbar spine

Type	Description of disruption
Compression	Failure of the anterior column with varying degrees of loss of height
Burst	Failure of anterior and middle columns from pure axial loading on vertebral body
Seat belt type	Failure of posterior and middle columns due to flexion forces
Fracture dislocations	Failure of anterior, middle, and posterior columns due to combined compression, rotation, tension, or shear forces resulting in varying degrees of subluxation or distraction

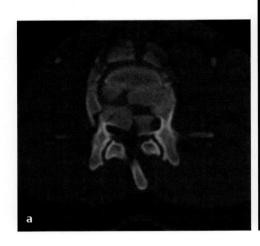
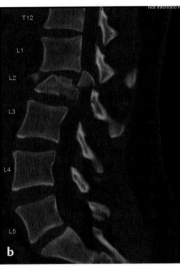

Fig. 24.5 **(a)** Axial computed tomography (CT) scan of an L2 burst fracture reveals disruption of both anterior and middle columns with displacement of bone into the spinal canal on the left. **(b)** Midsagittal CT scan of the same L2 burst fracture shows loss of vertebral body height and narrowing of the canal with distortion of the thecal sac from the retropulsed bone fragment.

Several injury classification systems based on the mechanism of injury, radiographic patterns of disruption, and neurologic status exist and continue to evolve.[36,37] The most common classification system is based on a three-column model, with the anterior column defined as the ALL to the anterior two thirds of the vertebral body; the middle column as the posterior one third of the vertebral body, including the anulus fibrosus and PLL; and the posterior column, encompassing all structures posterior to the PLL.[4,11] From this system, thoracic spine injuries may be divided into four broad categories[1]: compression fractures,[2] burst fractures,[3] seat belt–type injuries, and[4] fracture dislocations. According to this model, acute instability occurs with rupture of the middle and posterior columns (►Table 24.4).[4,36]

Compression fractures are defined as failure of the anterior column with an intact posterior column, are typically but not exclusively considered stable, and have no associated neurologic deficit.[36] These fractures occur with axial load forces to the vertebral body and result in wedging of the anterior vertebral body, causing varying degrees of kyphosis.[17] Upper thoracic compression fractures (T2–T10) deserve special consideration. Because the rib cage provides increased resistance to injury forces, much higher–energy forces are required to cause compression fractures in this region. Consequently, these fractures may have higher instances of progressive angulation and associated neurologic deficit and instability.[4,36]

Burst fractures (►Fig. 24.5a, b) are caused by axial compressive loading forces to the anterior and middle columns, causing injury to both.[17] These fractures have several subtypes, occur mainly at the thoracolumbar junction, and are frequently characterized by significant canal compromise due to bony

fragment retropulsion into the canal.[37] The presence or absence of posterior element injury helps to predict the stability of these injuries. Acute unstable burst fractures are characterized by posterior column disruption, which is a function of facet joint loading.[17]

Seat belt fractures or flexion distraction injuries result in failure of the middle and posterior columns, are not typically associated with neurologic deficit, but are considered unstable.[4,38] Fracture dislocations (►Fig. 24.6 and ►Fig. 24.7a, b) are high-energy translational/rotational injuries that disrupt all three columns and are considered very unstable.[11,17,36,37]

A more recent classification system, the Thoracolumbar Injury Classification and Severity Score (TLICS), has also been developed and is beginning to be more widely used. Like the SLIC, this system also takes into account injury morphology, posterior ligament integrity, and neurologic status. Also like the SLIC, each finding is assigned a point value and the sum guides the decision for surgical treatment. Injuries with a score of 1 to 3 are generally treated nonoperatively, whereas injuries with a score of 5 or higher are generally treated surgically. Treatment of injuries with a score of 4 is at the discretion of the treatment team.[37]

Initial radiographic assessment consists of anteroposterior (AP) and lateral radiographs, where the Cobb angle is a useful measurement of deformity. The upper thoracic column may be inadequately visualized on lateral plain films; thus, CT imaging is more sensitive in detecting fractures and permits a more detailed analysis of bony injury. MRI imaging remains useful for soft-tissue, ligamentous, intervertebral disk, and neural element assessment.[11,36]

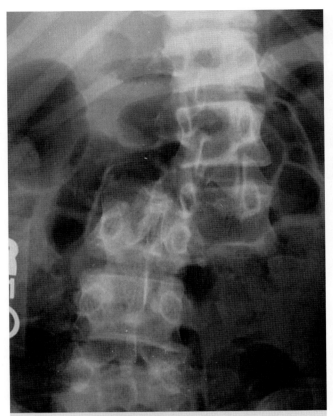

Fig. 24.6 Anteroposterior radiograph of the lumbar spine shows an L2–L3 fracture dislocation.

Management of thoracic and thoracolumbar fractures is often controversial; and although treatment algorithms have been proposed, the choice of operative versus nonoperative management remains based on maximizing biomechanical and neurologic stability.[4,37] Compression, stable burst, and isolated posterior column fractures are generally considered stable and may be treated nonoperatively with external immobilization, bed rest, and narcotics. Appropriate follow-up with weight-bearing radiographs and neurologic examination monitoring for delayed kyphosis, instability, or neurologic deterioration is imperative and may disclose individuals needing surgical stabilization.[39]

Indications for surgical stabilization include progressive neurologic deficit, disruption of the posterior ligamentous complex, dislocation, failure to maintain reduction, unacceptable deformity, and failure of conservative management.[4, 36] Surgical reduction and fixation/fusion is recommended in cases of three or more compression fractures in a row, loss of > 50% of height of a single compression fracture with angulation, kyphotic angulation > 40 degrees or 25%, or progressive kyphosis.[4,11,36] Operative management for unstable thoracic and thoracolumbar fractures aims to adequately decompress the spinal canal, optimize neurologic recovery, and provide spinal stability. Multiple approaches either in isolation or in combination are available and encompass anterior, lateral, and posterior decompression, reduction, fusion, and instrumentation techniques.[11,36,38]

24.14 Lumbar Column Injuries

Fractures of the lumbar and sacral spine are less common than cervical and thoracic injuries.[2,4] The upper lumbar spine, L1–L2, is considered part of the thoracolumbar complex and is addressed accordingly earlier in the chapter. Biomechanically, the lumbar spine has significantly greater flexion and extension compared with the thoracic spine; however, rotation is limited by the vertical orientation of the facets and anterior portion of the anulus compared with the thoracic spine.[11, 17] The three-column classification scheme and fracture categories described in detail earlier are also useful to identify, describe, and manage fractures of the lumbar spine.[36,37] Lumbosacral spondylolisthesis, characterized by anterolisthesis of L5 on S1,[40] is a rare injury thought to be caused by severe hyperflexion with high-energy rotational forces (▶Fig. 24.8 and ▶Fig. 24.9). Neurologic impairment is frequent, and surgical reduction and arthrodesis with instrumentation are recommended.[40]

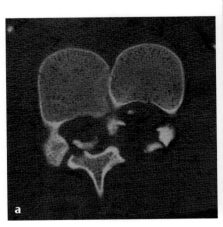
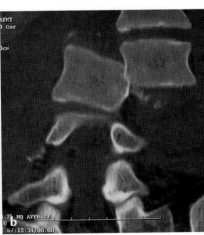

Fig. 24.7 (a) Coronal computed tomography (CT) scan reveals anterior and leftward displacement of L2 from L3 in the L2–L3 fracture dislocation shown in the previous radiograph (▶Fig. 24.6). (b) Axial CT scan shows the L2 and L3 vertebral bodies in the same plane, demonstrating the severe malalignment of the vertebral column at the injury site.

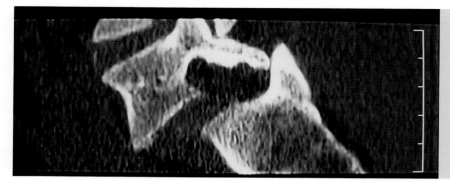

Fig. 24.8 Midsagittal computed tomography image shows anterolisthesis of L5 on S1 in a lumbosacral spondylolisthesis injury

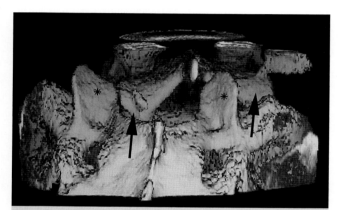

Fig. 24.9 Reformatted three-dimensional computed tomography image of the lumbosacral spondylolisthesis demonstrates a complete bilateral separation of L5 inferior facets (black arrows) from the superior facet processes of S1 (asterisks).

24.15 Conclusion

In all vertebral column injuries, the identification of instability and progressive neurologic deficit are often paramount in determining timing and type of intervention. Although definition of early and delayed surgical management is inconsistent, the principle objectives remain clear: to prevent secondary neurologic injury by decompressing compromised neural tissue, reducing deformity, and stabilizing the vertebral column with the aim of optimizing neurologic and medical outcomes.

References

[1] Nationwide Inpatient Sample (NIS). Healthcare Cost and Utilization Project (HCUP). 2013. Agency for Healthcare Research and Quality Web site. www.hcup-us.ahrq.gov/HCUPnet.jsp. Accessed March 31, 2016

[2] The National SCI Statistical Center. Spinal Cord Injury: Facts and Figures at a Glance. Birmingham, AL: University of Alabama at Birmingham National Spinal Cord Injury Center; 2015

[3] Carreon LY, Glassman SD, Campbell MJ. Pediatric spine fractures: a review of 137 hospital admissions. J Spinal Disord Tech. 2004; 17(6):477–482

[4] Benzel EC. Spine Surgery. 2nd ed. Philadelphia, PA: Elsevier Churchill Livingstone; 2005:512–571

[5] Goldberg W, Mueller C, Panacek E, Tigges S, Hoffman JR, Mower WR; NEXUS Group. Distribution and patterns of blunt traumatic cervical spine injury. Ann Emerg Med. 2001; 38(1):17–21

[6] Theodore N, Aarabi B, Dhall SS, et al. Transportation of patients with acute traumatic cervical spine injuries. Neurosurgery. 2013; 72(Suppl 2):35–39

[7] Hadley MN, Walters BC, Aarabi B, et al. Clinical assessment following acute cervical spinal cord injury. Neurosurgery. 2013; 72(Suppl 2):40–53

[8] Kerwin AJ, Frykberg ER, Schinco MA, Griffen MM, Murphy T, Tepas JJ. The effect of early spine fixation on non-neurologic outcome. J Trauma. 2005; 58(1):15–21

[9] Fehlings MG, Tator CH. An evidence-based review of decompressive surgery in acute spinal cord injury: rationale, indications, and timing based on experimental and clinical studies. J Neurosurg. 1999; 91(1, Suppl):1–11

[10] Gaebler C, Maier R, Kutscha-Lissberg F, Mrkonjic L, Vècsei V. Results of spinal cord decompression and thoracolumbar pedicle stabilisation in relation to the time of operation. Spinal Cord. 1999; 37(1):33–39

[11] Licina P, Nowitzke AM. Approach and considerations regarding the patient with spinal injury. Injury. 2005; 36(Suppl 2):B2–B12

[12] Albert TJ, Kim DH. Timing of surgical stabilization after cervical and thoracic trauma. Invited submission from the Joint Section Meeting on Disorders of the Spine and Peripheral Nerves, March 2004. J Neurosurg Spine. 2005; 3(3):182–190

[13] Theodore N, Aarabi B, Dhall SS, et al. The diagnosis and management of traumatic atlanto-occipital dislocation injuries. Neurosurgery. 2013; 72(Suppl 2):114–126

[14] Przybylski GJ, Clyde BL, Fitz CR. Craniocervical junction subarachnoid hemorrhage associated with atlanto-occipital dislocation. Spine. 1996; 21(15):1761–1768

[15] Chirossel JP, Passagia JG, Gay E, Palombi O. Management of craniocervical junction dislocation. Childs Nerv Syst. 2000; 16(10–11):697–701

[16] Hadley MN, Walters BC, Grabb PA, et al. Management of acute central cervical spinal cord injuries. Neurosurgery. 2002; 50(3, Suppl):S166–S172

[17] White AA, Panjabi MM. Clinical Biomechanics of the Spine. 2nd ed. Philadelphia, PA: JB Lippincott; 1990

[18] Dickman CA, Greene KA, Sonntag VKH. Injuries involving the transverse atlantal ligament: classification and treatment guidelines based upon experience with 39 injuries. Neurosurgery. 1996; 38(1):44–50

[19] Ryken TC, Aarabi B, Dhall SS, et al. Management of isolated fractures of the atlas in adults. Neurosurgery. 2013; 72(Suppl 2):127–131

[20] Hadley MN, Dickman CA, Browner CM, Sonntag VKH. Acute traumatic atlas fractures: management and long term outcome. Neurosurgery. 1988; 23(1):31–35

[21] Ochoa G. Surgical management of odontoid fractures. Injury. 2005; 36(Suppl 2):B54–B64

[22] Ryken TC, Hadley MN, Aarabi B, et al. Management of isolated fractures of the axis in adults. Neurosurgery. 2013; 72(Suppl 2):132–150

[23] German JW, Hart BL, Benzel EC. Nonoperative management of vertical C2 body fractures. Neurosurgery. 2005; 56(3):516–521, discussion 516–521

[24] Sasso RC. C2 dens fractures: treatment options. J Spinal Disord. 2001; 14(5):455–463

[25] Korres DS, Papagelopoulos PJ, Mavrogenis AF, Benetos IS, Kyriazopoulos P, Psycharis I. Chance-type fractures of the axis. Spine. 2005; 30(17):E517–E520

[26] Benzel EC, Hart BL, Ball PA, Baldwin NG, Orrison WW, Espinosa M. Fractures of the C-2 vertebral body. J Neurosurg. 1994; 81(2):206–212

[27] Ryken TC, Hadley MN, Aarabi B, et al. Management of acute combination fractures of the atlas and axis in adults. Neurosurgery. 2013; 72(Suppl 2):151–158

[28] Rozzelle CJ, Aarabi B, Dhall SS, et al. Management of pediatric cervical spine and spinal cord injuries. Neurosurgery. 2013; 72(Suppl 2):205–226

[29] Martinez-Lage JF, Martinez Perez M, Fernandez Cornejo V, Poza M. Atlanto-axial rotatory subluxation in children: early management. Acta Neurochir (Wien). 2001; 143(12):1223–1228

[30] Aarabi B, Walters BC, Dhall SS, et al. Subaxial cervical spine injury classification systems. Neurosurgery. 2013; 72(Suppl 2):170–186

[31] Patel AA, Hurlbert RJ, Bono CM, Bessey JT, Yang N, Vaccaro AR. Classification and surgical decision making in acute subaxial cervical spine trauma. Spine. 2010; 35(21, Suppl):S228–S234

[32] Vaccaro AR, Hulbert RJ, Patel AA, et al; Spine Trauma Study Group. The subaxial cervical spine injury classification system: a novel approach to recognize the importance of morphology, neurology, and integrity of the disco-ligamentous complex. Spine. 2007; 32(21):2365–2374

[33] Theodore N, Hadley MN, Aarabi B, et al. Prehospital cervical spinal immobilization after trauma. Neurosurgery. 2013; 72(Suppl 2):22–34

[34] Gelb DE, Aarabi B, Dhall SS, et al. Treatment of subaxial cervical spinal injuries. Neurosurgery. 2013; 72(Suppl 2):187–194

[35] Fehlings MG, Vaccaro A, Wilson JR, et al. Early versus delayed decompression for traumatic cervical spinal cord injury: results of the Surgical Timing in Acute Spinal Cord Injury Study (STASCIS). PLoS ONE. 2012; 7(2):e32037

[36] Vialle LR, Vialle E. Thoracic spine fractures. Injury. 2005; 36(Suppl 2):B65–B72

[37] Lee JY, Vaccaro AR, Lim MR, et al. Thoracolumbar injury classification and severity score: a new paradigm for the treatment of thoracolumbar spine trauma. J Orthop Sci. 2005; 10(6):671–675

[38] Stambough JL. Posterior instrumentation for thoracolumbar trauma. Clin Orthop Relat Res. 1997(335):73–88

[39] Mehta JS, Reed MR, McVie JL, Sanderson PL. Weight-bearing radiographs in thoracolumbar fractures: do they influence management? Spine. 2004; 29(5):564–567

[40] Vialle R, Wolff S, Pauthier F, et al. Traumatic lumbosacral dislocation: four cases and review of literature. Clin Orthop Relat Res. 2004(419):91–97

25 Athletic Injuries and Their Differential Diagnosis

Julian E. Bailes and Vincent J. Miele

Abstract

Participation in sporting activities promotes good health but also carries an inherent risk of injury to the athlete. This population presents a unique and complex array of issues relating to on-field management, diagnosis, and treatment. In the spectrum of sports-related injuries, those to the nervous system have a high potential for significant morbidity and mortality and have been described in virtually every sport from boxing to golf. This association often necessitates involvement of the neurosurgical community in the field of sports medicine. Differentiation between minor and serious injuries is the foundation of management of the athlete. A seemingly minor blow to the head may result in a slowly developing subdural hematoma (SDH), whereas, paradoxically, a more severe impact may cause a loss of consciousness but only a concussion. This chapter serves as a guide in this differentiation and outlines management strategies for neurologic injuries in the athlete.

Keywords: athletic injuries, concussion, head injuries, on-field management, spinal injuries

25.1 Head Injuries

One of the greatest threats to the athlete are high-speed encounters with other objects providing sufficient kinetic energy to result in major brain trauma. The possibility of major injury or death, despite their relative rarity, remains a constant in nearly every sport. During the last century, our level of understanding of the types of cerebral insults, their causes, and their treatment has advanced significantly. Research has better defined the epidemiologic issues related to sports injuries involving the central nervous system and has also led to classification and management paradigms that help guide decisions regarding athletes' return to play. Severe sports-related head injuries include epidural hematomas (EDHs), subdural hematomas (SDHs), brain contusions/parenchymal hemorrhages, diffuse axonal injury (DAI), traumatic subarachnoid hemorrhage (SAH), and cerebral edema. The short- and long-term effects of mild traumatic brain injury (mTBI) or concussion are becoming more understood. This common injury, once thought to be fairly benign, can result in persistant cognitive, behavioral, and psychiatric difficulties.[1] This poses difficulty with patient management, particularly when consideration for return to competition is necessary.

25.1.1 Incidence of Head Injury in Sports

Over 170 million adults and 38 million children participate in organized sports annually in the United States.[2] It is estimated that 3.8 million sports-related TBIs occur annually, including among those who do not seek medical care.[3] This would include a spectrum of injuries from concussion to more serious brain trauma. Over 18,000 adult and 11,000 pediatric brain injuries

related to sports are treated at level I or II trauma centers annually. Of these, 14% of the adult and 13% of the pediatric injuries were defined as moderate or severe in nature, with a mortality rate of 3.1% in adults and 0.8% in children.[4,5] A review of data from the United States National Registry of Sudden Death in Young Athletes from 1980 to 2009 found 261 deaths in athletes aged 21 years or younger due to trauma, most commonly to the head and neck.[6] One hundred and thirty-three nonprofessional American football players have died or endured incomplete neurologic recovery following catastrophic head and neck injury since 1982. Over 90% of these injuries occurred in high school athletes, 8% occurred in college participants, and 1% involved sandlot players.[7]

Injuries that are not immediately life-threatening are much more common. The Centers for Disease Control and Prevention estimates that 1.6 to 3.8 million concussions occur in sports and recreational activities annually in the United States.[2]

The incidence and severity of head injury vary greatly with the characteristics of the sport involved. It is beneficial to consider athletic endeavors in a category that allows the nature of the play and the participants to be defined in terms of types of sporting events and motivations of the players involved. The most useful classification is that of recreational and nonorganized sports versus organized, sanctioned sports. The former have little formal structure, fewer rules, no refereed officials, less use of protective equipment, and participation by a wide variety of people under a variable set of conditions. In contrast, organized sporting events have structure regarding training, rules and their enforcement, specialized equipment, and physicians and athletic trainers dedicated to the care of those who are injured.

American football, ice hockey, and boxing are commonly referred to when discussing sports-related head injury because of the frequent and obvious violent contact. However, head injuries are commonly observed in sporting activities considered less violent such as basketball, soccer, and lacrosse.[8,9,10] Bicycling and playground activities are examples of unorganized sports that have higher rates of serious head injuries than most organized sports.

Equestrian sports account for approximately 46,000 emergency room visits annually, with nearly 20% involving the head or neck and 70% of deaths related to head injuries.[11,12] Approximately seven fatalities occur annually related to skateboard injuries, with 90% involving severe injury to the head.[13] Recreational and commuter bicyclists younger than 20 years suffer an average of 247 TBI deaths and 140,000 head injuries each year in the United States.[14] Although sports such as gymnastics and cheerleading have traditionally been responsible for the highest number of head injuries in the female athlete,[15] women are now crossing into previously male-dominated sports such as boxing, and increasing numbers of serious head injuries are being incurred in contact/collision sports.[16]

Head injuries occur at one of the highest rates in downhill skiing and often occur as a result of collisions with trees and boulders as well as with other skiers.[17] Other recreational sports that are considered to be a high risk for head injury include snowboarding, hang-gliding, skydiving, mountaineering, and race-car driving.[18]

25.1.2 Epidural Hematoma

Epidural hematomas are an infrequent but emergent TBI in the athletic population, especially in sports in which the players do not wear helmets. They are classically associated with temporal skull fractures, which can tear the middle meningeal artery or vein. Although they are much more commonly identified in contact and collision sports, they have also been diagnosed in baseball players and golfers struck on the head by a high-velocity ball.[19,20] This lesion is usually associated with a brief loss of consciousness (LOC) followed by a lucid interval and then rapid deterioration. A typical example of this would be a pole vaulter whose head strikes the ground outside the landing pit. After being stunned for a brief period, the athlete may walk off the field fully alert. Within 15 to 30 minutes, a sudden excruciating headache is accompanied by progressive neurologic deterioration. Although this classic "lucid interval" presentation only occurs in one third of athletes with this condition, an understanding of this clinical picture is crucial for all caregivers, especially certified athletic trainers, coaches, and team physicians. It requires that an adequate observation period be planned for those athletes who display potential for delayed hematoma formation and neurologic deterioration. Early recognition and management are essential, and if treated early complete neurologic recovery can be expected because EDHs are not usually associated with other brain injuries.

25.1.3 Subdural Hematoma

Subdural hematomas are the most common form of sports-related intracranial bleeding and account for the majority of lethal brain injuries seen in both organized and recreational athletic activities.[18,21] It is important to understand that SDHs in athletes are not the same as those commonly seen in the elderly. The athlete usually does not have the large potential subdural space that an elderly patient possesses, so mass effect and increases in intracranial pressure occur more rapidly. In addition to injury from the mass effect of blood under the dura, there is often significant associated damage to the underlying brain (contusion or edema). Therefore, even with prompt treatment, prognosis is less favorable than for an EDH, with mortality rates as high as 60%. SDHs can occur at any location in the brain, and presentation is usually within 72 hours of injury. Athletes who suffer an SDH may become immediately unconscious and/or have focal neurologic deficits or may develop symptomatology insidiously over days or even weeks.

25.1.4 Brain Contusions/Parenchymal Hemorrhage

Brain contusions and parenchymal hemorrhages represent regions of primary neuronal and vascular injury. They contain edematous, punctate parenchymal hemorrhages that may extend into the white matter and the subdural and subarachnoid spaces and are most commonly the result of either direct trauma or acceleration/deceleration. The latter causes the brain to strike the skull, most commonly resulting in damage to the inferior frontal and temporal lobes. The areas of the brain adjacent to the floor of the anterior or posterior cranial fossa, the sphenoid wing, the petrous ridge, the convexity of the skull, and the falx or tentorium are also vulnerable. Contusions are also observed in the lateral midbrain, the inferior cerebellum and adjacent tonsil, and the midline superior cerebral cortex.

Importantly, these types of injuries often demonstrate progression over time with respect to the size and number of contusions and the amount of hemorrhage within the contusions. This progression most commonly occurs over the first 24 to 48 hours, with one fourth of cases demonstrating delayed hemorrhage in areas that were previously free of blood. Additionally, initial computed tomography (CT) findings can be normal or minimally abnormal because the partial volumes between the dense microhemorrhages and the hypodense associated edema can render contusions isoattenuating relative to the surrounding brain.

25.1.5 Diffuse Axonal Injury

Diffuse axonal injury plays a significant role in sports-related head injury. It occurs in nearly half of athletes who have suffered a severe head injury and is partially responsible for one third of all head injury–related fatalities.[22] Radiographically, DAI typically consists of several focal white matter lesions in a characteristic distribution.

The pathophysiology of DAI was first described in 1943. It is the result of the shearing of multiple axons secondary to rotational forces on the brain, commonly from lateral rotation of the head. These forces exert more effect on areas of the brain where tissue density is greatest, such as at the gray–white junction. DAI was classically believed to represent a primary injury (occurring at the instant of the trauma). However, it is apparent that the axoplasmic membrane alteration, transport impairment, and retraction ball formation may represent secondary (or delayed) components to the disease process. Although the initial trauma may not completely tear the axon, it can still produce focal alteration of the axoplasmic membrane, resulting in subsequent impairment of axoplasmic transport. This results in axoplasmic swelling and rupture. A retraction ball forms, which is a pathologic hallmark of shearing injury, followed by wallerian degeneration.

Although areas of the brain with different tissue densities have a predilection for DAI, the exact location depends on the plane of rotation and is independent of the distance from the center of rotation. The magnitude of injury depends on the distance from the center of rotation, the arc of rotation, and the duration and intensity of the force.

25.1.6 Traumatic Subarachnoid Hemorrhage

Sports-related head trauma can result in SAH. Some degree of SAH is usually present in any serious head injury. Although this usually results in meningeal irritation from blood between the pia and arachnoid, the condition is usually not life-threatening, and immediate treatment is not required for a good outcome. In large amounts, subarachnoid blood may lead to vasospasm. SAH may also result in the development of a communicating hydrocephalus, which can present clinically with a slower-than-expected recovery or late clinical deterioration.

25.1.7 Second-Impact Syndrome

In 1984, the death of a college football player was reported that seemed to have resulted from a second, seemingly minor, blow to the head. At the time, it was hypothesized that this fatality was the result of "a repeat blow to an already compliance-compromised brain which precipitated a catastrophic increase in intracranial pressure, perhaps through a loss of vasomotor tone."[23] The term *vascular congestion syndrome* was coined in 1991 following the death of a 17-year-old high school football player from an uncontrollable increase in intracranial pressure.[24] Both of these deaths are thought to have been the result of what is now known as second-impact syndrome (SIS). SIS is defined as a fatal uncontrollable increase in intracranial pressure secondary to diffuse brain swelling, which occurs after a blow to the head incurred before recovery from a previous blow to the head. Some controversy exists over the validity of this condition because of problems with documentation of the initial event, persistent symptoms, and severity of the second impact.[25]

The pathophysiology of SIS is thought to involve a sudden posttraumatic loss of autoregulation of the brain's blood supply as well as catecholamine release. This leads to vascular engorgement within the cranium, which in turn markedly increases intracranial pressure and a syndrome of uncal herniation, cerebellar herniation, or both. Animal research has shown that vascular engorgement in the brain after a mild head injury may be difficult, if not impossible, to control in this "double-impact" setting. From second impact to uncontrollable edema is rapid, usually taking 2 to 5 minutes.[18] There have been over 20 reported cases of this condition, all involving young athletes ranging in age from 10 to 24 years. Although the majority of the affected athletes have been American football players, 14% have occurred during boxing competition and isolated cases have been reported in association with karate, skiing, and ice hockey.[1]

Typically, the athlete experiences some degree of postconcussion symptoms after the first head injury. These may include visual, motor, or sensory changes and difficulty with cognitive and memory processes. Before these symptoms resolve, which may take days or weeks, the athlete returns to competition and receives a second blow to the head. The second blow may be minor, perhaps only involving a blow to the chest that jerks the athlete's head and indirectly imparts accelerative forces to the brain. Affected athletes may seem stunned but usually do not lose consciousness and often complete the play. They usually remain on their feet for 15 seconds to a minute or so but seem dazed, similar to a grade I concussion without LOC. Often, affected athletes remain on the playing field or walk off under their own power. What happens in the next few moments to several minutes sets this syndrome apart from a concussion or SDH. Usually, within seconds to minutes of the second impact, the athlete, who is conscious yet stunned, precipitously collapses to the ground and becomes comatose, with rapidly dilating pupils, loss of eye movement, and evidence of respiratory failure.

The condition is associated with a 50% mortality and nearly 100% morbidity rate.[18] It is important to understand this condition when making return-to-play decisions following a head injury in an athlete. Any athlete still symptomatic from a previous head injury should not be allowed to return to full practice or participation in a contact or collision sport.

25.1.8 Juvenile Head Trauma Syndrome

Juvenile head trauma syndrome has been reported primarily in children and may involve the same pathophysiology as SIS. It is defined as severe, cerebral edema and coma following a minor craniocerebral trauma.[1] The athlete may experience either immediate or delayed neurologic deterioration. Although the etiology of the condition is unknown, the sudden vasodilation and redistribution of blood into the brain parenchyma may involve a functional channelopathy or a disturbance of ion channel subunits. It has been linked to a mutation in the calcium channel subunit gene (*CACNA1A*) associated with familial hemiplegic migraine.[26] In some cases of juvenile head trauma syndrome, the rapidly developing cerebral edema occurs in a young athlete who experiences two head injuries, with the second injury occurring before complete recovery from the first impact, as seen in SIS.[27]

25.1.9 Concussion/Mild Traumatic Brain Injury

A concussion is defined as a traumatically induced transient disturbance of brain function resulting from a complex pathophysiologic process that is not yet fully understood. They are a subset of mTBIs, on the less severe end of the brain injury spectrum and are generally self-limited in duration and resolution.[28] Concussions are by far the most common type of sports-related head injury, with an estimated 1.6 to 3.8 million occurring annually in the United States. This accounts for 5 to 9% of all sport-related injuries and three fourths of all head injuries in this population.[29]

The recognition in the early 1980s that mTBI exists as an important clinical entity began to pave the way for an increased appreciation of concussion in sports. In the 1990s, there was an increased focus on defining and categorizing the athlete with mTBI, as more evidence suggested that concussion may be more common and serious than previously believed. The linking of concussion with long-term sequelae such as chronic traumatic encephalopathy (CTE) has brought both conditions to the forefront of research in diagnosis and management. The concept of mTBI or concussion has evolved, aided in great part by the application of formal neuropsychologic and cognitive studies.

Concussion results from the rapid acceleration, deceleration, and rotation of the brain. This results in the deformation/damage of individual components such as neurons, glial cells, and blood vessels and alterations of membrane permeability. Following the initial damage, a postconcussive hypermetabolic state occurs as well as period of diminished cerebral blood flow.

This causes a widening disparity between glucose supply and demand producing a cellular energy crisis.[30]

There are many characteristics and nuances of the sports-related mTBI population that make diagnosis and treatment difficult. One such difficulty is that athletes are the only group of patients who routinely and often fervently ask to be returned to play, thus invariably subjecting themselves to multiple future instances of head impact. Many of these impacts will result in at least subclinical (subconcussive) head injury. Although a single episode of mTBI seems to be well tolerated overall in the majority of athletes, long-term mental status morbidity can occur with multiple insults. Advances in the fields of diagnostic neuroradiology, neurobiology, neuropsychology, and neuropathology now provide the clinician with more accurate and objective methods of analyzing this population of patients.

Historically, there has been no universal agreement on the definition and grading of concussion, and attempts at classification have tended to focus on the presence or absence of a period of LOC and amnesia. Headache is the most commonly reported symptom and dizziness the second most common. Importantly, LOC only occurs in about 10% of concussions. The most recent consensus statement on the condition concludes that a concussion should be suspected when an individual has at least one of the following signs and symptoms[31]:

- Signs: physical signs (e.g., headache), cognitive signs (e.g., foggy feeling), emotional signs (e.g., uneasiness).
- Physical symptoms (e.g., LOC, amnesia).
- Behavioral changes (e.g., irritability).
- Cognitive impairment (e.g., slowed reaction time).
- Sleep disorder (e.g., insomnia).

25.1.10 On-the-Field Management

Athletes who suffer catastrophic injuries to the head or spinal cord are usually easy to identify, as are those who develop an immediate neurologic deficit. More challenging is the diagnosis of an injury with minimal initial symptomatology. There are five categories of on-field management: (1) preparation for any neurologic injury, (2) suspicion and recognition, (3) stabilization and safety, (4) immediate treatment and possible secondary treatment, and (5) evaluation for return to play.[32] It is mandatory that a spine board, cervical collar, and cardiopulmonary resuscitation equipment be on site and easily accessible during a contest. Specific equipment for protective gear removal (e.g., football face mask) should also be readily available. If a head or neck injury is suspected, an athlete should immediately be assessed for level of consciousness while still on the field. Following the initial evaluation, as in any head trauma patient, an athlete with a head injury should be assumed to have an associated cervical injury, and spinal stabilization is essential to limit any further injury. If an athlete is wearing protective gear with a face mask, the face mask should be removed. Although still not universally accepted, removal of all protective gear while on the field is becoming more common and is performed on a situational basis. Several situations have been identified that would require removal of the helmet and chinstrap. These include a loose-fitting helmet that would not hold the head securely so that if the helmet is immobilized the head will still be mobile, if the airway cannot be controlled or ventilation provided even after removal of the face mask, if the face mask cannot be removed after a reasonable period of time, and if the helmet prevents immobilization for transportation in an appropriate position. Helmet removal should be performed with concomitant occipital support or simultaneous removal of shoulder pads. If left in place following helmet removal, the shoulder pads may cause cervical hyperextension. Obviously, if the helmet is removed, cervical immobilization must be maintained during the procedure.

In a neurologically intact athlete with a normal mental status, once cervical spine involvement has been excluded, the athlete may be assisted to a sitting position and if stable in this position to a standing position. If able to stand, the athlete can then be walked off the field for further evaluation. Unconscious athletes need to be stabilized before any neurologic appraisal. Initial evaluation should begin with the airway, breathing, and circulation assessment of basic cardiopulmonary life support. If all of the athlete's protective equipment has not been removed, cardiopulmonary support can most often be accomplished by face mask removal for airway access and the front of the shoulder pads can be opened to allow compression or defibrillation. When sudden unconsciousness without preceding craniospinal trauma occurs, cardiac etiology should be considered. Immediate transfer to a facility with neurosurgical capabilities should be performed for an athlete with prolonged alteration of consciousness, worsening symptoms, or focal neurologic deficit. Transport should be performed under the assumption of a concomitant spinal cord injury (SCI), and spinal stabilization is mandatory.

Any athlete suspected of having a concussion should be immediately removed from play and assessed. This would include a focused physical examination to rule out more serious brain injury followed by a history, cognitive testing, and balance testing. Several standardized sideline concussion assessment tools are available and useful in reducing the subjectivity of the examination. The most common sideline measures include the use of symptoms scores, the Maddocks Questions, the Standardized Assessment of Concussion (SAC), and the Balance Error Scoring System (BESS) or modified BESS. The Sport Concussion Assessment Tool 2 (SCAT2) and the National Football League (NFL) Sideline Concussion Assessment Tool combine various assessment measures to give one score.[28]

25.1.11 Imaging

Specific guidelines on when to perform brain imaging on a head-injured athlete do not exist. Because of this, the physician needs to individualize when to perform imaging on a patient-to-patient basis. Those who exhibit focal neurologic deficits, persistent alterations in mental status, Glasgow Coma Scale score of 13 or less, and the concern for a skull fracture are common examples of when an athlete would require at least a CT scan. In cases that are not as clear-cut, the duration and severity of symptoms has been used to aid in this decision. CT does expose the brain to radiation and should be used judiciously. However, if there is any question of a life-threatening injury, CT imaging is a rapid and efficacious diagnostic modality.

Although standard CT and magnetic resonance imaging (MRI) do not detect concussions, newer imaging techniques such as functional MRI (fMRI), diffusion tensor imaging (DTI), and MR spectroscopy (MRS) are being investigated.[28] Functional MRI can be used to identify changes in regional blood flow patterns. DTI measures the movement of water within the brain and by doing so can provide structural images of white matter fiber tracts that can be damaged in a concussion. MRS measures changes in the ratio of neurometabolites in different areas of the brain.

25.1.12 Nontraumatic Sports-Related Brain Injury

Brain injuries to athletes can occur by mechanisms other than trauma. The two main causes of nontraumatic sports-related brain injury are cerebral air embolism and high-altitude cerebral edema (HACE). These conditions result from participation in underwater diving and mountaineering. Because of the increased number of people participating in these activities as well as an increase in access, it is imperative that the signs and symptoms of these conditions as well as management strategies be understood.

Recreational scuba diving has become a popular sport in the United States, with almost 9 million certified divers.[33] One of the most severe injuries that participants are at risk for is the development of cerebral air embolisms. Cerebral air embolisms are the most serious and rapidly fatal of all diving injuries and are second only to drowning as the leading cause of death associated with the sport.[34] Approximately 60% of divers with decompression sickness will have symptoms and signs of central nervous system involvement. The condition is most often the result of a rapid ascent from depths greater than 10 m when air-filled body spaces fail to equalize their pressure to changing ambient pressures. This results in air released from an overpressurized alveolus entering the pulmonary capillaries and traveling through the arterial circulation, causing occlusion of cerebral blood flow. In more than 80% of patients, symptoms develop within 5 minutes of reaching the surface, but they can also occur during ascent or after a longer surface interval. The athlete may complain of diplopia, tunnel vision, or vertigo or may display seizure activity, loss of memory and changes in affect, hemiplegia, or dysarthria. Importantly, this diagnosis should be high on the differential if a diver surfaces with an alteration in mental status—almost two thirds of patients have changes of consciousness (i.e., coma or obtundation).[35] Treatment consists of basic or advanced cardiac life support, 100% oxygen, rehydration, and transport to a recompression facility. Oxygen reduces ischemia in affected tissues and accelerates the dissolution of air emboli. Supportive care for seizures, shock, hyperglycemia, and pulmonary dysfunction should be anticipated. Recompression therapy should be initiated immediately using the United States Navy algorithm.[36] Recompression therapy reduces the size of air emboli by increasing ambient pressure. This expedites the passage of emboli through the vasculature and reestablishes blood flow to ischemic tissues.

HACE can result in significant increases in intracranial pressure and is responsible for up to 5% of deaths in climbers above 4000 m. Originally thought to be separate disorders, HACE is now largely considered to be the end stage of severe acute mountain sickness (AMS). AMS and HACE are likely on a continuum on the basis of a common underlying pathophysiologic process in an unacclimatized individual at high altitude. Affected athletes develop symptomatology most commonly within 72 hours that includes ataxia, vertigo, confusion, and hallucinations. The main contributor to high-altitude illness is hypoxia with resultant cerebral edema. Treatment consists of the immediate return to a lower elevation with the goal of reaching the lowest possible altitude,[37] oxygenation, and supportive care. Pharmacologic agents such as acetazolamide and dexamethasone have also been used to treat this condition, with varying success. Acetazolamide, a sulfonamide carbonic anhydrase inhibitor, enhances the renal excretion of bicarbonate, producing a mild acidosis. Ventilation increases in response to this acidosis, which is thought to mimic the process of acclimatization. Acetazolamide also lowers the cerebral spinal fluid volume and pressure by lowering production, increasing the minute ventilation oxygen saturation, and decreasing periodic breathing at night. Dexamethasone, a synthetic glucocorticoid, has been traditionally used in the treatment of altitude sickness. It is thought to be valuable in the treatment of HACE because of its ability to stabilize cerebral vascular integrity, thereby reducing vasogenic edema and lowering intracranial pressure.[38]

25.2 Spinal Injury

Each year, there are well over 10,000 cases of SCI in the United States. Sporting events are the fourth most common cause of these injuries (behind motor vehicle accidents, violence, and falls) and account for approximately 7.5% of the total injuries since 1990.[39,40] Sports-related SCIs also occur at a younger mean age of 24 and are the second most common cause of SCI in the first three decades of life.[41] A spectrum of soft-tissue, bony, and nervous system injury can occur to the spine of athletes that often result in significant disability and time lost from competition and can become the source of chronic pain with functional limitation. Injury to the spinal cord, however, is perhaps the most feared consequence of athletic activities, and no other sports injury is potentially more catastrophic.

A structural distortion of the cervical spinal column associated with actual or potential damage to the spinal cord is classified as a catastrophic cervical spine injury. Because this condition is fortunately rare, few physicians have extensive experience in the emergency care of these injuries. Improper handling of the patient on the field or during transport can worsen or precipitate spinal cord dysfunction. Failure to appropriately manage a catastrophic neck injury can result in compromise of the athlete's cardiac, respiratory, and neurologic status. Improved understanding of these injuries can facilitate early diagnosis and effective on-field management.

25.2.1 Incidence

Spinal injuries are more common in nonorganized sports such as diving and surfing.[42] The challenge in this population, which accounts for the majority of sports-related spinal injury, is that rules, supervision, and training are limited. This makes it difficult to improve injury patterns by enforcing safety guidelines and manufacturer standards.

Although less frequent, spinal injury in organized sports has a much higher public profile. Several organized sports have been identified as placing the participant at high risk for SCI. These include football, ice hockey, rugby, skiing, snowboarding, and equestrian sports.[43,44,45,46] Although American football has a lower per-participant rate of catastrophic cervical spine injuries than ice hockey or gymnastics, the huge number of participants translates into the largest overall number with catastrophic cervical spine injuries.[47]

A significant increase of catastrophic cervical trauma coincided with the development of the modern football helmet. Rule changes in 1976 prohibiting playing techniques that used the top of the helmet as the initial point of contact for blocking and tackling (spearing) have significantly reduced this trend. From 1976 to 1987, the rate of cervical injuries decreased 70% from 7.72 per 100,000 to 2.31 per 100,000 at the high school level.[48] Traumatic quadriplegia decreased approximately 82% over the same time period. The sport of ice hockey has experienced a marked increase in the occurrence of cervical spine injuries through its history.[49] Major vertebral column injury occurred at an increased rate between 1982 and 1993, with a mean of 16.8 fractures/dislocations per year during that time period. Checking an opponent from behind, which typically produces a head-first collision of the checked player with the boards, has been identified as an important causative factor of cervical spine trauma in hockey. Changes in the rules that prohibit checking from behind and checking of an opponent who is no longer controlling the puck seem to be decreasing the incidence of these injuries, and data suggest that fewer cases of complete quadriplegia have been caused by these playing techniques since the rule changes have been instituted.

25.2.2 Etiology

Cervical spine injury can be divided into several categories: unstable fractures and dislocations, transient quadriplegia, and acute central disk herniation. These produce neurologic symptoms and signs that involve the extremities in a bilateral distribution. Sports-related cervical spine injuries have been previously divided into three groups, which provide useful information when making return-to-play decisions.

Type I injuries are those in which the athlete sustains permanent SCI. This includes both immediate, complete paralysis and incomplete SCI syndromes. The incomplete injuries are of basically four types: Brown–Séquard syndrome, anterior spinal syndrome, central cord syndrome, and mixed types. Mixed types include the finding of crossed motor and sensory deficits with upper extremities more prominently involved, which is considered to be a central cord/Brown–Séquard variant. There are, in addition, a few individuals in whom the neurologic injury may be relatively minor but is associated with demonstrable spinal cord pathology on imaging studies. For example, a high-intensity lesion within the spinal cord seen on MRI documents a spinal cord contusion. Type II injuries occur in individuals with normal radiographic studies. These deficits completely resolve within minutes to hours, and eventually the athlete has a normal neurologic examination. An example of the type II injury is the "burning hands syndrome," a variant of central cord syndrome characterized by burning dysesthesias of the hands and associated weakness in the hands and arms.[50] Most of these patients have normal radiographic studies, and their symptoms completely resolve within approximately 24 hours. Type III injuries comprise players with radiographic abnormality without neurologic deficit. This category includes fractures, fracture–dislocations, ligamentous and soft-tissue injuries, and herniated intervertebral disks.

SCI can also be divided into upper (occiput, atlas, and axis) and lower (C3–T1) cervical spine. A thorough understanding of the normal anatomy and unique motion of the spine at various segments is mandatory when treating these injuries.

Unstable fracture and/or dislocation are the most common causes of catastrophic cervical spine trauma. The most common primary injury vector is axial loading with flexion in football and hockey. Eighty percent of injuries to the cervical spine result from the accelerating head and body striking a stationary object or another player.

The cervical spine is compressed between the instantly decelerated head and the mass of the continuing body when an axial force is applied to the vertex of the helmet. In neutral alignment, the cervical spinal column is slightly extended as a result of its normal lordotic posture, and it is believed that compressive forces can be effectively dissipated by the paravertebral musculature and vertebral ligaments. This buffering cervical lordosis is eliminated when the cervical spinal column is straightened and large amounts of energy are transferred directly along the spine's longitudinal axis. Under high enough loads, the cervical spine can respond to this compressive force by buckling.

Two major patterns of spinal column injury result from the compression injury vector. Compressive-flexion injury is the most common variant that results from the combination of axial loading and flexion. It results in shortening of the anterior column because of compressive failure of the vertebral body and lengthening of the posterior column because of tensile failure of the spinal ligaments. If the cervical vertebra is subjected to a relatively pure compression force, both the anterior and posterior columns shorten, resulting in a vertical compression (burst) fracture. The vertebral body essentially explodes, during which it is possible that disk material extrudes through the fractured end plate and retropulsion of osseous material into the spinal canal results in cord damage. Alternately, there may be significant SCI without major disruption of the spinal column's integrity. This type of injury is the result of transient spinal column distortion with energy transfer to the spinal cord.

Catastrophic cervical trauma caused by the primary disruptive vector flexion generally results from either a direct blow to the occipital region or rapid deceleration of the torso. Flexion–distraction injury most likely to result in spinal cord dysfunction is a bilateral facet dislocation. Unilateral facet dislocation that is associated with cord injury in up to 25% of cases can occur with the addition of axial rotation to the distractive force.[51] It should be recognized that unstable cervical fractures/dislocations do not always result in upper motor neuron dysfunction. A unilateral facet dislocation can cause a monoradiculopathy due to foraminal compression of a nerve root on the side of the dislocated articular process. In other cases, major osseous or ligamentous damage will produce no neurologic impairment. SCI in these scenarios is potential rather than actual based on the amount of loss of structural integrity of the vertebral column.[52]

25.2.3 Upper Cervical Spine Injury

For the purposes of sports-related injuries, the upper cervical spine is considered to be the occiput, atlas (C1), and axis (C2). The major function of the atlanto-occipital joint is motion in the sagittal plane, which accounts for 40% of normal flexion and extension of the spine and 5 to 10 degrees of lateral bending. The midline atlantodens articulation is stabilized by the transverse atlantal ligament, which prevents forward translation of the atlas. This specialized osseoligamentous anatomy allows the atlas to rotate in a highly unconstrained manner. The atlantoaxial complex is responsible for 40 to 60% of all cervical rotation.[53] This rotation is limited by the alar ligaments extending from the odontoid process to the inner borders of the occipital condyles. The apical ligaments attach the odontoid centrally to the anterior foramen magnum. Atlantoaxial joint strength is provided by the transverse ligament and the lateral joint capsules.

Spinal cord damage due to fractures or dislocations involving the upper cervical spine is rare because there is proportionately greater space available within the spinal canal compared with the lower cervical segments. Injuries that destabilize the atlantoaxial complex (fracture of the odontoid or rupture of the transverse atlantal ligament) are most likely to result in spinal cord dysfunction. Flexion is the most common cause of injury at the atlantoaxial joint. Odontoid fractures can also result from extension injuries. Unilateral rotary dislocations are usually the result of rotational forces. Cord compression is unusual with a burst fracture of the atlas or traumatic spondylolisthesis of the axis because these osseous injuries further expand the dimensions of the spinal canal. If anteroposterior radiographs are performed and there is spreading of the lateral masses of greater than 7 mm, the transverse ligament is likely torn. Bilateral pedicle fractures of the axis may occur from extension of the occiput on the cervical spine. Importantly, although these injuries can result in instability, they usually do not cause neurologic deficits secondary to the anatomically wide spinal canal, which is also present at this level. If an upper cervical cord injury does occur, diaphragmatic paralysis with acute respiratory insufficiency can occur along with quadriplegia because the phrenic nerve arises from three cervical nerve roots (C3–C5).

25.2.4 Lower Cervical Spine Injury

The lower cervical spine is composed of the C3 through C7 vertebrae. This area accounts for the remaining arcs of neck flexion, extension, lateral bending, and rotation and has several important anatomical differences with respect to the upper cervical spine. The spinal canal is not as wide at this level, and the facet joints are oriented at a 45-degree angle. Because of this angulation, axial rotation is somewhat limited. The facet articulations also restrain forward vertebral translation.

Each motion segment can be separated into an anterior and a posterior column. Stability of a cervical segment is derived mainly from the anterior spinal elements. Compression of the spinal column is primarily resisted by the vertebral bodies and intervertebral disk, whereas shearing forces are opposed primarily by paraspinal musculature and ligamentous support. Instability of the lower cervical spine has been defined radiographically as translatory displacement of two adjacent vertebrae greater than 3.5 mm or angulation of greater than 11 degrees between adjacent vertebrae.[54]

The majority of fractures and dislocations occur in the lower cervical region. Lower cervical spine injuries are defined by the forces acting on the area (i.e., flexion, extension, lateral rotation, axial loading). Dislocated joints are usually the result of a flexion mechanism with either distraction or rotation. The ligamentous structures are the primary restraints to distraction of the spine. Compression of the posterior structures as well as damage to the anterior structures is usually the result of extension or whiplash injuries. This mechanism of injury commonly results in tearing of the anterior longitudinal ligament and fractures of the posterior elements. Compressive forces usually result in vertebral body fractures. These are commonly seen in spear tackler's spine, which consists of four characteristics: reversal of cervical lordosis, radiographic evidence of previous healed minor vertebral body fractures, canal stenosis, and the habitual use of spear-tackling techniques. This population commonly has a flexed posture to the head and a loss of the protective cervical lordosis. Large axial loads can result in protrusion of disk material or fractured bone into the spinal canal. This is the most common mechanism for sports-related quadriplegia. The C3–C4 level is most commonly involved in cases of quadriplegia secondary to cervical dislocations.

25.2.5 Central Cord Syndrome/Burning Hands Syndrome

Injury to the lower cervical cord can result in a spectrum of neurologic dysfunction. Incomplete SCI can occur with partial preservation of sensory or motor function. Central cord syndrome is the most common manifestation of this, followed in frequency by the anterior cord syndrome.

Burning hands syndrome is considered to be a variant of central cord syndrome. It is characterized by burning dysesthesia in both upper extremities and is likely the result of vascular insufficiency affecting the medial aspect of the somatotopically arranged spinothalamic tracts.[55] The lower extremities may occasionally be involved, and weakness may occasionally be evident. Cervical spine fracture or soft-tissue injury is seen radiographically in 50% of the patients with this syndrome. Any athlete who exhibits this condition should be initially managed as an SCI.

25.2.6 Cervical Cord Neurapraxia/ Transient Quadriplegia

Neurapraxia of the cervical spinal cord resulting in transient quadriplegia has been estimated to occur in seven per 10,000 football players.[56] This alarming injury is characterized by a temporary loss of motor or sensory function and is thought to be the result of a physiologic conduction block without true anatomical disruption of neuronal tissue. The affected athlete may complain of pain, tingling, or loss of sensation bilaterally in the upper and/or lower extremities. A spectrum of muscle weakness is possible, varying from mild quadriparesis to complete quadriplegia. The athlete has a full, pain-free range of cervical motion and does not complain of neck pain. Hemiparesis or hemisensory loss is also possible.

This condition is thought to result from a pincer-type mechanism of compression of the cord between the posteroinferior portion of one vertebral body and the lamina of the vertebra below. The condition can also occur during hyperflexion, but usually with extension movements with infolding of the ligamentum flavum, which can result in a 30% or more reduction of the anteroposterior diameter of the spinal canal. The spinal cord axons become unresponsive to stimulation for a variable period of time, essentially creating a "postconcussive" effect.[57]

This condition is described by the neurologic deficit, the duration of symptoms, and the anatomical distribution. A continuum of neurologic deficits that range from sensory only, sensory disturbance with motor weakness, to episodes of complete paralysis may occur. These may be described as paresthesia, paresis, and plegia. An injury is defined as grade I if the cervical cord neurapraxia (CCN) symptoms do not persist for over 15 minutes. Grade II injuries are defined as lasting from 15 minutes to 24 hours. Grade III injuries persist for 24 to 48 hours. All four extremities may be involved; this is considered a "quad" pattern. Upper and lower extremity patterns may also be observed.[58]

By definition, this condition is transient, and complete resolution generally occurs within 15 minutes but may take up to 48 hours. Steroid administration in accordance with the Bracken protocol in this population is controversial. There have been no controlled studies reporting that the administration of steroids has altered the natural history of athletes who have suffered CCN.[59]

In players who return to football, the rate of recurrence has been reported to be as high as 56%.[58] A considerable amount of controversy exists regarding whether the presence of cervical stenosis makes an athlete more prone to sustaining permanent neurologic injury or transient quadriparesis. The anteroposterior diameter of the spinal canal (measured from the posterior aspect of the vertebral body to the most anterior point on the spinal laminar line) determined from lateral cervical spine radiographs is considered normal if more than 15 mm between C3 and C7. Cervical stenosis is considered to be present if the canal diameter is less than 13 mm. However, this measurement has significant variability secondary to variations in landmarks used for measurement, changes in target distances for making the radiographs, patient positioning, differences in the triangular cross-sectional shape of the canal, and magnification of the canal because of a patient's large body habitus. In an effort to eliminate this variability, Torg and Pavlov designed a ratio method for determining the presence of cervical stenosis, comparing the sagittal diameter of the spinal canal with the sagittal midbody diameter of the vertebral body at the same level.[60] A ratio of 1:1 was considered normal and less than 0.8 was indicative of significant cervical stenosis. This ratio was found to mislabel many athletes with adequately sized canals but large vertebral bodies as being stenotic. This observation, as well as an unprecedented ability to image the vertebral column, intervertebral disks, spinal canal, cerebrospinal fluid (CSF), and spinal cord directly, has made MRI, and not bone landmarks, currently the preferred method of choice for assessing "functional spinal stenosis." MRI assessment of CSF signal around the spinal cord, termed the functional reserve, can be determined and the visualization of the CSF signal, its attenuation in areas of stenosis,

and changes on dynamic sagittal flexion–extension MRI studies are paramount in the diagnosis of this condition. In cases involving an absent CSF pattern on axial and, particularly, sagittal MR images, functional stenosis is diagnosed.

Developmental or acquired cervical stenosis seems to predispose an athlete to CCN. It has been fairly well accepted that a young patient who suffered an episode of CCN was not predisposed to permanent neurologic injury. This assumption has been called into question now that a player who had experienced a CCN subsequently sustained a quadriplegic injury.[61]

25.2.7 Traumatic Intervertebral Disk Herniation

Acute herniation of an intervertebral disk can occur during participation in sports and in the athletic population. Extrusion of disk material into the central spinal canal can result in acute cord compression and a transient or permanent cord injury. Clinically, the athlete may present with acute paralysis of all four extremities and a loss of pain and temperature sensation. A traumatic central disk herniation is also typically accompanied by the sudden onset of posterior neck pain/paraspinal muscle spasm, as well as true radicular arm pain or referred pain to the periscapular area.

25.2.8 Stingers/Burners/Transient Brachial Plexopathy/Nerve Root Neurapraxia

This condition is one of the most common occurrences in collision sports and is not the result of an SCI. It was first described in 1965.[62] Because the mechanism was thought to be direct force applied to the shoulder with the neck flexed laterally away from the point of contact, the condition has also been referred to as cervical pinch syndrome. This is a transient neurologic event characterized by pain and paresthesia in a single upper extremity following a blow to the head or shoulder. The symptoms most commonly involve the C5 and C6 spinal roots. The affected athlete can experience burning, tingling, or numbness in a circumferential or dermatomal distribution. The symptoms may radiate to the hand or remain localized in the neck. These athletes often maintain a slightly flexed cervical spine posture to reduce pressure on the affected nerve root at the neural foramen or hold/elevate the affected limb in an attempt to decrease tension on the upper cervical nerve roots.

Weakness in shoulder abduction, external rotation, and arm flexion is a reliable indicator of the injury. If weakness is a component, it usually involves the C5–C6 neurotome. The radiating arm pain tends to resolve first (within minutes), followed by a return of motor function (within 24 to 48 hours). Although the condition is usually self-limiting, and permanent sensorimotor deficits are rare, a variable degree of muscle weakness can last up to 6 weeks in a small percentage of cases.

This injury is usually the result of downward displacement of the shoulder with concomitant lateral flexion of the neck toward the contralateral shoulder. This is thought to result in a traction injury to the brachial plexus. The condition may also result from ipsilateral head rotation with axial loading resulting in neural foramen narrowing and compression/impaction of the exiting nerve root within the foramen.[63] Direct blunt trauma at Erb's point, located superficially in the supraclavicular region, has also been reported to be an etiology for stingers. This can occur when an opponent's shoulder or helmet is driven into the affected athlete's shoulder pad and directly into this area.

This injury has been graded using Seddon's criteria. A grade I injury is essentially a neurapraxia defined as the transient motor or sensory deficit without structural axonal disruption. This type of injury usually completely resolves and full recovery can be expected within 2 weeks. Grade II injuries are equivalent to axonotmesis. This involves axonal disruption with an intact outer supporting epineurium. This results in a neurologic deficit for at least 2 weeks, and axonal injury may be demonstrated on electromyographic studies 2 to 3 weeks following the injury. Grade III injuries are considered neurotmesis or total destruction of the axon and all supporting tissue. These injuries persist for at least 1 year with little clinical improvement.

Cervical canal stenosis has been implicated as a risk factor for stingers.[64] The dimensions of the spinal cord remain relatively constant in the subaxial cervical spine, with an average midsagittal cord diameter in the range of 8 to 9 mm.[65] In contrast, the size of the vertebral canal in the lower cervical region shows significant individual variation. Determining the "functional reserve" (amount of CSF surrounding the spinal cord) can be accomplished using MRI and is currently the preferred method for assessing "functional spinal stenosis."

Stingers with prolonged neurologic symptoms are one of the most common reasons for high school and college athlete cervical spine evaluations in an emergency room. The athlete commonly demonstrates a full, pain-free arc of neck motion with no midline palpation tenderness on examination. If tenderness is present or unilateral neurologic symptoms persist, a paracentral disk herniation with associated nerve root compression should be considered. This is usually accompanied by the sudden onset of posterior neck pain and spasm. Monoradiculopathy characterized by radiating pain, paresthesias, or weakness in the upper extremity also occurs secondary to compression and inflammation of the cervical root.

25.2.9 On-the-Field Management

The immediate treatment of the player who has suffered an SCI should follow standard trauma protocols that address airway, breathing, and circulation. The initial objective in this primary survey is to assess the athlete for immediately life-threatening conditions and to prevent further injury. During this primary survey, appropriate resuscitation procedures are instituted and the emergency medical system is activated immediately on recognizing a life-threatening problem or serious spinal injury.

Following the primary survey, one of three clinical scenarios will become apparent: actual or impending cardiopulmonary collapse, altered mental status but no compromise of the cardiovascular or respiratory system, or normal level of consciousness and normal cardiopulmonary function.

If the athlete is experiencing cardiopulmonary collapse, the use of advanced cardiac life support principles is essential. An athlete lying prone must be carefully log-rolled into a supine position on a rigid backboard if available. Any face mask should be rapidly removed to provide adequate airway access. As mentioned earlier in this chapter, initial removal of the helmet and shoulder pads is becoming a more routine practice. If still in place, the mouthpiece should be taken out while manual stabilization of the neck in a neutral position is maintained. Airway evaluation should be performed with the understanding that obstruction can be secondary to a foreign body, facial fractures, or direct injury to the trachea or larynx. A depressed level of consciousness can also contribute to the inability to maintain an airway.

If breathing is of insufficient depth or rate, assisted ventilation is required. On the field, this is usually performed by using a bag–valve device and face mask. Hypoxia should be rapidly corrected by providing adequate ventilation with protection of the vertebral column at all times. In a patent airway, respiratory collapse could be the result of an upper cervical SCI due to paralysis of the diaphragm and accessory breathing muscles. Indications for definitive airway control by endotracheal intubation include apnea, inability to maintain oxygenation with face mask supplementation, and protection from aspiration. Circulation must also be addressed during the primary survey. Neurogenic shock secondary to SCI could result in diminished amplitude of the peripheral pulses in combination with bradycardia. If the femoral or carotid pulses are not palpable, cardiopulmonary resuscitation is required. If this is the case, the front of the shoulder pads can be opened to allow for chest compressions and defibrillation if they were not already removed.

If the athlete is found to have an altered mental status without cardiopulmonary compromise, a brief neurologic examination can be performed. The prevention of further injury to the cord is of primary importance, and once initial resuscitation and evaluation are performed, focus should be placed on immobilization. Neutral axial alignment and occipital support must be maintained. An unconscious player should be log-rolled into a supine position and the mouthpiece removed.

If, after completion of the primary survey, the athlete is found to have a normal mental status without cardiopulmonary compromise, a neurologic assessment should be performed. If the athlete exhibits symptoms or signs referable to cord damage, a catastrophic cervical cord trauma should be assumed. If the neurologic assessment is normal but the athlete exhibits cervicothoracic pain, focal spinal tenderness, or restricted neck motion, an unstable spinal column injury with potential cord compromise is assumed.

Removal from the field should be performed, with strict attention to immobilization of the spine. A rigid backboard with cervical collar or bolsters on the sides of the head should be used. It is important to remember that the athlete's helmet may cause unintended cervical flexion on a rigid spine board. Once the athlete arrives at the hospital, if still in place, the helmet and shoulder pads should be removed before radiographic examination.

Athletes who suffer a burner should be immediately removed from competition until symptoms have fully resolved. Management of the participant who receives this injury is often dependent on the presence of residual symptoms. They are usually considered an isolated benign injury. On-field evaluation should include palpation of the cervical spine to determine any points of tenderness or deformity. Evaluation of sensation and muscle strength should be performed, using the unaffected limb as a point of reference if necessary. Weakness in the muscles innervated by the upper trunk of the brachial plexus is often observed. These include the deltoid (C5), biceps (C56), supraspinatus (C56), and infraspinatus (C56). The shoulder of the affected limb should also be evaluated, with particular attention to the clavicle, acromioclavicular joint, and supraclavicular and glenohumeral regions. Percussion of Erb's point can be performed in an attempt to elicit radiating symptoms. Obviously, the athlete should be evaluated for other serious injuries such as cervical spine fractures and dislocations. It is unusual to find lower brachial trunk injury patterns involving the C7 or C8 nerve roots. It is also not common to see persistent sensory deficits involving either the lower or the upper extremities. This condition is always unilateral and has never been reported to involve the lower extremities. If bilateral upper extremity deficits are present, SCI should be at the top of the differential diagnosis. Localized neck stiffness or tenderness with apprehension toward active cervical movement should alert the examiner to a potentially serious injury and the subsequent initiation of full spinal precautions, including spine board immobilization and transport for advanced imaging.

If there are no complaints of neck pain, decreased range of motion, or residual symptoms, the player can usually return to competition. If symptoms do not resolve or there is persistent pain, prompt imaging of the brachial plexus via MRI is recommended. If the symptoms persist for over 2 weeks, electromyography can be performed to establish the distribution and degree of injury. Residual muscle weakness, cervical anomalies, and abnormal electromyographic studies are exclusion criteria for return to play.

By definition stingers and burners are transient phenomena. They usually do not require formal treatment. The athlete should be followed closely with repeat neurologic examinations because, although the condition usually resolves in minutes, motor weakness may develop hours to days following the injury. Repeated stingers may result in long-term muscle weakness with persistent paresthesias. Other options for participants to decrease the risk of future occurrences are to change their field position or modify their playing technique.

25.3 Conclusion

The health benefits of participation in sporting activities are undeniable. Unfortunately, there also exists the inherent risk of injury. Improvements in safety equipment and rule changes have led to a substantial drop in the number of catastrophic neurologic injuries suffered during athletic competition. When these injuries do occur, they must be treated promptly and correctly to optimize outcome. Less dramatic injuries such as stingers and concussions also require significant attention and management to prevent permanent long-term sequelae. It is hoped that this chapter will serve as a guide for the rapid diagnosis and treatment of neurologic emergencies in this population.

References

[1] McKee AC, Daneshvar DH, Alvarez VE, Stein TD. The neuropathology of sport. Acta Neuropathol. 2014; 127(1):29–51

[2] Daneshvar DH, Nowinski CJ, McKee AC, Cantu RC. The epidemiology of sport-related concussion. Clin Sports Med. 2011; 30(1):1–17, vii

[3] Langlois JA, Rutland-Brown W, Wald MM. The epidemiology and impact of traumatic brain injury: a brief overview. J Head Trauma Rehabil. 2006; 21(5):375–378

[4] Yue JK, Winkler EA, Burke JF, et al. Pediatric sports-related traumatic brain injury in United States trauma centers. Neurosurg Focus. 2016; 40(4):E3

[5] Winkler EA, Yue JK, Burke JF, et al. Adult sports-related traumatic brain injury in United States trauma centers. Neurosurg Focus. 2016; 40(4):E4

[6] Thomas M, Haas TS, Doerer JJ, et al. Epidemiology of sudden death in young, competitive athletes due to blunt trauma. Pediatrics. 2011; 128(1):e1–e8

[7] Mueller F, Cantu R. Catastrophic Football Injuries Annual Report. Chapel Hill, NC: National Center for Catastrophic Injury Research; 2009

[8] Buzas D, Jacobson NA, Morawa LG. Concussions from 9 youth organized sports: results from NEISS hospitals over an 11-year time frame, 2002–2012. Orthop J Sports Med. 2014; 2(4):2325967114528460

[9] Lincoln AE, Caswell SV, Almquist JL, Dunn RE, Norris JB, Hinton RY. Trends in concussion incidence in high school sports: a prospective 11-year study. Am J Sports Med. 2011; 39(5):958–963

[10] Centers for Disease Control and Prevention (CDC). Nonfatal traumatic brain injuries from sports and recreation activities—United States, 2001–2005. MMWR Morb Mortal Wkly Rep. 2007; 56(29):733–737

[11] Barone GW, Rodgers BM. Pediatric equestrian injuries: a 14-year review. J Trauma. 1989; 29(2):245–247

[12] Ingemarson H, Grevsten S, Thorén L. Lethal horse-riding injuries. J Trauma. 1989; 29(1):25–30

[13] Retsky J, Jaffe D, Christoffel K. Skateboarding injuries in children. A second wave. Am J Dis Child. 1991; 145(2):188–192

[14] Sosin DM, Sacks JJ, Webb KW. Pediatric head injuries and deaths from bicycling in the United States. Pediatrics. 1996; 98(5):868–870

[15] Miele VJ, Bailes JE. Neurological injuries in miscellaneous sports. In: Bailes JE, Day A, eds. Neurological Sports Medicine. Vol. 1. Lebanon, NH: American Association of Neurological Surgeons; 2000:181–250

[16] Miele VJ, Carson L, Carr A, Bailes JE. Acute on chronic subdural hematoma in a female boxer: a case report. Med Sci Sports Exerc. 2004; 36(11):1852–1855

[17] Levy AS, Hawkes AP, Hemminger LM, Knight S. An analysis of head injuries among skiers and snowboarders. J Trauma. 2002; 53(4):695–704

[18] Bailes JE, Cantu RC. Head injury in athletes. Neurosurgery. 2001; 48(1):26–45, discussion 45–46

[19] Pennycook AG, Morrison WG, Ritchie DA. Accidental golf club injuries. Postgrad Med J. 1991; 67(793):982–983

[20] Pasternack JS, Veenema KR, Callahan CM. Baseball injuries: a Little League survey. Pediatrics. 1996; 98(3 Pt 1):445–448

[21] Cantu RC, Mueller FO. Brain injury-related fatalities in American football, 1945–1999. Neurosurgery. 2003; 52(4):846–852, discussion 852–853

[22] Ghiselli G, Schaadt G, McAllister DR. On-the-field evaluation of an athlete with a head or neck injury. Clin Sports Med. 2003; 22(3):445–465

[23] Saunders RL, Harbaugh RE. The second impact in catastrophic contact-sports head trauma. JAMA. 1984; 252(4):538–539

[24] Kelly JP, Nichols JS, Filley CM, Lillehei KO, Rubinstein D, Kleinschmidt-DeMasters BK. Concussion in sports. Guidelines for the prevention of catastrophic outcome. JAMA. 1991; 266(20):2867–2869

[25] McCrory P. Does second impact syndrome exist? Clin J Sport Med. 2001; 11(3):144–149

[26] Kors EE, Terwindt GM, Vermeulen FL, et al. Delayed cerebral edema and fatal coma after minor head trauma: role of the CACNA1A calcium channel subunit gene and relationship with familial hemiplegic migraine. Ann Neurol. 2001; 49(6):753–760

[27] McQuillen JB, McQuillen EN, Morrow P. Trauma, sport, and malignant cerebral edema. Am J Forensic Med Pathol. 1988; 9(1):12–15

[28] Harmon KG, Drezner J, Gammons M, et al; American Medical Society for Sports Medicine. American Medical Society for Sports Medicine position statement: concussion in sport. Clin J Sport Med. 2013; 23(1):1–18

[29] Jordan BD. The clinical spectrum of sport-related traumatic brain injury. Nat Rev Neurol. 2013; 9(4):222–230

[30] Giza CC, Hovda DA. The new neurometabolic cascade of concussion. Neurosurgery. 2014; 75(Suppl 4):S24–S33

[31] McCrory P, Meeuwisse W, Aubry M, et al. Consensus statement on concussion in sport—the 4th International Conference on Concussion in Sport held in Zurich, November 2012. Phys Ther Sport. 2013; 14(2):e1–e13

[32] Kleiner DM; Inter-Association Task Force for Appropriate Care of the Spine-Injured Athlete. Prehospital care of the spine-injured athlete: monograph summary. Clin J Sport Med. 2003; 13(1):59–61

[33] Dean GdL, Uguccioni D, Denoble P, Dean G de L, Uguccioni DM, Denoble PJ, et al. Underwater and Hyperbaric Medicine, abstracts from the literature. Undersea Hyperb Med. 2000; 27:51

[34] Dick AP, Massey EW. Neurologic presentation of decompression sickness and air embolism in sport divers. Neurology. 1985; 35(5):667–671

[35] Greer HD, Massey EW. Neurologic injury from undersea diving. Neurol Clin. 1992; 10(4):1031–1045

[36] United States Navy. Recompression treatments when chamber available. Revision 1 c, rev. 15th ed. 0994-LP-001-9110. In: U.S. Navy Diving Manual. Vol. 1 (Air Diving). Washington, DC: Naval Sea Systems Command Publication; 1993

[37] Clarke C. High altitude cerebral oedema. Int J Sports Med. 1988; 9(2):170–174

[38] Meurer LN, Slawson JG. Which pharmacologic therapies are effective in preventing acute mountain sickness? J Fam Pract. 2000; 49(11):981

[39] Bailes JE, Hadley MN, Quigley MR, Sonntag VK, Cerullo LJ. Management of athletic injuries of the cervical spine and spinal cord. Neurosurgery. 1991; 29(4):491–497

[40] National Spinal Cord Injury Statistical Center. Spinal Cord Information Network: Facts and Figures at a Glance. Birmingham, AL: University of Alabama at Birmingham; 2003

[41] DeVivo MJ. Causes and costs of spinal cord injury in the United States. Spinal Cord. 1997; 35(12):809–813

[42] Maroon JC, Bailes JE. Athletes with cervical spine injury. Spine. 1996; 21(19):2294–2299

[43] Levy AS, Smith RH. Neurologic injuries in skiers and snowboarders. Semin Neurol. 2000; 20(2):233–245

[44] Quarrie KL, Cantu RC, Chalmers DJ. Rugby union injuries to the cervical spine and spinal cord. Sports Med. 2002; 32(10):633–653

[45] Schmitt H, Gerner HJ. Paralysis from sport and diving accidents. Clin J Sport Med. 2001; 11(1):17–22

[46] Tator CH, Carson JD, Cushman R. Hockey injuries of the spine in Canada, 1966–1996. CMAJ. 2000; 162(6):787–788

[47] Cantu RC, Mueller FO. Catastrophic spine injuries in American football, 1977–2001. Neurosurgery. 2003; 53(2):358–362, discussion 362–363

[48] Torg JS, Truex R, Jr, Quedenfeld TC, Burstein A, Spealman A, Nichols C, III. The National Football Head and Neck Injury Registry. Report and conclusions 1978. JAMA. 1979; 241(14):1477–1479

[49] Tator CH, Provvidenza CF, Lapczak L, Carson J, Raymond D. Spinal injuries in Canadian ice hockey: documentation of injuries sustained from 1943–1999. Can J Neurol Sci. 2004; 31(4):460–466

[50] Maroon JC, Abla AA, Wilberger JI, Bailes JE, Sternau LL. Central cord syndrome. Clin Neurosurg. 1991; 37:612–621

[51] Coelho DG, Brasil AV, Ferreira NP. Risk factors of neurological lesions in low cervical spine fractures and dislocations. Arq Neuropsiquiatr. 2000; 58(4):1030–1034

[52] Banerjee R, Palumbo MA, Fadale PD. Catastrophic cervical spine injuries in the collision sport athlete, part 2: principles of emergency care. Am J Sports Med. 2004; 32(7):1760–1764

[53] Ghanayem A, Zdeblich T, Dvorak J. Functional anatomy of joints, ligaments, and discs. In: Cervical Spine Research Society, ed. The Cervical Spine. Philadelphia, PA: Lippincott-Raven; 1998:45–52

[54] White AA, III, Johnson RM, Panjabi MM, Southwick WO. Biomechanical analysis of clinical stability in the cervical spine. Clin Orthop Relat Res. 1975(109):85–96

[55] Wilberger JE, Abla A, Maroon JC. Burning hands syndrome revisited. Neurosurgery. 1986; 19(6):1038–1040

[56] Torg JS, Guille JT, Jaffe S. Injuries to the cervical spine in American football players. J Bone Joint Surg Am. 2002; 84-A(1):112–122

[57] Zwimpfer TJ, Bernstein M. Spinal cord concussion. J Neurosurg. 1990; 72(6):894–900

[58] Torg JS, Corcoran TA, Thibault LE, et al. Cervical cord neurapraxia: classification, pathomechanics, morbidity, and management guidelines. J Neurosurg. 1997; 87(6):843–850

[59] Castro FP, Jr. Stingers, cervical cord neurapraxia, and stenosis. Clin Sports Med. 2003; 22(3):483–492

[60] Torg JS. Cervical spinal stenosis with cord neurapraxia and transient quadriplegia. Sports Med. 1995; 20(6):429–434

[61] Cantu RC. Cervical spine injuries in the athlete. Semin Neurol. 2000; 20(2):173–178

[62] Chrisman OD, Snook GA, Stanitis JM, Keedy VA. Lateral-flexion neck injuries in athletic competition. JAMA. 1965; 192:613–615

[63] Weinberg J, Rokito S, Silber JS. Etiology, treatment, and prevention of athletic "stingers". Clin Sports Med. 2003; 22(3):493–500, viii

[64] Kelly JD, IV, Aliquo D, Sitler MR, Odgers C, Moyer RA. Association of burners with cervical canal and foraminal stenosis. Am J Sports Med. 2000; 28(2):214–217

[65] Okada Y, Ikata T, Katoh S, Yamada H. Morphologic analysis of the cervical spinal cord, dural tube, and spinal canal by magnetic resonance imaging in normal adults and patients with cervical spondylotic myelopathy. Spine. 1994; 19(20):2331–2335

26 Penetrating Spine Trauma

Michael D. Martin and Christopher E. Wolfla

Abstract

Penetrating spinal trauma often occurs in and as a result of violent situations, either as the result of an assault or accident of some kind. Management of these sometimes complex injuries must take into account the repercussions to the neurologic elements of the spine, the bony anatomy with its biomechanical concerns, and injuries to the patient's body in general that so often accompany this type of trauma. This chapter discusses the epidemiology, proper evaluation, and management of penetrating injuries that result in spinal trauma.

Keywords: gunshot wound, penetrating trauma, spinal instability

26.1 Introduction

Penetrating spine trauma encompasses injury caused by firearms, both military and civilian, as well as foreign bodies, including knives and a myriad of other implements. It is in essence largely a social problem, and perhaps summarized best in a quote from the *Lancet*, ca. 1962: "In an instant—and often for a negligible reason—an otherwise healthy man is incapacitated, either permanently or for many months."[1] Reports vary widely as to the proper management of such injuries, but certain guiding principles can be gleaned from the available data. This chapter distills what is known about these injuries, as well as provides a logical approach to the management of penetrating spinal trauma. Finally, we will discuss the outcome of these often devastating injuries with respect to neurologic recovery.

26.2 Epidemiology

The incidence of spinal cord injury in penetrating neck injuries is between 3.7 and 15.0%.[2,3] The average age of victims of civilian-type gunshot wounds in one series was approximately 32 years, with 89% of the victims being male.[4] Not surprisingly, the same series of 92 patients revealed that the thoracic region was the most often injured (59%), followed by the cervical spine (31%), and finally the lumbar spine (10%). Seventy-five percent of these had complete injuries, whereas 25% had incomplete injuries. With regard to military gunshot wounds, a large review of injuries from World War II revealed that most wounds were located near the midline and at the cervicothoracic junction.[5] Literature from the Vietnam conflict cited the thoracic spine as the most common location.[6] Spinal injury from stab wounds also occurred more frequently in males (84% compared with 16% females in a large series).[7] A very interesting series from South Africa reported that this injury was caused most commonly by knives (84.2%), although a surprising number of implements may be involved.[7] Complete motor deficits in stab wounds range from 20 to 43%.[7,8]

26.3 Initial Evaluation and Imaging

In all types of penetrating spinal injury, initial history and physical examination are important in guiding both the need for further investigation and the proper type of treatment. History must be obtained to best delineate the probable mechanism by which the spinal cord has been injured. Nowhere is this more evident than in the difference between a wound from a civilian versus a military firearm. Wounding patterns differ between these two types of weapons because of ballistics.[9,10] As a bullet passes through tissue, a sonic pressure wave precedes the projectile without causing injury in and of itself.[10] As expected, bullets are rapidly slowed as they enter tissue, and this rapid deceleration creates a temporary cavity in the tissue. This process is often referred to as cavitation.[10] The amount of cavitation is related to the velocity of the projectile involved, with wounding capacity quadrupling as velocity is doubled.[9] Physical examination is important in all patients, and documentation of motor and sensory levels is important in any spinal cord injury. By convention, spinal cord injuries are identified by the lowest level of antigravity motor function. Assessment of entrance and exit wounds can be useful in determining trajectory, which has been shown to be an important factor in the severity of injury suffered.[11] A statistically significant difference has been found in the degree of spinal cord injury suffered by those in whom a bullet has traversed the spinal canal and those in whom it did not (88% complete injuries if the bullet traversed the canal, 78% incomplete if it did not).[11]

Stab wounds most often (63.8%) involve the thoracic spine, followed by the cervical spine (29.6%) and finally the lumbar region (6.7%). Complete cord injury also occurred in a higher percentage of patients stabbed in the thoracic spine (24%) than in the cervical (15.8%) or lumbar (10%) spine.[7] In this type of nonmissile penetrating trauma, the bony elements of the spine seem to deflect injuries to either side of the midline, decreasing the chance of complete cord injury[1,12] (▶ Fig. 26.1). The implement used may directly injure the spinal cord, may injure arterial supply or venous drainage, or may cause a contrecoup type of cord contusion.[1,7] This may lead to injury patterns that do not follow the classic Brown–Séquard pattern, even in the case of a knife causing anatomical hemisection of the cord.[7] Laminar fractures have been reported if the instrument used was of sufficient size and mass.[1]

Initial imaging should include complete spine X-rays, computed tomography (CT), and magnetic resonance imaging (MRI) when available and clinically feasible.[13,14] Some have suggested that it is unnecessary to use cervical spine immobilization in fully conscious patients with isolated penetrating trauma,[15,16,17] although it must be remembered that cervical spine fractures in gunshot wounds to the neck may occur in 14.6 to 43.0% of patients.[18] Cervical instability is a possible, albeit rare, sequel of penetrating neck trauma.[19] Although MRI is an important tool in spinal cord injury, quality may be decreased by ferromagnetic

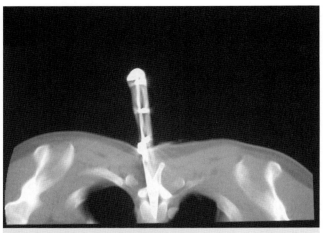

Fig. 26.1 Axial computed tomography scan demonstrating a knife in the spinal canal. It has been deflected from the midline somewhat by the bony spinous process.

artifact from foreign body residue.[12] MRI is not recommended in the case of a known retained metallic foreign body. Penetrating trauma may cause neurologic deficit from epidural or subdural hematoma, disk herniation, foreign bodies within the spinal canal, or displaced bony elements of the spinal column.[14] Cord contusions may appear as high-signal-intensity areas on proton density–weighted and T2-weighted MR images, whereas T2-weighted images are probably the best sequence for evaluating cord edema.[14] Acute or subacute hemorrhage can be represented by a focus of low signal intensity on T2-weighted and proton density–weighted images, or an area of high signal intensity on T1-weighted, T2-weighted, and proton density–weighted sequences.[14] Intramedullary knife tracts are best demonstrated as high-signal-intensity lesions on T2-weighted and proton density–weighted images[14] (▶ Fig. 26.2). Subdural hematomas usually demonstrate a concave surface facing the cord and a convex surface toward the adjacent vertebral body, whereas epidural hematomas are often biconvex (as in intracranial epidural hematomas).[14]

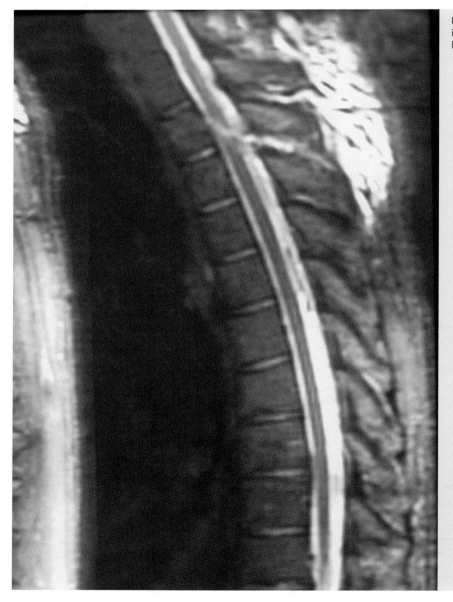

Fig. 26.2 T2-weighted magnetic resonance image of the spine following knife injury. The knife tract is hyperintense on this sequence.

A review of the literature finds that the incidence of vertebral artery injury in penetrating cervical trauma is 1.0 to 8.0%.[2,20,21,22] In most cases, physical examination and CT of the bony elements of the cervical spine provide reliable evaluation of vascular insult in the neck and should be used to guide the decision for further vascular imaging[23,24,25,26] (▶Fig. 26.3). Injury may include occlusion, arteriovenous fistula, intimal tear, and pseudoaneurysm.[27,28] Up to 20% of patients may have no signs at all,[22] and vertebral artery injury in the absence of cervical spine fracture is rare. Angiography has been the standard evaluation tool for suspected vertebral artery injury, although modern noninvasive imaging is likely of similar benefit.[29,30]

Magnetic resonance angiography (MRA) and computed tomographic angiography (CTA) hold the promise of noninvasive diagnosis in evaluating vertebral artery trauma.[31,32] CT and CTA are useful in detecting other indirect signs of vascular injury, including bullet and bone fragments less than 5 mm from a major vessel, injury path through a vessel, and hematoma around the vessel.[31] Direct signs of vascular injury visible on CTA include changes in vessel caliber, irregularities in the vessel wall, extravasation of contrast, and lack of enhancement.[31] MRA has a reported specificity of 98 to 100% but a sensitivity of 20 to 60% (depending on the sequence used) in detecting vertebral artery injury.[31] MRA has lower resolution than arteriography and at present is not recommended over arteriography for diagnosing vertebral artery injury.[33]

Vertebral arteriovenous fistula (AVF) is a rare complication of penetrating spine or neck trauma and may develop some time after the initial injury.[34] The most common symptom is tinnitus, present in 39% of patients in one series.[35] Other symptoms include headache, vertigo, diplopia, cervical neuralgia, and neck mass.[34,35] Roughly 41% of patients have no neurologic symptoms and present with only a cervical bruit. Heart failure is one possible sequela of any AVF, including those arising from the vertebral artery.[35,36] Another rare presentation is cervical cord or nerve root compression from draining veins arising from the AVF.[35,37]

Headache has been noted as a sequel of gunshot wounds to the spine.[38] A rare but interesting late-onset symptom is that of plumbism from retained bullet fragments in the disk space, which should resolve with removal of the fragments.[39] Others have reported osteomyelitis or sepsis following gunshot wounds to the spine that traversed the gastrointestinal tract, but larger series suggest that this is a rare entity.[40,41,42,43]

26.4 Treatment

Treatment of victims of penetrating spinal trauma is dependent on both the mechanism of injury and the patient's early postinjury course. Methylprednisolone increases complications but does not improve outcomes in patients who are victims of penetrating spinal trauma.[44,45] Some series have recommended aggressive surgical treatment for all gunshot victims,[46] and one larger series showed improvement after bullet removal only in lesions at T12 or below.[42] Other series have shown, however, that operating on all victims of civilian gunshot wounds conveys no significant improvement over conservative management and may increase the risk of infection, cerebrospinal fluid leakage, pseudomeningocele, and spinal instability.[4,45,47,48,49]

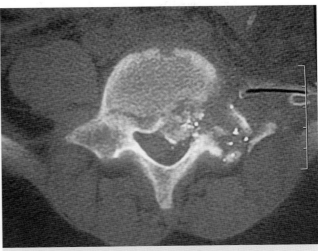

Fig. 26.3 Axial computed tomography scan following gunshot wound to the spine demonstrating disruption of bony elements.

Indications for surgical intervention in civilian gunshot wounds to the spine therefore include progressive neurologic deficit and persistent spinal fluid leakage, although most authors feel that these are rare entities.[4,45,48,50] Although technically difficult, surgery may be beneficial in the case of incomplete injury with evidence of continued neural compression (▶Fig. 26.4), instability, or decline in neurologic examination.[45,51,52] A smaller series of patients with incomplete injuries of the cauda equina showed a worse outcome with surgery (47% improvement) compared with conservative management (71% improvement).[53] Victims of shotgun injuries to the spinal cord have demonstrated no significant improvement following laminectomy[54] and have an overall increased mortality when compared with other gunshot victims.[55]

Experience in the military literature has been quite different. Although some studies have found results similar to the civilian data,[56,57] many authors advocate an aggressive approach to management of penetrating spinal trauma from military (i.e., high-velocity) weapons.[58,59,60,61,62] Laminectomy, foreign body removal, and dural repair, if possible, in all patients with neurologic deficit and without irrefutable evidence of complete anatomical transection has been shown in the military literature to provide some measure of recovery in 47.6 to 52.4% of patients.[58,60,61] Side-to-side bullet trajectories have been shown to be the most unstable and often require stabilization.[63] Not surprisingly, victims of penetrating spinal trauma in a combat setting do not fair as well as those suffering from blunt spinal trauma.[64]

Stab wounds inflicted by knives or other foreign bodies are best treated with the same general approach as gunshot wounds. Indications for surgery in the case of nonmissile penetrating trauma include retained foreign body material, persistent cerebrospinal fluid leakage, and development of sepsis from a sinus tract or epidural abscess.[1,7] In a very large series, spinal fluid leakage was encountered in only 4% of cases, and it almost always resolved spontaneously. The development of sepsis did not occur.[7] Other authors advocate routine exploration for all nonmissile penetrating trauma, albeit from a small series of patients.[65]

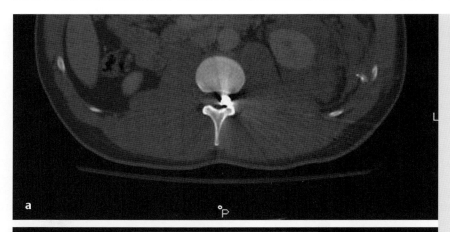

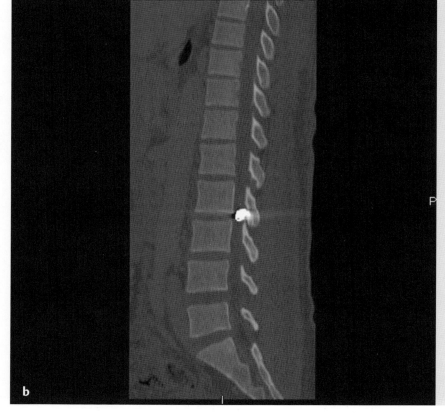

Fig. 26.4 (a) Axial and (b) sagittal computed tomography scan demonstrating retained bullet fragment in the spinal canal. This was removed because of persistent left-sided radicular pain.

Open surgical reconstruction of the injured vertebral artery has been advocated and described by some authors,[66] with a mortality of 4.7 to 22.0%.[67,68] The development of effective endovascular techniques, however, has led to their use for the treatment of most injuries to the vertebral artery, including AVF, dissection, and pseudoaneurysm.[35,69,70,71,72,73] Emergency intervention is sometimes indicated because of active bleeding or hemodynamic instability.[71] Attention should be paid to the patency of the contralateral vertebral artery as well as the location of any arteries feeding AVFs[74] because a patent artery on the opposite side is a good indicator of the safety of ligation of the injured vertebral artery.[75] Pseudoaneurysms should be treated with coiling, stent-assisted coiling or open surgery.[27,73]

26.5 Neurologic Outcomes

A large series comparing surgically versus conservatively managed penetrating trauma patients found no differences between the two groups in terms of neurologic outcome.[49] Those with complete injuries from gunshot wounds showed mild improvement in 13 to 15% and worsening of their deficit in 3 to 6%. Incomplete injuries improved in 40 to 58% of patients and worsened in 18 to 20% of cases. Similar results were seen in stab wounds. Overall morbidity from penetrating spinal injuries in the military literature has decreased since the early 20th century and was reported as 2.3% in one paper from the Vietnam era.[52] A large body of data from the Korean conflict (in which almost all patients had operations) divided outcome data by the level of injury.[60] All of those with incomplete lesions of the cervical spine had some recovery following laminectomy (28.6% full recovery, 71.4% partial recovery). Thirty-five percent of those with complete cervical injuries showed no improvement, 60% had partial recovery, and 5% made a complete recovery. Incomplete lesions in the thoracic region were similar, with 20% achieving full recovery and 80% partial recovery, but patients with complete lesions in the thoracic region recovered function only 9% of the time (90% partial recovery, 10% full recovery). Partial injuries to the lumbar spine resulted in full recovery only 14.2% of the time, and complete injuries in this region showed some recovery in 18.8% of patients. A review of 450 cases of stab wounds to the spine demonstrated that recovery was good (meaning able to ambulate with minimal support) in 65.6% of patients.[7] The vast majority of the patients (95.6%) in this series were not treated surgically. The authors went on to say that 17.1% of their patients made a "fair" recovery (walking with moderate assistance) and 17.3% made no functional recovery.

26.6 Conclusion

Penetrating spinal trauma can cause devastating injury to otherwise healthy and most often young individuals. Neurosurgeons must use the clinical history, when available, as well as detailed physical examination and appropriate imaging to guide treatment and evaluate for other injuries such as vascular deformation. Although intervention may help patients who suffer wounds from high-velocity weapons or those resulting in spinal instability or vascular insult, the majority of patients seen in the urban trauma center will not require operative intervention. Perhaps advances in spinal cord rehabilitation and research will add to the somewhat limited armamentarium with which neurosurgeons currently treat these devastating injuries.

References

[1] Lipschitz R, Block J. Stab wounds of the spinal cord. Lancet. 1962; 2(7248):169–172

[2] Flax RL, Fletcher HS, Joseph WL. Management of penetrating injuries of the neck. Am Surg. 1973; 39(3):148–150

[3] Almskog BA, Angerås U, Hall-Angerås M, Malmgren S. Penetrating wounds of the neck. Experience from a Swedish hospital. Acta Chir Scand. 1985; 151(5):419–423

[4] Kupcha PC, An HS, Cotler JM. Gunshot wounds to the cervical spine. Spine. 1990; 15(10):1058–1063

[5] Klemperer WW. Spinal cord injuries in World War II. I. Examination and operative technic in 201 patients. U S Armed Forces Med J. 1959; 10(5):532–552

[6] Jacobson SA, Bors E. Spinal cord injury in Vietnamese combat. Paraplegia. 1970; 7(4):263–281

[7] Peacock WJ, Shrosbree RD, Key AG. A review of 450 stabwounds of the spinal cord. S Afr Med J. 1977; 51(26):961–964

[8] McCaughey EJ, Purcell M, Barnett SC, Allan DB. Spinal Cord Injury caused by stab wounds: incidence, natural history and relevance for future research. J Neurotrauma. 2016; 33(15):1416–1421

[9] Ordog GJ, Wasserberger J, Balasubramanium S. Wound ballistics: theory and practice. Ann Emerg Med. 1984; 13(12):1113–1122

[10] Hollerman JJ, Fackler ML, Coldwell DM, Ben-Menachem Y. Gunshot wounds: 1. Bullets, ballistics, and mechanisms of injury. AJR Am J Roentgenol. 1990; 155(4):685–690

[11] Waters RL, Sie I, Adkins RH, Yakura JS. Injury pattern effect on motor recovery after traumatic spinal cord injury. Arch Phys Med Rehabil. 1995; 76(5):440–443

[12] Takhtani D, Melhem ER. MR imaging in cervical spine trauma. Clin Sports Med. 2002; 21(1):49–75, vi

[13] Splavski B, Sarić G, Vranković D, Glavina K, Mursić B, Blagus G. Computed tomography of the spine as an important diagnostic tool in the management of war missile spinal trauma. Arch Orthop Trauma Surg. 1998; 117(6–7):360–363

[14] Moyed S, Shanmuganathan K, Mirvis SE, Bethel A, Rothman M. MR imaging of penetrating spinal trauma. AJR Am J Roentgenol. 1999; 173(5):1387–1391

[15] Connell RA, Graham CA, Munro PT. Is spinal immobilisation necessary for all patients sustaining isolated penetrating trauma? Injury. 2003; 34(12):912–914

[16] Eftekhary N, Nwosu K, McCoy E, Fukunaga D, Rolfe K. Overutilization of bracing in the management of penetrating spinal cord injury from gunshot wounds. J Neurosurg Spine. 2016; 25(1):110–113

[17] Vanderlan WB, Tew BE, Seguin CY, et al. Neurologic sequelae of penetrating cervical trauma. Spine. 2009; 34(24):2646–2653

[18] Arishita GI, Vayer JS, Bellamy RF. Cervical spine immobilization of penetrating neck wounds in a hostile environment. J Trauma. 1989; 29(3):332–337

[19] Apfelbaum JD, Cantrill SV, Waldman N. Unstable cervical spine without spinal cord injury in penetrating neck trauma. Am J Emerg Med. 2000; 18(1):55–57

[20] Carducci B, Lowe RA, Dalsey W. Penetrating neck trauma: consensus and controversies. Ann Emerg Med. 1986; 15(2):208–215

[21] Demetriades D, Charalambides D, Lakhoo M. Physical examination and selective conservative management in patients with penetrating injuries of the neck. Br J Surg. 1993; 80(12):1534–1536

[22] Roberts LH, Demetriades D. Vertebral artery injuries. Surg Clin North Am. 2001; 81(6):1345–1356, xiii

[23] Menawat SS, Dennis JW, Laneve LM, Frykberg ER. Are arteriograms necessary in penetrating zone II neck injuries? J Vasc Surg. 1992; 16(3):397–400, discussion 400–401

[24] Klyachkin ML, Rohmiller M, Charash WE, Sloan DA, Kearney PA. Penetrating injuries of the neck: selective management evolving. Am Surg. 1997; 63(2):189–194

[25] Sekharan J, Dennis JW, Veldenz HC, Miranda F, Frykberg ER. Continued experience with physical examination alone for evaluation and management of penetrating zone 2 neck injuries: results of 145 cases. J Vasc Surg. 2000; 32(3):483–489

[26] Azuaje RE, Jacobson LE, Glover J, et al. Reliability of physical examination as a predictor of vascular injury after penetrating neck trauma. Am Surg. 2003; 69(9):804–807

[27] Larsen DW. Traumatic vascular injuries and their management. Neuroimaging Clin N Am. 2002; 12(2):249–269

[28] Mwipatayi BP, Jeffery P, Beningfield SJ, Motale P, Tunnicliffe J, Navsaria PH. Management of extra-cranial vertebral artery injuries. Eur J Vasc Endovasc Surg. 2004; 27(2):157–162

[29] Roon AJ, Christensen N. Evaluation and treatment of penetrating cervical injuries. J Trauma. 1979; 19(6):391–397

[30] Diaz-Daza O, Arraiza FJ, Barkley JM, Whigham CJ. Endovascular therapy of traumatic vascular lesions of the head and neck. Cardiovasc Intervent Radiol. 2003; 26(3):213–221

[31] LeBlang SD, Nunez DB, Jr. Noninvasive imaging of cervical vascular injuries. AJR Am J Roentgenol. 2000; 174(5):1269–1278

[32] Hollingworth W, Nathens AB, Kanne JP, et al. The diagnostic accuracy of computed tomography angiography for traumatic or atherosclerotic lesions of the carotid and vertebral arteries: a systematic review. Eur J Radiol. 2003; 48(1):88–102

[33] Mascalchi M, Bianchi MC, Mangiafico S, et al. MRI and MR angiography of vertebral artery dissection. Neuroradiology. 1997; 39(5):329–340

[34] Ammirati M, Mirzai S, Samii M. Vertebral arteriovenous fistulae. Report of two cases and review of the literature. Acta Neurochir (Wien). 1989; 99(3–4):122–126

[35] Vinchon M, Laurian C, George B, et al. Vertebral arteriovenous fistulas: a study of 49 cases and review of the literature. Cardiovasc Surg. 1994; 2(3):359–369

[36] Davis JM, Zimmerman RA. Injury of the carotid and vertebral arteries. Neuroradiology. 1983; 25(2):55–69

[37] Ross DA, Olsen WL, Halbach V, Rosegay H, Pitts LH. Cervical root compression by a traumatic pseudoaneurysm of the vertebral artery: case report. Neurosurgery. 1988; 22(2):414–417

[38] Spierings EL, Foo DK, Young RR. Headaches in patients with traumatic lesions of the cervical spinal cord. Headache. 1992; 32(1):45–49

[39]   Scuderi GJ, Vaccaro AR, Fitzhenry LN, Greenberg S, Eismont F. Long-term clinical manifestations of retained bullet fragments within the intervertebral disk space. J Spinal Disord Tech. 2004; 17(2):108–111

[40]   Craig JB. Cervical spine osteomyelitis with delayed onset tetraparesis after penetrating wounds of the neck. A report of 2 cases. S Afr Med J. 1986; 69(3):197–199

[41]   Miller BR, Schiller WR. Pyogenic vertebral osteomyelitis after transcolonic gunshot wound. Mil Med. 1989; 154(2):64–66

[42]   Waters RL, Adkins RH. The effects of removal of bullet fragments retained in the spinal canal. A collaborative study by the National Spinal Cord Injury Model Systems. Spine. 1991; 16(8):934–939

[43]   Velmahos GC, Degiannis E, Hart K, Souter I, Saadia R. Changing profiles in spinal cord injuries and risk factors influencing recovery after penetrating injuries. J Trauma. 1995; 38(3):334–337

[44]   Levy ML, Gans W, Wijesinghe HS, SooHoo WE, Adkins RH, Stillerman CB. Use of methylprednisolone as an adjunct in the management of patients with penetrating spinal cord injury: outcome analysis. Neurosurgery. 1996; 39(6):1141–1148, discussion 1148–1149

[45]   Heary RF, Vaccaro AR, Mesa JJ, Balderston RA. Thoracolumbar infections in penetrating injuries to the spine. Orthop Clin North Am. 1996; 27(1):69–81

[46]   Turgut M, Ozcan OE, Güçay O, Sağlam S. Civilian penetrating spinal firearm injuries of the spine. Results of surgical treatment with special attention to factors determining prognosis. Arch Orthop Trauma Surg. 1994; 113(5):290–293

[47]   Yashon D, Jane JA, White RJ. Prognosis and management of spinal cord and cauda equina bullet injuries in sixty-five civilians. J Neurosurg. 1970; 32(2):163–170

[48]   Heiden JS, Weiss MH, Rosenberg AW, Kurze T, Apuzzo ML. Penetrating gunshot wounds of the cervical spine in civilians. Review of 38 cases. J Neurosurg. 1975; 42(5):575–579

[49]   Simpson RK, Jr, Venger BH, Narayan RK. Treatment of acute penetrating injuries of the spine: a retrospective analysis. J Trauma. 1989; 29(1):42–46

[50]   Comarr AE, Kaufman AA. A survey of the neurological results of 858 spinal cord injuries; a comparison of patients treated with and without laminectomy. J Neurosurg. 1956; 13(1):95–106

[51]   Beaty N, Slavin J, Diaz C, Zeleznick K, Ibrahimi D, Sansur CA. Cervical spine injury from gunshot wounds. J Neurosurg Spine. 2014; 21(3):442–449

[52]   Klimo P, Jr, Ragel BT, Rosner M, Gluf W, McCafferty R. Can surgery improve neurological function in penetrating spinal injury? A review of the military and civilian literature and treatment recommendations for military neurosurgeons. Neurosurg Focus. 2010; 28(5):E4

[53]   Robertson DP, Simpson RK. Penetrating injuries restricted to the cauda equina: a retrospective review. Neurosurgery. 1992; 31(2):265–269, discussion 269–270

[54]   Simpson RK, Jr, Venger BH, Fischer DK, Narayan RK, Mattox KL. Shotgun injuries of the spine: neurosurgical management of five cases. Br J Neurosurg. 1988; 2(3):321–326

[55]   Sherman RT, Parrish RA. Management of shotgun injuries: a review of 152 cases. J Trauma. 1963; 3:76–86

[56]   Jacobs GB, Berg RA. The treatment of acute spinal cord injuries in a war zone. J Neurosurg. 1971; 34(2 Pt 1):164–167

[57]   Hammoud MA, Haddad FS, Moufarrij NA. Spinal cord missile injuries during the Lebanese civil war. Surg Neurol. 1995; 43(5):432–437, discussion 437–442

[58]   Pool JL. Gunshot wounds of the spine; observations from an evacuation hospital. Surg Gynecol Obstet. 1945; 81:617–622

[59]   Haynes WG. Acute war wounds of the spinal cord. Am J Surg. 1946; 72:424–433

[60]   Wannamaker GT. Spinal cord injuries; a review of the early treatment in 300 consecutive cases during the Korean Conflict. J Neurosurg. 1954; 11(6):517–524

[61]   Splavski B, Vranković D, Sarić G, Blagus G, Mursić B, Rukovanjski M. Early management of war missile spine and spinal cord injuries: experience with 21 cases. Injury. 1996; 27(10):699–702

[62]   Louwes TM, Ward WH, Lee KH, Freedman BA. Combat-related intradural gunshot wound to the thoracic spine: significant improvement and neurologic recovery following bullet removal. Asian Spine J. 2015; 9(1):127–132

[63]   Duz B, Cansever T, Secer HI, Kahraman S, Daneyemez MK, Gonul E. Evaluation of spinal missile injuries with respect to bullet trajectory, surgical indications and timing of surgical intervention: a new guideline. Spine. 2008; 33(20):E746–E753

[64]   Blair JA, Possley DR, Petfield JL, Schoenfeld AJ, Lehman RA, Hsu JR; Skeletal Trauma Research Consortium (STReC). Military penetrating spine injuries compared with blunt. Spine J. 2012; 12(9):762–768

[65]   Thakur RC, Khosla VK, Kak VK. Non-missile penetrating injuries of the spine. Acta Neurochir (Wien). 1991; 113(3–4):144–148

[66]   Robbs JV, Human RR, Rajaruthnam P, Duncan H, Vawda I, Baker LW. Neurological deficit and injuries involving the neck arteries. Br J Surg. 1983; 70(4):220–222

[67]   Demetriades D, Stewart M. Penetrating injuries of the neck. Ann R Coll Surg Engl. 1985; 67(2):71–74

[68]   Reid JD, Weigelt JA. Forty-three cases of vertebral artery trauma. J Trauma. 1988; 28(7):1007–1012

[69]   Richardson A, Soo M, Fletcher JP. Percutaneous transluminal embolization of vertebral artery injury. Aust N Z J Surg. 1984; 54(4):361–363

[70]   Ben-Menachem Y, Fields WS, Cadavid G, Gomez LS, Anderson EC, Fisher RG. Vertebral artery trauma: transcatheter embolization. AJNR Am J Neuroradiol. 1987; 8(3):501–507

[71]   Demetriades D, Theodorou D, Asensio J, et al. Management options in vertebral artery injuries. Br J Surg. 1996; 83(1):83–86

[72]   Hung CL, Wu YJ, Lin CS, Hou CJ. Sequential endovascular coil embolization for a traumatic cervical vertebral AV fistula. Catheter Cardiovasc Interv. 2003; 60(2):267–269

[73]   Greer LT, Kuehn RB, Gillespie DL, et al. Contemporary management of combat-related vertebral artery injuries. J Trauma Acute Care Surg. 2013; 74(3):818–824

[74]   Albuquerque FC, Javedan SP, McDougall CG. Endovascular management of penetrating vertebral artery injuries. J Trauma. 2002; 53(3):574–580

[75]   Jeffery P, Immelman E, Beningfield S. A review of the management of vertebral artery injury. Eur J Vasc Endovasc Surg. 1995; 10(4):391–393

27 Spinal Cord Compression Secondary to Neoplastic Disease: Epidural Metastasis and Pathologic Fracture

James A. Smith, Roy A. Patchell, and Phillip A. Tibbs

Abstract

Spinal cord compression from metastatic disease frequently presents as a medical emergency with neurologic compromise. Historically, prior to accurate radiographic imaging and advances in neurosurgical technique, radiotherapy and corticosteroids were the mainstay treatment for patients with spinal metastases and cord compression. Now, newer studies show that radical surgery plus conformal radiation is the superior modality and primary treatment of choice. With the development of stereotactic radiosurgery, local tumor control may also be achieved by delivering high-dose radiation using image guidance in selected patients. Onset of neurologic deficits requires emergent treatment for the best chance in preservation and recovery of neurologic function. Given the advances in technique, neurosurgeons will be consulted frequently and earlier in the management of patients with spinal cord compression from metastatic disease, and they must be knowledgeable about decompressive and surgical reconstruction techniques and role of stereotactic radiosurgery in these patients.

Keywords: cervical, spine, corticosteroids, decompressive laminectomy, Denny–Brown motor examination, metastatic epidural spinal cord compression (MESCC), pathologic fracture, radiotherapy, stereotactic radiosurgery, thoracic spine

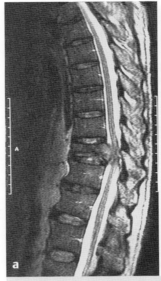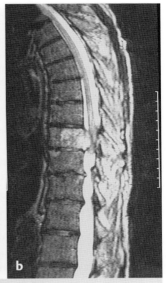

Fig. 27.1 **(a)** Midthoracic vertebral metastasis with pathologic fracture of bone compressing spinal cord. **(b)** Upper thoracic vertebral metastasis with collapse of the vertebral body and large epidural tumor mass anterior to the cord.

27.1 Introduction

Spinal cord compression frequently presents as a medical emergency with rapidly progressive loss of neurologic control of the extremities, bladder, and bowel (▶Fig. 27.1a, b).[1] The patient may or may not have a known diagnosis of cancer. In many cases, the onset of paraparesis or quadriparesis from cord compression may be the first evidence of occult malignancy.[2] Pain is the universal harbinger of cord compression and, all too often, patients are managed with escalating doses of narcotic analgesics to treat a pain of unknown origin until the expanding tumor causes devastating neurologic consequences. It has been reported that in cancer patients with acute onset of back pain, rates of spinal metastasis may exceed 25%.[3,4]

For many years, radiotherapy and corticosteroids were the standard of care for patients with spinal metastases and cord compression.[5] This was an era prior to accurate radiographic imaging of the spine and prior to advances in neurosurgical technique allowing direct decompression and reconstruction of the affected vertebral segments and before the advent of stereotactic radiosurgery. Newer studies, including an extensive meta-analysis of the literature and the first reported prospective randomized trial of radical surgery plus conformal external beam radiotherapy versus conformal external beam radiotherapy alone, have convincingly demonstrated that surgical therapy is the superior modality and the primary treatment of choice in selected patients with metastatic epidural spinal cord compressions (MESCCs).[3,6,7] With the development of stereotactic radiosurgery, and its proven superior results in local tumor control versus conformal external beam radiation, it is now possible to deliver high-dose radiation using image guidance to safely decompress the spinal cord in select patients.[3,8] Neurosurgeons therefore will be consulted more frequently and earlier in the course of management of these patients and must be prepared to advise regarding operability and case selection as well as be knowledgeable about decompressive and surgical reconstruction techniques and the role of stereotactic radiation in this group of patients. Acute onset of neurologic deficit requires immediate treatment if optimal clinical outcome with preservation and recovery of neurologic functions is to be achieved.[1]

27.2 Epidemiology

MESCC is a frequent complication of cancer, occurring in 5 to 14% of cancer patients and causing over 20,000 cases of cord compression per year in the United States.[5] When cancer spreads, the spine is its most common target, and up to 40% of cancer patients develop this complication of systemic malignancy, causing debilitating pain even in the absence of paralysis.[9] As life expectancies are lengthened because of improvements in cancer care, it is likely that an increasing number of patients will survive long enough to develop MESCC.

The osseous vertebral column is affected in 85% of cases, paravertebral sites in 10 to 15%, and there are rare cases of isolated epidural or intramedullary metastasis.[10] ▶ Fig. 27.2 depicts the most common locations of spinal metastases. Approximately 75% of spinal metastases occur in the thoracic spine, 20% in the lumbar spine, and 10% in the cervical spine.[11] In the 20 to 40% of patients with spinal metastases, multiple noncontiguous sites of involvement can be found.[10]

Breast, lung, and prostate cancers account for about half of spinal metastases.[5] The remaining 50% include (in decreasing order of frequency) renal cell carcinoma, gastrointestinal (GI) malignancy, thyroid cancer, lymphoma, and multiple myeloma. Some primary tumor types have a very high incidence of spinal metastasis in the course of the disease, including prostate cancer at 90%, breast cancer at 75%, melanoma at 55%, and lung cancer at 45%.[12]

27.3 Evolution of the Standard of Care for Metastatic Epidural Spinal Cord Compression

Well into the 1990s, an extensive body of medical literature has supported the notion that the combination of radiotherapy and corticosteroids (RT+CS) is the initial treatment of choice for MESCC.[13,14] Numerous articles showed no benefit of surgery for cord decompression over external beam radiotherapy and steroid administration.[11,14,15] In this literature, "surgery"

essentially equaled laminectomy. Laminectomy does not allow direct access and decompression for the majority of cases of MESCC where the metastatic deposit is anterior to the cord. Laminectomy not only does not provide adequate surgical exposure to allow reconstruction of the damaged vertebra, it also may destabilize the spine, resecting the only intact column of stability.[11,14,16]

This treatment standard of RT+CS kept only about 50% of patients ambulatory, and few nonambulatory patients ever regained functional independence.[11,14] These reports were retrospective analyses in an era where the quality of radiographic imaging was limited and surgery consisted mostly of decompressive laminectomy. Often the extent of systemic disease and spinal involvement was poorly understood, there was little thought given to the biomechanics of spinal stability, and the revolution of instrumentation for spinal reconstruction was embryonic.

Because of this discouraging literature, there has been a natural reluctance to consider surgery as an option. Neurosurgeons were most commonly consulted when neurologic deficit progressed despite radiotherapy, when delayed recurrence developed in a spinal region that had received prior maximum radiation dosage, or when the destruction of the vertebral body had progressed to the point of pathologic fracture with obvious instability. In this clinical setting, where surgery is relegated to a salvage role in late-stage cases, high morbidity and poor outcome are expected. A heavily radiated surgical field in a patient on high-dose steroids is a prescription for surgical complications, including wound infection, wound dehiscence, failure of instrumented stabilization, and nonunion.

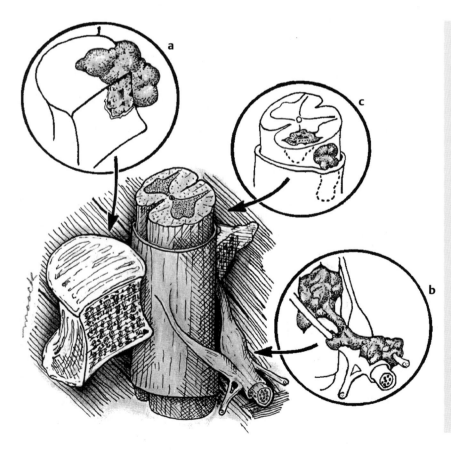

Fig. 27.2 (a) Locations of metastases to the spine. Most tumor emboli seed the vertebral column surrounding the spinal cord, with the posterior half of the vertebral body being the most common initial focus. **(b)** Tumor can also originate in a paravertebral location and track along the spinal nerves to enter the spinal column by way of the neural foramina. Both of these mechanisms can lead to epidural spinal cord compression. **(c)** Intramedullary, subdural/leptomeningeal, and isolated epidural metastatic deposits are rarely encountered. (Reproduced with permission from Klimo P Jr, Schmidt MH. Surgical management of spinal metastases. Oncologist 2004;9:188–196.)

Beginning in the 1980s, with improved cancer staging and spinal imaging by computed tomography (CT) and ultimately magnetic resonance imaging (MRI), the possibility of direct attack on the metastatic tumor was explored by several surgeons.[17,18] The fact that in the majority of cases of MESCC the epicenter of the tumor is anterior to the spinal cord necessitated development of surgical teams that include a thoracic or general surgeon to provide anterior access and a neurosurgeon to perform decompression and stabilization. Complex instrumentation systems that were initially conceived to treat scoliosis, vertebral fracture, and degenerative spinal conditions were adapted and improved to allow reduction of cancer-related pathologic fracture and correction of spinal instability (▶ Fig. 27.3a, b).[19,20]

Starting in the early 1990s, there has been development of new technologies, including the ability to deliver targeted radiation to a specific area in the body, defined by the physician, based on imaging studies.[3] With the advancement in this field, direct attack on single or multiple spinal metastatic tumors now not only can be achieved with traditional surgery; it can also be achieved with stereotactic radiosurgery. This has been further studied by several surgeons and radiation oncologists and with the progress in spinal imaging (CT and MRI) and advances in image-guided delivery of focal high-dose radiation, stereotactic radiosurgery has the potential to change the way spine metastasis and spinal cord compression is managed.[8]

Changing the standard of care for such a complex clinical problem requires more than anecdotal or retrospective reports. Oncologists, radiotherapists, patients, and surgeons themselves have needed objective data to properly direct therapy toward surgery, RT+CS, and/or stereotactic radiosurgery on the basis of rigorous analysis of the literature and methodologically sound trials.

Klimo et al published a detailed meta-analysis of 1,542 patients who had undergone radiation or surgery plus radiation for MESCC.[6] Patients treated with surgery plus RT+CS achieved an 85% rate of ambulation (recovery from paraparesis or preservation of ambulation) versus 64% for the patients receiving conventional external beam radiotherapy alone. Citing the work done by Patchell et al as the first randomized clinical trial to be presented on this subject, they concluded that the option of surgery should be considered as the primary modality in patients with MESCC with conventional radiation postoperatively as adjuvant therapy.5 By providing much shorter fractionation, less side effects, and potentially greater chances of disease control as well as less damage to the spinal cord itself, stereotactic radiotherapy also may provide superior results than conventional RT + CS alone as well. In 2014, a systematic literature review by McCaighy et al, no randomized clinical trials or meta-analyses were identified; therefore, until such a study is done; stereotactic radiosurgery is usually reserved for patients who are inoperable or those who are not found to be good candidates for conventional radiation.[21]

The authors have completed a multi-institutional, National Institutes of Health (NIH)–funded, prospective, randomized trial of direct decompressive surgical resection of epidural metastasis followed by radiotherapy versus radiotherapy alone.5 Their study demonstrates that the combination of surgery plus radiation is superior to radiation alone in preserving intact neurologic function, recovering lost ambulatory capacity, preservation

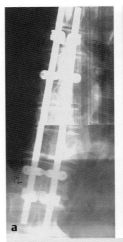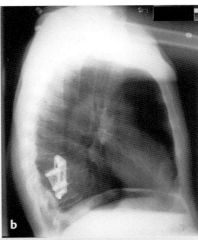

Fig. 27.3 **(a)** Midthoracic epidural metastasis localized to the lamina, pedicle, and dorsal cord after decompressive laminectomy, stabilization by a compression rod construct to reconstitute the dorsal tension band. **(b)** Thoracic corpectomy for metastasis reconstructed with a titanium cage and transvertebral screw and plate fixation.

of bladder and bowel function, maintaining quality of life, and improving pain control.[7] Furthermore, patients initially randomized to radiotherapy who failed treatment and crossed over to surgery had poorer outcomes and more complications than patients receiving surgery as a primary therapy; however, their outcomes were still superior to radiotherapy alone. This emphasizes that surgery should be the first treatment in appropriate patients and not used as a salvage procedure.

27.4 Clinical Evaluation

Comprehensive clinical evaluation includes the recording of a thorough and accurate history, an understanding of risk factors particular to each individual patient, a careful neurologic and musculoskeletal examination, and review of definitive radiographic imaging. The neurologic examination should include a segmental motor examination of the extremities using the Denny–Brown system, evaluation of deep tendon reflexes looking for hyperreflexia or pathologic reflexes indicating upper motor neuron involvement, and careful sensory examination to define a discrete sensory level. Assessment of bladder and bowel function can be made through history and a rectal examination.

Radiographic evaluation includes enhanced total spinal MRI to determine whether more than one area of vertebral involvement may be responsible for neurologic deficit.[22] Likewise, imaging the brain is usually worthwhile because a negative study is reassuring, whereas a study positive for brain metastasis may not only explain some of the patient's neurologic deficit but also impact upon the decision to operate given that the intracranial lesion will limit life expectancy. Anteroposterior (AP) and lateral spine radiographs reveal spinal deformity due to pathologic fracture and high-resolution CT of the spine with sagittal reconstruction often reveals details of bony destruction surpassing MRI and assisting with the decision to surgically stabilize a severely weakened vertebral segment.

27.5 Patient Selection for Surgery

Although there is increasing evidence that the advanced surgical techniques available today are superior to RT+CS in many cases, not all patients with MESCC are candidates for surgery. It is the responsibility of the consulting neurosurgeon to make a recommendation for surgery based upon sound clinical criteria deriving from the current literature and surgical experience.

Key factors in determining whether an individual will potentially benefit from surgery include the following:

- Operability—Is the metastatic lesion accessible within a reasonable degree of safety?[20,23] This depends not only on the site of the lesion but the availability of a thoracic or general surgeon to provide access and the experience of the neurosurgeon. In some patients, an anterior approach, although technically ideal to achieve optimal decompression and stabilization, may be impossible because of the severe pulmonary disease or other factors, and an alternative such as a dorsolateral approach may be necessary.[24] In patients in whom surgery is not an option secondary to medical comorbidities or surgically inaccessible areas, stereotactic radiotherapy may be an option.
- Radiosensitivity of the lesion—In general, tissue diagnoses exquisitely sensitive to radiotherapy need not have surgery. The exception to this rule is when the metastatic disease has progressed to pathologic fracture or such fracture appears imminent when the disease involves two or three of the structural columns of the vertebra.[23] In some cases where tissue diagnosis is unknown in a patient presenting with apparent MESCC and neurologic deficit, we have performed CT-guided needle biopsy of the spinal lesion or fine-needle aspirate biopsy of an easily accessible mass (e.g., breast lesions or lung mass) to guide this decision-making process. Radioresistant tumors such as renal cell carcinoma, sarcoma, primary colon cancer, and certain lung carcinomas are more likely candidates for surgical treatment when alternative modalities have little to offer.[25]
- Life expectancy—In general, we have not considered or encouraged surgery when life expectancy is predicted by the attending oncologist to be less than 3 months. In such cases, stereotactic radiotherapy may be an option to provide safer palliative relief of pain and symptoms to selected patients.
- Duration of neurologic deficit—Patients who have total and complete cord deficit for 24 hours or more have little hope of benefiting from surgery.

27.6 Preoperative Care

On confirming the diagnosis of spinal cord compression due to metastatic tumor, the patient is given a loading dose of dexamethasone followed by a maintenance regimen. In the study by Gerszten and Welch, 100 mg dose of dexamethasone was initially administered followed by 24 mg every 6 hours.[7] These large doses were selected because they appear to be the highest dose known to have therapeutic benefit. Diabetic patients and patients with a history of sensitivity to or adverse affect from high-dose steroids should be given lesser dosages.

Appropriate antibiotic prophylaxis is essential. In general, intravenous administration of a cephalosporin covers Staphylococcus and most other organisms that complicate clean surgical cases.[26] If the patient in question has been septic or has known urinary tract infection or other organ system infection, coverage should be extended to cover any identified bacterial organism particularly if instrumentation systems are to be implanted.

Preoperative laboratory work-up must include coagulation studies and complete blood count. Patients with systemic malignancy are often anemic and should be transfused to a hematocrit of greater than 30 prior to beginning a major neurosurgical procedure, and type- and cross-matched blood must be immediately available because some metastatic tumors such as renal cell carcinoma and melanoma are notoriously vascular. Likewise, cancer patients, especially patients with lymphoreticular malignancy, may require platelet transfusions or fresh frozen plasma administration before it is safe to proceed with surgery.

27.7 Surgical Management

If surgery is the appropriate therapy for a patient with MESCC, time is of the essence. Neurologic function may deteriorate rapidly by progressive tumor expansion and suddenly by either pathologic collapse of the vertebra or vascular compromise to the cord (▶ Fig. 27.4). Moreover, if the paresis progresses to plegia and the total deficit persists for more than 24 hours, the prognosis is dismal for neurologic recovery even with excellent surgical intervention. It is clear therefore that intervention should be expedited and handled as an emergency.[13] The decision on timing is tempered by the fact that preoperative preparations must be completed. The team of access surgeon and neurosurgeon must be assembled, and necessary operating room staff and instrumentation systems must be available for the case to begin.

The goals of surgical therapy for MESCC are circumferential decompression of the spinal cord by direct attack on the lesion plus definitive reconstruction and stabilization of the spine (▶ Fig. 27.5a, b). These goals may not be achievable in a single operation. Staged procedures or combined anterior and posterior approaches may be required.[2] The specific surgical technique chosen is dependent on two critical factors:

1. Location of the lesion.
2. Assessment of biomechanical stability.

In the authors' study, 60% of metastatic lesions were located anterior to the spinal cord, 20% were lateral, and 20% were posterior.[5] The authors recommend a direct approach to the tumor (▶ Fig. 27.6). Metastatic lesions entirely within the vertebral body with extension into the anterior epidural space with or without pathologic fracture are optimally treated through an anterolateral transthoracic or retroperitoneal approach (▶ Fig. 27.2). The decision to utilize such approaches must take into consideration the presence of mediastinal, pulmonary, or retroperitoneal disease and the capacity of the patient to tolerate pneumothorax, ileus, and so forth.[2,23] That being said, the authors had lower 30-day operative mortality in 32 patients who underwent anterior approaches (6%) than in the 28 patients undergoing radiation therapy for anterior

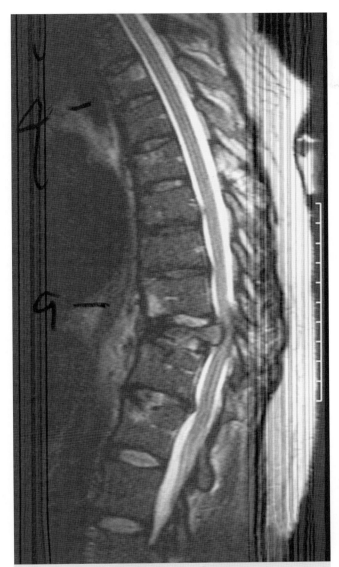

Fig. 27.4 Thoracic vertebral metastasis with pathologic fracture, anterior cord compression, and kyphotic angulation.

disease (14%).[7] These patients also did not have a longer length of stay than patients managed with RT+ CS. Although patients undergoing transthoracic and retroperitoneal approaches required more narcotic pain medication in the immediate postoperative period, in the long term they required considerably less opiates because of improved tumor control and spinal stability.

The surgical "no man's land" from T2 to T6 provides a particular surgical challenge for anterior metastatic lesions. In rare cases, the cardiothoracic surgeons have performed sternotomy to provide very satisfactory access. In cases where the cancer is lateralized, for the most part, a very satisfactory resection can be achieved by a dorsolateral approach that may or may not require rib resection.[24]

In the cervical spine, the results of cervical corpectomy and reconstruction for cervical cord compression from MESCC are particularly gratifying.[27] The approach is very familiar to most neurosurgeons and is very well tolerated by patients. Aggressive tumor resection and reconstruction in this spinal region can yield superb long-term results (▶Fig. 27.7). It must be emphasized, however, that if malignancy extends into the pedicle and facet joint, a supplementary posterior decompression and stabilization may be needed using lateral mass instrumentation.[2]

Laminectomy, although inappropriate as a universal approach to metastatic disease of the spine, remains a well-tolerated option when the tumor bulk derives from the lamina or facet, where the tumor occupies the dorsal or dorsolateral epidural space, and in cases where shifting of the cord from one side to the other by a laterally placed mass allows an access plane into the lateral aspect of the vertebral body (▶Fig. 27.8).[15]

In all cases, the neurosurgeon must make an assessment as to whether decompression alone is sufficient to deal with an individual patient's circumstances or whether the decompression must be supplemented with devices to replace a resected vertebral body or increase loading capacity through screw and rod systems either anteriorly or posteriorly.[10,28] Selected patients with MESCC may be able to be managed with less invasive techniques such as vertebroplasty, minimally invasive surgery, and focal stereotactic radiosurgery.[8,29,30] The latter three approaches are a rapidly expanding and exciting direction that will, hopefully, allow the benefits of less invasive methods of treatment to be offered to a larger group of patients and reduce surgical morbidity.

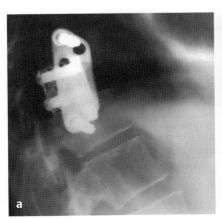
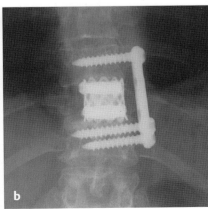

Fig. 27.5 (a) Lateral view of thoracic metastasis reconstructed by anterolateral approach with corpectomy and insertion of titanium cage with screw and plate system. **(b)** Anteroposterior view.

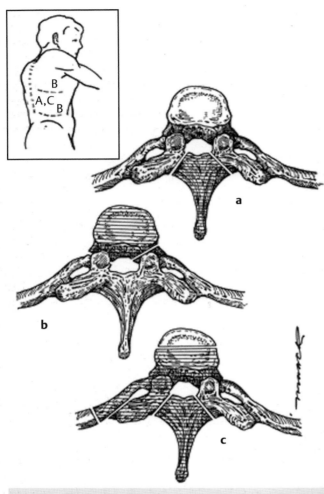

Fig. 27.6 Surgical approaches to the spine. The shaded areas indicate the bone removed in each of the approaches. **(a)** Laminectomy. The spinous process and the adjacent lamina are removed up to the junction of the pedicles. This was the standard surgical procedure for many years regardless of where the tumor was actually located within the vertebra. It can still be used for disease isolated to the posterior elements. **(b)** Transthoracic or retroperitoneal. These anterior approaches provide direct access to the vertebral body in the thoracic (transthoracic) and thoracolumbar/lumbar regions (retroperitoneal). **(c)** Posterolateral. For patients who cannot tolerate an anterior approach or have significant posterior extension of their disease, a posterolateral approach provides excellent access to both the anterior and posterior elements. Inset. Skin incisions for each of the approaches. The laminectomy and posterolateral approaches can be taken through a midline incision. The transthoracic (upper B line) and retroperitoneal (lower B line) approaches require flank incisions. (Reproduced with permission from Klimo P Jr, Schmidt MH. Surgical management of spinal metastases. Oncologist 2004;9:188–196.)

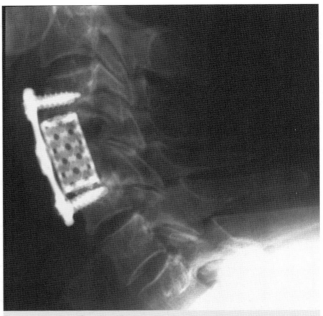

Fig. 27.7 Metastatic renal cell carcinoma to C4 vertebral body with cord compression and pathologic fracture treated by complete corpectomy, insertion of interbody titanium cage, and plating C3 to C5.

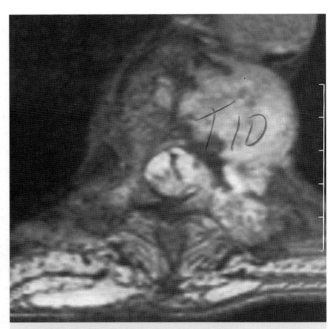

Fig. 27.8 Metastatic breast tumor involving left hemivertebra and shifting the cord from left to right. A dorsolateral approach is possible through the tumor bed.

27.8 Complications of Surgery

The list of potential complications from major spinal neurosurgery in cancer patients can be very intimidating, especially when considering the large transthoracic and retroperitoneal procedures.[28] The superior degree of preservation and recovery of neurologic function, however, eclipses these risks.[20] In the authors' series of 101 patients with MESCC, the 30-day mortality in the surgery patients was 6%, and for the RT+CS patients, 30-day mortality was 14%.5

One of the most common postoperative complications is wound infection. Contributing factors include need for high-dose steroids and complex and lengthy surgery. Malnutrition, obesity, and incontinence are additional risk factors.[26,29] We recommend antibiotic coverage, as noted in Preoperative Care. It has also been found that dexamethasone dosage could be more rapidly weaned in the surgical patients because they had good cord decompression.[7] In patients with long upper thoracic posterior incisions, it was found that placing heavy retention sutures through large buttons at several levels along the incision reduced the incidence of wound dehiscence. This trick, learned from abdominal surgery colleagues, is good to remember because patients with normal upper extremities but upper thoracic paraparesis can place tremendous stress on their wound closures as they attempt to transfer themselves.

Gokaslan et al have shown that transthoracic vertebrectomy and reconstruction can be accomplished with an acceptable rate of morbidity and mortality.[20] They described a variety of complications, including atelectasis, wound infection, and pulmonary embolism in 21 of 72 patients, with a 3% 30-day mortality rate. This excellent result emphasizes the importance of an experienced surgeon in these major reconstruction cases.

Hardware failure with loss of stability occurs in a small number of cases and is best treated by reoperation to reinsert the instrumentation plus consideration of supplementary stabilization, usually from a posterior approach.

27.9 Role of Stereotactic Radiotherapy

Because stereotactic radiotherapy is relatively new, there have been few to no published treatment algorithms that take into account spinal stereotactic radiotherapy. Ryu et al has suggested that the goal of spine stereotactic radiotherapy is for preservation and improvement of neurologic status, much different than what's in practice today.31 It has been suggested that radiosurgery is comparable to surgery in neurologic outcomes in patients who are neurologically intact, ambulatory, or with minor deficit.[8] Safety in stereotactic spinal radiotherapy has also been established as demonstrated in a case-series review by Hall et al.32 A pool of almost 1,400 patients showed a local tumor control rate of 90%, pain reduction of 79%, and an incidence of myelopathy of less than 0.5%.[3] Spinal stereotactic radiosurgery is a safe and effective modality that should be considered when deciding treatment options for patients with spinal epidural metastasis. The surgeon should make clear to the patient and radiotherapist that rapidly progressive neurologic deterioration despite targeted radiotherapy is an indication for emergency salvage surgical decompression or stabilization. Further review and randomized trials are helpful to change clinical practice; however, the results from these two studies show a promising future for the change in clinical practice for the management of spine metastasis and cord compression.

27.10 Conclusion

Advances in spinal imaging and surgical techniques have progressed to the point that surgical decompression of the spinal cord and stabilization of the vertebral column constitute the treatment of choice in patients with MESCC whose lesions are operable, whose general condition will tolerate major surgery, and whose life expectancy is at least 3 months. A neurosurgeon should be consulted to determine if the patient's lesion is amenable and appropriate for surgery. When pathologic fracture with instability is the major cause of cord compression, traditional radiotherapy or stereotactic radiotherapy is not sufficient to achieve restoration of mechanical instability. If stereotactic radiosurgery is elected, careful monitoring of the patient's neurologic condition is mandatory, with a backup plan to intervene surgically if deterioration occurs. If surgery is indicated, the patient should have careful preoperative preparation, and the completion of the surgery should be expedited. In these appropriate patients, surgery should be the primary therapy, followed by adjuvant radiotherapy (conventional or stereotactic). Surgery is less effective as a salvage treatment after failed radiotherapy. A direct approach to the tumor with a goal of circumferential cord decompression and stabilization of the vertebral column is advised. The patient's outcome is best served by a treatment plan coordinated by the patient's oncologist and neurosurgeon. Optimizing neurologic function is a critical goal of modern cancer care for patients with MESCC.

References

[1] Klimo P, Jr, Schmidt MH. Surgical management of spinal metastases. Oncologist. 2004; 9(2):188–196

[2] Sundaresan N, Steinberger AA, Moore F, et al. Indications and results of combined anterior-posterior approaches for spine tumor surgery. J Neurosurg. 1996; 85(3):438–446

[3] Byrne TN. Spinal cord compression from epidural metastases. N Engl J Med. 1992; 327(9):614–619

[4] Klimo P, Jr, Thompson CJ, Kestle JRW, Schmidt MH. A meta-analysis of surgery versus conventional radiotherapy for the treatment of metastatic spinal epidural disease. Neuro-oncol. 2005; 7(1):64–76

[5] Patchell RA, Tibbs PA, Regine WF, et al. Direct decompressive surgical resection in the treatment of spinal cord compression caused by metastatic cancer: a randomised trial. Lancet. 2005; 366(9486):643–648

[6] Böhm P, Huber J. The surgical treatment of bony metastases of the spine and limbs. J Bone Joint Surg Br. 2002; 84(4):521–529

[7] Gerszten PC, Welch WC. Current surgical management of metastatic spinal disease. Oncology (Williston Park). 2000; 14(7):1013–1024, discussion 1024, 1029–1030

[8] Gilbert RW, Kim JH, Posner JB. Epidural spinal cord compression from metastatic tumor: diagnosis and treatment. Ann Neurol. 1978; 3(1):40–51

[9] Wong DA, Fornasier VL, MacNab I. Spinal metastases: the obvious, the occult, and the impostors. Spine. 1990; 15(1):1–4

[10] Loblaw DA, Laperriere NJ. Emergency treatment of malignant extradural spinal cord compression: an evidence-based guideline. J Clin Oncol. 1998; 16(4):1613–1624

[11] Black P. Spinal metastasis: current status and recommended guidelines for management. Neurosurgery. 1979; 5(6):726–746

[12] Greenberg HS, Kim JH, Posner JB. Epidural spinal cord compression from metastatic tumor: results with a new treatment protocol. Ann Neurol. 1980; 8(4):361–366

[13] Young RF, Post EM, King GA. Treatment of spinal epidural metastases. Randomized prospective comparison of laminectomy and radiotherapy. J Neurosurg. 1980; 53(6):741–748

[14] Siegal T, Siegal T, Robin G, Lubetzki-Korn I, Fuks Z. Anterior decompression of the spine for metastatic epidural cord compression: a promising avenue of therapy? Ann Neurol. 1982; 11(1):28–34

[15] Harrington KD. Anterior cord decompression and spinal stabilization for patients with metastatic lesions of the spine. J Neurosurg. 1984; 61(1):107–117

[16] Cybulski GR. Methods of surgical stabilization for metastatic disease of the spine. Neurosurgery. 1989; 25(2):240–252

[17] Gokaslan ZL, York JE, Walsh GL, et al. Transthoracic vertebrectomy for metastatic spinal tumors. J Neurosurg. 1998; 89(4):599–609

[18] Ghogawala Z, Mansfield FL, Borges LF. Spinal radiation before surgical decompression adversely affects outcomes of surgery for symptomatic metastatic spinal cord compression. Spine. 2001; 26(7):818–824

[19] Cook AM, Lau TN, Tomlinson MJ, Vaidya M, Wakeley CJ, Goddard P. Magnetic resonance imaging of the whole spine in suspected malignant spinal cord compression: impact on management. Clin Oncol (R Coll Radiol). 1998; 10(1):39–43

[20] Cooper PR, Errico TJ, Martin R, Crawford B, DiBartolo T. A systematic approach to spinal reconstruction after anterior decompression for neoplastic disease of the thoracic and lumbar spine. Neurosurgery. 1993; 32(1):1–8

[21] McCaighy S. What type of patients with lesions of the pancreas and spine are suitable candidates for treatment with the CyberKnife robotic radiosurgical system? J Radiotherapy Pract. 2014; 13:106–114

[22] Boriani S, Biagini R, De Iure F, et al. En bloc resections of bone tumors of the thoracolumbar spine. A preliminary report on 29 patients. Spine. 1996; 21(16):1927–1931

[23] McPhee IB, Williams RP, Swanson CE. Factors influencing wound healing after surgery for metastatic disease of the spine. Spine. 1998; 23(6):726–732, discussion 732–733

[24] Adams M, Sonntag VKN. Surgical treatment of metastatic cervical spine disease. Contemp Neurosurg. 2001; 23(5):1–5

[25] Fourney DR, Abi-Said D, Lang FF, McCutcheon IE, Gokaslan ZL. Use of pedicle screw fixation in the management of malignant spinal disease: experience in 100 consecutive procedures. J Neurosurg. 2001; 94(1, Suppl):25–37

[26] Fourney DR, Schomer DF, Nader R, et al. Percutaneous vertebroplasty and kyphoplasty for painful vertebral body fractures in cancer patients. J Neurosurg. 2003; 98(1, Suppl):21–30

[27] McLain RF. Spinal cord decompression: an endoscopically assisted approach for metastatic tumors. Spinal Cord. 2001; 39(9):482–487

[28] Wise JJ, Fischgrund JS, Herkowitz HN, Montgomery D, Kurz LT. Complication, survival rates, and risk factors of surgery for metastatic disease of the spine. Spine. 1999; 24(18):1943–1951

[29] Olsen MA, Mayfield J, Lauryssen C, et al. Risk factors for surgical site infection in spinal surgery. J Neurosurg. 2003; 98(2, Suppl):149–155

[30] McLain RF. Spinal cord decompression: an endoscopically assisted approach for metastatic tumors. Spinal Cord. 2001; 39(9):482–487

[31] Ryu S, Yoon H, Stessin A, Gutman F, et al. Contemporary treatment with radiosurgery for spine metastasis and spinal cord compression in 2015. Radiat Oncol J. 2015; 33(1):1–11

[32] Hall WA, Stapleford LJ, Hadjipanayis CG, Curran WJ, et al. Stereotactic body radiosurgery for spinal metastatic Disease: An evidence-based review. Int J Surg Oncol. 2011; 2011:979214

28 Intraspinal Hemorrhage

Kenneth A. Follett and Linden E. Fornoff

Abstract

Acute spinal cord and cauda equina compression from intraspinal hemorrhage can be neurosurgical emergencies and may lead to profound neurologic deficits even if identified and treated promptly. Hemorrhagic etiologies are numerous and include trauma, iatrogenesis, secondary origins such as underlying tumor, vascular pathology, and anticoagulation, as well idiopathic causes. Spinal hemorrhages can be epidural, subdural, subarachnoid, and/or intramedullary in location. This entity spans all ages and is imperative to consider in the differential diagnosis for symptoms of acute pain and/or neurologic deficit until appropriately ruled out. Prompt surgical intervention is warranted in many or most cases of symptomatic intraspinal hemorrhage.

Keywords: anticoagulation, decompressive laminectomy, neurologic deficit, spinal epidural hemorrhage, spinal intramedullary hemorrhage, spinal subarachnoid hemorrhage, spinal subdural hemorrhage

28.1 Etiology

Intraspinal hemorrhages have a multitude of different causes. As many as 43% are idiopathic with unknown identifiable causes.[1] Secondary causes for intraspinal hemorrhage include trauma, coagulopathies, vascular anomalies, tumor, and iatrogenesis.

28.1.1 Pathogenesis of Idiopathic Spinal Epidural Hematoma

Idiopathic spinal epidural hematoma (SEH) has been studied and reviewed extensively in the literature.[1] Current opinion is that the hemorrhage originates from the valveless venous epidural plexus on the basis of SEH's propensity to form in the posterior spinal canal as a segmented hemorrhagic collection. This plexus permits the transmission of pressure waves that are generated in the systemic circulation (e.g., Valsalva maneuver), leading to plexus rupture and subsequent SEH formation.[1,2] There have been several case reports describing posttussive SEH and also SEH following extended breath-holding during underwater spear-fishing.[3,4]

28.1.2 Pathogenesis of Idiopathic Spinal Subdural and Subarachnoid Hematoma

Spinal subdural hematoma (SSH) of idiopathic origin is postulated to arise secondary to hemorrhage from valveless radiculomedullary veins traversing both the subarachnoid and subdural spaces.[1,5] Rupture secondary to a sudden increase in venous pressure results in subarachnoid hemorrhage that dissects the subdural space to form a SSH with/without spinal subarachnoid hemorrhage.[5,6]

28.1.3 Secondary Causes of Intraspinal Hemorrhage

Secondary hemorrhages are most often related to the use of anticoagulation medications, including thrombolytics.[7,8,9,10] As many as 30% of intraspinal hemorrhages are attributed to anticoagulant administration.[1] Disease processes such as hemophilia, blood dyscrasias, and vasculitidies, including systemic lupus erythematosus (SLE), may also cause coagulopathy and may be associated with intraspinal hemorrhage.[1,11]

Major spinal column trauma is an unusual cause of hematoma formation that is, by itself, symptomatic.[1,12] Intraspinal hemorrhage associated with trauma may be only a single component of a patient's injuries, may not be responsible for neurologic deficits, and should be evaluated in the context of other injuries. When present, traumatic hematomas are typically epidural and may occur in the absence of other structural abnormalities.[13] Kreppel et al found that trauma-associated hemorrhage accounted for only 1 to 1.7% of intraspinal hemorrhage.[1] Minor trauma such as vigorous massage and prolonged Valsalva have also been implicated in SEH formation.[3,14] There have also been numerous case reports describing minor trauma with subacute presentation of progressive neurologic symptoms attributed to hemorrhage within the ligamentum flavum.[15]

Vascular malformations, the most common being hemangiomas, comprise 9.1% of intraspinal hemorrhages.[1] Other vascular malformations associated with intraspinal hemorrhage include cavernous angiomas,[16] arteriovenous (AV) fistulas, true aneurysms,[17] and pseudoaneurysms.[18]

Pregnancy, parturition, rheumatologic disorders (ankylosing spondylitis, rheumatoid arthritis, neurosarcoidosis, systemic lupus erythematosus),[1,19,20] spinal cord vasculitis,[11] illicit stimulant use,[21] exercise,[22] and coarctation of the aorta[23] have all been described in association with intraspinal hemorrhage. Of note, Groen and Hoogland have found that arterial hypertension is not a cause for intraspinal hemorrhage, but merely coincidental.[24] Bleeding may also occur from intraspinal tumors, including ependymoma, nerve sheath tumor, meningioma, metastatic tumor, astrocytoma, hemangioblastoma, and sarcoma.[1] Several case reports have identified juxtafacet synovial cysts as sources of intraspinal hemorrhage.[25] Vertebral body abnormalities such as Paget's disease may also lead to SEH formation.[1]

Iatrogenic causes include spinal surgery[26] (with a reported incidence of clinically relevant SEH post spinal surgery of up to 1%),[27] ventriculoperitoneal shunting,[28] neuraxial anesthesia,[1] neuraxial radiation therapy,[29] and lumbar puncture (LP).[1] The risk of clinically significant intraspinal hemorrhage following LP is increased if the tap is traumatic, if anticoagulation is started earlier than 1 hour post LP, or if the patient is on antiplatelet therapy.[30]

Medication-induced coagulopathies are an area of increasing concern as irreversible/partially reversible anticoagulants come into greater clinical use. This includes direct factor Xa inhibitors that are being used to replace the vitamin K antagonists and heparin.[8,10] Wide usage of clopidogrel for neurologic and cardiac issues has also been implicated in intraspinal hemorrhage.[7,9] In regards to post–spine surgery pharmacologic deep venous thrombosis (DVT) prophylaxis, starting such medication 24 to 36 hours postoperatively does not increase the risk for SEH.[31]

28.2 Presentation

Intraspinal hematomas occur in individuals of any age, from in utero[32] to the elderly.[1] There appears to be two peaks in age frequency: 15 to 20 years old and 45 to 75 years old.[1] Bleeding is most commonly epidural (75% of intraspinal hemorrhages) and typically localized to the dorsal or dorsolateral portion of the canal.[1] Males are affected more commonly by intraspinal hemorrhage in general (2:1); however, the male:female distribution is equal with respect to spinal subdural hemorrhage.[1] Spinal subarachnoid hemorrhage represents 15.7% of cases, with spinal subdural hemorrhage and intramedullary hemorrhage representing 4.1% and 0.82%, respectively.[1] Children are more likely to experience intraspinal hemorrhage in the cervicothoracic region versus adults (ages 45–75), in whom hemorrhages tend to occur more often in lower thoracic and lumbar regions.[1]

Pain is usually the first symptom of intraspinal hemorrhage, followed by signs and symptoms of neural element compression.[1] Patients may present with subacute or chronic pain symptoms, or even with a remitting/relapsing course.[1] Signs of neurologic dysfunction generally evolve over the span of hours, but progression may be very rapid. Deficits typically include sensory loss with paraparesis or paraplegia, urinary retention, cauda equina syndrome, and priapism.[1] Patients may present with Brown–Séquard,[1] central cord,[33] or anterior cord syndrome.[34] Of note, there are reports of patients' intraspinal hemorrhage presenting like an acute coronary syndrome.[35]

28.3 Evaluation

The differential diagnosis includes a variety of causes of acute spinal cord dysfunction, including disk herniation, spinal fracture (pathologic or traumatic), infection (e.g., epidural abscess), transverse myelitis, infarction, tumor, trauma, and dissecting abdominal aortic aneurysm. The history and physical examination provide a foundation for establishing a diagnosis, but radiographic evaluation is required for definitive diagnosis.

Magnetic resonance imaging (MRI) with susceptibility-weighted imaging is the preferred modality secondary to its noninvasiveness and ability to delineate the spinal cord and vertebral column contents, as well as ability to determine the age of hemorrhage.[1,36] The MRI appearance of hematomas varies with the age of the hematoma. On T1- and T2-weighted images, respectively, blood is iso-/hypointense and hyperintense hyperacutely; iso-/hypointense and hypointense acutely; hyperintense and hypointense early subacutely; hyperintense and hyperintense late subacutely (►Fig. 28.1, ►Fig. 28.2); and iso-/hypointense and hypointense chronically.[37] SSHs are concave relative to the cord, whereas SEHs are convex in relation to the cord on sagittal imaging (►Fig. 28.3, ►Fig. 28.4).[38] Gadolinium may help in identification of structural lesions such as tumors, infections, or slow-flow vascular malformations. The dural sac may enhance because of hyperemia in the subacute stages after a hemorrhage, providing better demarcation between the thecal sac and hematoma.[39] Of note, when viewing the axial T2-weighted images in the lumbar spine, the Mercedes Benz star sign may be evident. It is associated with an intradural as opposed to an extradural hemorrhage. The Mercedes Benz star sign is secondary to blood products both anterior and posterior to the nerve roots, causing them to congregate towards midline.[40]

Myelography was the procedure of choice prior to the advent of MRI. It still remains relevant, especially in conjunction with postmyelogram computed tomography (CT) scanning. This is primarily utilized in patients for whom it is unsafe to perform MRI (e.g., non–MRI-compatible implanted medical devices or metal). Myelography is contraindicated in patients with coagulopathy, however, and necessitates a delay of evaluation while coagulation parameters are checked and possibly corrected. The LP for myelography may be "dry" or technically difficult in the presence of clot.[41]

CT is noninvasive and may be used in patients with coagulopathy and those with contraindications to MRI scanning. It may be especially useful in cases involving spinal column bone pathology by virtue of its sensitivity in detecting bone abnormalities (e.g., fractures and osteolytic or -blastic changes). Its sensitivity in demonstrating hematoma is limited, however. Blood appears hyperdense acutely, whereas subacute and chronic hemorrhages appear isodense (►Fig. 28.5) The sensitivity and specificity of CT scanning are improved with intrathecal contrast (►Fig. 28.6); however, as previously stated, LP is contraindicated in those patients with coagulopathy.

Angiography is not routinely performed in the preoperative setting unless the MRI or other diagnostic information suggests the presence of a vascular malformation.[26] In the acute setting, it may be impractical to take time to obtain a spinal angiogram. If the initial studies (e.g., MRI), history, or physical examination suggests a vascular abnormality as the cause for hemorrhage, then angiography is appropriate. In some instances, emergent decompressive surgery is required and the angiogram must be deferred until the patient has been stabilized.[1]

Coagulation parameters (e.g., prothrombin time with international normalized ratio [INR], partial thromboplastin time, platelet count) should be obtained in each patient to determine the presence of a coagulopathy. Specialized studies may be required to identify a coagulation factor deficiency, and it should be noted whether the patient has been taking aspirin, clopidogrel, nonsteroidal anti-inflammatory medication, or other agents that interfere with platelet function. Newer anticoagulants may not alter the coagulation studies; therefore, care should be taken to obtain a thorough medication history. Complete blood count (CBC), erythrocyte sedimentation rate, and C-reactive protein may indicate infectious or inflammatory causes underlying a hemorrhage.

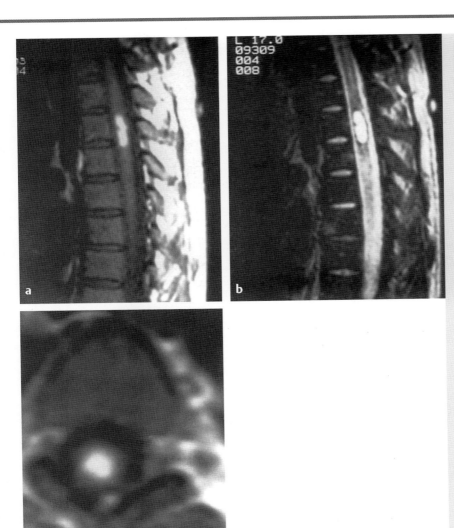

Fig. 28.1 **(a)** T1-weighted sagittal, **(b)** T2-weighted sagittal, and **(c)** T1-weighted axial magnetic resonance images demonstrating a subacute hyperintense intramedullary hematoma.

28.4 Treatment

Prompt surgical evacuation of the hematoma for decompression of the spinal cord and/or cauda equina is the standard treatment for patients presenting acutely with neurologic deficit, especially in those with progressive deterioration. Coagulopathies should be corrected with fresh frozen plasma, vitamin K, protamine sulfate, aminocaproic acid, platelets, or factor infusion. Prothrombin complex concentrate is commonly used to aid in total/partial reversal of anticoagulants in the acute setting where emergent neurosurgical intervention is warranted. Prothrombotic complications are low and justify usage in this setting.[8] Clotting studies should be obtained regularly during the operative and postoperative periods because of the short half-lives of some of the agents used for correction of coagulopathy. It is generally not necessary to maintain 100% normal levels of the missing factor in patients with factor deficiencies. Factor replacement should be continued for several days postoperatively to prevent rebleeding.

The operative procedure typically involves laminectomy for decompression and exploration because hematomas are often located posteriorly/posterolaterally and are accessed easily via laminectomy.[1,42,43] If the clot is tenacious, care must be taken not to limit the exposure such that evacuation is incomplete or underlying pathology missed or inadequately treated. In cases of ventral hemorrhage (extra- or intradural), it may be possible to remove the hematoma with careful irrigation through a small-diameter catheter (e.g., 8 French) and suction. Subarachnoid hemorrhage in the cauda equina may require careful microdissection to mobilize clot adherent to nerve roots.[1] Intramedullary hemorrhages should be removed through a myelotomy, typically overlying the hematoma if it lies very close to the cord surface or via midline myelotomy.[1] Care must be taken to remove as much clot as possible within the realm of patient safety. The surgeon should be prepared to deal with underlying structural abnormalities such as tumor or vascular malformation that may not have been apparent on preoperative studies.

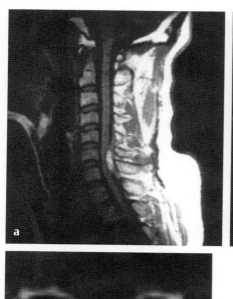
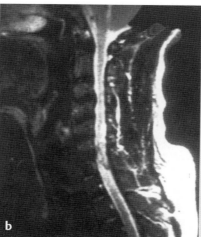
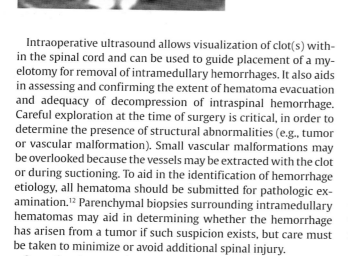

Fig. 28.2 **(a)** T1-weighted sagittal, **(b)** T2-weighted sagittal, and **(c)** T1-weighted axial magnetic resonance images demonstrating a subacute hyperintense posterolateral epidural hematoma with moderate signal inhomogeneity.

Intraoperative ultrasound allows visualization of clot(s) within the spinal cord and can be used to guide placement of a myelotomy for removal of intramedullary hemorrhages. It also aids in assessing and confirming the extent of hematoma evacuation and adequacy of decompression of intraspinal hemorrhage. Careful exploration at the time of surgery is critical, in order to determine the presence of structural abnormalities (e.g., tumor or vascular malformation). Small vascular malformations may be overlooked because the vessels may be extracted with the clot or during suctioning. To aid in the identification of hemorrhage etiology, all hematoma should be submitted for pathologic examination.[12] Parenchymal biopsies surrounding intramedullary hematomas may aid in determining whether the hemorrhage has arisen from a tumor if such suspicion exists, but care must be taken to minimize or avoid additional spinal injury.

Operative intervention provides rapid decompression and aids in establishing a pathologic diagnosis. In some cases (e.g., tumor), proper diagnosis can have a substantial impact on the patient's long-term care. Equally important, operative management can permit definitive treatment of a vascular malformation, preventing rehemorrhage that may have devastating consequences.[16] Histologic examinations of some spinal vascular lesions removed during clot evacuation show evidence of previous hemorrhage.[44]

Patients too medically unstable to tolerate operative intervention may be treated with less invasive techniques. Occasionally, a hematoma can be successfully aspirated with a Tuohy needle or other catheter placed percutaneously into the clot, permitting irrigation through the catheter.[45] These approaches are more likely to be effective in instances of chronic hematoma formation, when the clot is liquefied. There are case reports describing effective management of intraspinal hemorrhage with LP.[46]

Conservative management is advocated for patients demonstrating early improvement in pain and neurologic deficit, or in patients presenting with pain in the absence of neurologic deficit.[47] Conservative care is best suited for improving patients

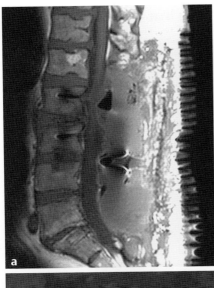
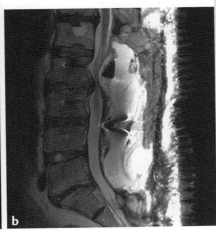
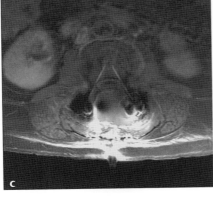

Fig. 28.3 **(a)** T1-weighted sagittal, **(b)** T2-weighted sagittal, and **(c)** T1-weighted postcontrast axial magnetic resonance images demonstrating a large posterior lumbar epidural hematoma that developed 10 days after a fusion procedure. Note the minimal enhancement of the hematoma.

who have suffered a secondary hemorrhage that is not felt to be surgically treatable (e.g., hemorrhage secondary to excessive anticoagulation).[1] Operative intervention should be undertaken in any conservatively treated patient who deteriorates neurologically and as a means of diagnosing and definitively treating an underlying structural abnormality felt to be responsible for the hemorrhage.[1]

28.5 Outcome

Recovery of function is related generally to the severity of preoperative deficit and time to surgery.[1,26,48] In general, if patients with incomplete lesions undergo timely decompression, there is a high likelihood of meaningful recovery.[1] Complete deficit does not preclude functional recovery[26,32]; therefore, patients should undergo operative decompression expeditiously.[1,32] In their meta-analysis, Kreppel et al found that studies where patients were treated within 12 hours of symptom onset had the best rate of recovery.[1] Those patients with subarachnoid hematoma[49] or traumatic hematomyelia[50] are unlikely to recover from severe deficits, however.

Mortality ranges from 3 to 24% in operative series.[19,26] Mortality is highest in patients with complete deficits (23%) compared with patients with incomplete deficits (7% mortality).[51] Death is more likely to occur in conservatively managed patients, who typically have other serious medical disorders that make them poor surgical candidates,[41] and in patients with cervical hemorrhages.[43]

28.6 Conclusion

Intraspinal hemorrhage may be a neurosurgical emergency and should be suspected in any patient with symptoms and signs of spinal cord dysfunction, especially if associated with acute onset of pain and/or the presence of coagulopathies. MRI is the preferred methods of evaluation. Surgical decompression can be readily accomplished and is associated with good recovery of function in many patients, including those with complete sensorimotor dysfunction. Identifiable etiologies for intraspinal hemorrhage should be ruled out meticulously prior to labeling hemorrhage as idiopathic.

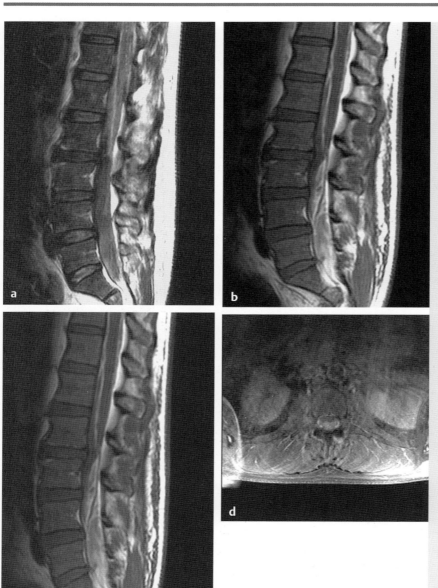

Fig. 28.4 **(a)** T2-weighted sagittal, **(b)** T1-weighted sagittal, **(c)** T1-weighted postcontrast sagittal, and **(d)** T1-weighted axial magnetic resonance images demonstrating a large lumbar subdural hematoma induced during lumbar puncture.

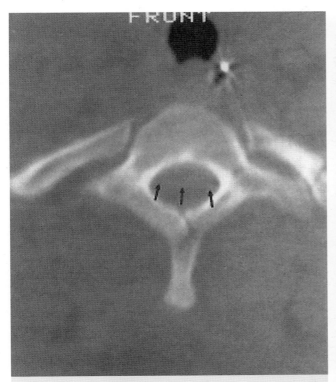

Fig. 28.5 Unenhanced axial computed tomography (CT) scan through the upper thoracic spine reveals a slightly hyperdense mass occupying the ventral half of the canal (posterior aspect delineated by arrows), consistent with acute epidural hematoma. Even when hyperdense, hematomas can be difficult to distinguish from surrounding structures on CT imaging.

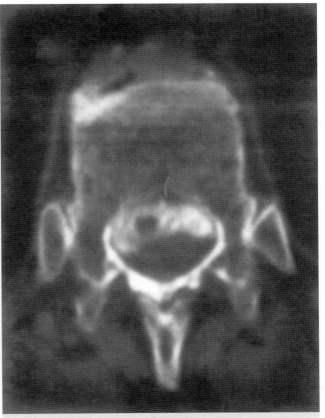

Fig. 28.6 Axial computed tomography imaging following intrathecal administration of metrizamide clearly demonstrates a large dorsal extradural defect at the thoracolumbar junction, consistent with epidural hematoma.

References

[1] Kreppel D, Antoniadis G, Seeling W. Spinal hematoma: a literature survey with meta-analysis of 613 patients. Neurosurg Rev. 2003; 26(1):1–49

[2] Groen RJ, Ponssen H. The spontaneous spinal epidural hematoma. A study of the etiology. J Neurol Sci. 1990; 98(2–3):121–138

[3] Oji Y, Noda K, Tokugawa J, Yamashiro K, Hattori N, Okuma Y. Spontaneous spinal subarachnoid hemorrhage after severe coughing: a case report. J Med Case Reports. 2013; 7:274

[4] Tremolizzo L, Patassini M, Malpieri M, Ferrarese C, Appollonio I. A case of spinal epidural haematoma during breath-hold diving. Diving Hyperb Med. 2012; 42(2):98–100

[5] Haines DE, Harkey HL, al-Mefty O. The "subdural" space: a new look at an outdated concept. Neurosurgery. 1993; 32(1):111–120

[6] Morandi X, Riffaud L, Chabert E, Brassier G. Acute nontraumatic spinal subdural hematomas in three patients. Spine. 2001; 26(23):E547–E551

[7] Bhat KJ, Kapoor S, Watali YZ, Sharma JR. Spontaneous epidural hematoma of spine associated with clopidogrel: a case study and review of the literature. Asian J Neurosurg. 2015; 10(1):54

[8] El Ahmadieh TY, Aoun SG, Daou MR, et al. New-generation oral anticoagulants for the prevention of stroke: implications for neurosurgery. J Clin Neurosci. 2013; 20(10):1350–1356

[9] Moon HJ, Kim JH, Kim JH, Kwon TH, Chung HS, Park YK. Spontaneous spinal epidural hematoma: an urgent complication of adding clopidogrel to aspirin therapy. J Neurol Sci. 2009; 285(1–2):254–256

[10] Zaarour M, Hassan S, Thumallapally N, Dai Q. Rivaroxaban-induced non-traumatic spinal subdural hematoma: an uncommon yet life-threatening complication. Case Rep Hematol. 2015; 2015:275380

[11] Fu M, Omay SB, Morgan J, Kelley B, Abbed K, Bulsara KR. Primary central nervous system vasculitis presenting as spinal subdural hematoma. World Neurosurg. 2012; 78(1–2):E5–E8

[12] Wittebol MC, van Veelen CW. Spontaneous spinal epidural haematoma. Etiological considerations. Clin Neurol Neurosurg. 1984; 86(4):265–270

[13] Cuenca PJ, Tulley EB, Devita D, Stone A. Delayed traumatic spinal epidural hematoma with spontaneous resolution of symptoms. J Emerg Med. 2004; 27(1):37–41

[14] Maste P, Paik SH, Oh JK, et al. Acute spinal subdural hematoma after vigorous back massage: a case report and review of literature. Spine. 2014; 39(25):E1545–E1548

[15] Wild F, Tuettenberg J, Grau A, Weis J, Krauss JK. Ligamentum flavum hematomas of the cervical and thoracic spine. Clin Neurol Neurosurg. 2014; 116:24–27

[16] Badhiwala JH, Farrokhyar F, Alhazzani W, et al. Surgical outcomes and natural history of intramedullary spinal cord cavernous malformations: a single-center series and meta-analysis of individual patient data. J Neurosurg Spine. 2014; 21(4):662–676

[17] Nakagawa I, Park HS, Hironaka Y, Wada T, Kichikawa K, Nakase H. Cervical spinal epidural arteriovenous fistula with coexisting spinal anterior spinal artery aneurysm presenting as subarachnoid hemorrhage—case report. J Stroke Cerebrovasc Dis. 2014; 23(10):e461–e465

[18] Tanweer O, Woldenberg R, Zwany S, Setton A. Endovascular obliteration of a ruptured posterior spinal artery pseudoaneurysm. J Neurosurg Spine. 2012; 17(4):334–336

[19] Penar PL, Fischer DK, Goodrich I, Bloomgarden GM, Robinson F. Spontaneous spinal epidural hematoma. Int Surg. 1987; 72(4):218–221

[20] Pegat B, Drapier S, Morandi X, Edan G. Spinal cord hemorrhage in a patient with neurosarcoidosis on long-term corticosteroid therapy: case report. BMC Neurol. 2015; 15(1):123

[21] Ray WZ, Krisht KM, Schabel A, Schmidt RH. Subarachnoid hemorrhage from a thoracic radicular artery pseudoaneurysm after methamphetamine and synthetic cannabinoid abuse: case report. Global Spine J. 2013; 3(2):119–124

[22] Yang JC, Chang KC. Exercise-induced acute spinal subdural hematoma: a case report. Kaohsiung J Med Sci. 2003; 19(12):624–627

[23] Devara KV, Joseph S, Uppu SC. Spontaneous subarachnoid haemorrhage due to coarctation of aorta and intraspinal collaterals: a rare presentation. Images Paediatr Cardiol. 2012; 14(4):1–3

[24] Groen RJ, Hoogland PV. High blood pressure and the spontaneous spinal epidural hematoma: the misconception about their correlation. Eur J Emerg Med. 2008; 15(2):119–120

[25] Machino M, Yukawa Y, Ito K, Kanbara S, Kato F. Spontaneous hemorrhage in an upper lumbar synovial cyst causing subacute cauda equina syndrome. Orthopedics. 2012; 35(9):e1457–e1460

[26] Lawton MT, Porter RW, Heiserman JE, Jacobowitz R, Sonntag VK, Dickman CA. Surgical management of spinal epidural hematoma: relationship between surgical timing and neurological outcome. J Neurosurg. 1995; 83(1):1–7

[27] Glotzbecker MP, Bono CM, Wood KB, Harris MB. Postoperative spinal epidural hematoma: a systematic review. Spine. 2010; 35(10):E413–E420

[28] Wurm G, Pogady P, Lungenschmid K, Fischer J. Subdural hemorrhage of the cauda equina. A rare complication of cerebrospinal fluid shunt. Case report. Neurosurg Rev. 1996; 19(2):113–117

[29] Agarwal A, Kanekar S, Thamburaj K, Vijay K. Radiation-induced spinal cord hemorrhage (hematomyelia). Neurol Int. 2014; 6(4):5553

[30] Ruff RL, Dougherty JH, Jr. Complications of lumbar puncture followed by anticoagulation. Stroke. 1981; 12(6):879–881

[31] Strom RG, Frempong-Boadu AK. Low-molecular-weight heparin prophylaxis 24 to 36 hours after degenerative spine surgery: risk of hemorrhage and venous thromboembolism. Spine. 2013; 38(23):E1498–E1502

[32] Babayev R, Ekşi MŞ. Spontaneous thoracic epidural hematoma: a case report and literature review. Childs Nerv Syst. 2016; 32(1):181–787

[33] Mavroudakis N, Levivier M, Rodesch G. Central cord syndrome due to a spontaneously regressive spinal subdural hematoma. Neurology. 1990; 40(8):1306–1308

[34] Foo D, Chang YC, Rossier AB. Spontaneous cervical epidural hemorrhage, anterior cord syndrome, and familial vascular malformation: case report. Neurology. 1980; 30(3):308–311

[35] Estaitieh N, Alam S, Sawaya R. Atypical presentations of spontaneous spinal epidural hematomas. Clin Neurol Neurosurg. 2014; 122:135–136

[36] Wang M, Dai Y, Han Y, Haacke EM, Dai J, Shi D. Susceptibility weighted imaging in detecting hemorrhage in acute cervical spinal cord injury. Magn Reson Imaging. 2011; 29(3):365–373

[37] Liebeskind D. Intracranial hemorrhage. EMedicine [serial online]. June 29, 2004. Updated May 2015, accessed December 20, 2015.

[38] Domenicucci M, Ramieri A, Ciappetta P, Delfini R. Nontraumatic acute spinal subdural hematoma: report of five cases and review of the literature. J Neurosurg. 1999; 91(1, Suppl):65–73

[39] Crisi G, Sorgato P, Colombo A, Scarpa M, Falasca A, Angiari P. Gadolinium-DTPA-enhanced MR imaging in the diagnosis of spinal epidural haematoma. Report of a case. Neuroradiology. 1990; 32(1):64–66

[40] Krishnan P, Banerjee TK. Classical imaging findings in spinal subdural hematoma—"Mercedes-Benz" and "Cap" signs. Br J Neurosurg. 2016; ; 30(1):99–100

[41] Russell NA, Benoit BG. Spinal subdural hematoma. A review. Surg Neurol. 1983; 20(2):133–137

[42] Pereira BJA, de Almeida AN, Muio VM, et al. Predictors of outcome in non-traumatic spontaneous acute spinal subdural hematoma: case report and literature review. World Neurosurg. 2016; 89:574–577

[43] Groen RJ, van Alphen HA. Operative treatment of spontaneous spinal epidural hematomas: a study of the factors determining postoperative outcome. Neurosurgery. 1996; 39(3):494–508, discussion 508–509

[44] Müller H, Schramm J, Roggendorf W, Brock M. Vascular malformations as a cause of spontaneous spinal epidural haematoma. Acta Neurochir (Wien). 1982; 62(3–4):297–305

[45] Schwerdtfeger K, Caspar W, Alloussi S, Strowitzki M, Loew F. Acute spinal intradural extramedullary hematoma: a nonsurgical approach for spinal cord decompression. Neurosurgery. 1990; 27(2):312–314

[46] Lee JI, Hong SC, Shin HJ, Eoh W, Byun HS, Kim JH. Traumatic spinal subdural hematoma: rapid resolution after repeated lumbar spinal puncture and drainage. J Trauma. 1996; 40(4):654–655

[47] Groen RJ. Non-operative treatment of spontaneous spinal epidural hematomas: a review of the literature and a comparison with operative cases. Acta Neurochir (Wien). 2004; 146(2):103–110

[48] Dziedzic T, Kunert P, Krych P, Marchel A. Management and neurological outcome of spontaneous spinal epidural hematoma. J Clin Neurosci. 2015; 22(4):726–729

[49] Scott EW, Cazenave CR, Virapongse C. Spinal subarachnoid hematoma complicating lumbar puncture: diagnosis and management. Neurosurgery. 1989; 25(2):287–292, discussion 292–293

[50] Bondurant FJ, Cotler HB, Kulkarni MV, McArdle CB, Harris JH, Jr. Acute spinal cord injury. A study using physical examination and magnetic resonance imaging. Spine. 1990; 15(3):161–168

[51] Foo D, Rossier AB. Preoperative neurological status in predicting surgical outcome of spinal epidural hematomas. Surg Neurol. 1981; 15(5):389–401

29 Emergent Presentation and Management of Spinal Dural Arteriovenous Fistulas and Vascular Lesions

Michael P. Wemhoff, Asterios Tsimpas, and William W. Ashley Jr.

Abstract

Spinal vascular malformations are complex lesions that may not be immediately recognized by their clinical presentation. Although symptoms are usually insidious in onset, they can present acutely with sudden myelopathy, pain, or severe neurologic deficit due to vascular steal or various types of hemorrhage. Prompt radiographic work-up can expedite the diagnosis and pave the way for angiographic characterization and subsequent treatment of these lesions. Both endovascular and surgical management have been used to treat these lesions, with outcomes dependent on the individual characteristics, and thus classification, of the lesions. Prompt recognition and management can improve neurologic outcomes.

Keywords: dural arteriovenous fistulas, spinal cord injury, spinal hemorrhage, vascular malformations

29.1 Introduction

Spinal vascular malformations are rare lesions, but they carry a potential risk for devastating neurologic consequences, both from insidious and acute loss of neurologic function that may be irreversible. Given the complex and varied anatomical basis for spinal vascular malformations, a classification scheme has evolved as more radiographic and angiographic data have been gathered. Originally managed with surgery alone, their endovascular treatment has evolved as well with increasingly durable results.

29.2 Anatomy and Pathophysiology

The radiculomedullary artery supplies the feeder vessel to the dural arteriovenous fistula (dAVF), usually within the nerve root sleeve of the dura.[1] The dAVF is drained by the medullary vein via retrograde flow. This vein anastomoses with the venous plexus, where sluggish flow causes venous congestion. This congestion leads to venous hypertension and the manifestation of symptoms from the mass effect of the dilated venous system on the spinal cord. Venous hypertension may also result in hemorrhage of a vein or venous plexus, which may produce epidural hematoma, subdural hematoma, subarachnoid hemorrhage, or intramedullary hemorrhage depending on the type and location of the involved lesion. Given the slow-flow nature of these lesions, hemorrhage does not occur frequently, but cervical lesions have been reported to hemorrhage more frequently than thoracolumbar lesions. When high flow in the form of a shunt directs arterial blood away to the venous phase, a steal phenomenon may occur, leading to symptoms of spinal cord ischemia and myelomalacia that may manifest clinically as myelopathy.

29.3 Classification Schemes

Spinal vascular malformations are frequently classified on the basis of their anatomy in a scheme developed by Di Chiro.[2] Type I spinal arteriovenous malformation (AVM) refers to a spinal dAVF that has a direct connection between the radicular feeding artery and a dural vein at the nerve root sleeve. Type II spinal AVMs are intramedullary lesions, also known as glomus AVMs. Type III lesions are juvenile AVMs and show intra- or extradural extension, sometimes over more than one spinal level. Type IV AVMs are intradural extramedullary lesions that are fed via the anterior spinal artery (or, rarely, from the posterior spinal artery).

A three-point anatomical classification for spinal dAVFs was proposed by Borden et al.[3] Type I dAVFs drain into Batson's epidural plexus. Type II lesions drain into both the epidural and perimedullary venous plexuses. Type III lesions receive blood supply via branches of the radicular artery and drain into the coronal venous plexus.

In an effort to be more comprehensive, Spetzler et al[4] have subsequently proposed an alternative classification scheme based on the anatomy and pathophysiology of the different lesion types (▶Table 29.1).

Extradural AVFs are uncommon lesions that contain a direct anastomosis between the radicular artery and epidural venous plexus. These are high-flow lesions with engorgement that can cause mass effect on the nerve roots, spinal cord, or both, leading to symptoms corresponding to the compressed structure(s).

Intradural dorsal AVFs constitute the most common class of spinal AVFs. Similar to the Di Chiro type I spinal AVMs, the intradural dorsal AVFs result from a direct connection between a radicular artery and a dural vein. They are typically located in the thoracic spinal cord.

Intradural ventral AVFs involve a direct connection between the anterior spinal artery (ASA) and the coronal venous plexus. These midline lesions exist within the ventral subarachnoid space. The size of these lesions determines their type: type A are small shunts with slow blood flow with a moderate amount of venous hypertension; types B and C are larger, often resulting in a significantly dilated coronal venous plexus. Larger shunts beget more flow through the fistula, thus increasing the phenomenon of vascular steal, clinically resulting in progressive myelopathy.

Extradural–intradural AVMs are analogous to the Di Chiro type III juvenile AVMs and are quite rare. As their name implies, they are typically found in children, although cases are reported in adult patients as well.

Intramedullary AVMs are located within the spinal cord parenchyma and receive arterial input from the ASA and the posterior spinal artery (PSA), and this blood may be supplied via multiple branches. These lesions may be referred to as compact or diffuse depending on the morphology of the nidus. Given the

Table 29.1 Classification of spinal vascular malformations based on the scheme developed by Spetzler et al[4]

Classification	Description
Extradural AVFs	Uncommon, direct anastomosis between radicular artery and epidural venous plexus; high-flow lesions that may cause symptoms from mass effect from engorgement
Intradural dorsal AVFs	Most common, similar to Di Chiro type I spinal AVM, direct anastomosis between a radicular artery and a dural vein; commonly in thoracic spinal cord
Intradural ventral AVFs	Midline lesions with direct anastomosis between ASA and coronal venous plexus; type A are small, slow-flow lesions; types B and C are larger, higher-flow lesions
Extradural–intradural AVMs	Rare lesions, analogous to Di Chiro type III juvenile AVMs
Intramedullary AVMs	Seated within the spinal cord parenchyma; receive arterial input from the ASA and the PSA; high-pressure, high-flow lesions associated with aneurysm formation; analogous to Di Chiro type II lesions
Conus medullaris AVMs	Complex nidus with multiple shunts from ASA, PSA, and radicular arteries

Abbreviations: ASA, anterior spinal artery; AVF, arteriovenous fistula; AVM, arteriovenous malformation; PSA, posterior spinal artery.

presence of multiple feeding vessels, these lesions have high pressure and high flow, making their association with aneurysm formation more common.

Lastly, conus medullaris AVMs are considered in their own category because they exhibit "complex nidal angioarchitecture" resulting from multiple shunts from the ASA, PSA, and radicular arteries, and they may drain into both anterior and posterior venous plexuses. Typically, these lesions will contain a pial-based, extramedullary glomus–type nidus. In other cases, the nidus is intramedullary.[5]

29.4 Demographics

The majority of patients with Di Chiro type I dAVFs present between the fifth and eighth decades of life.[6] Very few patients present before the fourth decade of life, and this has been thought to support the suggestion that these lesions may be acquired rather than congenital. There is sex predisposition of these lesions such that 80% of patients with Di Chiro type I dAVFs are male. No family history has been found to correlate with their development. Di Chiro type II and III AVMs, on the other hand, often appear in adult patients before the fifth decade of life and do not share a male predominance.

29.5 Clinical Presentation

Clinical symptoms and presentation vary depending on the type and location of the lesion involved. Classically, the clinical symptom noted first is pain of variable location—often either local or radicular. Subsequently, patients may notice leg weakness leading to a spastic paraparesis along with loss of pain and temperature sensation. A sensory level may correspond to the nidus of the lesion. These symptoms tend to be insidious in onset and slowly progressive, and most patients will present with stepwise neurologic deterioration. Only 10 to 15% of patients have acute onset of symptoms with Di Chiro type I lesions; however, over 50% of patients with Di Chiro type II or III AVMs experience acute onset of symptoms.[7] Because of the low-flow nature of these lesions, hemorrhage is considered unlikely, although the exact incidence is unknown.[8] Case reports have described hemorrhage rates varying from 30 to 68%, although mainly occurring intracranially or in the cervical region. The reported hemorrhage rate of thoracolumbar dAVFs has been described

as only 0.89%, markedly lower than other regions of the spinal cord.[9] On occasion, these vascular lesions may present with subdural or subarachnoid hemorrhage.[10] Lesions located in the cervical spine can present with intracranial subarachnoid hemorrhage either by extension of subarachnoid blood from the spinal to the intracranial level or the rostral transmission of venous hypertension from a valveless coronal plexus to an engorged, stretched perimesencephalic vein that ruptures during physical strain or Valsalva.[11,12,13,14] Intramedullary hemorrhage of dAVFs is remarkably rare, and only two cases have been reported to date.[15,16] Although the flow dynamics of these lesions has yet to be fully characterized, this may be a contributing factor to the likelihood of hemorrhage. Kinouchi et al[17] found that 77.8% of patients with hemorrhage from cervical dAVFs had increase venous flow within the lesion and 55.6% had a venous varix. In the same study, no patients who presented without hemorrhage demonstrated the presence of a venous varix.

One recent study found that 75% of patients with spinal vascular malformations presented with insidious onset of symptoms; 26.4% had evidence of hemorrhage, and this was noted to be more common in AVMs than AVFs. The highest rupture rates were found in intramedullary and extradural AVMs.

In the case of spinal AVM rupture, the patient may present in neurogenic shock that is characterized by acute hypotension and bradycardia due to loss of sympathetic tone and skeletal muscle reflexes with unopposed vagal tone.[18,19] Injuries above the T1 level have the ability to disrupt the spinal cord tracts that direct the entire sympathetic system. Injuries that occur from the level of T1 to T3 may only partially interrupt the sympathetic outflow. With more rostral injuries, patients are more likely to exhibit severe symptoms. Appropriate resuscitation with intravenous fluid boluses and chemical blood pressure augmentation are usually required during the acute phase. Current central nervous system (CNS) guidelines for acute cervical spinal cord injury recommend resuscitation based on the following parameters: correction of hypotension in spinal cord injury (defined as systolic blood pressure less than 90 mm Hg) when possible and as soon as possible; and maintenance of mean arterial blood pressure between 85 and 90 mm Hg for the first 7 days following an acute spinal cord injury.[20]

Neurogenic pulmonary edema (NPE) is a clinical syndrome characterized by acute pulmonary edema occurring shortly after a central neurologic insult.[21] Multiple etiologies have been speculated for the syndrome, including neurocardiac, neurohemodynamic, "blast theory" (which states that the edema is the result of a high-pressure hydrostatic influence and pulmonary endothelial injury), and pulmonary venule adrenergic hypersensitivity. The common denominator in all cases of NPE is likely an endogenous serum catecholamine surge, which can lead to changes in cardiopulmonary hemodynamics. Despite this commonality, the clinical presentation may differ, with some patients presenting predominately with cardiac dysfunction, and others may have capillary leak as the main sign. Treatment is therefore individualized, with implications for cardiac evaluation, fluid management, and choice of inotropic or vasoactive substances such as an α-adrenergic blockade. One case is reported in which a patient with a ruptured cervical spinal AVM presenting with stunned myocardium along with NPE and neurogenic shock.[22]

Sudden onset of symptoms can also be from an acute, necrotizing myelitis referred to as Foix–Alajouanine syndrome, which historically has been thought to be a result of thrombosis within the draining medullary veins.[23] Spinal venous thrombosis, however, is quite rare and not part of any common spinal vascular syndromes. Review and translation of the original paper suggests that the inclusion of thrombosis in the clinical picture of this syndrome is incorrect, and patients included in the original paper may have in fact had progressive myelopathy from Di Chiro type I dAVFs.[24]

The natural history of spinal vascular malformations has been previously described by Aminoff et al,[1] who noted that at 6 months after symptom onset, only 56% of patients had unrestricted activity and 19% were severely disabled. At 36 months after symptom onset, only 9% were without activity restriction and 50% were severely disabled.

29.6 Imaging Studies

Imaging modalities to visualize spinal vascular malformations have evolved over recent decades to include noninvasive techniques. Although digital subtraction angiography remains the gold standard, these newer modalities provide a safe adjunct within the diagnostic algorithm.[25] Computed tomography angiography (CTA) has the advantage of being noninvasive and relatively faster in the acquisition of images than magnetic resonance angiography (MRA), while also possessing capabilities of increased resolution of the vasculature involved. Magnetic resonance imaging (MRI) and MRA remain the preferred modalities for noninvasive evaluation of spinal vascular malformations at this time. This modality can demonstrate spinal cord edema and flow voids from aberrant arterial or venous anatomy such as enlarged coronal venous plexus, arterialized venous plexus, and serpentine pattern of T2 flow voids. MRI also carries the additional advantage of being able to evaluate the spinal cord for signs of neurologic compromise secondary to the lesion. MRA protocols have been developed that allow for a larger field of view and improved acquisition time to enhance the ability to diagnose these lesions.[26]

The gold standard modality of radiographic study of these lesions is selective spinal angiography.[25] This is accomplished via contrast injection into the bilateral radiculomedullary vessels with biplanar angiography. This technique allows the precise location, extension, hemodynamic qualities, and venous drainage to be ascertained. The vast majority of dAVFs are located in the midthoracic to thoracolumbar segments of the spinal cord, typically along the dorsal aspect of the cord. This location is unique to dAVFs of the spinal cord in comparison with AVMs, which may be found anywhere within the spinal cord, with equal distribution. Depending on the clinical suspicion for additional lesions, additional segments must be evaluated to ensure that the entire lesion has been visualized, as well as any accompanying lesions. Furthermore, all possible feeding vessels must be injected (and this is dependent upon the segment of the cord involved).

In spinal dAVFs, selective spinal angiography will typically reveal a radiculomedullary feeding vessel transforming into a group of smaller pathologic vessels at the dural sheath within, or near, the neuroforamen. Within this clustering of vessels exists the AVF itself. After passing through this group of vessels containing the abnormal anastomosis, contrast is then seen to enter a dilated dorsal venous plexus, which will usually extend through multiple spinal segments.[27]

29.7 Management

The goal of management for dAVF is to achieve occlusion or obliteration of the arterialized draining vein at its fistulous connection—namely, the feeding vessel and the proximal efferent intradural arterialized vein.[28] The decision to utilize surgical or endovascular management for the treatment of spinal dAVFs should take into account the angiographic anatomy and feasibility of embolization. Particularly, situations in which the segmental artery that supplies the dAVF also supplies the anterior or posterior spinal artery will not be amenable to endovascular treatment because of the high disk of spinal cord ischemia post embolization. The treatment of Di Chiro type I lesions has been most frequently discussed in the literature, and this management is discussed below. Treatment of other types of dAVF relies on similar principles, but their management is more complex; they require highly individualized treatment, and treatment may be palliative rather than curative.

29.7.1 Endovascular Treatment

Technically, endovascular treatment of spinal dAVFs involves the insertion of a microcatheter in the distal radiculomeningeal artery, close to the fistula between the artery and draining vein, and subsequently injecting the embolic agent of choice.[28] The main hurdles that must be overcome with endovascular treatment include unfavorable vascular anatomy and vascular recanalization. In cases where there is a common origin of the radiculomedullary artery of Adamkiewicz and the radiculomedullary arterial feeder of the spinal dAVF, there is a risk of embolization of the ASA with possible occlusion, leading to stroke. Surgical management is favored in these patients. Other limitations from the vascular anatomy that may inhibit endovascular treatment include the tortuosity or stenosis of the vessels, which may prevent appropriate delivery of embolic material to the lesion. Intradural AVFs composed of pial–medullary arteries communicating directly with pial veins must be recognized, as endovascular treatment may harbor the potential for disastrous thromboembolic complications and require a separate treatment algorithm.

With the advent of use of liquid embolization materials such as N-butyl cyanoacrylate (NBCA) and Onyx, the rate of successful endovascular treatment of these lesions has been reported to be between 70 and 89%.[29] Advanced techniques such as balloon-assisted transarterial embolization of a Di Chiro type I dAVF have also been used and offer additional tools for the treatment of these complex lesions.

Even with the advances and successful initial treatment achieved with endovascular approaches, resilience of these treatments has been variable. Early endovascular treatment strategies using polyvinyl alcohol demonstrated higher rates of vessel recanalization compared with surgical management, but this technique is rarely used today. Still, recurrence rates of endovascular treatment have been reported to be higher than surgically treated patients, even with the advances of treatment with Onyx embolization. The endovascular treatment objective of spinal dAVF is complete closure of the arteriovenous shunt by obliteration of the fistula and the first 1 to 2 cm of draining vein while avoiding any compromise of spinal venous drainage.[28] Indeed, making sure that there is adequate venous penetration has been linked to durable fistula obliteration, whereas those lesions that only receive treatment of arterial pedicles tend to recur. Prerequisite identification of the artery of Adamkiewicz and spinal cord arterial supply should be made prior to embolization.

Even when the decision is made to pursue open surgical management, preoperative embolization has increasingly become favored for both dAVFs and AVMs. Rangel-Castilla et al[30] report a series of 110 patients treated with this multidisciplinary approach; they found complete angiographic obliteration in 83.6% of lesions treated (95.5% for dAVFs and 75.7% for AVMs).

29.7.2 Surgical Management

Historically, dAVFs have been treated surgically with high cure rates. Earlier surgical management focused on resection of the posterior perimedullary veins because of an erroneous understanding of the pathophysiology of these lesions. Current microsurgical approaches call for the disruption of the arterialized vein within the dural sleeve.[31] The draining vein must be exposed from its connection to the fistula and is coagulated and then cut. Disruption of flow at this location is crucial for effective and durable treatment. Previous surgical techniques involving stripping away the dilated venous structures from the dorsal surface of the spinal cord are in fact contraindicated, as this may result in postoperative neurologic deficits. Prior to this approach, preoperative angiography must be correlated with the direct intraoperative findings to identify the correct level of dural penetration of the fistula. A meta-analysis of the surgical management of dAVFs reported a 98% rate of successful obliteration of these lesions, and subsequent studies have confirmed this result.

For surgical management of AVMs,[30] the vascular anatomy may be more difficult to ascertain than with dAVFs, and a thorough inspection of the spinal cord is necessary. This can be assisted intraoperatively with the use of indocyanine green (ICG) angiography. The use of ICG can help to identify arterial pedicle feeders and draining veins, and its subsequent use in later portions of the case can help identify any residual vessels. If preoperative embolization is used, material from this procedure

can also be located intraoperatively to identify feeding vessels. Although myelotomy was previously performed by convention, its recommended role is now limited to intramedullary lesions or evacuation of an intraparenchymal hematoma or syrinx. In the pial resection technique developed by Spetzler,[32] subpial dissection is minimized by identifying feeding arteries and draining veins, coagulating and dividing them along the surface of the spinal cord. Although remaining at the pial surface, the disruption of these vessels devascularizes the lesion sufficiently to alleviate the venous hypertension.

29.8 Conclusion

Spinal vascular malformations may not be in the clinician's initial differential diagnosis because of their rarity and presenting symptoms that may be confused for myelopathy or radiculopathy from spondylosis. Subsequently, patients may erroneously undergo decompressive spinal procedures without improvement. Thus, clinicians must maintain a high level of suspicion for spinal vascular malformations in patients with appropriate clinical signs and symptoms. Proper imaging with careful attention to any observed abnormalities in or around the spinal cord is paramount to the correct diagnosis of these lesions. Further investigation with noninvasive angiography can be obtained safely and quickly. Patients will invariably require catheter angiography to elucidate the anatomy of the lesion, and this will guide further treatment, endovascularly, or surgically, or both. A comprehensive multidisciplinary approach is critical in order to ensure optimal outcomes for patients with these complex leisons. Current research has mainly focused on improving endovascular outcomes and durability, and new embolic agents and techniques have shown promise in the successful treatment of these complex lesions.

References

[1] Aminoff MJ, Barnard RO, Logue V. The pathophysiology of spinal vascular malformations. J Neurol Sci. 1974; 23(2):255–263

[2] Di Chiro G, Doppman J, Ommaya AK. Selective arteriography of arteriovenous aneurysms of spinal cord. Radiology. 1967; 88(6):1065–1077

[3] Borden JA, Wu JK, Shucart WA. A proposed classification for spinal and cranial dural arteriovenous fistulous malformations and implications for treatment. J Neurosurg. 1995; 82(2):166–179

[4] Spetzler RF, Detwiler PW, Riina HA, Porter RW. Modified classification of spinal cord vascular lesions. J Neurosurg. 2002; 96(2, Suppl):145–156

[5] Wilson DA, Abla AA, Uschold TD, McDougall CG, Albuquerque FC, Spetzler RF. Multimodality treatment of conus medullaris arteriovenous malformations: 2 decades of experience with combined endovascular and microsurgical treatments. Neurosurgery. 2012; 71(1):100–108

[6] Koch C. Spinal dural arteriovenous fistula. Curr Opin Neurol. 2006; 19(1):69–75

[7] Cho WS, Kim KJ, Kwon OK, et al. Clinical features and treatment outcomes of the spinal arteriovenous fistulas and malformation. J Neurosurg Spine. 2013; 19(2):207–216

[8] Rosenblum B, Oldfield EHE, Doppman JLJ, Di Chiro G. Spinal arteriovenous malformations: a comparison of dural arteriovenous fistulas and intradural AVM's in 81 patients. J Neurosurg. 1987; 67(6):795–802

[9] Hamdan A, Padmanabhan R. Intramedullary hemorrhage from a thoracolumbar dural arteriovenous fistula. Spine J. 2015; 15(2):e9–e16

[10] Kitazono M, Yamane K, Toyota A, Okita S, Kumano K, Hashimoto N. [A case of dural arteriovenous fistula associated with subcortical and subdural hemorrhage] No Shinkei Geka. 2010; 38(8):757–762

[11] Aviv RI, Shad A, Tomlinson G, et al. Cervical dural arteriovenous fistulae manifesting as subarachnoid hemorrhage: report of two cases and literature review. AJNR Am J Neuroradiol. 2004; 25(5):854–858

[12] Do HM, Jensen ME, Cloft HJ, Kallmes DF, Dion JE. Dural arteriovenous fistula of the cervical spine presenting with subarachnoid hemorrhage. AJNR Am J Neuroradiol. 1999; 20(2):348–350

[13] Fassett DR, Rammos SK, Patel P, Parikh H, Couldwell WT. Intracranial subarachnoid hemorrhage resulting from cervical spine dural arteriovenous fistulas: literature review and case presentation. Neurosurg Focus. 2009; 26(1):E4

[14] Morimoto T, Yoshida S, Basugi N. Dural arteriovenous malformation in the cervical spine presenting with subarachnoid hemorrhage: case report. Neurosurgery. 1992; 31(1):118–120, discussion 121

[15] Mascalchi M, Mangiafico S, Marin E. [Hematomyelia complicating a spinal dural arteriovenous fistula. Report of a case] [in French]. J Neuroradiol. 1998; 25(2):140–143

[16] Minami M, Hanakita J, Takahashi T, et al. Spinal dural arteriovenous fistula with hematomyelia caused by intraparenchymal varix of draining vein. Spine J. 2009; 9(4):e15–e19

[17] Kinouchi H, Mizoi K, Takahashi A, Nagamine Y, Koshu K, Yoshimoto T. Dural arteriovenous shunts at the craniocervical junction. J Neurosurg. 1998; 89(5):755–761

[18] Guly HR, Bouamra O, Lecky FE; Trauma Audit and Research Network. The incidence of neurogenic shock in patients with isolated spinal cord injury in the emergency department. Resuscitation. 2008; 76(1):57–62

[19] Shaikh N, Raza A, Rahman A, Sabana A, Malmstrom F, Al Sulaiti G. Prolonged bradycardia, asystole and outcome of high spinal cord injury patients. Panam J Trauma Crit Care Emerg Surg. 2014; 3(3):87–92

[20] Ryken TC, Hurlbert RJ, Hadley MN, et al. The acute cardiopulmonary management of patients with cervical spinal cord injuries. Neurosurgery. 2013; 72(Suppl 2):84–92

[21] Davison DL, Terek M, Chawla LS. Neurogenic pulmonary edema. Crit Care. 2012; 16(2):212

[22] Mehesry TH, Shaikh N, Malmstrom MF, Marcus MA, Khan A. Ruptured spinal arteriovenous malformation: presenting as stunned myocardium and neurogenic shock. Surg Neurol Int. 2015; 6(Suppl 16):S424–S427

[23] Criscuolo GR, Oldfield EH, Doppman JL. Reversible acute and subacute myelopathy in patients with dural arteriovenous fistulas. Foix-Alajouanine syndrome reconsidered. J Neurosurg. 1989; 70(3):354–359

[24] Ferrell AS, Tubbs RS, Acakpo-Satchivi L, Deveikis JP, Harrigan MR. Legacy and current understanding of the often-misunderstood Foix-Alajouanine syndrome. Historical vignette. J Neurosurg. 2009; 111(5):902–906

[25] Donghai W, Ning Y, Peng Z, et al. The diagnosis of spinal dural arteriovenous fistulas. Spine. 2013; 38(9):E546–E553

[26] Amarouche M, Hart JL, Siddiqui A, Hampton T, Walsh DC. Time-resolved contrast-enhanced MR angiography of spinal vascular malformations. AJNR Am J Neuroradiol. 2015; 36(2):417–422

[27] Takai K, Komori T, Taniguchi M. Microvascular anatomy of spinal dural arteriovenous fistulas: arteriovenous connections and their relationships with the dura mater. J Neurosurg Spine. 2015; 23(4):526–533

[28] Su IC, terBrugge KG, Willinsky RA, Krings T. Factors determining the success of endovascular treatments among patients with spinal dural arteriovenous fistulas. Neuroradiology. 2013; 55(11):1389–1395

[29] Agarwal V, Zomorodi A, Jabbour P, et al. Endovascular treatment of a spinal dural arteriovenous malformation (DAVF). Neurosurg Focus. 2014; 37(1, Suppl):1

[30] Rangel-Castilla L, Russin JJ, Zaidi HA, et al. Contemporary management of spinal AVFs and AVMs: lessons learned from 110 cases. Neurosurg Focus. 2014; 37(3):E14

[31] Ropper AE, Gross BA, Du R. Surgical treatment of Type I spinal dural arteriovenous fistulas. Neurosurg Focus. 2012; 32(5):E3

[32] Velat GJ, Chang SW, Abla AA, Albuquerque FC, McDougall CG, Spetzler RF. Microsurgical management of glomus spinal arteriovenous malformations: pial resection technique. J Neurosurg Spine. 2012; 16(6):523–531

30 Spinal Infections

Edward K. Nomoto, Eli M. Baron, Joshua E. Heller, and Alexander R. Vaccaro

Abstract

Spinal infections represent a considerable source of morbidity and mortality even in the era of modern neuroimaging, antibiotics, and surgical treatment strategies. Their infectious etiologies are traditionally divided into pyogenic and nonpyrogenic organisms. The classification, clinical presentation, diagnosis, and treatment of spinal infections are reviewed. Medical versus surgical treatment is considered. The management of spine surgical wound infections is also reviewed.

Keywords: diskitis, epidural abscess, osteomyelitis, Pott's disease, spinal wound infection

30.1 Introduction

Spinal infections represent a serious source of morbidity and mortality for patients. Sequelae include pain, neurologic deficit, and spinal instability. Even with modern day treatment modalities, including surgical débridement, spinal reconstruction, and antibiotic therapy, a mortality rate of 20% has been reported in some variants of spinal infection.[1] We review pyogenic and nonpyogenic infections of the spine. We also review postoperative wound infections, as these may be the most common spinal infection requiring surgery. Excluded from this discussion are infectious entities that may involve the spinal cord or its coverings that are generally treated medically, such as human immunodeficiency virus (HIV)–related myelopathy and meningitis.

30.2 Classification

Spinal infections can be classified as pyogenic versus nonpyogenic.[2] Pyogenic spinal infections refer to infections of the spine resulting in purulence and predominantly a neutrophilic response.[3] These are typically caused by bacteria but may also occur as a result of parasitic or fungal organisms. Nonpyogenic infections result in a granulomatous response and are usually caused by mycobacteria, parasites, or fungi.[4]

Spinal infections can also be categorized by their anatomical location in relation to the spinal column, dura, and spinal cord. Vertebral osteomyelitis refers to infection of the vertebra or bone of the spine.[5] Alternatively, this is referred to as infectious spondylitis. Diskitis refers to infection of the disk space. Combined infection of the disk and adjacent bone is referred to as spondylodiskitis. Septic arthritis of the facet joint may be seen in isolation or in combination with adjacent osteomyelitis or epidural abscess.[6,7,8,9,10,11]

Epidural abscess can be seen alone but is usually seen in combination with diskitis or spondylodiskitis. Subdural infection is much more rare but has been reported.[12,13] Intramedullary abscess of the spinal cord may also be seen.[14,15,16,17,18,19]

30.3 Organisms

The most common organism seen causing pyogenic infections is *Staphylococcus aureus* (about 60% of infections), followed by enterobacter (30%). Less commonly, *Salmonella*, *Klebsiella*, *Pseudomonas*, and *Serratia* are involved[4] Epidural abscess is caused most often by *Staphylococcus aureus* (63% of cases). Species are usually methicillin sensitive (MSSA). Cases of methicillin-resistant organisms (MRSA), however, can also occur. Other less common causative bacteria are *Streptococcus* species, *Pseudomonas*, *Escherichia coli*, and *Lactobacillus*. Mixed flora with combinations of the above organisms also occurs, as well as infection with oral flora such as *Prevotella oris* and *Peptostreptococcus micros*.[20,21,22,23,24]

Nonpyogenic infections of the spine are most commonly caused by *Mycobacterium tuberculae*, followed by *Brucella* species. Fungal pathogens are seen in normal hosts and immunocompromised hosts. Those seen in normal hosts include *Blastomyces dermatitis*, *Coccidioides immitis*, and *Histoplasma capsulatum*, whereas opportunistic fungi, including *Aspergillus*, *Candida*, *Cryptococcus*, and *Mucor*, are seen in immunocompromised hosts.[4,25] Reports of other unusual fungal organisms, such as *Scedosporium* (*Pseudallescheria*) species, causing vertebral osteomyelitis also exist.[26,27] Echinococcosis, onchocerciasis, toxoplasmosis, and toxocariasis all can cause nonsuppurative spondylodiskitis.[4] *Taenie solium*, the causative agent of cysticercosis, may cause epidural, subarachnoid, or intramedullary spinal infection.[28,29,30,31,32,33,34] Nocardial species have also been reported to cause nonpyogenic spondylodiskitis and epidural abscess.[35,36,37,38]

30.4 Risk Factors, Epidemiology, and Pathophysiology

Spinal infections are caused by direct inoculation, contiguous spread, or by hematogenous spread. Multiple theories exist for spread through the venous and arterial systems, as described by Batson. The Batson plexus is a valveless retrograde system allows back flow and stasis.[5] This is implicated in the spread of infection to the vertebral body and seeding from distant sites as seen in bacterial endocarditis. Multiple risk factors exist that predispose patients to the development of spinal infections, including advanced age, malnutrition, immunocompromise, human immunodeficiency virus/acquired immunodeficiency syndrome (HIV/AIDS), chronic steroids, renal failure, cancer, renal failure, septicemia, history of spinal surgery, and presence of foreign bodies.[39] Endocarditis can be found in almost 30% of hematogenous spinal infections and must be ruled out as a source when spinal infection is found.

Pyogenic spinal epidural abscess is a relatively rare condition. The incidence of this potentially devastating infection appears to have increased in recent years. Current best estimates of incidence in the United States is two hospitalizations per 10,000,[20] higher than original estimates of 2 to 25 patients per 100,000.[22,40]

Table 30.1 Predisposing conditions for spinal epidural abscess

Systematic condition	Potential source of infection	Local vertebral predisposing factor
Alcoholism	Vertebral osteomyelitis/diskitis	Spondylosis
Liver cirrhosis	Pulmonary/mediastinal infections	Previous spinal operations
Chronic renal insufficiency	Sepsis	Previous spinal trauma
Crohn's disease	Urinary tract infection	Epidural anesthesia
SLE	Paraspinal abscess	Paravertebral injections
Neoplasm	Pharyngitis	Lumbar puncture
Immunodeficiency syndrome	Wound infection	
Advanced age	Endocarditis	
	Upper respiratory tract infection	
	Sinusitis	
	HIV infection	
	Soft-tissue infection	
	Intravenous drug abuse	
	Vascular catheter	

Abbreviations: HIV, human immunodeficiency virus; SLE, systemic lupus erythematosus.

Adapted with permission from Bremer and Darouiche.[42]

Spinal epidural abscess occurs most commonly in males over the age of 30, with most patients being in their 60s. The male-to-female ratio in epidural abscess is 2.5 to 1.[24] Epidural infection in the pediatric population is very unusual, although rare case reports exist.[41] Probably the most frequent risk factor for spinal epidural abscess is intravenous drug use (27% of cases).[20] Additional risk factors are listed in ► Table 30.1.[42]

Nonspinal infections may lead to epidural abscess via hematogenous spread (45%) or by direct extension (55%).[43] Cellulitis can lead to hematogenous seeding of the epidural space, whereas retropharyngeal abscess, often after surgery (21% of cases), can extend directly posteriorly, leading to osteomyelitis and epidural abscess. Diabetes mellitus is a well-known risk factor for the development of infection and is identified in approximately 20% of cases. Disease states and therapies that lead to an immunocompromised state such as HIV, malignancy, and chronic steroid use also predispose patients to the development of epidural abscess.[20] Hemodialysis and indwelling catheters (which often become infected) can predispose patients with end-stage renal disease to the formation of epidural abscesses, often with methicillin-resistant *S. aureus*.[44,45,46] Other important risk factors include preexisting or synchronous nonspinal infections and spine trauma.[20,24]

Spinal epidural abscess after epidural steroid injection has been described, but its incidence is very low, estimated at 1 case per 70 to 400,000. More commonly, epidural abscess develops following infection of indwelling catheters, such as those used in epidural anesthesia.[47] Recent spinal trauma has also been identified as a risk factor for the development of epidural infection. It is theorized that blunt trauma leads to a focal area of decreased immunologic resistance, facilitating the implantation of infection by a hematogenous route.[24]

Spinal epidural abscesses most commonly occur in the lumbar spine, followed by the thoracic spine where they are usually confined to one or two levels.[24] They are often associated with vertebral osteomyelitis and/or diskitis.[3] The most common organism seen in one series was *S. aureus*, followed by *Mycobacterium tuberculosis*, *E. coli*, and *Staphylococcus epidermidis*.[24]

Vertebral osteomyelitis represents roughly 2 to 7% cases of osteomyelitis and in developed countries ranks third in frequency only to femoral and tibial osteomyelitis.[48] Given its relative rarity, and often nonspecific presentation, diagnosis is often delayed. Additionally, given the common presentations of neck or of back pain, and nearly universal occurrence of these symptoms in the general population, the diagnosis is often delayed for weeks to months.[49,50,51] Pyogenic vertebral osteomyelitis appears to be on the rise. This is probably due to an increase in the elderly population and immunocompromised population, including human immunodeficiency virus (HIV) and intravenous drug abuse. Additionally, more invasive diagnostic and therapeutic medical procedures may be associated with pyogenic infections, especially urologic procedures. Concurrent infection of the skin, respiratory tract, or genitourinary tract is often seen as sources of spinal infection. These may be present in roughly 40% of patients who have vertebral osteomyelitis.[52] Other common risk factors include intravenous drug abuse, which occurs in roughly 40% of cases, diabetes mellitus in 10 to 30% of cases, and concurrent medical illness in 20 to 23% of cases.[52,53,54]

The pathophysiology of pyogenic osteomyelitis and diskitis remains uncertain. Controversy exists as to the precise route of infection spread. Although local diskitis usually occurs in children and young adults, primary involvement of the vertebrae is significantly more common in adulthood.[49] Given the highly vascular nature of the intervertebral disks in children, where there is direct profusion of the nucleus pulposus, the blood supply may be a source of hematogenous seeding of the disk. In a mature spine, however, the vasculature is limited to that anulus fibrosis. Thus, in the adult, the initial infection may start in the metaphysis of the vertebral body, with subsequent spread to the disk space.[55] Infection can also spread directly into the spinal canal and form an epidural abscess. Prolonged infection can result in fracture causing instability.

Staphylococcus aureus is the most common organism seen with vertebral osteomyelitis, accountable for 50 to 65% of cases. Additionally, *S. aureus* was nearly responsible for all osteomyelitis cases in the preantibiotic era.[39,48,56] Less commonly, other organisms are seen, including *E. coli* and other enteric bacteria.

Intramedullary spinal cord abscess is significantly rarer than the above entities. Since 1950, an average of one case per year has been reported in the literature. Intramedullary abscess seems to occur with a male preponderance, with a mean age of 28.9 years and most commonly involving the thoracic cord.[57] Usually abscesses occur secondary to a primary focus of infection. More common foci of infection associated with intramedullary abscess include pneumonitis, genitourinary tract infection, skin infections, endocarditis, and meningitis. Immunocompromised state is also a risk factor.[58,59] There is also an association with dermoids, epidermoids, infected dermal sinus tracts, and dysraphism.[57,60,61,62]

Typically, intramedullary abscesses start in the gray matter and extend into the white matter. Afterwards, the infection may extend rostrocaudally separating fiber tracts.[57] Organisms may enter the spinal cord via a variety of routes, including hematogenous spread, septic emboli, and contiguous spread from an adjacent infection or by continuity with an infected dermal sinus tract.

Tuberculosis of the spine, also known as Pott's disease, had decreased markedly in incidence in developed countries with the advent of improved treatment. Since the 1980s, however, there appears to be an increase in incidence largely due to its association with HIV. The majority of cases of Pott's disease are likely hematogenous in origin, with an original pulmonary focus.[63] Spinal tuberculosis represents 1% of all *M. tuberculosis* infections and 25 to 60% of all osteomyelitis and joint infections caused by *M. tuberculae*.[4,64] Lower thoracic and lumbar vertebrae are most frequently involved, whereas the sacrum and cervical region are involved less frequently.[65]

Tuberculosis has been noted to spread in three major patterns: peridiskal, central, and anterior. The most common form of spread is the peridiskal type, which starts in a single end plate and spreads peripherally around the disk. Contiguous spread tracks deep to the anterior longitudinal ligament, sparing the disk. In the central type, an abscess forms in the middle of the vertebral body, which can lead to collapse and eventual spinal deformity. The anterior type begins with seeding of the anterior vertebrae and spread along the anterior longitudinal ligament, leading to the classic finding of scalloping of the vertebral body or bodies if the spread is across multiple levels.[66]

Brucellosis of the spine occurs in 2 to 30% of all cases of brucellosis with bone involvement.[65] Brucellosis, is a zoonotic infection, occurs most commonly amongst farmers, veterinarians, dairy workers, and other people working with grazing domestic mammals.[4] The main methods of transmission are through ingestion of unpasteurized milk products. However, airborne transmission can be also through inhalation of aerosolized particles.[67] Spinal involvement occurs more frequently in elderly patients, patients with a delay in diagnosis, and spinal brucellosis patients have an elevated erythrocyte sedimentation rate (ESR) compared with brucellosis patients without spondylitis.[68] The most common presentation is isolated single-level lumbar disease, although it can be diffuse.[68] Cervical or thoracic involvement usually is associated with more neurologic deficits.[69]

Fungal spinal infections also tend to be more common in immunocompromised hosts and usually result from hematogenous seeding.[50,70,71] Nevertheless, as mentioned above, certain regional endemic fungi may affect immunocompetent hosts and, rarely, result in spinal infection. *Coccidioides immitis* infections are endemic to the dry soil of the American Southwest and Central and South America, and its disease prevalence is increasing. One hundred thousand new infections are diagnosed yearly, of which 34% are symptomatic. Amongst symptomatic individuals, 5 to 10% will develop a serious pulmonary infection, and of those who have a serious infection, less than 1% will develop chronic pulmonary disease and/or extrapulmonary dissemination including spinal involvement.[72] *Histoplasma capsulatum* is endemic to Missouri and the Ohio and Mississippi river valleys and usually causes a benign and self-limited disease. Normal host defense mechanisms tend to limit or prevent disseminated spread from its initial pulmonary focus. When disseminated histoplasmosis occurs, only very rarely does it cause an intramedullary abscess.[73] Other *Histoplasma* species have been reported to rarely cause spondylodiskits.[74,75,76] *Blastomyces dermatitidis* is a dimorphic fungus endemic to the soil of the Mississippi and Ohio river basins and also midwestern states that border the Great Lakes. Infection has also been reported in Central and South America, Africa, and the Middle East. Infection likely occurs by inhalation of conidia. Extrapulmonary dissemination may occur, with the skin being the most common site of involvement.[25] Osseous involvement may occur in as many as 10 to 60% of those patients with disseminated disease.[77] When it occurs in the spine, it most likely causes a spondylodiskitis in the lower thoracic or lumbar spine, where the anterior vertebral body is affected initially.[25]

Pathogenic fungi that typically invade immunocompromised hosts include *Cryptococcus*, *Candida*, *Aspergillus*, and *Mucor* species. These exist worldwide. *Cryptococcus* is found in soil and pigeon feces and is common amongst patients with HIV and amongst organ transplant recipients. Infection is usually acquired by inhalation. Spread is usually hematogenous.[25] Roughly 5 to 10% of patients with cryptococcal infection will have spinal vertebral involvement, where the lumbar spine is most frequently involved, followed by the cervical spine.[78,79] *Aspergillus* spores typically are found in water soil, decaying plant matter, and grains. Like the other fungi, infection most commonly occurs by hematogenous spread, usually from the lungs. *Aspergillus* vertebral osteomyelitis is similar to pyogenic vertebral osteomyelitis in that there is a male preponderance, usually the lumbar spine is involved, and the most common symptom is back pain. *Candida* species are amongst the normal flora of the gastrointestinal tract and skin and female genital tract.[25] The lower thoracic or lumbar spine is most frequently involved.[80]

Parasitic infection may also occur in the spine. *Echinococcus* species are found worldwide amongst carnivorous mammals and live within their intestines, and their ova are passed with stool. Subsequently, intermediate hosts such as livestock ingest the ova, which hatch in the duodenum, and these embryos reproduce asexually, forming multiloculated cysts. Human infection occurs when contact with ova occur through contaminated food or direct contact with feces. Osseous involvement with hydatid cyst disease is unusual, but when it does occur, it involves the spine 44% of the time.[81] Spinal infection most likely occurs through vertebral–portal venous anastomosis.[82] Spinal infection with *Echinococcus* can occur as primary intramedullary cyst, intradural extramedullary cyst, extradural intraspinal hydatid cyst, hydatid disease of the vertebrae, and paravertebral involvement.[83]

Neurocysticercosis is worldwide the most common parasitic infection effecting the central nervous system. Spinal neurocysticercosis is unusual even in endemic regions. Infection occurs as a result of ingestion of the eggs of the pork tapeworm, *Taenia soleum*. The larvae are released from the eggs in the stomach after ingestion. The larvae then penetrate the intestinal mucosa and gain access to the blood stream, and central nervous system involvement then may occur. Spinal neurocysticercosis can occur in either the subarachnoid space or in the parenchyma of the cord.[84] Extradural and bony involvement may also occur but are extremely rare.[33,85]

30.5 Diagnosis

The most common presenting symptom of spinal epidural abscess is back pain, which nearly always occurs, followed by fevers, which occurs about two thirds of the time. Cervical epidural abscess may present with neck pain, fever, and some degree of neurologic dysfunction. Radiculopathy may also be seen. Fever, defined as temperature greater than 101°F, is a presenting sign approximately 50% of the time and is clearly not required for diagnosis. Neurologic dysfunction, including weakness, sensory loss, and bowel or bladder dysfunction, may also be seen.[86]

The diagnosis of pyogenic spondylodiskitis is often delayed due to the presentation of the patient with nonspecific signs and symptoms. Additionally, given the relative rarity of these conditions, diagnostic delays of weeks to months are quite common.[55] Most commonly, patients present with back pain, which occurs in 60 to 95% of patients.[87] Other symptoms include muscle weakness (33–68% of patients), difficulties with ambulation (55%), sensory disturbance (49%), fevers (43%), and sphincteric disturbance is (25%).[51,87,88] On examination, patients may have a limited range of motion, severe paraspinal muscle spasm, and tenderness over the infected level.[49] Pyogenic vertebral osteomyelitis should also be strongly considered in any patients with pleural effusion of undetermined cause, especially in the presence of back pain.[89]

Patients with intramedullary spinal cord abscess most commonly present with neurologic deficits, followed by pain and fever. Patients with an acute intramedullary abscess may present with a clinical picture similar to transverse myelitis, whereas those with a more subacute abscess may present with deficits similar to an expanding intramedullary spinal cord tumors.[57]

Blood cultures are positive in one half to two thirds of cases of epidural abscess. Blood and abscess cultures are nearly 100% concordant when both are positive and thus are very helpful in focusing antibiotic therapy.[20] Laboratory studies useful in the diagnosis include complete blood count with differential, ESR, and C-reactive protein (CRP). Leukocytosis with a moderate elevation in white blood cell count (WBC) greater than 15,000/mm[3] often accompanies spinal epidural abscess, but a normal WBC is not uncommon. ESR is consistently elevated (95%) in the presence of epidural abscess.[90] Elevation greater than 30 mm/h is common even without fever or leukocytosis.[91]

Elevations greater than 100 mm/h in a patient with neck pain is highly suggestive of epidural infection.[92] CRP is also often elevated. Both ESR and CRP can also be used to follow a response to treatment.

Laboratory studies are also useful in the diagnosis and management of pyogenic vertebral osteomyelitis. Elevated WBC is seen only in approximately 55% of patients. Elevation in the inflammatory markers CRP and ESR, however, have been reported to have sensitivities of 98% and 100%, respectively.[93] Elevated ESR (> 20 mm per hour as found in > 95% of cases) and an elevated CRP may be found in nearly all cases.[51,87,88] Nevertheless, these markers normally may rise after an invasive procedure where there is no infection. Most often ESR will peak between postoperative days 4 and 6 and will typically normalize within 14 days. The CRP level typically normalizes by postoperative day 6.[48]

Blood cultures are also useful in the laboratory work up of osteomyelitis. They may be positive in 50 to 75% of cases.[51,94] These should be drawn in an attempt to isolate the infected organism. Some organisms may be difficult to culture, and a more rapid diagnosis may be obtained by techniques such as polymerase chain reaction (PCR). Although a diagnosis of a vertebral osteomyelitis may be suspected on the basis of examination and imaging, the actual diagnosis should be made using definitive tissue studies, such as blood culture, PCR, or a vertebral body biopsy.[55] Biopsy, whether open or computed tomography (CT) guided, can identify an organism in approximately 80% of cases where the patient has not yet been started on antibiotics. The yield decreases to 48%, however, if antibiotics were started prior to biopsy.[94] Although a urinalysis may be useful in suggestive source of infection, certainly other sources should be sought after, as a biopsy may actually identify infection related to a different organism.[49,56]

For spinal infections, magnetic resonance imaging (MRI) with contrast is the diagnostic imaging modality of choice.[95] Typical MRI characteristics of spinal epidural abscess are a heterogeneously enhancing epidural collection that is isointense/hypointense on T1-weighted images and hyperintense on T2-weighted images[20] (▶ Fig. 30.1). Liquid pus in a spinal epidural abscess typically has low signal intensity on T1-weighted imaging, whereas granulation tissue typically has a rim of enhancement after gadolinium injection.[96] In cases of a nontuberculosis bacterial abscess, there is often associated spondylodiskitis where hypointense signal changes are seen in the disk and adjacent vertebral bodies on T1-weighted images and a high signal is seen on T2-weighted images. There is usually marked enhancement of the affected vertebral body. In cases attributable to tuberculosis, both epidural involvement and spondylodiskitis have been described with an isointense or hypointense appearance on T1-weighted MRI and a hyperintense appearance on T2-weighted imaging. Additionally large paraspinal masses are often seen with similar MRI characteristics.[97] In patients whom a MRI cannot be obtained, a CT myelogram can demonstrate the lesion well but carries with it the added risks of myelography, including the risk of seeding infection into the subarachnoid space if concomitant lumbar epidural abscess exists. MRI with contrast and CT myelogram has been shown to have equivalent sensitivities (91–92%) in detecting epidural abscess.[20]

For vertebral osteomyelitis, plain radiographs may show changes in the vertebral body or the disk by week 4 of infection; these are often not seen until 8 weeks of infection.[98,99] Radiographic

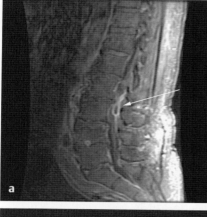

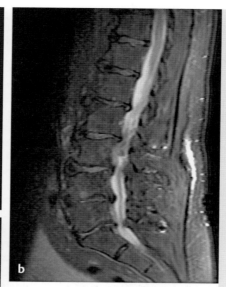

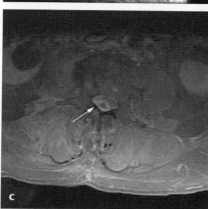

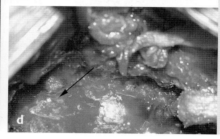

Fig. 30.1 Spinal epidural abscess. **(a)** T1 sagittal image post contrast administration demonstrating a lumbar dorsal epidural abscess at L2–L3 (arrow). Note the rim enhancement with a central hypointense area, suggestive of granulation tissue. **(b)** On T2-weighted imaging, the lesion is hyperintense to the neural elements but less intense than CSF. **(c)** Axial T1 image post contrast administration demonstrating significant thecal sac compression secondary to the posteriorly situated mass (arrow). The patient who presented with back pain, fever, lower extremity weakness, and bladder dysfunction was treated with L2–L3 laminectomy and evacuation of the abscess. **(d)** At surgery, the patient was noted to have minimal pus but thick granulation tissue compressing the dura (arrow).

findings in osteomyelitis include disk space narrowing, parting of the end plates, and evidence of soft-tissue swelling. By weeks 8 to 12, osteosclerosis may be seen (▶ Fig. 30.2).[99] More sensitive are radionuclide bone scans with technetium methylene diphosphonate. These, however, may be positive in bone-forming process and are not specific for inflammatory disorders.[98,99] More specific for inflammatory processes are bone scans with gallium 67 or indium 3. A combination of gallium and technetium may have increased sensitivity and specificity than either scan alone.[98] Nevertheless, given the lack of sensitivity and specificity overall of plain radiographs, other modalities including CT scan and MRI have been used as the mainstay of radiologic diagnosis.[54,98,99] MRI is considered the imaging method of choice, as it has a sensitivity of greater than 80% and specificity between 53 and 94%.[54,98] MRI is particularly useful, as it demonstrates suspected lesions as decreased signal on T1-weighted images and hyperintensity on T2-weighted imaging.[98] The administration of gadolinium may result in enhancement of infection on T1-weighted imaging.[54,98,100] As discussed later on, postoperative MRI changes may be difficult to assess, especially in the setting of suspected vertebral osteomyelitis. MRI changes may be normal or they may be indicative of infection, especially if there is evidence of changes involving both the nucleus pulposus and adjoining vertebral marrow, or changes in the consistency of the disk space when the disk was not removed surgically.[55] **(d)** Sagittal CT reconstruction clearly demonstrating retropulsion of diseased bone into the spinal canal. Osteosclerotic changes and disease of the inferior T12 end plate are also seen. **(e)** T1 sagittal imaging post contrast infusion demonstrating enhancement of

the infected retropulsed L1 vertebral body. Also note enhancement of the inferior T12 vertebral body and involvement of the adjacent disk spaces. **(f)** T2-weighted sagittal MRI demonstrates increased signal in the involved bone/disk. **(g)** T2-weighted axial imaging through the T12/L1 facet joints demonstrates septic arthritis (arrow) of the right joint. This is seen as increased signal intensity in the affected joint. The patient underwent L1 vertebrectomy, placement of an autogenous iliac crest bone graft strut and placement of T12–L2 staples/rods. The body of T12 was found to be hard at surgery without any evidence of significant erosion or disease. Postoperative imaging is shown in (h, i, and j). This was followed by delayed posterior spinal fusion with pedicle screws, rods, and allograft/autograft extending from T10 to L4 (l, m).

CT can be used to assess the amount of bony destruction and bony changes. Changes on CT scan appear earlier than they do on plain films. Soft-tissue visualization is poor compared with MRI. Paraspinal abscesses, however, can be visualized well, and CT can be used to assess bony involvement for surgical planning.

For intramedullary spinal cord abscess, plain films may reveal associated vertebral osteomyelitis. Although myelogram may demonstrate a block or a widened spinal cord, MRI has become the imaging modality of choice for intramedullary abscesses. MRI typically shows a low-intensity lesion on T1-weighted imaging and high signal on T2-weighted imaging. Early T1 imaging with contrast reveals a poorly defined area of marginal enhancement, whereas follow-up imaging may show well-defined enhancement of a spinal cord lesion with a central hypointensity.[57,101]

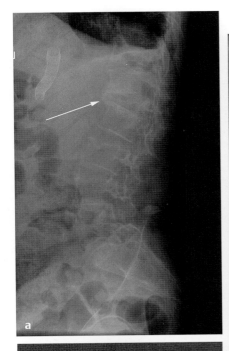

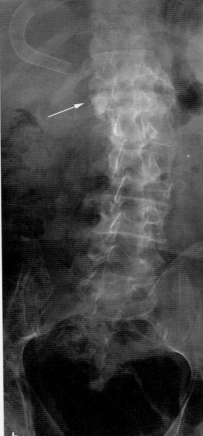

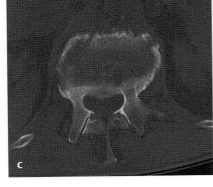

Fig. 30.2 Pyogenic vertebral osteomyelitis. **(a, b)** Lateral and anteroposterior lumbar radiographs demonstrating collapse of the L1 vertebrae (arrow). Note the osteosclerosis adjacent to the collapsed level, but also in the remaining L1 vertebral body. Also note the severe osteopenia seen in this 56-year-old male with cirrhosis. **(c)** Axial computed tomography (CT) scan through the diseased L1 vertebral body. Note the erosions through the involved end plate.

Tuberculosis-related spinal infections tend to be more indolent and of more gradual onset than pyogenic osteomyelitis. The most common presentation is back pain, which is usually in the thoracic region. Other associated symptoms include fever, malaise, night sweats, and weight loss. With cervical involvement, dysphagia, hoarseness, or cervical lymphadenopathy may occur.[4] Because of slow and insidious progression, nonspecific presentation, and the mildness of its associated back pain, considerable delay in diagnosis may occur. Chronic untreated infections can present with kyphotic deformity, cutaneous sinuses, and neurologic deficits (10–61%).[102,103] Neurologic deficit can occur by direct compression from infectious material or from progressive kyphotic deformity. On examination, patients with spinal tuberculosis may have spinal tenderness with spasm in the region of the pain. Range of motion testing may elicit severe pain. With advanced disease, the patient may have a Pott's kyphosis in the thoracic or lumbar spine, with collapse of the involved vertebral body resulting in sharp angulation and subsequent prominence of the spinous process at that level. Some patients may demonstrate a psoas sign on examination because of an anterior abscess tracking into the psoas muscle. Patients with a psoas sign lie flat with their hips flexed; when their hips are extended, they experience severe pain.[104]

Radiologic finding usually support the diagnosis earlier than laboratory testing. Plain radiographs may reveal vertebral body collapse. Occasionally, a lytic lesion may be seen within an involved vertebral body or within the posterior elements.[63] Plain radiographs may also reveal osteoporosis, a gibbus deformity, and scoliosis.[4] Most frequently, however, plain films are within normal limits.[63] CT examination frequently shows destruction at the level of the vertebral end plates, paravertebral abscesses that may have calcifications, and epidural collections. The cortical definition of the affected vertebral body is frequently lost; this is in distinction from pyogenic vertebral osteomyelitis where their cortical borders tend to be preserved. Rim enhancement of a paraspinal mass with calcifications within the mass is highly suggestive of spinal tuberculosis.[4] MRI is considered the imaging modality of choice for spinal tuberculosis (▶ Fig. 30.3). T1-weighted images may show homogenous low signal in the body with contiguous subligamentous spread. T2-weighted images can display increased signal is a similar patter. MRI may reveal

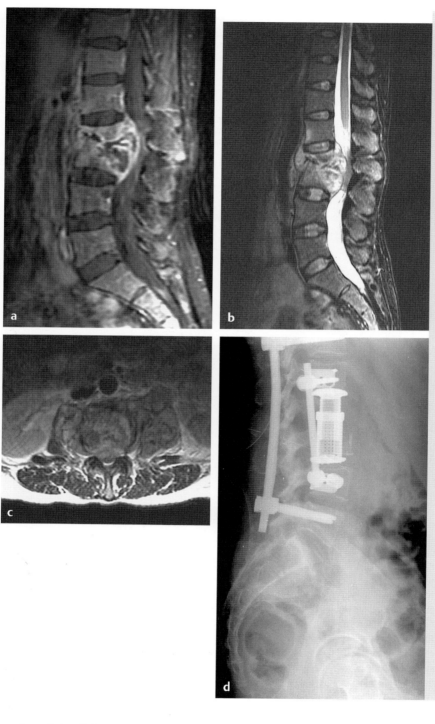

Fig. 30.3 Pott's disease. **(a)** T1-weighted sagittal magnetic resonance imaging post contrast administration demonstrating marked rim enhancement of spinal tuberculosis. Disease of the L2–L3 vertebral bodies is seen with relative sparing of the L2–L3 disk space. **(b)** T2-weighted sagittal imaging demonstrates extension of the tuberculosis abscess anteriorly and superiorly along the anterior longitudinal ligament. **(c)** Axial T2 image demonstrating bilateral involvement of the abscess in the paraspinal musculature. **(d)** Postoperative lateral radiography, post L2–L3 vertebrectomy and placement of an expandable cage/allograft bone/staples/rod followed by posterior spinal fusion/allograft/autograft. Note the restoration of lumbar lordosis.

sparing of the disk space with involvement of the vertebral body on either side of the disk, an unusual finding if malignancy is a consideration.[104] Additionally, an epidural mass with a bilobed configuration may be seen. MRI also is very useful for demonstrating bony involvement with infection, paraspinal masses/masses, and fistula formation.[4] MRI can also demonstrate enhancing intradural and/or intramedullary tuberculomas.[63] Intravenous gadolinium contrast is often added to assist with the diagnosis of an infectious process by showing peripheral enhancement.

The diagnosis of spinal tuberculosis should be confirmed by biopsy, as the treatment regimen varies drastically from other similarly presenting processes such as pyogenic or neoplastic involvement. Acid-fast bacillus organisms may or may not be seen on stain and may take 6 to 8 weeks to grow on traditional Lowenstein–Jensen medium. However, this has been improved with Middlebrook medium, which may decrease the diagnosis to within 2 weeks. PCR testing can be used for diagnosis and can be done within 6 hours, with a sensitivity of 75% and specificity greater than 99%.[105,106] Nevertheless, it is only approved for pulmonary tuberculosis. Additional supportive evidence may come from chest radiographs, purified protein derivative, and sputum/urine culture.[104] These tests support the diagnosis but are not definitive when compared with biopsy and culture of the spinal involvement. Although ESR may be elevated and may be useful for following treatment, it is often within normal limits.[4,63]

Spinal brucellosis usually presents with nonspecific symptoms and is diagnostically a challenge, often associated with a delay in diagnosis. Back pain, fever, and malaise in patients exposed to livestock and other animals in regions were the disease is endemic should raise suspicion for spinal brucellosis. Radiologically, early signs of the disease include osteoporosis of the affected vertebrae followed by erosion of the anterior aspect of the superior end plate. The disease may be characterized as *focal* or *diffuse*, where the focal disease limits itself to the anterior vertebral body and superior end plate, whereas the diffuse form can involve the entire spinal segment, extending into the posterior elements and adjacent paravertebral and epidural spaces. There is usually no necrosis or central caseation. As bone healing soon begins after its destruction, an anterior osteophyte, known as a parrot's beak, may form. On CT, air may be seen trapped between the disk and the superior end plate. Paraspinal muscle masses occur about 12% of the time, as opposed to tuberculosis where they occur 50% of the time. Epidural involvement is common. MRI may demonstrate mild enhancement of the affected disk space on postcontrast T1 imaging. In advanced stages of the disease, complete ankylosis of the affected vertebra may occur, where the affected vertebrae may be mistaken for a congenital segmentation anomaly. Collapsed vertebral bodies, gibbus deformity, and scoliosis are very unusual and suggest spinal tuberculosis; usually the infected vertebra in spinal brucellosis maintains its morphology.[4] The diagnosis of spinal brucellosis may be corroborated by serologic studies. These include a *Brucella* antibody of 1:160 (sensitivity between 68 and 91%) and the Rose Bengal test (sensitivity 92.9%).[68,107] Neurobrucellosis is confirmed by cerebrospinal fluid (CSF) serology.[69] ESR and CRP may be mildly elevated. Given the specificity of laboratory examinations, biopsy is rarely needed (5% patients).[108] Definite diagnosis may be made by biopsy.[65]

Symptoms of spinal fungal disease are also nonspecific, with back pain, fever, malaise, and night sweats being common presenting complaints. Some patients also present with neurologic deficits. On examination, local tenderness may be present. Radiologic findings may be similar to tuberculosis where relative sparing of the disk space, anterior involvement of the vertebral body, and large paraspinal abscesses are seen. Some patterns are commonly seen with specific fungal infections. Coccidioidomycosis infections may cause paravertebral swelling, with involvement of the posterior spinal elements. Gibbus deformity/vertebral body collapse is common with blastomyces. Lytic lesions maybe seen in cryptococcal spinal infections within the vertebral bodies.[25] Spinal cryptococcosis may manifest with an intraspinal granulomatous mass (infiltrating extradural lesion, intradural extramedullary granuloma), resulting in spinal cord compression. Candidal infection may involve the vertebral body or paravertebral regions. A macroabscess or mass mimicking a granuloma may be seen without disk space involvement.[4] These may resemble those in coccidioidomycosis or the cystic form of tuberculosis, with discrete margins and surrounding abscess formation. Both CT and MRI maybe useful in the diagnosis. CT

may show erosion in the bones, with small islands of bone preserved. This may be a useful characteristic to help differentiate these lesions from neoplastic disease. The diagnosis of fungal spinal involvement is made with biopsy and histopathologic assessment. Additionally, there are numerous commercially available kits that use immunoassay and PCR technologies to identify specific fungi. Although inflammatory markers and white count maybe elevated, these are useful for following infection and are nonspecific for diagnostic purposes.[25]

Spinal hydatid cyst disease most commonly presents in adults as a slow-onset progressive paraparesis. Other common symptoms include back pain, radiculopathy, sensory loss, sphincteric disturbances, and even paraplegia. MRI is typically highly suggestive of hydatid spinal involvement. T1-weighted imaging demonstrates cystic, often multiloculated structures adjacent to or involving the spinal canal. CT scan may demonstrate subtle osteolytic changes but does not demonstrate the relationship of cysts to the dura as would MRI. The diagnosis is confirmed with surgical specimen.[81]

Spinal neurocysticercosis most commonly presents as progressive paraparesis or weakness secondary to cord or cauda equina compression. Neurocysticercosis should be considered on the differential for anyone presenting with these symptoms who lives or traveled in areas where cysticercosis is endemic. Whereas extramedullary lesion may grow very large and patients exhibit symptoms very late, intramedullary lesions are often symptomatic early when at a small size. MRI is the neuroradiologic modality of choice for studying these lesions. T1-weighted imaging is useful for demonstrating the cyst wall, whereas T2-weighted imaging demonstrates the contents of the cyst itself and possibly pericystic edema. Occasionally, a mural nodule can be seen on MRI. Although CT scan may demonstrate calcifications in cases of degenerated organisms, the role of CT is lesser than MRI in the diagnosis of spinal neurocysticercosis. Myelography may be useful in detecting small lesions in the subarachnoid space; nevertheless, its role is limited with the advent of MRI and the possibility of cysticerca-related arachnoid scarring, limiting dye flow. Enzyme-linked immunoassay of CSF and serum are highly sensitive and specific for confirming the diagnosis.[84]

30.6 Treatment

30.6.1 Pyogenic Epidural Abscess

The goals of therapy for spinal epidural include preservation of normal neurologic function, as well as improving or stabilizing existing or progressive neurologic deficits.[20,109] Treatment options often consist of decompression and evacuation of the abscess with or without spinal reconstruction followed by a course if antibiotics versus antibiotics alone. Additionally, in the presence of bony destruction or instability, a concurrent or delayed stabilization procedure maybe considered. Urgent surgery remains the treatment of choice; however, some have had success with conservative therapy,[12,21,110,111] as well as with percutaneous procedures.[112,113]

For infection where the abscess is predominantly dorsal to the thecal sac or spinal cord, surgery usually involves laminectomy and evacuation of the abscess. If the infection is acute (< 12–16 days), frank pus is usually encountered. More chronic collections often have a more granulation tissue–like consistency, which can be tightly adherent to the dura. Caution must be exerted when attempting to remove granulation tissue; a dural tear in the face of epidural infection may have a high rate of associated meningitis. In instances where the lesion involves multiple spinal levels, some have advocated the use of irrigation devices to be passed sublaminarly so as to avoid too much bony disruption. In a similar fashion, if the lesion is acute, i.e., pus, and involves multiple levels, the judicious use of laminotomies and catheters for evacuation of the collection and irrigation has had some success.[112] These techniques should only be attempted in cases where there is enough room between the dura and the lamina to safely place the catheter. For many cases, traditional laminectomy may be technically easier and possibly safer. Regardless of technique, copious amounts of irrigation should be used and drains should be left in place postoperatively. Infections resulting in masses predominantly anterior to the cord or thecal sac are usually treated via an anterior approach. The use of bone graft and instrumentation in this setting is discussed below.

With improvements in neuroradiologic imaging and increased access to health care, the diagnosis of abscess may occur earlier in the disease process. In these instances, there are those who have advocated conservative therapy in patients for whom a causative organism has been identified who do not present with any neurologic deficits.[110,114] It must be recognized that this treatment plan often fails. Approximately one half of patients initially treated nonoperatively with antibiotics alone eventually experience neurologic decline requiring surgical decompression. Although antibiotics followed by delayed surgery, should conservative management fail, is an option, the outcome is usually not as good as with early surgery.[20] Harrington et al eloquently reviewed both the surgical and medical management of spinal epidural abscess.[115] They concluded that surgery was indicated, and medical management inappropriate, for the following indications: persistent pyrexia or raised inflammatory markers, failure to identify causative organisms, persistent severe pain, the presence of associated spinal deformity or instability, deteriorating neurologic examination related to the abscess, the presence of greater than 50% compression of the thecal sac on MRI, inability to follow a patient with serial MRI imaging, lack of availability of facilities for emergent spinal surgery if needed, failure of an abscess to resolve despite greater than 6 weeks of intravenous antibiotic treatment, and an immuno-compromised host.

30.6.2 Pyogenic Vertebral Osteomyelitis

Generally, the treatment of vertebral osteomyelitis involves medical treatment with spinal immobilization, early ambulation, and intravenous antibiotics. Greater than 75% of patients will experience relief and often fuse spontaneously. Patients under the age of 60 who are normal immunologically with a decreasing ESR followed by serial evaluation often respond well to nonsurgical therapy.[48,87,116] Should a patient fail medical treatment, surgical intervention may be necessary. Surgical

treatment includes evacuation of the abscess and possible spinal reconstruction.

With antibiotic treatment, outcomes of vertebral osteomyelitis have improved dramatically. In clinically stable patients, a 4- to 6-week regimen of high-dose parenteral antibiotic followed by oral antibiotic treatment may be sufficient. The antibiotic treatment may be shortened if the ESR has declined to one half of the pretreatment value.[55] However, patients with abscess may need a longer course of treatment.

For staphylococcal infection, high-dose penicillin is usually recommended. This, of course, precludes methicillin-resistant *S. aureus*, which is treated with vancomycin. Patients allergic to penicillin may be treated with first- or second-generation cephalosporins. For pseudomonal infections, generally two drugs are recommended. These include third-generation cephalosporins and possibly an aminoglycoside.[117,118] In a series of 111 patients treated, where 72 were initially treated with antibiotics alone, one third of patients failed conservative treatment, with final outcomes most related to the patient's immunologic status and their age.[87] Indications for operative therapy include static or progressive neurologic impairment, the presence of an abscess that fails to clear with medical therapy, sepsis from the locus of infection, persistent pain despite external immobilization, progressive spinal deformity, severe instability, failure to identify an organism, and the failure of nonoperative treatment.[48] Three surgical principles are sought: débridement of all necrotic and infected tissues, the provision of an adequate blood supply to the area of infection, and creation of immediate spinal stability.[55]

An anterior approach is most commonly used for infections involving the vertebral body and/ or disk. Débridement and decompression can be performed anteriorly. Likely instability will result after débridement; therefore, stability will need to be achieved by anterior reconstruction by strut or cage with or without a plate.[119] Titanium mesh cages have been shown to achieve good results without increased risk of chronic infection.[120,121] Posterior instrumentation can also be performed to increase stability.[122] Rarely is isolated posterior decompression indicated in the presence of vertebral osteomyelitis. Only in the unusual setting of an isolated epidural abscess with minimal vertebral body involvement is laminectomy indicated (▶ Fig. 30.1). Otherwise, laminectomy alone may result in a poor clinical outcome, including progressive deformity, increasing pain, worsening of instability, and possible worsening neurologic insult. Eismont et al reviewed 61 patients with vertebral osteomyelitis where 7 patients were treated by laminectomy alone: 3 worsened and 4 remained unchanged neurologically.[123] Usually the anterior vertebral column is involved, where the posterior column is typically uninvolved; thus, resection of the posterior element with a posterior decompression often fails to address the primary pathology and results in disruption of the stabilizing posterior structures.[48,123]

As a result of the above considerations, posterior débridement of any abscess followed by delayed placement of posterior instrumentation and bone graft has been advocated by some.[124] This may be done via a strict posterior approach or an extracavitary approach/costotransversectomy may be used. An extracavitary approach or costotransversectomy may, however, be technically challenging, as it may be difficult to place an adequate anterior structural graft. Other surgeons have advocated primary placement of posterior instrumentation during the time of the index débridement procedure, providing the posterior soft-tissue epidural space or bony elements are not involved. Rath et al reviewed 43 surgically managed patients with vertebral osteomyelitis, including 18 patients who underwent initial posterior débridement with concurrent autologous bone graft and instrumentation placement, where 94% achieved successful fusion.[88] Alternatively, anterior decompression with or without autologous bone graft may be performed. In general, anterior decompression without bone grafting is rarely indicated given the benefits of placing a graft in these patients.[125] Cahill et al[126] reviewed 10 patients who underwent anterior débridement and fusion without instrumentation with subsequent casting or bracing. Although their patients did well, the authors suggested that instrumentation may have reduced the need for a prolonged external immobilization. Similarly, Lifeso[127] reported good results in 11 patients who underwent anterior débridement and fusion for osteomyelitis.

The benefits of autologous bone grafting include minimizing the risk of rejection and improved and more rapid bony consolidation as compared with an allograft source. Adding posterior instrumentation to a noncontaminated posterior field may further optimize treatment by reducing the incidence of graft displacement and a collapse while conferring enough support to allow early mobilization and perhaps improve functional outcome.[48,124,126,128] Posterior stabilization following anterior débridement and placement of a bone graft therefore reduces the morbidity associated with prolonged bed rest. This may actually result in improved patient satisfaction and functional outcome.[48,129,130] Krödel et al[131] reported excellent results with 41 patients treated in this manner.

As far as using anterior instrumentation in the same surgical field as an active pyogenic vertebral osteomyelitis, this is more controversial. Some have advocated avoiding this to reduce the risk of hardware contamination and subsequent clinical reinfection at the same site.[132] Others, however, have argued that in the cervical spine, anterior cervical plating immediately following débridement and grafting confers immediate stabilization, prevents graft dislodgment, and potentially avoids another surgical procedure.[3,133] Lee et al reported good outcomes for a heterogeneous group of 29 patients who had osteomyelitis in the cervical, thoracic, or lumbar spine where many patients had titanium cages or allograft and plates placed during their index procedure.[2] Similarly, Ogden and Kaiser concluded in their series of 16 patients and a review of the literature that primary débridement and placement of instrumentation is safe without a significant risk of reinfection.[134] Some cases of osteomyelitis may benefit from the adjunctive use of a vascular tissue graft during débridement and reconstruction.[135] This affords immediate continuous blood supply to the donor graft, may protect against failure of the graft substance, and potentially increases the rate of successful graft incorporation.[136,137] This may be in the form of bringing omentum to the graft or, in selective cases, to a cage field while bone graft. Additionally, the external oblique muscle may provide a robust source of blood supply for an iliac crest graft used from T8 to the sacrum. A less robust source is the internal oblique muscle supplied by the deep circumflex iliac artery. The rib and the fibula provide alternative vascularized grafting options. Vascularized grafts, however, are not without their complications, including femoral nerve palsy, donor site hematoma, and hernia formation.[48]

Some have advocated the use of antibiotics beads as a method for the local delivery of antibiotics to the surrounding soft tissues and bone. Unfortunately, persistent bead contamination, persistent infection, and possible impairment of leukocyte function have been associated with the use of methylmethacrylate in this manner.[133,138]

Others have advocated percutaneous techniques for the treatment of vertebral osteomyelitis. Jeanneret and Magerl[129] reported on 23 patients with osteomyelitis managed either with percutaneous stabilization alone or in conjunction with a secondary anterior débridement. The patients all received external posterior spinal stabilization. Twelve of 15 patients were managed successfully with this strategy.

In summary, vertebral osteomyelitis may be successfully treated in most cases with antibiotics, immobilization, and initially bed rest alone. Nevertheless, there are patients who will certainly require further surgical intervention. Anterior débridement and bone grafting coupled with posterior stabilization seems to be a method of choice for a majority of cases requiring surgery (▶ Fig. 30.2). Some cases may benefit from anterior instrumentation in the setting of primary infections. It remains controversial whether a two-stage procedure is needed as far as placement of posterior instrumentation and when a posterior decompression/débridement is performed. Nevertheless, if the posterior elements are not grossly infected, many have advocated placement of instrumentation during the index procedure.

30.6.3 Diskitis

Similar to vertebral osteomyelitis, antibiotic therapy is the mainstay of treatment. Broad-spectrum antibiotics are given if an organism cannot be identified. Length of antibiotic therapy has been found to be critical in preventing recurrence. Treatment less than 8 weeks has shown recurrence rates greater than 10%, whereas treatment greater than 12 weeks has a less than 5% rate.[122,139] Surgery for diskitis without epidural abscess is rarely indicated. Indications include failure of medical management with progression of infection and development of osteomyelitis.

30.6.4 Intramedullary Abscess

An intramedullary spinal cord abscess is a surgical emergency. Once recognized, a decompressive laminectomy followed by myelotomy and abscess drainage should ensue. Antibiotics should be tailored to organisms grown from intraoperative culture.[57] Bartels et al reported a 13.6% mortality rate in those undergoing surgery for spinal intramedullary abscess.[140] Steroids are probably not beneficial in the postoperative period. With early recognition and early surgery followed by antibiotic therapy, most patients have a good prognosis, even when neurologic deficits are present.

30.6.5 Spinal Tuberculosis

Multidrug therapy remains the primary treatment for most cases of spinal tuberculosis. Disease amenable to medical treatment alone includes patients with early disease and those without deformity or neurologic deficit. First-line drugs include isoniazid, rifampin, ethambutol, and pyrazinamide. Additionally, pyridoxine is administered concurrently with isoniazid to reduce the risk of peripheral neuropathy. Second-line agents include cycloserine, quinolones, and amikacin.[104] However, antibiotic resistance is an emerging problem, with up to 25% patients having multidrug-resistant (MDR) tuberculosis.[127,141] This has been attributed to insufficient duration of antibiotic regimen or inappropriate regimen at the initiation of treatment. Principles of management of MDR tuberculosis have been proposed, which include attaining a culture and sensitivities, never adding a single drug to a failing regimen, regimens should consist of four drugs not used previously, and an injectable aminoglycoside should be used for at least 2 months. The recommended duration of pharmacotherapy is at least 24 months.[142]

Although medical treatment remains the first-line therapy for treatment of spinal tuberculosis, surgery may be necessary for patients with neurologic deficit, those who fail medical management, and patients with instability or deformity. Patients with significant neurologic deficit have improved outcomes with surgery.[127,143,144]

The goal of surgical intervention for neurologic deficit involves decompression of the spine by removal of purulent material and sequestered fragment compressing neural structures. Bone fragments that are noncompressive need not be removed because they will reconstitute after treatment with medications. When instability or deformity are present, the goal of surgery is not only to eradicate infection but also to correct or prevent deformity.[144,145] If the spine is at risk for deformity, then earlier surgical intervention may be warranted.[146] In general, most cases of Pott's disease treated surgically should initially be treated anteriorly with débridement/vertebrectomy and placement of a structural graft, including autograft, allograft, or cages.[143,145,146] Anterior rod/plate instrumentation has been used on numerous occasions successfully, but its use remains controversial. Alternatively, some have advocated the use of titanium cages[147] (▶ Fig. 30.3). Surgery for tuberculosis may be easier and achieve better results if it is performed early in the disease process before scarring and fibrosis develops, possibly resulting in adhesions to the great vessels and other organs, making surgery more dangerous and difficult. Patients also seem to respond better and more completely when they undergo surgery in the acute phase rather than when they have chronic disease and deformity.[104] After anterior decompression and fusion, many have advocated delayed supplemental posterior instrumentation. This may facilitate earlier mobilization of the patient. A delay of 1 to 2 weeks may allow an interval course of antibiotics and optimization of medical and nutritional parameters.[147]

Posterior spinal decompression alone is indicated when there is an isolated epidural mass compressing the thecal sac. Laminectomy alone is generally contraindicated, as it may lead to progressive deformity and neurologic decline. More recently, posterior-only approaches have been performed, including vertebral column resection with cage placement and posterior stabilization.[146,148] No difference was noted between anterior-posterior and posterior-only approaches when looking at new neurologic deficit or neurologic recovery. However, kyphosis was improved in combined approaches as opposed to posterior-only approach. The posterior-only group did have significant decrease in surgical time, estimated blood loss, and length of stay. Either approach appears to be acceptable as long as the surgical goals of decompression, removal of infected material, and spinal reconstruction and stabilization are achieved.[148]

Minimally invasive approaches have also been advocated for patients who cannot tolerate a thoracotomy when indicated. Thoracoscopic treatment of tuberculosis has recently been performed.[149,150] Alternatively, a transpedicular approach followed by bracing can be performed.[151]

30.6.6 Spinal Brucellosis

Numerous reports exist for successful treatment of spinal brucellosis with antibiotics alone.[69,152] These include combinations of doxycycline and rifampin or doxycycline and streptomycin. Fluoroquinolones also may be effective.[69] Surgical intervention, ranging from abscess drainage to spinal reconstruction, is required in approximately 10.7% of cases.[153] In cases of deformity, cord compression or disease progression surgery may be indicated with an approach similar to that for tuberculosis. Intramedullary abscess caused by *Brucella* species should be treated with laminectomy, myelotomy, drainage, and antibiotics.[154]

30.6.7 Treatment of Fugal Spinal Infection

Treatment of fungal spinal infections involves therapy with appropriate antifungal agents and possibly surgical intervention. Nonoperative treatment also consists of bracing, early ambulation, and correction of factors leading to fungal infection, i.e., nutritional support and addressing any underlying immunocompromised state. Amphotericin B is often used as an agent of choice for treating spinal fungal infections. Although its liposomal formulation has less toxicity, it is notorious for its nephrotoxicity. The azoles, including itraconazole, fluconazole, and ketoconazole, are alternatives that may be consider first-line drugs for some fungi, including *Coccidioides*, *Blastomycoces*, and *Candida* species. Newer agents, including echinocandin and caspofungin, may also have a role in the treatment of spinal fungal disease.[25]

Indications for surgery are similar to those for other nonpyogenic spinal infections. These include relief of neural compression, instability/deformity, lack of a diagnosis, and progressive infection despite adequate medical treatment.[25] As with other causes of osteomyelitis, usually anterior decompression provides the most thorough decompression (as pathology is usually located in the vertebral body) and allows height restoration through strut grafting. Additionally, posterior spinal instrumentation is usually required. Although a single procedure performed posteriorly may be considered (via a transpedicular approach or via transpedicular/lateral extracavitary approach), débridement is often not as thorough and should a mycotic aneurysm be encountered, bleeding may be very difficult or impossible to control. Advantages of a posterior circumferential decompression is that the thoracic cavity is not entered and a single incision is required.[25] Given, however, the higher rate of recurrence[26,155] of fungal spinal infections necessitating serial débridements, an anterior approach for anterior infections may be more appropriate.

Fungal intramedullary abscess is a neurosurgical emergency that usually requires laminectomy, myelotomy, and drainage.[156] Nevertheless, selective cases have been managed conservatively,[157] and patients should be assessed on a case-by-case basis.

30.6.8 Treatment of Parasitic Spinal Infections

Surgery is usually the treatment modality of choice for hydatid cyst disease. Laminectomy is performed with cyst removal, followed by antihelmintic drugs such as albendazole or mebendazole. Intraoperative rupture may occur with spillage of the cyst's contents and result in recurrence of multiple cysts and/or anaphylactic reaction. Although the operating microscope may help, no specific technique is known to completely avoid this problem.[81] Some have advocated intraoperative irrigation with hypertonic saline or povidone iodine solutions with the hopes of parasites being destroyed by osmotic disruption; nevertheless, this strategy remains unproven.[81,158,159]

Spinal neurocysticercosis has been treated both medically and surgically. Medical treatment consists of antihelmintics, such as albendazole or praziquantel. Steroid therapy may also be administered to reduce the inflammatory reaction seen with death of the cysts. Nevertheless, if any neurologic deficits are seen, surgery is usually recommended. This may require intraoperative microscopic intradural dissection and intraoperative ultrasonography. Meticulous sharp dissection, with gentle irrigation and Valsalva maneuvers, may assist in cyst removal. Subarachnoid scarring may require duraplasty to reestablish CSF flow if there is obstruction. Systemic cysticercosis may need concurrent treatment.[84]

30.6.9 Postoperative Wound Infections

Postoperative wound infections may occur in as often as 0.7 to 16% of patients undergoing spine surgery. They continue to be a source of morbidity and compromise outcomes with increased hospital stay, increased mortality, and higher reoperation rates. All contributing to an increase in cost, which was estimated to be $200,000 per patient. Risk factors for postoperative infections can be divided into unchangeable factors, which are patient related, and changeable factors, which are procedure related. Patient-related risk factors include age (older than 70), American Society of Anesthesiologists (ASA) score of 2, and medical comorbidities such as diabetes mellitus and obesity, malnutrition, long-term steroid use, smoking, previous surgery, and immunologic competency.[160,161,162] It should be stressed that malnutrition may be a very important risk factor for postoperative spinal infection. Protein malnutrition and calorie malnutrition are both associated with difficulties with wound healing and an increased incident of wound infection and immunosuppression.[163] Malnourished patients are 15 times more likely to acquire an infection after spinal procedures.

Procedure-related risk factors include duration of surgery, estimated blood loss, blood transfusion, use of instrumentation, number of levels, multiple-staged interventions, and length of hospitalization.[161] Another very significant variable affecting the rate of infection is the type of operation.[164] Although risk factors cannot be completely eliminated, modifiable risk factors should be considered to minimize overall risk.

Wound infections are often diagnosed when a patient presents with the new onset of peri-incisional pain after experiencing relief of their initial surgical pain. This is typically about 15 days from the index procedure. Also, wound drainage is present in the majority of cases.[165] Most commonly, fever is not present. The wound is often reddish in appearance. Additionally, the ESR may be elevated.[165] Nevertheless, low virulence wound infections may present years after the index procedure with the sudden onset of local pain and swelling without fever after the patient being pain-free for years.[166] In these cases, patients may have both a have normal ESR and CRP.[166]

Radiographic imaging is often of limited value. There may be confusion on both CT and MRI in terms of whether a postoperative fluid collection is a sterile seroma versus an infected collection. Additionally, instrumentation-related medical artifact may confuse the issue further.[164] *Staphylococcus aureus* is the most common organism implicated, followed by *S. epidermidis*. Although these organisms are usually responsible for postoperative wound infection, mixed gram-positive and gram-negative organisms may be involved.[164] Recently, *Propionibacterium acnes* and other slow-growing organisms have been implicated in chronic indolent spinal surgery infections.[166,167]

Wound infectious should be a thought of as a surgical problem. Medical therapy alone is rarely indicated for postoperative spinal wound infections. When a patient presents with early signs and symptoms of a wound infection, all too often a clinician may attempt treatment with oral antibiotics in the hopes of eradicating a potential infection. Rarely is this strategy useful. Less aggressive therapies may be indicated for patients who are immunocompromised or too debilitated to tolerate an extensive procedure. Yet these patients, too, at the least will require bedside opening of their wounds, irrigation, and débridement. Irrigation and débridement is the mainstay of treatment and should be considered in the majority of patients. Débridement consists of aggressive removal of necrotic tissue and foreign materials, including sutures. The vast majority of time the fascia should be opened. In terms of spinal instrumentation and bone graft, these could be left in place. Only in situations where the infection fails to clear after multiple débridements should consideration of removal of instrumentation and bone graft be made.[164]

Serial débridements are often necessary. Additionally, drainage with copious amounts of antibiotic containing saline solution may be useful.[165] Others have advocated inflow–outflow-type drainage systems. Massie et al[168] reported healing of postoperative wound infections with such as system. Additionally, Levi, et al[169] reported using such systems to clear infections in patients after spinal instrumentation was placed. Others have reported success with vacuum-assisted wound closure following wound infection.[170] These may be especially useful after serial wound débridements.[171] Plastics surgery consultation and closure may be necessary, especially with infection post deformity procedures. Closure of thoracolumbar wounds and vertebral osteomyelitis after scoliosis surgery often proves difficult because of tissue tautness and lack of usable tissue. Latissimus dorsi myocutaneous flaps may be useful in closure and providing blood supply to open incisions in the lower thoracic and thoracolumbar areas, whereas incisions involving the lumbosacral area may be better covered with a latissimus dorsi flap with an additional transposed gluteus maximus muscle flap to obtain coverage over the caudal extent of the wound. This may allow healing of once-infected wounds and allow preservation of initially placed spinal instrumentation and bone graft.[172]

Addressing preoperative risk factors before surgery may prevent wound infections. Patients can have their nutritional status optimized following a wound infection. Additionally, a single dose of antibiotics before skin incision is made may be of benefit in reducing infections.[173] Further does of antibiotics may be given intraoperatively if the procedure lasts beyond 4 hours. Postoperative doses and doses to "cover" drains/catheters, etc., may increase the risk of secondary infections.[174] Ultraclean air (vertical exponential filtered airflow system) operating rooms may also have a role.[175] Additionally, frequent intraoperative irrigation, with a solution containing dilute iodine (20–50 ppm), may be of benefit in reducing infection.[174] Recently, intrawound vancomycin has been used for prophylaxis and has appeared to have lower the incidence of spine surgical infections from 4.1% to 1.3% in retrospective studies.[176,177] Adverse events, although rare (0.3%), have been reported with its use, including classic adverse effects such as ototoxicity and renal dysfunction. Spinal surgery–related complications have been noted with increased rates of culture negative seroma.[178] Vancomycin also has been noted to negatively impact osteoblastic function in a dose-dependent fashion, which may potentially lead to pseudoarthrosis.[179]

30.7 Conclusion

Spinal infections are potentially fatal neurosurgical emergencies. A high index of suspicion is required for their diagnosis. Although many infections are treated medically, there should be a low threshold for surgical intervention, especially in cases of symptomatic neural compression, instability, and deformity. Familiarity with rare causes of spinal infection such as fungi and parasites may aid the clinician in appropriate selection of treatment. Wound infections should be treated surgically with débridement, irrigation, and appropriate antimicrobial therapy.

References

[1]   Quiñones-Hinojosa A, Jun P, Jacobs R, Rosenberg WS, Weinstein PR. General principles in the medical and surgical management of spinal infections: a multidisciplinary approach. Neurosurg Focus. 2004; 17(6):E1
[2]   Lee MC, Wang MY, Fessler RG, Liauw J, Kim DH. Instrumentation in patients with spinal infection. Neurosurg Focus. 2004; 17(6):E7
[3]   Acosta FL, Jr, Chin CT, Quiñones-Hinojosa A, Ames CP, Weinstein PR, Chou D. Diagnosis and management of adult pyogenic osteomyelitis of the cervical spine. Neurosurg Focus. 2004; 17(6):E2
[4]   Tali ET. Spinal infections. Eur J Radiol. 2004; 50(2):120–133
[5]   Batson OV. The vertebral system of veins as a means for cancer dissemination. Prog Clin Cancer. 1967; 3:1–18
[6]   Alcock E, Regaard A, Browne J. Facet joint injection: a rare form cause of epidural abscess formation. Pain. 2003; 103(1–2):209–210
[7]   Baltz MS, Tate DE, Glaser JA. Lumbar facet joint infection associated with epidural and paraspinal abscess. Clin Orthop Relat Res. 1997(339):109–112
[8]   Halpin DS, Gibson RD. Septic arthritis of a lumbar facet joint. J Bone Joint Surg Br. 1987; 69(3):457–459

[9]   Heenan SD, Britton J. Septic arthritis in a lumbar facet joint: a rare cause of an epidural abscess. Neuroradiology. 1995; 37(6):462–464
[10] Ogura T, Mikami Y, Hase H, Mori M, Hayashida T, Kubo T. Septic arthritis of a lumbar facet joint associated with epidural and paraspinal abscess. Orthopedics. 2005; 28(2):173–175
[11] Okazaki K, Sasaki K, Matsuda S, et al. Pyogenic arthritis of a lumbar facet joint. Am J Orthop. 2000; 29(3):222–224
[12] Nussbaum ES, Rigamonti D, Standiford H, Numaguchi Y, Wolf AL, Robinson WL. Spinal epidural abscess: a report of 40 cases and review. Surg Neurol. 1992; 38(3):225–231
[13] Butler EG, Dohrmann PJ, Stark RJ. Spinal subdural abscess. Clin Exp Neurol. 1988; 25:67–70
[14] Vora YA, Raad II, McCutcheon IE. Intramedullary abscess from group F Streptococcus. Surg Infect (Larchmt). 2004; 5(2):200–204
[15] Elmaci I, Kurtkaya O, Peker S, et al. Cervical spinal cord intramedullary abscess. Case report. J Neurosurg Sci. 2001; 45(4):213–215, discussion 215
[16] Kumar R. Spinal tuberculosis: with reference to the children of northern India. Childs Nerv Syst. 2005; 21(1):19–26
[17] Erşahin Y. Intramedullary abscess of the spinal cord. Childs Nerv Syst. 2003; 19(10–11):777
[18] Sverzut JM, Laval C, Smadja P, Gigaud M, Sevely A, Manelfe C. Spinal cord abscess in a heroin addict: case report. Neuroradiology. 1998; 40(7):455–458
[19] Tacconi L, Arulampalam T, Johnston FG, Thomas DG. Intramedullary spinal cord abscess: case report. Neurosurgery. 1995; 37(4):817–819
[20] Curry WT, Jr, Hoh BL, Amin-Hanjani S, Eskandar EN. Spinal epidural abscess: clinical presentation, management, and outcome. Surg Neurol. 2005; 63(4):364–371, discussion 371
[21] Siddiq F, Chowfin A, Tight R, Sahmoun AE, Smego RA, Jr. Medical vs surgical management of spinal epidural abscess. Arch Intern Med. 2004; 164(22):2409–2412
[22] Hadjipavlou AG, Mader JT, Necessary JT, Muffoletto AJ. Hematogenous pyogenic spinal infections and their surgical management. Spine. 2000; 25(13):1668–1679
[23] Frat JP, Godet C, Grollier G, Blanc JL, Robert R. Cervical spinal epidural abscess and meningitis due to Prevotella oris and Peptostreptococcus micros after retropharyngeal surgery. Intensive Care Med. 2004; 30(8):1695
[24] Pereira CE, Lynch JC. Spinal epidural abscess: an analysis of 24 cases. Surg Neurol. 2005; 63(Suppl 1):S26–S29
[25] Kim CW, Perry A, Currier B, Yaszemski M, Garfin SR. Fungal infections of the spine. Clin Orthop Relat Res. 2006; 444(444):92–99
[26] German JW, Kellie SM, Pai MP, Turner PT. Treatment of a chronic Scedosporium apiospermum vertebral osteomyelitis. Case report. Neurosurg Focus. 2004; 17(6):E9
[27] Lonser RR, Brodke DS, Dailey AT. Vertebral osteomyelitis secondary to Pseudallescheria boydii. J Spinal Disord. 2001; 14(4):361–364
[28] Sheehan JP, Sheehan J, Lopes MB, Jane JA, Sr. Intramedullary spinal cysticercosis. Case report and review of the literature. Neurosurg Focus. 2002; 12(6):e10
[29] Delobel P, Signate A, El Guedj M, et al. Unusual form of neurocysticercosis associated with HIV infection. Eur J Neurol. 2004; 11(1):55–58
[30] Sheehan JP, Sheehan JM, Lopes MB, Jane JA. Intramedullary cervical spine cysticercosis. Acta Neurochir (Wien). 2002; 144(10):1061–1063
[31] Parmar H, Shah J, Patwardhan V, et al. MR imaging in intramedullary cysticercosis. Neuroradiology. 2001; 43(11):961–967
[32] Lau KY, Roebuck DJ, Mok V, et al. MRI demonstration of subarachnoid neurocysticercosis simulating metastatic disease. Neuroradiology. 1998; 40(11):724–726
[33] Mohanty A, Das S, Kolluri VR, Das BS. Spinal extradural cysticercosis: a case report. Spinal Cord. 1998; 36(4):285–287
[34] Garza-Mercado R. Intramedullary cysticercosis. Surg Neurol. 1976; 5(6):331–332
[35] Atalay B, Azap O, Cekinmez M, Caner H, Haberal M. Nocardial epidural abscess of the thoracic spinal cord and review of the literature. J Infect Chemother. 2005; 11(3):169–171
[36] Graat HC, Van Ooij A, Day GA, McPhee IB. Nocardia farcinica spinal osteomyelitis. Spine. 2002; 27(10):E253–E257
[37] Lakshmi V, Sundaram C, Meena AK, Murthy JM. Primary cutaneous nocardiosis with epidural abscess caused by Nocardia brasiliensis: a case report. Neurol India. 2002; 50(1):90–92
[38] Siao P, McCabe P, Yagnik P. Nocardial spinal epidural abscess. Neurology. 1989; 39(7):996

[39] Sampath P, Rigamonti D. Spinal epidural abscess: a review of epidemiology, diagnosis, and treatment. J Spinal Disord. 1999; 12(2):89–93

[40] Durack DT, Scheld WM, Whitley RJ. Infections of the Central Nervous System. 2nd ed. Philadelphia, PA: Lippincott-Raven; 1997

[41] Marks WA, Bodensteiner JB. Anterior cervical epidural abscess with pneumococcus in an infant. J Child Neurol. 1988; 3(1):25–29

[42] Bremer AA, Darouiche RO. Spinal epidural abscess presenting as intra-abdominal pathology: a case report and literature review. J Emerg Med. 2004; 26(1):51–56

[43] Zimmerer SM, Conen A, Müller AA, et al. Spinal epidural abscess: aetiology, predispoent factors and clinical outcomes in a 4-year prospective study. Eur Spine J. 2011; 20(12):2228–2234

[44] Kovalik EC, Raymond JR, Albers FJ, et al. A clustering of epidural abscesses in chronic hemodialysis patients: risks of salvaging access catheters in cases of infection. J Am Soc Nephrol. 1996; 7(10):2264–2267

[45] Obrador GT, Levenson DJ. Spinal epidural abscess in hemodialysis patients: report of three cases and review of the literature. Am J Kidney Dis. 1996; 27(1):75–83

[46] Philipneri M, Al-Aly Z, Amin K, Gellens ME, Bastani B. Routine replacement of tunneled, cuffed, hemodialysis catheters eliminates paraspinal/vertebral infections in patients with catheter-associated bacteremia. Am J Nephrol. 2003; 23(4):202–207

[47] Huang RC, Shapiro GS, Lim M, Sandhu HS, Lutz GE, Herzog RJ. Cervical epidural abscess after epidural steroid injection. Spine. 2004; 29(1):E7–E9

[48] Khan IA, Vaccaro AR, Zlotolow DA. Management of vertebral diskitis and osteomyelitis. Orthopedics. 1999; 22(8):758–765

[49] Blumberg KD, Silveri CP, Balderston RA. Presentation and treatment of pyogenic vertebral osteomyelitis. Semin Spine Surg. 1996; 8(2):115–125

[50] Broner FA, Garland DE, Zigler JE. Spinal infections in the immunocompromised host. Orthop Clin North Am. 1996; 27(1):37–46

[51] Rezai AR, Woo HH, Errico TJ, Cooper PR. Contemporary management of spinal osteomyelitis. Neurosurgery. 1999; 44(5):1018–1025, discussion 1025–1026

[52] Lestini WF, Bell GR. Spinal infection: patient evaluation. Semin Spine Surg. 1996; 8(2):81–94

[53] Calderone RR, Larsen JM. Overview and classification of spinal infections. Orthop Clin North Am. 1996; 27(1):1–8

[54] Maiuri F, Iaconetta G, Gallicchio B, Manto A, Briganti F. Spondylodiscitis. Clinical and magnetic resonance diagnosis. Spine. 1997; 22(15):1741–1746

[55] Vaccaro AR, Harris BM. Presentation and treatment of pyogenic vertebral osteomyelitis. Semin Spine Surg. 2000; 12:183–191

[56] Currier BL. Spinal infections. In: An HS, ed. Principles and Techniques of Spine Surgery. Baltimore, MD: Lippincott Williams & Wilkins; 1996:567–603

[57] Desai KI, Muzumdar DP, Goel A. Holocord intramedullary abscess: an unusual case with review of literature. Spinal Cord. 1999; 37(12):866–870

[58] Byrne RW, von Roenn KA, Whisler WW. Intramedullary abscess: a report of two cases and a review of the literature. Neurosurgery. 1994; 35(2):321–326, discussion 326

[59] Koppel BS, Daras M, Duffy KR. Intramedullary spinal cord abscess. Neurosurgery. 1990; 26(1):145–146

[60] Benzil DL, Epstein MH, Knuckey NW. Intramedullary epidermoid associated with an intramedullary spinal abscess secondary to a dermal sinus. Neurosurgery. 1992; 30(1):118–121

[61] Cokça F, Meço O, Arasil E, Unlü A. An intramedullary dermoid cyst abscess due to Brucella abortus biotype 3 at T11–L2 spinal levels. Infection. 1994; 22(5):359–360

[62] Hardwidge C, Palsingh J, Williams B. Pyomyelia: an intramedullary spinal abscess complicating lumbar lipoma with spina bifida. Br J Neurosurg. 1993; 7(4):419–422

[63] Almeida A. Tuberculosis of the spine and spinal cord. Eur J Radiol. 2005; 55(2):193–201

[64] Sharif HS, Morgan JL, al Shahed MS, al Thagafi MY. Role of CT and MR imaging in the management of tuberculous spondylitis. Radiol Clin North Am. 1995; 33(4):787–804

[65] Tekkök IH, Berker M, Ozcan OE, Ozgen T, Akalin E. Brucellosis of the spine. Neurosurgery. 1993; 33(5):838–844

[66] Tay BK, Deckey J, Hu SS. Spinal infections. J Am Acad Orthop Surg. 2002; 10(3):188–197

[67] Pappas G, Akritidis N, Bosilkovski M, Tsianos E. Brucellosis. N Engl J Med. 2005; 352(22):2325–2336

[68] Solera J, Lozano E, Martínez-Alfaro E, Espinosa A, Castillejos ML, Abad L. Brucellar spondylitis: review of 35 cases and literature survey. Clin Infect Dis. 1999; 29(6):1440–1449

[69] Tur BS, Suldur N, Ataman S, Ozturk EA, Bingol A, Atay MB. Brucellar spondylitis: a rare cause of spinal cord compression. Spinal Cord. 2004; 42(5):321–324

[70] Chia SL, Tan BH, Tan CT, Tan SB. Candida spondylodiscitis and epidural abscess: management with shorter courses of anti-fungal therapy in combination with surgical debridement. J Infect. 2005; 51(1):17–23

[71] Abu Jawdeh L, Haidar R, Bitar F, et al. Aspergillus vertebral osteomyelitis in a child with a primary monocyte killing defect: response to GM-CSF therapy. J Infect. 2000; 41(1):97–100

[72] Lewicky YM, Roberto RF, Curtin SL. The unique complications of coccidioidomycosis of the spine: a detailed time line of disease progression and suppression. Spine. 2004; 29(19):E435–E441

[73] Hott JS, Horn E, Sonntag VK, Coons SW, Shetter A. Intramedullary histoplasmosis spinal cord abscess in a nonendemic region: case report and review of the literature. J Spinal Disord Tech. 2003; 16(2):212–215

[74] Musoke F. Spinal African histoplasmosis simulating tuberculous spondylitis. Afr Health Sci. 2001; 1(1):28–29

[75] N'dri Oka D, Varlet G, Kakou M, Zunon-Kipre Y, Broalet E, Ba Zeze V. [Spondylodiscitis due to Histoplasma duboisii. Report of two cases and review of the literature] Neurochirurgie. 2001; 47(4):431–434

[76] Lecamus JL, Ribault L, Floch JJ. [A new case of African histoplasmosis with multiple localizations in the bones] Med Trop (Mars). 1986; 46(3):307–309

[77] Goldman AB, Freiberger RH. Localized infectious and neuropathic diseases. Semin Roentgenol. 1979; 14(1):19–32

[78] Jain M, Sharma S, Jain TS. Cryptococcosis of thoracic vertebra simulating tuberculosis: diagnosis by fine-needle aspiration biopsy cytology—a case report. Diagn Cytopathol. 1999; 20(6):385–386

[79] Liu PY. Cryptococcal osteomyelitis: case report and review. Diagn Microbiol Infect Dis. 1998; 30(1):33–35

[80] Miller DJ, Mejicano GC. Vertebral osteomyelitis due to Candida species: case report and literature review. Clin Infect Dis. 2001; 33(4):523–530

[81] Schnepper GD, Johnson WD. Recurrent spinal hydatidosis in North America. Case report and review of the literature. Neurosurg Focus. 2004; 17(6):E8

[82] Iplikçioğlu AC, Kökeş F, Bayar A, Doğanay S, Buharali Z. Spinal invasion of pulmonary hydatidosis: computed tomographic demonstration. Neurosurgery. 1991; 29(3):467–468

[83] Braithwaite PA, Lees RF. Vertebral hydatid disease: radiological assessment. Radiology. 1981; 140(3):763–766

[84] Alsina GA, Johnson JP, McBride DQ, Rhoten PR, Mehringer CM, Stokes JK. Spinal neurocysticercosis. Neurosurg Focus. 2002; 12(6):e8

[85] Kurrein F, Vickers AA. Cysticercosis of the spine. Ann Trop Med Parasitol. 1977; 71(2):213–217

[86] Heller JE, Baron EM, Weaver MW. Cervical epidural abscess. In: Lee JY, Lim MR, Albert TA, eds. Challenges in Cervical Spine Surgery. New York, NY: Thieme; 2007

[87] Carragee EJ. Pyogenic vertebral osteomyelitis. J Bone Joint Surg Am. 1997; 79(6):874–880

[88] Rath SA, Neff U, Schneider O, Richter HP. Neurosurgical management of thoracic and lumbar vertebral osteomyelitis and discitis in adults: a review of 43 consecutive surgically treated patients. Neurosurgery. 1996; 38(5):926–933

[89] Bass SN, Ailani RK, Shekar R, Gerblich AA. Pyogenic vertebral osteomyelitis presenting as exudative pleural effusion: a series of five cases. Chest. 1998; 114(2):642–647

[90] Rigamonti D, Liem L, Wolf AL, et al. Epidural abscess in the cervical spine. Mt Sinai J Med. 1994; 61(4):357–362

[91] Wong D, Raymond NJ. Spinal epidural abscess. N Z Med J. 1998; 111(1073):345–347

[92] Mehta SH, Shih R. Cervical epidural abscess associated with massively elevated erythrocyte sedimentation rate. J Emerg Med. 2004; 26(1):107–109

[93] Khan MH, Smith PN, Rao N, Donaldson WF. Serum C-reactive protein levels correlate with clinical response in patients treated with antibiotics for wound infections after spinal surgery. Spine J. 2006; 6(3):311–315

[94] Rothman SL. The diagnosis of infections of the spine by modern imaging techniques. Orthop Clin North Am. 1996; 27(1):15–31

[95] Cornett CA, Vincent SA, Crow J, Hewlett A. Bacterial spine infections in adults: evaluation and management. J Am Acad Orthop Surg. 2016; 24(1):11–18

[96] Klekamp J, Samii M. Extradural infections of the spine. Spinal Cord. 1999; 37(2):103–109

[97] Parkinson JF, Sekhon LH. Spinal epidural abscess: appearance on magnetic resonance imaging as a guide to surgical management. Report of five cases. Neurosurg Focus. 2004; 17(6):E12

[98] Thurnher MM, Post MJ, Jinkins JR. MRI of infections and neoplasms of the spine and spinal cord in 55 patients with AIDS. Neuroradiology. 2000; 42(8):551–563

[99] Boutin RD, Brossmann J, Sartoris DJ, Reilly D, Resnick D. Update on imaging of orthopedic infections. Orthop Clin North Am. 1998; 29(1):41–66

[100] Küker W, Mull M, Mayfrank L, Töpper R, Thron A. Epidural spinal infection. Variability of clinical and magnetic resonance imaging findings. Spine. 1997; 22(5):544–550, discussion 551

[101] Murphy KJ, Brunberg JA, Quint DJ, Kazanjian PH. Spinal cord infection: myelitis and abscess formation. AJNR Am J Neuroradiol. 1998; 19(2):341–348

[102] Kim CJ, Song KH, Jeon JH, et al. A comparative study of pyogenic and tuberculous spondylodiscitis. Spine. 2010; 35(21):E1096–E1100

[103] Boachie-Adjei O, Squillante RG. Tuberculosis of the spine. Orthop Clin North Am. 1996; 27(1):95–103

[104] McLain RF, Isada C. Spinal tuberculosis deserves a place on the radar screen. Cleve Clin J Med. 2004; 71(7):537–539, 543–549

[105] Colmenero JD, Ruiz-Mesa JD, Sanjuan-Jimenez R, Sobrino B, Morata P. Establishing the diagnosis of tuberculous vertebral osteomyelitis. Eur Spine J. 2013; 22(Suppl 4):579–586

[106] Cheng VC, Yam WC, Hung IF, et al. Clinical evaluation of the polymerase chain reaction for the rapid diagnosis of tuberculosis. J Clin Pathol. 2004; 57(3):281–285

[107] Ruiz-Mesa JD, Sánchez-Gonzalez J, Reguera JM, Martín L, Lopez-Palmero S, Colmenero JD. Rose Bengal test: diagnostic yield and use for the rapid diagnosis of human brucellosis in emergency departments in endemic areas. Clin Microbiol Infect. 2005; 11(3):221–225

[108] Colmenero JD, Jiménez-Mejías ME, Sánchez-Lora FJ, et al. Pyogenic, tuberculous, and brucellar vertebral osteomyelitis: a descriptive and comparative study of 219 cases. Ann Rheum Dis. 1997; 56(12):709–715

[109] Krauss WE, McCormick PC. Infections of the dural spaces. Neurosurg Clin N Am. 1992; 3(2):421–433

[110] Wheeler D, Keiser P, Rigamonti D, Keay S. Medical management of spinal epidural abscesses: case report and review. Clin Infect Dis. 1992; 15(1):22–27

[111] Godeau B, Brun-Buisson C, Brugières P, Roucoules J, Schaeffer A. Complete resolution of spinal epidural abscess with short medical treatment alone. Eur J Med. 1993; 2(8):510–511

[112] Panagiotopoulos V, Konstantinou D, Solomou E, Panagiotopoulos E, Marangos M, Maraziotis T. Extended cervicolumbar spinal epidural abscess associated with paraparesis successfully decompressed using a minimally invasive technique. Spine. 2004; 29(14):E300–E303

[113] Lyu RK, Chen CJ, Tang LM, Chen ST. Spinal epidural abscess successfully treated with percutaneous, computed tomography-guided, needle aspiration and parenteral antibiotic therapy: case report and review of the literature. Neurosurgery. 2002; 51(2):509–512, discussion 512

[114] Moriya M, Kimura T, Yamamoto Y, Abe K, Sakoda S. Successful treatment of cervical spinal epidural abscess without surgery. Intern Med. 2005; 44(10):1110

[115] Harrington P, Millner PA, Veale D. Inappropriate medical management of spinal epidural abscess. Ann Rheum Dis. 2001; 60(3):218–222

[116] Carragee EJ. The clinical use of magnetic resonance imaging in pyogenic vertebral osteomyelitis. Spine. 1997; 22(7):780–785

[117] Sapico FL. Microbiology and antimicrobial therapy of spinal infections. Orthop Clin North Am. 1996; 27(1):9–13

[118] Savoia M. An overview of antibiotics in the treatment of bacterial, mycobacterial, and fungal osteomyelitis. Semin Spine Surg. 1996; 8(2):105–114

[119] Singh K, DeWald CJ, Hammerberg KW, DeWald RL. Long structural allografts in the treatment of anterior spinal column defects. Clin Orthop Relat Res. 2002(394):121–129

[120] Kuklo TR, Potter BK, Bell RS, Moquin RR, Rosner MK. Single-stage treatment of pyogenic spinal infection with titanium mesh cages. J Spinal Disord Tech. 2006; 19(5):376–382

[121] Robinson Y, Tschoeke SK, Kayser R, Boehm H, Heyde CE. Reconstruction of large defects in vertebral osteomyelitis with expandable titanium cages. Int Orthop. 2009; 33(3):745–749

[122] Friedman JA, Maher CO, Quast LM, McClelland RL, Ebersold MJ. Spontaneous disc space infections in adults. Surg Neurol. 2002; 57(2):81–86

[123] Eismont FJ, Bohlman HH, Soni PL, Goldberg VM, Freehafer AA. Pyogenic and fungal vertebral osteomyelitis with paralysis. J Bone Joint Surg Am. 1983; 65(1):19–29

[124] McGuire RA, Eismont FJ. The fate of autogenous bone graft in surgically treated pyogenic vertebral osteomyelitis. J Spinal Disord. 1994; 7(3):206–215

[125] A 15-year assessment of controlled trials of the management of tuberculosis of the spine in Korea and Hong Kong. Thirteenth Report of the Medical Research Council Working Party on Tuberculosis of the Spine. J Bone Joint Surg Br. 1998; 80(3):456–462

[126] Cahill DW, Love LC, Rechtine GR. Pyogenic osteomyelitis of the spine in the elderly. J Neurosurg. 1991; 74(6):878–886

[127] Lifeso RM. Pyogenic spinal sepsis in adults. Spine. 1990; 15(12):1265–1271

[128] Fang D, Cheung KM, Dos Remedios ID, Lee YK, Leong JC. Pyogenic vertebral osteomyelitis: treatment by anterior spinal debridement and fusion. J Spinal Disord. 1994; 7(2):173–180

[129] Jeanneret B, Magerl F. Treatment of osteomyelitis of the spine using percutaneous suction/irrigation and percutaneous external spinal fixation. J Spinal Disord. 1994; 7(3):185–205

[130] Redfern RM, Miles J, Banks AJ, Dervin E. Stabilisation of the infected spine. J Neurol Neurosurg Psychiatry. 1988; 51(6):803–807

[131] Krödel A, Krüger A, Lohscheidt K, Pfahler M, Refior HJ. Anterior debridement, fusion, and extrafocal stabilization in the treatment of osteomyelitis of the spine. J Spinal Disord. 1999; 12(1):17–26

[132] Liebergall M, Chaimsky G, Lowe J, Robin GC, Floman Y. Pyogenic vertebral osteomyelitis with paralysis. Prognosis and treatment. Clin Orthop Relat Res. 1991(269):142–150

[133] Heary RF, Hunt CD, Wolansky LJ. Rapid bony destruction with pyogenic vertebral osteomyelitis. Surg Neurol. 1994; 41(1):34–39

[134] Ogden AT, Kaiser MG. Single-stage debridement and instrumentation for pyogenic spinal infections. Neurosurg Focus. 2004; 17(6):E5

[135] Hsieh PC, Wienecke RJ, O'Shaughnessy BA, Koski TR, Ondra SL. Surgical strategies for vertebral osteomyelitis and epidural abscess. Neurosurg Focus. 2004; 17(6):E4

[136] Hayashi A, Maruyama Y, Okajima Y, Motegi M. Vascularized iliac bone graft based on a pedicle of upper lumbar vessels for anterior fusion of the thoraco-lumbar spine. Br J Plast Surg. 1994; 47(6):425–430

[137] Yelizarov VG, Minachenko VK, Gerasimov OR, Pshenisnov KP. Vascularized bone flaps for thoracolumbar spinal fusion. Ann Plast Surg. 1993; 31(6):532–538

[138] Heggeness MH, Esses SI, Errico T, Yuan HA. Late infection of spinal instrumentation by hematogenous seeding. Spine. 1993; 18(4):492–496

[139] Grados F, Lescure FX, Senneville E, Flipo RM, Schmit JL, Fardellone P. Suggestions for managing pyogenic (non-tuberculous) discitis in adults. Joint Bone Spine. 2007; 74(2):133–139

[140] Bartels RH, Gonera EG, van der Spek JA, Thijssen HO, Mullaart RA, Gabreëls FJ. Intramedullary spinal cord abscess. A case report. Spine. 1995; 20(10):1199–1204

[141] Pawar UM, Kundnani V, Agashe V, Nene A, Nene A. Multidrug-resistant tuberculosis of the spine—is it the beginning of the end? A study of twenty-five culture proven multidrug-resistant tuberculosis spine patients. Spine. 2009; 34(22):E806–E810

[142] Rajasekaran S, Khandelwal G. Drug therapy in spinal tuberculosis. Eur Spine J. 2013; 22(Suppl 4):587–593

[143] Zhang X, Ji J, Liu B. Management of spinal tuberculosis: a systematic review and meta-analysis. J Int Med Res. 2013; 41(5):1395–1407

[144] Jain AK, Dhammi IK. Tuberculosis of the spine: a review. Clin Orthop Relat Res. 2007; 460(460):39–49

[145] Rajasekaran S. Kyphotic deformity in spinal tuberculosis and its management. Int Orthop. 2012; 36(2):359–365

[146] Sun L, Song Y, Liu L, Gong Q, Zhou C. One-stage posterior surgical treatment for lumbosacral tuberculosis with major vertebral body loss and kyphosis. Orthopedics. 2013; 36(8):e1082–e1090

[147] Swanson AN, Pappou IP, Cammisa FP, Girardi FP. Chronic infections of the spine: surgical indications and treatments. Clin Orthop Relat Res. 2006; 444(444):100–106

[148] Wang X, Pang X, Wu P, Luo C, Shen X. One-stage anterior debridement, bone grafting and posterior instrumentation vs. single posterior debridement, bone grafting, and instrumentation for the treatment of thoracic and lumbar spinal tuberculosis. Eur Spine J. 2014; 23(4):830–837

[149] Kapoor SK, Agarwal PN, Jain BK, Jr, Kumar R. Video-assisted thoracoscopic decompression of tubercular spondylitis: clinical evaluation. Spine. 2005; 30(20):E605–E610

[150] Huang TJ, Hsu RW, Chen SH, Liu HP. Video-assisted thoracoscopic surgery in managing tuberculous spondylitis. Clin Orthop Relat Res. 2000(379):143–153

[151] Chacko AG, Moorthy RK, Chandy MJ. The transpedicular approach in the management of thoracic spine tuberculosis: a short-term follow up study. Spine. 2004; 29(17):E363–E367

[152] Bodur H, Erbay A, Colpan A, Akinci E. Brucellar spondylitis. Rheumatol Int. 2004; 24(4):221–226

[153] Erdem H, Elaldi N, Batirel A, et al. Comparison of brucellar and tuberculous spondylodiscitis patients: results of the multicenter "Backbone-1 Study". Spine J. 2015; 15(12):2509–2517

[154] Vajramani GV, Nagmoti MB, Patil CS. Neurobrucellosis presenting as an intra-medullary spinal cord abscess. Ann Clin Microbiol Antimicrob. 2005; 4:14

[155] Gupta PK, Mahapatra AK, Gaind R, Bhandari S, Musa MM, Lad SD. Aspergillus spinal epidural abscess. Pediatr Neurosurg. 2001; 35(1):18–23

[156] Parr AM, Fewer D. Intramedullary blastomycosis in a child: case report. Can J Neurol Sci. 2004; 31(2):282–285

[157] Lindner A, Becker G, Warmuth-Metz M, Schalke BC, Bogdahn U, Toyka KV. Magnetic resonance image findings of spinal intramedullary abscess caused by Candida albicans: case report. Neurosurgery. 1995; 36(2):411–412

[158] Bavbek M, Inci S, Tahta K, Bertan V. Primary multiple spinal extradural hydatid cysts. Case report and review of the literature [corrected]. Paraplegia. 1992; 30(7):517–519

[159] Erşahin Y, Mutluer S, Güzelbağ E. Intracranial hydatid cysts in children. Neurosurgery. 1993; 33(2):219–224, discussion 224–225

[160] Pull ter Gunne AF, Cohen DB. Incidence, prevalence, and analysis of risk factors for surgical site infection following adult spinal surgery. Spine. 2009; 34(13):1422–1428

[161] Koutsoumbelis S, Hughes AP, Girardi FP, et al. Risk factors for postoperative infection following posterior lumbar instrumented arthrodesis. J Bone Joint Surg Am. 2011; 93(17):1627–1633

[162] Olsen MA, Lefta M, Dietz JR, et al. Risk factors for surgical site infection after major breast operation. J Am Coll Surg. 2008; 207(3):326–335

[163] Klein JD, Garfin SR. Nutritional status in the patient with spinal infection. Orthop Clin North Am. 1996; 27(1):33–36

[164] Beiner JM, Grauer J, Kwon BK, Vaccaro AR. Postoperative wound infections of the spine. Neurosurg Focus. 2003; 15(3):E14

[165] Weinstein MA, McCabe JP, Cammisa FP, Jr. Postoperative spinal wound infection: a review of 2,391 consecutive index procedures. J Spinal Disord. 2000; 13(5):422–426

[166] Muschik M, Lück W, Schlenzka D. Implant removal for late-developing infection after instrumented posterior spinal fusion for scoliosis: reinstrumentation reduces loss of correction. A retrospective analysis of 45 cases. Eur Spine J. 2004; 13(7):645–651

[167] Hahn F, Zbinden R, Min K. Late implant infections caused by Propionibacterium acnes in scoliosis surgery. Eur Spine J. 2005; 14(8):783–788

[168] Massie JB, Heller JG, Abitbol JJ, McPherson D, Garfin SR. Postoperative posterior spinal wound infections. Clin Orthop Relat Res. 1992(284):99–108

[169] Levi AD, Dickman CA, Sonntag VK. Management of postoperative infections after spinal instrumentation. J Neurosurg. 1997; 86(6):975–980

[170] Yuan-Innes MJ, Temple CL, Lacey MS. Vacuum-assisted wound closure: a new approach to spinal wounds with exposed hardware. Spine. 2001; 26(3):E30–E33

[171] Mehbod AA, Ogilvie JW, Pinto MR, et al. Postoperative deep wound infections in adults after spinal fusion: management with vacuum-assisted wound closure. J Spinal Disord Tech. 2005; 18(1):14–17

[172] Mitra A, Mitra A, Harlin S. Treatment of massive thoracolumbar wounds and vertebral osteomyelitis following scoliosis surgery. Plast Reconstr Surg. 2004; 113(1):206–213

[173] Savitz MH, Katz SS. Rationale for prophylactic antibiotics and neurosurgery. Neurosurgery. 1981; 9(2):142–144

[174] Brown EM, Pople IK, de Louvois J, et al; British Society for Antimicrobial Chemotherapy Working Party on Neurosurgical Infections. Spine update: prevention of postoperative infection in patients undergoing spinal surgery. Spine. 2004; 29(8):938–945

[175] Gruenberg MF, Campaner GL, Sola CA, Ortolan EG. Ultraclean air for prevention of postoperative infection after posterior spinal fusion with instrumentation: a comparison between surgeries performed with and without a vertical exponential filtered air-flow system. Spine. 2004; 29(20):2330–2334

[176] Kang DG, Holekamp TF, Wagner SC, Lehman RA, Jr. Intrasite vancomycin powder for the prevention of surgical site infection in spine surgery: a systematic literature review. Spine J. 2015; 15(4):762–770

[177] Chiang HY, Herwaldt LA, Blevins AE, Cho E, Schweizer ML. Effectiveness of local vancomycin powder to decrease surgical site infections: a meta-analysis. Spine J. 2014; 14(3):397–407

[178] Ghobrial GM, Cadotte DW, Williams K, Jr, Fehlings MG, Harrop JS. Complications from the use of intrawound vancomycin in lumbar spinal surgery: a systematic review. Neurosurg Focus. 2015; 39(4):E11

[179] Eder C, Schenk S, Trifinopoulos J, et al. Does intrawound application of vancomycin influence bone healing in spinal surgery? Eur Spine J. 2016; 25(4):1021–1028

31 Summary of Spine Injury Treatment Guidelines

Kevin N. Swong, Russell P. Nockels, and G. Alexander Jones

Abstract
The Joint Section on Disorders of the Spine and Peripheral Nerves periodically reviews the literature, and publishes recommendations, on the diagnosis and management of acute cervical spine and spinal cord injuries. Following is a summary of the most recent recommendations.

Keywords: central cord syndrome, SCIWORA, spinal cord injury, spine fracture, spine trauma, vertebral dissection

31.1 Overview

In 2013, the Joint Section on Disorders of the Spine and Peripheral Nerves, comprising members of the American Association of Neurological Surgeons and the Congress of Neurological Surgeons, released revised guidelines for the management of acute cervical spine and spinal cord injuries. The authors systematically screened the English-language medical literature for relevant articles, which they then reviewed and categorized on the basis of the strength of evidence presented. From this, they crafted recommendations for diagnosis and treatment. These recommendations were, likewise, stratified on the basis of the supporting evidence.

In the previous iteration,[1] these recommendations were termed Standards, Guidelines, and Options, in order of decreasing strength of supporting evidence. In the current version,[2] the authors have used a similar but distinct system with recommendations labeled Level I (for Standard), Level II (for Guideline), and Level III (for Option). The first article in this series provides an excellent overview of the methodology used in developing these guidelines. As of the time of this writing, the guidelines are available for download in their entirety, without charge, at the Congress of Neurological Surgeons Web site at www.cns.org.

In developing these guidelines, the working group from the Joint Section has distilled a great deal of information into a number of concise articles. In this chapter, we have further reduced that information to its component parts, namely, the recommendations presented in the Joint Section guidelines. This chapter is not, in any way, meant to replace the information presented in the original guidelines articles. Rather, we hope it will serve as a basic framework for understanding the scope and content of the guidelines and stimulate the readers' interest to read in more detail about these important topics in the guidelines, and the source literature.

31.2 Prehospital Cervical Spinal Immobilization after Trauma

For the prehospital evaluation and management of suspected cervical spine injury, three topics were addressed: immobilization, transport, and neurologic assessment. There are no Level I recommendations. On the basis of class II and III evidence, several Level II recommendations are offered, including triage and evaluation of trauma patients in the field by experienced and trained personnel, and immobilization of those patients with an injury mechanism sufficient to cause cervical spine injury. Immobilization of patients who meet certain clinical criteria, and thus have very low risk of cervical spine injury, is not recommended. As a Level III recommendation, the use of a rigid collar with blocks is recommended, but the use for sandbags is not, as they do not appear to decrease unwanted cervical spine motion. For penetrating neck injuries, rigid collars should not be applied, as they decrease resuscitation efforts.[3]

31.3 Transportation of Patients with Acute Traumatic Cervical Spine Injuries

There is no class I evidence to recommend ground or air transport as the ideal transport method. The best method of transport depends on the distance that needs to be traversed, location, and availability of these methods and takes into account the other injuries that have been sustained. On the basis of several class III studies, two Level III recommendations are offered: those who have suffered an acute spine injury should be transported in the most expeditious manner available to a facility capable of providing definitive care; and transfer to a center with a dedicated spinal cord injury center has been shown to improve outcomes and is recommended when possible.[4]

31.4 Clinical Assessment Following Acute Cervical Spinal Cord Injury

Clinical assessment of patients with spinal cord injury relies on standardized measures to assess given parameters. Ideally, such an instrument should be clinically validated and possess excellent intra- and interobserver reliability. Numerous scales exist to evaluate spinal cord injury. Some assess neurologic ability, some functional capacity, and others pain and disability. The ability to evaluate each of these dimensions is critical, as the effectiveness of treatment can best be determined when measured by such valid, reproducible means.

On the basis of Level II evidence, the American Spinal Injury Association (ASIA) score again had the highest intra- and interobserver reliability, and its use carries a Level II recommendation. To measure functional outcome, class I evidence supports use of the Spinal Cord Independence Measure III (SCIM III). Finally, to determine the type and amount of pain associated with a spinal cord injury, class I evidence supports the International Spinal Cord Injury Basic Pain Data Set.[5] The use of these latter two are offered as Level I recommendations.

31.4.1 Radiographic Assessment

Since the original guidelines were published in 2002, imaging of acute trauma patients has evolved substantially. High-quality computed tomography (CT) scanning has become widely available and has proven to be safe, efficient, and accurate. The literature published in the interim, as well as the latest guidelines, now reflect the value of this technology.

Robust class I evidence supports that radiographic assessment is not indicated for trauma patients who are awake, alert, without distracting injuries, are not intoxicated, without neck pain and have a normal neurologic examination.[4] Management of these patients carries Level I recommendations that imaging is not recommended, and that discontinuation of immobilization or collar is recommended without imaging.

For awake but symptomatic patients, and for obtunded or unevaluable patients, the Level I recommendation is to obtain a CT scan instead of routine radiographs (anteroposterior [AP], lateral, and odontoid views) when possible. For awake patients with neck pain, but a normal neurologic examination, several treatment recommendations are offered at Level III: (1) continuation of a rigid cervical collar until the patient is asymptomatic; (2) discontinue collar on the basis of normal and adequate flexion–extension radiographs; (3) if an magnetic resonance imaging (MRI; with STIR [short-tau inversion recovery] imaging, performed within 48 hours of injury) does not demonstrate any ligamentous injury, then the cervical collar may be removed even if neck pain persists; or (4) removal of the collar at the discretion of the treating physician.

For obtunded patients with a normal CT scan but high index of suspicion for injury, the Level II recommendation is for further management to involve physicians trained in the diagnosis and management of spinal injuries. As Level III recommendations, several options exist for continued bracing in obtunded patients with a normal CT: (1) continue bracing until asymptomatic; (2) discontinue bracing on the basis of a normal MRI scan (with STIR images, obtained within 48 hours of injury); or (3) discontinue bracing at the discretion of the treating physician. In obtunded patients, there is no clear evidence to support the use of dynamic imaging under live fluoroscopy, and this practice is not recommended.[6]

31.5 Initial Closed Reduction of Cervical Spinal Fracture–Dislocation Injuries

The available evidence on this topic includes a number of Class III studies, and as such, the recommendations are all Level III.

In awake patients, early closed reduction with craniocervical traction is recommended to restore anatomical alignment. Closed reduction in patients with an additional rostral injury is not recommended. MRI is recommended for patients who cannot be examined, or before anterior or posterior open reduction in patients whose fracture–dislocation cannot be reduced prior to operation. Although prereduction MRI imaging will show disk herniation or disruption in one third to one half of patients with facet subluxation injuries, these findings do not seem to influence clinical outcomes of awake patients undergoing closed reduction. Thus, the value of MRI in this setting has not been established.[7]

31.6 Acute Cardiopulmonary Management of Patients with Cervical Spinal Cord Injuries

On this topic, class III data serve as the basis for several Level III recommendations. These include transferring patients to an intensive care unit or similar monitored setting. Use of monitoring to assess for cardiopulmonary dysfunction is recommended. Hypotension (systolic blood pressure < 90 mm Hg) should be corrected as soon as possible, with a goal of mean arterial pressures of 85 to 90 mm Hg for 7 days, to maximize spinal cord perfusion.[8]

31.7 Pharmacologic Therapy for Acute Spinal Cord Injury

Over the past generation, few topics have been more controversial than the administration of high-dose corticosteroids in the setting of acute spinal cord injury. The rationale for the use of steroids is to provide protection against secondary injury. The original National Acute Spinal Cord Injury Study (NASCIS I) demonstrated no benefit in higher-dose steroids, when compared with lower dose.[9]

As a Level I recommendation, the administration of methylprednisolone (MP) is not recommended for the treatment of acute spinal cord injury. Inconsistent class III evidence supports the use of MP, whereas class I, II, and III evidence exists to show that administration of high-dose steroids is associated with serious complications and death. As an additional Level I recommendation, the administration of GM-1 ganglioside (Sygen) is not recommended.

Prospectively, NASCIS II demonstrated no benefit to the administration of MP.[10] However, there was some benefit in short- and long-term motor outcomes when a post hoc analysis applied an 8-hour treatment cutoff to the administration of MP. The guidelines authors downgrade the positive results of this study to class III on the basis of this, and other, methodological flaws.[11] Similar concerns plagued NASCIS III.

Several other class I studies have been published, showing no benefit to MP administration, and with evidence of varying strength showing increased complication rates in the MP group[12,13]; a number of other class II and III studies show a trend toward increased complications in the MP group as well. These include respiratory complications, gastrointestinal bleeding, infection, death, hyperglycemia, increased length of intensive care unit (ICU) stay, and pulmonary embolus.

31.8 Occipital Condyle Fractures

Imaging recommendations include the routine use of CT when available to diagnose and classify occipital condyle fractures (Level II) and MRI to assess the integrity of the craniocervical ligaments (Level III). In terms of treatment, evidence supports the use (Level III) of a rigid cervical collar for most injuries, with consideration of a halo for bilateral injuries. Halo immobilization or instrumented fusion is recommended for those with evidence of ligamentous injury or instability.[14]

31.9 Diagnosis and Management of Traumatic Atlanto-occipital Dislocation Injuries

For suspected atlanto-occipital dislocation (AOD), use of the condyle–C1 interval to diagnose AOD in the pediatric population is offered as a Level I recommendation; it has not been studied yet in adults. A number of Level III recommendations are available. The use of radiographs in adults is recommended; if a radiographic measurement is used to evaluate for AOD, the basion axial interval–basion dental interval (BAI–BDI) is recommended for diagnosis. The presence of upper cervical soft-tissue swelling should prompt a CT scan to evaluate for AOD. Traction is not recommended and is associated with a 10% risk of neurologic deterioration. Internal fixation is the preferred treatment modality.[15]

31.10 Management of Isolated Fractures of the Atlas in Adults

For these fractures, the evidence supports several Level III recommendations. Treatment decisions should be based on the specific fracture type and on the integrity of the transverse atlantal ligament in particular. Fractures with an intact transverse atlantal ligament should be managed with immobilization, whereas those with disruption of the ligament may be managed with immobilization alone or with fixation and fusion.[16]

These fractures are considered in three main groupings, based on mechanism and fracture morphology: odontoid fractures, traumatic C2–C3 spondylolisthesis (i.e., hangman's fracture), and C2 body fractures.

For patients over the age of 50 years with a type II odontoid fracture, consideration of internal fixation is recommended (Level II). As a Level III recommendation, initial management of type I, II, or III odontoid fracture with external immobilization is recommended, with the understanding that the nonunion rate is higher in type II fractures than in the others. If surgical stabilization is chosen, either anterior or posterior approach is recommended. In type II and III fractures, surgical stabilization and fusion is recommended in those patients with > 5 mm displacement of the dens, those with a comminuted fracture, or those in whom alignment cannot be maintained with external bracing.

For hangman's fractures, initial management with external immobilization is recommended, except in the case of severe angulation at C2–C3, traumatic disruption of the C2–C3 disk space, or inability to maintain alignment with immobilization, in which cases surgical stabilization and fusion are recommended (Level III).

Similarly, for C2 vertebral body fractures, treatment with external immobilization is recommended, except in cases of severe ligamentous disruption or inability to maintain alignment with bracing. In these cases, consideration should be given to surgical stabilization. In the case of a comminuted C2 vertebral body fracture, the vertebral arteries should be evaluated for injury. All of these recommendations are Level III.[17]

31.11 Management of Acute Combination Fractures of the Atlas and Axis in Adults

Several Level III recommendations exist. Treatment of combination C1–C2 fractures should be based primarily on the characteristics of the C2 fracture. Treatment of most of these fractures with external bracing is recommended. Surgical stabilization should be considered for C1 hangman's fractures with angulation of C2 on C3 > 11 degrees, and for C1 type II odontoid fractures with atlanto-dental ratio of > 5 mm.[18]

31.12 Os Odontoideum

To diagnose an os odontoideum, radiographs, including open-mouth and flexion–extension views, should be obtained with or without CT or MRI. This is a Level III recommendation, as are all the others regarding this pathologic entity.

If asymptomatic, these may be managed with operative fixation and fusion or followed conservatively. If treated nonoperatively, regular follow-up with imaging should be obtained. If there is evidence of increased instability, or progressive neurologic decline, then surgical fixation should be pursued. If there is ventral or dorsal cervicomedullary compression, this should be addressed with appropriate decompression at the time of operation.[19]

31.13 Subaxial Cervical Spine Injury Classification Systems

Classification of cervical spine injuries is important, in order to guide treatment and to communicate information about the nature of the injury. The ideal classification system would be clinically validated, logical, simple enough to use in clinical practice, account for structural and neurologic instability, guide surgical treatment decisions, and would have high interobserver reliability. As Level I recommendations, the authors endorse the use of the Subaxial Injury Classification (SLIC) system, and the Cervical Spine Injury Severity Score (CSISS), with the caveat that the latter is "somewhat complicated" and may not be suitable for daily practice.

As a Level III recommendation, the authors recommend against the use of the Harris classification system for describing the bony and soft-tissue characteristics on imaging studies. They also recommend against use of the Allen classification for describing mechanistic and injury findings. Both of these recommendations are due to low reliability in these classification systems.[20] However, it is worth noting that neither system was validated when it was initially published, and that these observations were published as part of the validation of the SLIC system.[21]

31.14 Treatment of Subaxial Cervical Spinal Injuries

Reviewed data support a number of Level III recommendations. Open or closed reduction of fractures or dislocations is recommended, with the goal of decompression of the cord. Stable immobilization (internal or external) allows for early rehabilitation; anterior or posterior approach is recommended if neither one is specifically required for decompression of the spinal cord. If more contemporary measures (i.e., surgical intervention) are not available, traction and bed rest are recommended. For patients with ankylosing spondylitis, a CT and MRI scan should be obtained even after minor trauma given the high chance of injury. These patients usually require posterior long-segment fixation and fusion, or an anterior fusion with posterior supplementation, given the high rate of failure with anterior stabilization alone.[22]

31.15 Management of Acute Traumatic Central Cord Syndrome

A number of Class III studies have been published on this topic. There is still significant debate in the literature regarding the management of some subgroups of acute traumatic central cord syndrome (ATCCS) patients, including those with long-segment cord compression and those with stenosis and no bony injury. A total of four recommendations, all at Level III, are offered.

These include intensive care unit management of patients with ATCCS, particularly those with severe neurologic deficits; medical management, including maintenance of mean arterial pressure (MAP) of 85 to 90 mm Hg; early reduction of fracture-dislocation injuries; and surgical decompression of the compressed spinal cord, especially if the compression is focal and anterior.[23]

31.16 Management of Pediatric Cervical Spine and Spinal Cord Injuries

In pediatric spine injury, evidence supports a Level I recommendation to measure the C1–condylar interval to diagnose AOD. Paralleling the recommendations for adults at very low risk of spine injury, there is a Level II recommendation to avoid imaging for children who are > 3 years of age, awake, without pain, neurologically intact, and without evidence of intoxication, distracting injuries, or unexplained hypotension. Similarly, for children < 3 years with Glasgow Coma Scale (GCS) score > 13 and no pain or neurologic deficit, no imaging is required. However, if the child was involved in a motor vehicle collision, had a fall > 10 feet, or has unexplained hypotension, or there is suspected nonaccidental trauma (NAT), imaging should be obtained with radiographs or CT scan.

Three-position CT with C1–C2 motion analysis is recommended to confirm and classify atlantoaxial rotary fixation (AARF). Level III recommendations for imaging include AP and lateral radiographs or CT for children < 9 years of age. For children > 9

years of age, open-mouth views may be added. Flexion–extension radiographs should be considered to evaluate for dynamic instability and an MRI may be obtained to evaluate the soft tissues.

Regarding treatment, only Level III recommendations are supported by the evidence. Owing to the relative large head size, occipital recess or thoracic elevation should be used for children < 8 years. If there is injury to the C2 synchondrosis, it should be treated with closed reduction and a halo vest for children < 7 years. Closed reduction is recommended for acute AARF < 4 weeks that does not spontaneously reduce. If > 4 weeks, reduce with halter tongs/halo vest and consider surgery if AARF is irreducible or recurrent. If there is evidence of ligamentous instability or irreducible fractures, or for cases that fail conservative management, surgical intervention should be considered. Spinal cord birth trauma is not addressed in the literature. The condition may be diagnosed by symptoms of spinal shock: flaccidity, hypotension, and lack of deep tendon reflexes. No recommendations can be made regarding treatment because of the lack of data.[24]

31.17 Spinal Cord Injury without Radiographic Abnormality

For instances where there is evidence of myelopathy from trauma without objective signs of fracture or ligamentous injury, spinal cord injury without radiographic abnormality (SCIWORA), several Level III recommendations are supported by the literature.

MRI of the area of suspected injury is recommended, as is radiographic imaging of the entire spine. Flexion–extension radiographs may be helpful in determining if there is dynamic instability. These should be performed in the acute setting, and in a delayed fashion, even in the case of an MRI showing no evidence of discoligamentous injury. Neither spinal angiography nor myelogram is helpful in making the diagnosis, and these procedures are thus not recommended.

The injured segment should be kept in external immobilization for up to 12 weeks. Bracing may be discontinued earlier at the discretion of the treating physician if the patient has become asymptomatic and there is confirmed dynamic stability on repeat flexion–extension radiographs. "High-risk" activities should be avoided for up to 6 months.[25]

31.18 Management of Vertebral Artery Injuries Following Nonpenetrating Cervical Trauma

In blunt injuries to the cervical spine, the incidence of vertebral artery injuries may be as high as 11%. The data support a Level I recommendation to obtain a CT angiogram if Denver screening is positive (infarct on head CT, nonexpanding cervical hematoma, massive epistaxis, anisocoria or a Horner's syndrome, GCS score < 8 without imaging correlation on head CT, cervical spine fracture, basilar skull fracture, Le Fort II or III fracture, seat belt sign above clavicle, or a cervical bruit or thrill). As a Level III recommendation, a formal angiogram should be obtained if CT angiogram is unavailable, or if there is high suspicion that an endovascular intervention will need to take place. MRI is recommended in the setting of complete spinal cord injury or vertebral body subluxation. Treatment of vertebral artery injury, including the use of antiplatelet or anticoagulant medications, should be tailored to the nature of the injury, as well as any associated injuries, and risk of bleeding (Level III). The role for endovascular therapy has not been established at this point; therefore, no recommendations are warranted.[26]

31.19 Deep Venous Thrombosis and Thromboembolism in Patients with Cervical Spinal Cord Injuries

For prophylaxis, several Level I recommendations are supported by the available evidence, including the general use of prophylactic treatment of venous thromboembolism (VTE) in patients with severe motor deficits from spinal cord injury. Low-molecular-weight heparin (LMWH), rotating beds, or combination therapy is recommended. Low-dose heparin in conjunction with sequential compression device (SCD) boots or electrical stimulation is likewise recommended.

As Level II recommendations, neither low-dose heparin nor oral anticoagulation alone is sufficient for deep vein thrombosis (DVT) prevention. DVT prophylaxis should be started within 72 hours. A 3-month prophylactic treatment is recommended. At Level III, inferior vena cava (IVC) filters should not be placed as routine and should be reserved for patients who cannot have or have failed anticoagulation. Physical examination, Doppler ultrasound, and other tests including plethysmography are recommended to evaluate for DVT.[27]

31.20 Nutritional Support after Spinal Cord Injury

As a Level II recommendation, indirect calorimetry is recommended as the best means to establish the caloric needs of a patient with spinal cord injury. At Level III, nutritional support should be started as soon as possible, preferably within 72 hours. However, initiating enteral support has not been shown to affect neurologic outcome, length of stay, or complication rate in patients with spinal cord injury.[28]

31.21 Conclusion

The treatment of spine injuries, as with other neurosurgical conditions, is based on an understanding of the underlying anatomy and pathophysiology and guided by the available scientific literature. The Joint Section guidelines are a particularly robust and useful summary of the literature because of the rigorous, uniform, and transparent methodology used to screen and evaluate published studies, followed by a clear and logical statement of treatment recommendations based on this review.

References

[1] Hadley MN, Walters BC, Grabb PA, et al. Guidelines for the management of acute cervical spine and spinal cord injuries. Clin Neurosurg. 2002; 49:407–498

[2] Walters BC. Methodology of the guidelines for the management of acute cervical spine and spinal cord injuries. Neurosurgery. 2013; 72(Suppl 2):17–21

[3] Theodore N, Hadley MN, Aarabi B, et al. Prehospital cervical spinal immobilization after trauma. Neurosurgery. 2013; 72(Suppl 2):22–34

[4] Theodore N, Aarabi B, Dhall SS, et al. Transportation of patients with acute traumatic cervical spine injuries. Neurosurgery. 2013; 72(Suppl 2):35–39

[5] Hadley MN, Walters BC, Aarabi B, et al. Clinical assessment following acute cervical spinal cord injury. Neurosurgery. 2013; 72(Suppl 2):40–53

[6] Ryken TC, Hadley MN, Walters BC, et al. Radiographic assessment. Neurosurgery. 2013; 72(Suppl 2):54–72

[7] Gelb DE, Hadley MN, Aarabi B, et al. Initial closed reduction of cervical spinal fracture-dislocation injuries. Neurosurgery. 2013; 72(Suppl 2):73–83

[8] Ryken TC, Hurlbert RJ, Hadley MN, et al. The acute cardiopulmonary management of patients with cervical spinal cord injuries. Neurosurgery. 2013; 72(Suppl 2):84–92

[9] Bracken MB, Collins WF, Freeman DF, et al. Efficacy of methylprednisolone in acute spinal cord injury. JAMA. 1984; 251(1):45–52

[10] Bracken MB, Shepard MJ, Collins WF, et al. A randomized, controlled trial of methylprednisolone or naloxone in the treatment of acute spinal-cord injury. Results of the Second National Acute Spinal Cord Injury Study. N Engl J Med. 1990; 322(20):1405–1411

[11] Hurlbert RJ, Hadley MN, Walters BC, et al. Pharmacological therapy for acute spinal cord injury. Neurosurgery. 2013; 72(Suppl 2):93–105

[12] Pointillart V, Petitjean ME, Wiart L, et al. Pharmacological therapy of spinal cord injury during the acute phase. Spinal Cord. 2000; 38(2):71–76

[13] Matsumoto T, Tamaki T, Kawakami M, Yoshida M, Ando M, Yamada H. Early complications of high-dose methylprednisolone sodium succinate treatment in the follow-up of acute cervical spinal cord injury. Spine. 2001; 26(4):426–430

[14] Theodore N, Aarabi B, Dhall SS, et al. Occipital condyle fractures. Neurosurgery. 2013; 72(Suppl 2):106–113

[15] Theodore N, Aarabi B, Dhall SS, et al. The diagnosis and management of traumatic atlanto-occipital dislocation injuries. Neurosurgery. 2013; 72(Suppl 2):114–126

[16] Ryken TC, Aarabi B, Dhall SS, et al. Management of isolated fractures of the atlas in adults. Neurosurgery. 2013; 72(Suppl 2):127–131

[17] Ryken TC, Hadley MN, Aarabi B, et al. Management of isolated fractures of the axis in adults. Neurosurgery. 2013; 72(Suppl 2):132–150

[18] Ryken TC, Hadley MN, Aarabi B, et al. Management of acute combination fractures of the atlas and axis in adults. Neurosurgery. 2013; 72(Suppl 2):151–158

[19] Rozzelle CJ, Aarabi B, Dhall SS, et al. Os odontoideum. Neurosurgery. 2013; 72(Suppl 2):159–169

[20] Aarabi B, Walters BC, Dhall SS, et al. Subaxial cervical spine injury classification systems. Neurosurgery. 2013; 72(Suppl 2):170–186

[21] Vaccaro AR, Hulbert RJ, Patel AA, et al; Spine Trauma Study Group. The subaxial cervical spine injury classification system: a novel approach to recognize the importance of morphology, neurology, and integrity of the disco-ligamentous complex. Spine. 2007; 32(21):2365–2374

[22] Gelb DE, Aarabi B, Dhall SS, et al. Treatment of subaxial cervical spinal injuries. Neurosurgery. 2013; 72(Suppl 2):187–194

[23] Aarabi B, Hadley MN, Dhall SS, et al. Management of acute traumatic central cord syndrome (ATCCS). Neurosurgery. 2013; 72(Suppl 2):195–204

[24] Rozzelle CJ, Aarabi B, Dhall SS, et al. Management of pediatric cervical spine and spinal cord injuries. Neurosurgery. 2013; 72(Suppl 2):205–226

[25] Rozzelle CJ, Aarabi B, Dhall SS, et al. Spinal cord injury without radiographic abnormality (SCIWORA). Neurosurgery. 2013; 72(Suppl 2):227–233

[26] Harrigan MR, Hadley MN, Dhall SS, et al. Management of vertebral artery injuries following non-penetrating cervical trauma. Neurosurgery. 2013; 72(Suppl 2):234–243

[27] Dhall SS, Hadley MN, Aarabi B, et al. Deep venous thrombosis and thromboembolism in patients with cervical spinal cord injuries. Neurosurgery. 2013; 72(Suppl 2):244–254

[28] Dhall SS, Hadley MN, Aarabi B, et al. Nutritional support after spinal cord injury. Neurosurgery. 2013; 72(Suppl 2):255–259

32 Penetrating Injuries of Peripheral Nerves

James Tait Goodrich

Abstract

Peripheral nerve injury and its surgical repair can be a daunting task for the neurosurgeon. With the advancements of microsurgical techniques, better instrumentation, and improved radiologic diagnosis, neurosurgeons are now better able to assess peripheral nerve injuries. We are now able to better discuss the timing of the repair in the sense of an acute versus delayed repair. Discussed in this chapter are the techniques available for repair of an acute penetrating nerve injury. Surgical imaging and graphics are provided to assist the neurosurgeon in the various repair techniques.

Keywords: epineural repair, nerve repair, nerve trauma, perineural repair, peripheral nerve injury, peripheral nerve trauma

32.1 Introduction

With increasing interest on the part of plastic and orthopedic surgeons in the field of peripheral nerve surgery, fewer neurosurgeons are becoming involved in managing such problems, even though historically, the treatment of the acutely injured nerve was primarily the province of the neurosurgeon. The basic microsurgical principles underlying the care of peripheral nerve injuries are taught to all neurosurgeons. This chapter will review these principles and summarize the concepts relevant to the management of the acutely injured peripheral nerve. The primary emphasis is on management of a penetrating nerve injury in the acute setting; for the sake of completeness, the principles of treating the penetrating injury for which delayed surgery is indicated are also reviewed.

It is of historical interest that the concept of what a "nerve" is, and what its physiologic function is, is a very recent development dating just back to the first half of the 19th century. Nerves and tendons were often confused anatomically and also in their functions. One of the earliest illustrations of peripheral nerves appeared in a 19th century monograph by Ernest Burdach (1801–1870)[1,2,3] (▶Fig. 32.1).

32.2 Anatomical Considerations and Their Clinical Implications

It is imperative that the surgeon who intends to operate on a peripheral nerve has a thorough understanding of the anatomy of the nerve and its surrounding vascular and muscular structures. The aim of any peripheral nerve repair is coaptation of neural elements in the most anatomically accurate fashion achievable, and this presupposes a thorough understanding of the anatomical structures being dealt with (▶Fig. 32.2). The neurosurgical operative principles of meticulous technique, careful handing of tissues, and hemostasis apply just as rigorously to the repair of a peripheral nerve injury as to any other neurosurgical procedure.

▶Fig. 32.2 shows an illustrated rendering of a "typical" peripheral nerve. The nerve axon is enclosed within a sheath of perineurium, and in turn multiple axons form the fascicle. A typical adult human peripheral nerve can contain as many as 10,000 axons. Contrary to what many believe, axons do not follow a direct, linear pathway but often cross over and anastomose at a number of different points along the various pathways of the nerve. Another important concept often overlooked by the surgeon concerns the anatomical segregation of the motor and sensory components within a major nerve. In the proximal portion of the nerve, the motor and sensory units are diffusely scattered, and it is only distally that they segregate into discrete motor and sensory components.

The surgeon must keep these concepts in mind; they justify the principle that exact matching of two cut ends of a nerve is theoretically impossible.[4,5] This point should be clearly made in a preoperative discussion with the patient and family so that their expectations as to the possibilities for recovery are appropriate. The surgeon must not neglect to deal with other dimensions of recovery from the injury. On the one hand, patients and families commonly do not understand how a long a nerve takes to recover function; on the other, they are likely to be overly optimistic about the degree of function a repaired nerve will eventually provide. Careful and detailed explanations of the nature of the nerve repair and the length of the expected recovery period can go a long way toward reducing the postoperative depression and anxiety that patients often present.

32.3 Basic Considerations of Peripheral Nerve Repair

Several basic considerations must be kept in mind with dealing with a peripheral nerve injury. In 1978, Sir Sydney Sunderland (1910–1993), one of the great pioneers in peripheral nerve surgery,[6,7] defined what he considered to be the key determinants of the outcome of peripheral nerve repair; they remain highly relevant to this day:

1. the specific nerve injury;
2. the level of the injury;
3. the severity and extent of the injury;
4. the severity of the injury to the surrounding tissues;
5. the cellular response of the nerve to injury; and
6. the timing and technique of the repair.

Sunderland's list clearly indicates the relatively small extent to which the surgeon can influence the outcome—i.e., only in the timing and technique of the repair: the recovery depends in greatest part on the natural response of the nerve to injury.

In urban centers, a common cause of peripheral nerve injury is the missile (e.g., bullet, shrapnel, etc.). In this type of injury the ballistic details need to be worked out and the anatomical path of the injury determined. An acute, sharply cut nerve presents a different injury from that caused by a blast (i.e., gunshot) injury. In a bullet or high-impact missile injury, the initial blast effect will often cause a complete paralysis of the nerve. This type of injury results in the injury sequelae of neuropraxia and axonotmesis (see below). It has been my experience that many

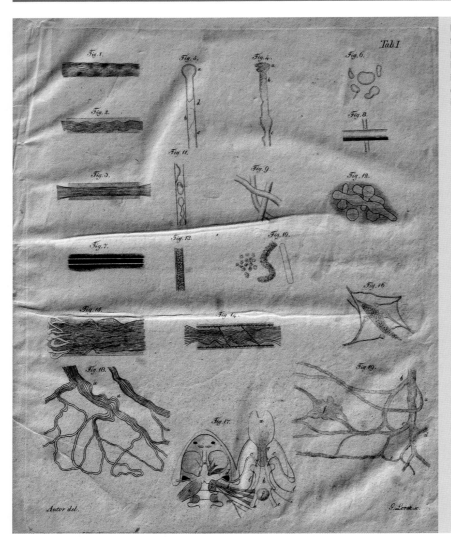

Fig. 32.1 This illustration comes from one of the earliest monographs to deal with a detailed peripheral nerve anatomy, which was authored by Ernest Burdach, a German anatomist. This illustration comes from his work, and the details of the nerve anatomy including the fascicles are illustrated here for the first time.

patients with such injuries recover on their own and that acute intervention is not always indicated. An exception to this principle arises when a vessel in proximity to the damaged nerve has been injured, leading to a compressive hematoma. This situation often requires urgent treatment. If the missile track is sufficiently disruptive, then intraneural fibrosis can develop, causing a neural conduction deficit. In this group, later intervention is often required. In my experience, missile injuries are less likely to cause permanent nerve injury than injury by a knife or glass.

In carrying out peripheral nerve repair, the surgeon and the operating-room team have to keep in mind that the only elements susceptible to control are the alignment of the severed nerves, including the fascicles, the tension at the suture line (which should be minimal), and the risk of infection; all else depend on the forces of nature.[8,9,10] The surgeon can only deal with the technical details. The team's involvement in the biological response to nerve injury and reparative procedures is restricted to understanding and applying the principles that enhance recovery. A number of ongoing studies are addressing the goal of enhancing the environmental milieu of a regenerating nerve, but those are beyond the scope of this chapter. Immune suppression, growth factors, electrical field stimulation, and the

like have been tried, but their reported success has been at best marginal. In the anatomical reconstruction of an injured nerve, fibrin glue, different suture materials, and steroids have also been used but have so far have met with only limited success. The optimal environment for a regenerating nerve has yet to be determined. An often-overlooked concept in treating a peripheral nerve injury, key to any reconstruction, is that an injured nerve should be considered not a degenerating element but rather one undergoing regeneration. To allow a regenerating nerve the best options for recovery, it behooves us to continue to search for ways to enhance its environmental milieu. In what follows, the major emphasis will be on the important parameters of surgical technique and treatment planning, which, as already noted, are the only ones within the surgeon's control.

32.3.1 Classification of Traumatic Nerve Injuries

A number of classifications have been introduced to describe the different types of nerve injuries. It is important to be familiar with them, as they are used consistently throughout the

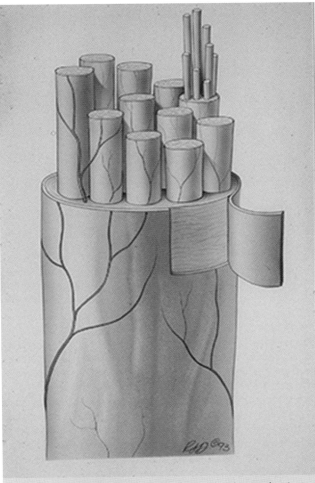

Fig. 32.2 A schematic reconstruction of a peripheral nerve showing the pertinent anatomical details.

tubes remain intact, allowing the regenerating axons to regain their peripheral connections.

* *Neurotmesis*: severe injury, in which a nerve has been completely disrupted or is so severely damaged that spontaneous regeneration cannot occur. As a result of wallerian degeneration and neuroma formation, it is impossible for axons to regenerate distally.

Sunderland, in 1951, expanded Seddon's classification (▶ Table 32.1), taking into consideration more of the possible intraoperative surgical findings in peripheral nerve injury.[6,7]

Over the years, other classifications have been proposed, but their details are well beyond the scope of this chapter. The reader is referred to an excellent article by Gentili and Hudson[12] that presents a number of the classification systems and their electrophysiologic correlates. Mackinnon and Dellon have also reviewed the various classifications and their anatomical correlates, employing a diagrammatic format of presentation.[13]

32.3.2 Timing of Nerve Repair

The issue of when to perform nerve repair continues to generate controversy, as attested by the peripheral nerve literature. Significant disagreement as to timing, i.e., acute versus delayed, has prevailed since World War I. For purposes of this chapter, repair is classed as acute (within 24–48 hours), delayed (3–6 weeks), and prolonged delayed (more than 4–6 months).

When the patient is first seen, it is important to determine the mechanism of injury. This evaluation will determine the type of repair that is appropriate and its timing. A nerve that has been sharply cut by glass or a knife is often easier to acutely repair than one injured by a missile (bullet, shrapnel, and the like).

Acute Repair

When the mechanism of injury is a clean, sharp laceration— as in injuries due to domestic violence or motor vehicle accidents—performance of nerve repair within the first 24 to 48 hours, i.e., acutely, should always be considered. The absence of scar tissue and relatively normal anatomical planes (i.e., because soft-tissue damage is slight) usually make the repair straightforward. Early repair also allows for anastomosis of endoneural tubes that are of the same caliber, which is more appropriate than the joining of tubes of different caliber, often the only resort in delayed repairs. Acute repair of the sharply lacerated brachial plexus and of the proximal sciatic nerve should also be considered, as here the ability to mobilize the nerve is only marginal. To avoid the natural retraction

peripheral nerve literature. Although some believe that classification systems have been overemphasized, they remain extremely useful. Two classifications are presented here.

In 1946, Seddon introduced a classification that has remained both reliable and useful.[11] In fact, Seddon's terminology has become a fundamental part of the peripheral nerve repair literature:

* *Neuropraxia*: a temporary disruption of nerve conduction associated with minimal injury, marked by ischemic demyelination that usually is local in extent.
* *Axonotmesis*: moderate injury characterized by interruption of axons and their myelin sheaths. The endoneural

Table 32.1 Sunderland classification of nerve injury

Classification	Description
Grade 1	Loss of axonal conduction
Grade 2	Loss of continuity of axons with intact endoneurium
Grade 3	Transection of nerve fiber (axon and sheath) with intact perineurium
Grade 4	Loss of perineurium and fascicular continuity
Grade 5	Loss of continuity of the entire nerve trunk

of a cut nerve, injuries of these types need to be dealt with very early; on my service they are typically treated within the first 24 to 48 hours.

Another factor that must be kept in mind is the length of the nerve that needs to be regenerated. In the case of a brachial plexus or a sciatic nerve injury, the sooner the repair, the more quickly the nerve can start to regenerate. These nerves have to cover long regenerating pathways, and unnecessary delays can only lead to further atrophy of the distal muscles.

Delayed Repair

In open contaminated or multiply contused wounds, on the other hand, delayed repair should always be considered. If there is extensive local tissue damage and contamination, as in electrical or blast injuries, delay is also recommended (contaminated wounds are discussed further in the section on gunshot wounds). The relevant reasoning is straightforward: repaired nerves heal much better when their environment is not disrupted by foreign material, contused tissue, and potentially infected material. Another advantage of delaying the repair in a multiply contused nerve is that the injured portions tend to demarcate with time, enabling more effective interposition fascicle grafting.

On the other hand, there are also disadvantages to a delayed repair. Working in a scarred, fibrotic wound in which anatomical demarcations have been lost is certainly more difficult than in freshly injured tissue. In addition, the natural anatomical response of an injured nerve is to retract, and when this occurs in a fibrotic scar, the nerve endings can be tediously difficult to locate, mobilize, and repair. If there is any question as to the extent or nature of the injury, it is never unreasonable to carry out a preliminary exploration to assist in treatment planning. If the wound is contaminated or a vessel injured, these immediate urgent problems can be managed and nerve repair deferred. Severed nerve endings can also be identified and tacked down to prevent retraction, making for easier identification later.

Prolonged Delay

Prolonged-delay repairs have been most commonly advocated in military medicine. They were devised to manage typical injuries encountered in a war zone; one might argue that with the recent introduction of high-powered weapons into urban areas, these should also be classed as war zones. War (and urban) injuries typically involve high-energy missile wounds that are often been multiply contaminated by dirt, clothing, and surface debris.[14]

32.4 Repair Techniques

32.4.1 General Principles

In dealing with the repair of an injured nerve or nerves, a number of principles and techniques have to be kept in mind. An old adage in surgery is that exposure is key. This adage holds true in a peripheral nerve repair. In any nerve exploration, the anatomy of the injury has to be worked out first. It is always a good rule to start from undisrupted anatomical sites and work towards

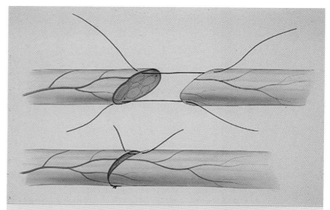

Fig. 32.3 An epineural repair. Note how the surgical realignment attempts to restore the pattern of the nerve's surface vasculature.

the injury. Accordingly, the dissection of the injury site should be deferred until the nerve has been exposed from above and below the injury. Blunt dissection for exposure is contraindicated because it often subjects the injured nerve to unacceptable torsion forces. The no. 15 or no. 11 scalpel blade and even ophthalmologic iris knives are in my experience the most useful for sharp dissection. Because the nerve is an "electrical" element, electrophysiologic monitoring is essential throughout the exposure and the repair. The nerve needs to be fully dissected on both sides of the injury so that stimulating and recording leads can be easily placed for monitoring. Any nerve is wholly dependent on its vascular supply for nutrients. The surgeon must therefore identify and attempt to preserve any large feeding vessels. Factors in the design and equipment of the operating room will make for optimal surgery (see ▶ Box 32.1).

Box 32.1 Operating room requirements and instrumentation

Magnification loupes for initial anatomical dissection of nerve
Operative magnification with illumination for fascicle repairs
Comfortable chair with armrest
Electrophysiologic monitoring for both stimulation and recording
Spring-loaded needle holders
Diamond or sapphire knives (ophthalmic cataract knives also useful)
8–0 nylon with 75-mm needle for epineural repair
10–0 nylon with 50-mm needle for fascicular repair

32.4.2 Epineural Repair

Among the most common ways of dealing with an acute penetrating nerve injury is the epineural repair. This is a useful technique for repairing a sharply lacerated nerve in an acute setting. The anatomical aspects of this repair are straightforward and are diagramed in ▶ Fig. 32.3. Once an adequate exposure has been achieved, as discussed above,

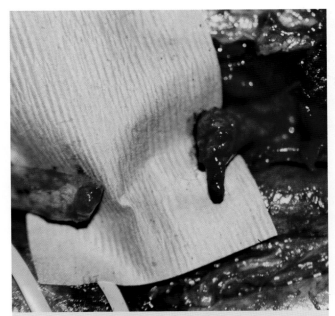

Fig. 32.4 An acutely lacerated nerve showing the typical "mushroom" that occurs at each end.

the traumatized nerve endings have to be prepared. Laceration typically causes the nerve endings to "mushroom" at the point of division (▶ Fig. 32.4). The "mushroom" has to be removed prior to the repair by trimming it back to the epineurium. This is easily done by laying each dissected end on a sterile tongue blade and excising the "mushroomed" portion with a fresh unused scalpel blade.

Proper realignment of the nerve endings is key. The nerve's surface vascularity pattern offers a visual guide to anatomical alignment if the tissue has not been too severely disrupted. Once the alignment has been determined, two 8–0 nylon sutures are placed in the epineurium 180 degrees apart. The two nerve ends are juxtaposed, taking care that tension is minimal. Sometimes additional proximal and distal dissection is required to further relax the nerve. Once the ends have been approximated and the tension on the nerve checked, several 9–0 or 10–0 nylon sutures are placed in the epineural plane, taking care to pass them through full-thickness epineurium without injuring the underlying fascicles. After the wound is closed, the limb is splinted for 3 to 4 weeks to prevent undo tension on the nerve anastomosis. This is the time required for a healing nerve to obtain an adequate tensile strength to sustain movement without disruption. After 3 to 4 weeks, the splint is removed and a rehabilitation regimen begun.

Excellent postoperative care is crucially important. Physical therapy and rehabilitation are required after any peripheral nerve repair. In addition to the one to two daily exercise sessions typically conducted by the rehabilitation team, I advise the patient to continue range-of-motion (ROM) and muscle straightening exercises throughout the day. The patient must be encouraged to actively participate in his/her recovery. Nothing will inhibit a good repair faster than a frozen joint or an atrophied muscle: both need to be avoided.

Complications of Epineural Repair

Although epineural repair is an excellent technique, one has to keep its anatomical aftermath in mind. This concept was discussed by Edshage in a paper dealing with complications of healing.[15] The surgeon will often be able to fashion an anastomosis whose external appearance is satisfactory. This external appearance, however, can be misleading. It can happen that if a section through a nerve repaired by the epineural technique is placed under a microscope, the fascicles are seen to be disrupted, buckled, and poorly aligned. The gaps we leave behind often fill with connective tissue and block neural regeneration. Despite such difficulties, the epineural repair remains useful. But it is important to keep in mind the findings reviewed by Edshage: they emphasize how important the principles of magnification, illumination, and attention to fascicular alignment are; these are the only aspects of technique under the surgeon's control in an acute repair.

32.4.3 Fascicle Repair

In both acute and delayed repairs, a technique that has been used with increasing frequency is the fascicle repair (▶ Fig. 32.5a, b). First introduced in 1953 by Sunderland,[6,16] it has become technically feasible only with the introduction of the operating microscope in the mid-1960s by Smith.[17] The requirement for painstaking attention to the microanatomical details of the fascicle repair calls for patience on the part of the surgeon, high magnification, and adequate microinstrumentation. It is the best form of repair in those cases in which only a few large fascicles are identifiable. The technique is also particularly useful for repairing the distal portion of a nerve in instances in which severed components typically can be mobilized and juxtaposed with minimal tension. In the urban environment, where a knife or glass is often involved in a nerve injury, a not uncommon situation is one in which the nerve is only partially severed, with some fascicles left intact. This is an ideal situation for a fascicle repair. In some cases—in particular those in which a delayed repair is elected—one finds a nerve with disrupted fibrotic ends that require resection, with resultant foreshortening of the fascicles. In such instances, placement of an interfascicular graft (discussed below) rather than a fascicle repair is more appropriate.

Method

The injured nerve is exposed until both severed ends have been identified. The anatomical dissection is carried out in such a fashion as to assure that both ends are sufficiently mobile to be approximated without tension. The superficial epineurium is then excised 3 to 4 mm on each end to expose the fascicles. The fascicles that are to be anastomosed are then teased

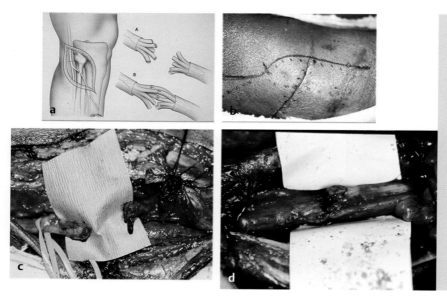

Fig. 32.5 **(a)** A fascicular nerve repair on the peroneal nerve. A and B, schematic details of a fascicle repair. **(b)** The injury here occurred because of self-inflicted knife injuries. **(c)** An acute laceration of a peroneal nerve, the cut ends, which have already retracted (in an injury just at 24 hours), are seen just below the rectangular rubber dam. **(d)** The sutured and repaired nerve.

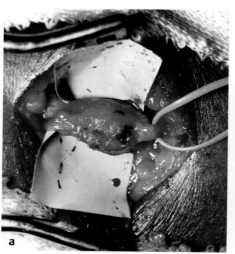

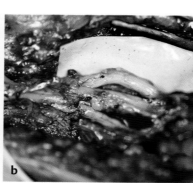

Fig. 32.6 Interfascicular nerve graft repair. **(a)** A traumatic neuroma in continuity. Electromyography done post injury showed no return of function or axonal conduction. **(b)** The neuroma was resected an interfascicular grafts were placed, using the sural nerve as a donor site. **(c)** Schematic of the technique of the interfascicular nerve graft. The epineurium cuff is rolled back to expose the fascicles. The grafts are matched to size and sutured into place.

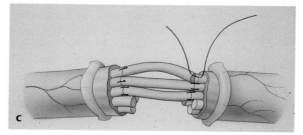

out under the microscope from the surrounding interfascicular connective tissue. Using a 10–0 nylon suture with a small needle (typically, 50 mm), a full bite of perineurium is taken, using care not to injure the underlying fascicles. A good rule of thumb is that if the sutures break, the tension is too great. Occasionally the fascicles will "mushroom" out and need to be trimmed back to the perineurium before closure. In some cases, the fascicles cannot be identified, and here an epineural repair is more easily performed.

32.4.4 Group Fascicle Repairs

In management of the more severely disrupted nerve from which individual fascicles cannot be teased out, a useful technique is the group fascicle repair (▶ Fig. 32.6). This technique is similar to that described for the fascicle repair, except that groups of fascicles are selected for repair. In such cases, interposing fascicular epineurium is typically present, and it is in its plane that the dissection is carried out. The same technique described for fascicle repair is then performed using whatever epineurium can be located.

32.4.5 Interfascicular Nerve Grafting— Nerve Grafts

Over the years, a number of investigators have shown that one of the greatest impediments to a good recovery is excess tension on a repaired nerve. To overcome this problem, the use of nerve grafts harvested from other regions has been introduced. Historically, nerve grafts have waxed and waned in popularity but are now considered essential in some repairs, particularly those involving significant gaps between the nerve ends. There is no question that with better techniques and a clearer understanding of when to use them, grafts have proved effective in enhancing the recovery of appropriately selected injured nerves. The excellent clinical studies of Millesi and Samii[5 and others18,19,20,21] have reintroduced the use of nerve grafts. It is beyond the scope of this chapter to review studies of graft physiology; the interested reader is referred to the work of Millesi, Samii, and others.[13,19,20,21]

32.4.6 Useful Donor Sites

A number of criteria apply to the selection of a donor nerve graft site. Nerves that have been identified as potential donor sites and the indications for their usage are as follows:

- *Sural nerve.* The most frequently used donor nerve for a repair is the sural nerve. Easy to locate, it provides a long graft (typically 20–30 cm) and its removal causes minimal morbidity. It can usually be located just behind and below the lateral malleolus and then followed up the calf. By "gently" tugging on the nerve during the dissection, it can be seen in outline and followed up the leg. Its removal can cause some sensory loss to the base of the foot, but most patients do not find this a problem; this outcome should, of course, be described to the patient prior to surgery.
- *Superficial radial nerve.* This nerve was once frequently used, but the risk of partial sensory loss to the hand has made it acceptable only as a last resort. Its short length may restrict the amount of nerve available for the repair.
- *Medial or lateral cutaneous nerve of the forearm.*
- *Lateral cutaneous nerve of the femur.*
- *Medial cutaneous nerve of the arm.* Each of the latter three nerves can be particularly useful for a nearby injury. Their disadvantages include small caliber and short graft length. In any procedure that requires a graft of significant length or multiple grafts, the sural nerve remains the best source.

32.4.7 Techniques

A number of technical points need to be kept in mind.

- The cross-sectional size of an interfascicular graft should be the same size as, or larger (so that one can "fishmouth" over the endings) than, the nerve elements at the host site.

- As part of the repair, the fibrotic nerve endings are removed and the dissection carried back to normal nerve. About 1 cm of the epineurium is removed to provide an adequate exposure of the internal anatomy.
- The fascicles are dissected as previously described.
- Fascicles from the graft are matched according to size to the host site fascicles.
- The grafts typically "shrink," and to allow for this, the graft is trimmed to a length 10 to 15% longer than the distance between the host nerve segments. If this is not done adequately, undue tension can develop at the repair site.
- Another key point is to make the various fascicle repairs at different locations so that the suture lines do not all lie within the same plane. To provide approximation, usually two 10–0 nylon sutures are needed; occasionally one suffices. As has been mentioned above, special care must be taken not to traumatize the nerve during suture placement.
- A natural fibrin "glue" is given off by the exposed nerve endings. We not uncommonly use this glue to help in achieving approximation.

Depending on the size of the harvested graft, very large fascicles may require placement of two grafts (▶ Fig. 32.7). In our experience four to six grafts will typically be needed to repair a medium-sized nerve such as the medial or ulnar nerve. Occasionally, after dissecting the injured nerve, the surgeon will find a poor demarcation of the fascicle groupings. In these cases, it is often easier to arbitrarily divide the groupings with the grafts placed in an approximate manner. After a graft is placed, the extremity is splinted or otherwise immobilized for 3 to 4 weeks to allow healing without undue tension. As mentioned earlier (Section 32.4.1), after this healing time has elapsed, it is extremely important to get the limb mobilized and an exercise regimen started, especially in those cases where a joint is involved.

To repeat a critically important point and the ultimate reason for performing a nerve graft: while providing an anatomical track, it assures that the tension along the suture line is not excessive. It is now well established that a regenerating axon will not cross a line of tension; furthermore, tension increases connective tissue proliferation, which becomes a barrier to a regenerating nerve. The use of a nerve graft will provide additional length, prevent tension, and with appropriate attention to the anatomical repair serve as an excellent medium for repair and growth.

32.4.8 Dealing with Nerve Gaps

As has already been discussed, the application of tension to a healing nerve will only cause further fibrosis and retard healing. Nerves are inherently elastic and when cut will immediately retract up to 1 to 2 cm. In the acute period, such retraction is readily overcome with further anatomical dissection and additional relaxation of the nerve. As the interval of time since the injury increases, the natural response of the nerve is to form an intraneural fibrosis, permanently foreshortening the nerve endings. Nerve grafting as a means of overcoming this problem

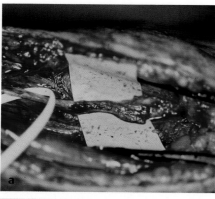

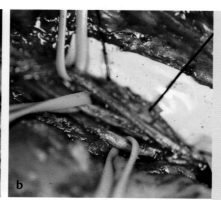

Fig. 32.7 **(a)** The case of a patient with a traumatic injury to the median nerve. Intraoperative recordings showed a partial injury with some fascicles intact and some disrupted. **(b)** A typical intrafascicular dissection and then electrical monitoring was done to isolated out those fascicles which were not conducting. This concept is shown schematically in **(c)**.

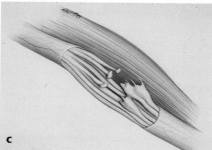

has already been discussed. Several other techniques may be of help in dealing with this problem.[22]

Useful Techniques to Overcome Gaps

- *Transposition*. The principle underlying the transposition of a nerve is straightforward. In rerouting the nerve (i.e., transposing it), the anatomical course becomes straighter, increasing the nerve's effective length. There are natural limitations to this technique, as it can be applied only in a few of anatomical locations. The ulnar nerve can be transposed at the elbow over the epicondyle, providing an additional 3 to 5 cm of length. The median nerve can be transposed just anterior to the pronator teres, allowing up to 2 cm of additional length. When the radial nerve has been transected in a humerus injury, it can be transposed anteriorly and placed between the biceps and the brachialis. In appropriate circumstances, transposition can avoid the necessity of placing a graft.
- *Mobilization*. Mobilization is useful in the instance of nerves without multiple proximal motor branches, which tether the nerve. In mobilizing a nerve, one must be careful not to devascularize it. A nerve is typically supplied along its length by an incoming palisade of vessels, which can be easily identified. If possible, palisading vessels should be mobilized along with the nerve. A generous dissection will usually allow mobilization of an additional 2 to 4 cm of nerve. The main disadvantage to this technique is that the nerve may be required to survive on the basis of its internal

vascular supply, its external supply often being disrupted by the mobilization. Also, as a result of the anatomical dissection, the surgical bed becomes scarred, sometimes impeding a regenerating nerve. Nevertheless, this is a useful technique where only small gaps need to be overcome and avoids the use of grafting.
- *Nerve stretching*. This technique is of only historical interest and to be avoided at all costs except in acute repairs, where only the natural retraction of the severed nerve needs to be overcome.
- *Joint flexion*. The technique of flexing the joint closest to the nerve injury has been frequently used to shorten the course a repaired nerve must traverse. After the repair site has been allowed to heal, the joint is slowly reextended. Although in principle this technique might be sound, studies have yielded disturbing evidence that no matter how slowly the joint is extended, tension is subsequently applied to the nerve, causing intraneural fibrosis and eventual disruption of the repair. As has already been pointed out, a frozen or immobile joint is of no use to a healing nerve and will only retard regeneration. However, in those cases where only mild flexion (10–15 degrees) is used, the technique can be useful; if greater flexion is required or a long immobilization time is predicted, then the use of interposition nerve grafts is a better alternative.[23]
- *Skeletal shortening*. The technique of skeletal shortening was introduced in the Great War and further popularized during World War II and the Vietnam War as a way to deal with foreshortened nerves. Because of the morbidity associated with this technique, it is now primarily of historical

interest. The risk of injury to the surrounding soft tissue more than offsets the benefits of the additional nerve length. As a result, the technique has for the most part been abandoned.

32.5 Surgical Management of Problematic Injuries

32.5.1 Gunshot Nerve Injury

The treatment of nerve injuries caused by gunshot wounds is discussed as a separate category in recognition of their distinctive problems. Formerly restricted to the battlefield, handguns are now a common cause of injury in the urban community. National statistics indicate that 2,500,000 new handguns are legally purchased in the United States each year; how many illegal ones are purchased is unknown. Our hospital admits, on the average, at least two to three patients with gunshot injuries a week. As adolescents and drug suppliers have become more sophisticated in the use of firearms (e.g., 9-mm rapid-repeating weapons, and the like), the emergency room demographics have changed. In the Bronx, most victims of such weapons are dead on arrival. It must be kept in mind that the injury due to the gunshot wound differs from the clean laceration caused by a knife or glass. A high-velocity bullet carries with it both mass and energy. As the bullet travels through soft tissue, it typically exerts a crushing effect on any nerve exposed to its effects; direct impact is unusual. In most cases, as the bullet passes through the soft tissue, the energy is dispersed, the tissue distorted, and the nerve stretched secondary to a cavitation effect. The extent of tissue and nerve disruption depends on the projectile's mass and the striking velocity. Wounds from handguns fired within 2.5 feet of the body have additional unique features to consider, namely, the introduction into the wound of expelled gases formed by the combustion of gunpowder and clothing debris that overlies the bullet entry point (▶ Fig. 32.8a, b).[24]

Principles of Initial Care of Gunshot Wounds

In the treatment of gunshot wounds, certain considerations reflecting the nature of this type of injury must always be kept in mind. Débridement and removal of necrotic tissue are essential, along with incision of any surrounding fascial sheets that might otherwise inhibit circulation as a result of swelling and edema. Because of the large forces applied to the tissues and the resultant energy propagation, nearby neurovascular structures should be directly visualized and any damaged vessels that have the potential to provide blood supply repaired. Perfusion is key to reducing ischemia and providing nutrients to both the nerve and the surrounding tissue. By restoring circulation to the extent possible, the surgical team will enhance the environmental milieu of a regenerating nerve. If during the initial exploration the nerve is noted to be transected and repair deferred, then the nerve endings should be identified and tacked down to the adjacent

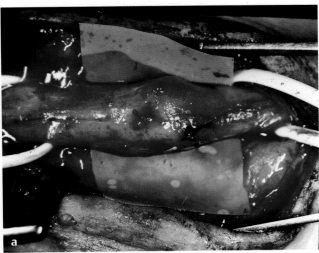

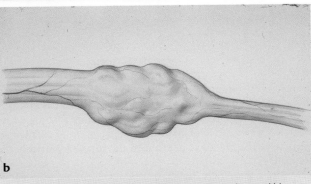

Fig. 32.8 This patient had a gunshot wound injury with partial blow injury to the medial nerve; **(a)** a large neuroma formed at the site of the injury, which can be seen between the two vessels loops. **(b)** A schematic showing a neuroma in continuity from a blunt or cavitation injury.

tissue; doing so reduces the extent of retraction and makes it easier to identify the ending later.

Achieving a clean, débrided wound with adequate circulation and proper skin closure takes priority over performing the repair as an acute procedure. Neurorrhaphy should be undertaken only when the clinical situation and the environmental milieu of the nerve are as close to optimal as possible. Nerves never heal, much less regenerate, in a dirty, contaminated, poorly vascularized wound. Waiting a week or longer for a more optimal environment for healing is not uncommon in gunshot wounds (▶ Fig. 32.9a, b).

32.5.2 Injection Injury

A not uncommon and often overlooked nerve injury in the hospital setting is damage to a peripheral nerve secondary to drug injection. Such injuries range from blunt trauma to direct through-and-through penetration of the nerve. Depending on the extent of the injury and the amount of scar formed, significant functional nerve loss can occur. Other important factors that determine the degree of injury are the anatomical level of injection within the nerve and the neurotoxicity of the drug. For example, intrafascicular injections of diazepam, tetanus toxoid,

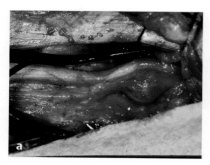

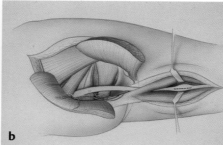

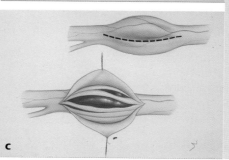

Fig. 32.9 **(a)** This is a case of a taxi driver who was shot in the thigh with immediate partial loss of sciatic nerve function. At acute exploration, exposure of the sciatic nerve showed it to be acutely swollen and discolored, directly in the trajectory of the bullet. **(b)** An internal neurolysis was done and a hematoma was found within the nerve —diagrammatically illustrated in **(b)** and **(c)**. The fascicles were split along their longitudinal axes and the hematoma removed. The patient had an excellent return of function.

or hydrocortisone sodium succinate are much more destructive to the internal milieu of the nerve than potassium chloride, bupivacaine, or dexamethasone. A number of clinical studies have examined the toxicity of injectable drugs; for more detailed information, the reader is referred to the report by Gentili and Hudson.[12]

Despite a seemingly benign anatomical location, even extrafascicular drug injection can cause a significant degree of damage to axons. The main factor that will determine the amount of injury is once again the type of drug injected. Therefore, in evaluating a patient with an injection injury, the nerve involved and the potential degree of drug toxicity should be taken into account in predicting the potential severity of the lesion. In most cases of drug injection, recovery from the injury and regeneration of the nerve will occur; the earlier the recovery, the better the prognosis. This is one of the few types of peripheral nerve injury in which early operative intervention is rarely, if ever, indicated. If significant signs of recovery have not been detected by 6 months, an intraoperative exploration is indicated. Intraoperative electrical monitoring is essential to map out the length of the lesion. In injection injuries, it is not uncommon to find that the nerve is normal in external appearance or perhaps surrounded by fibrosis and scarring. In some cases, the only finding noted is that the nerve appears a bit shriveled in its external caliber. In these cases, an internal neurolysis is indicated, as only by opening the nerve and exploring the intrafascicular region can the extent and degree of damage be assessed. The releasing of scar and performance of neurolysis will in some cases enhance the regeneration potential and allow some return of function.

32.5.3 Penetrating Injuries of the Brachial Plexus

There are only a few areas in neurosurgery as challenging as the brachial plexus. For this reason, many neurosurgeons have

either not attempted or have abandoned surgery of the brachial plexus (▶Fig. 32.10). Although the management of a single nerve laceration within the brachial plexus usually is not a daunting challenge to the neurosurgeon, few are enthusiastic about dealing with it, because of the potential complexity of the anatomical reconstruction. Nevertheless, surgery within this region remains fairly straightforward. The anatomy of the brachial plexus has been well worked out, and its not unusual anatomical variants have long been appreciated. Successful outcomes depend on the same factors that govern most of neurosurgery: thorough knowledge of the anatomy, an understanding of the causation of the injury and potential effects, and finally technique—careful, gentle reapproximation of the injured nerves, whether by primary reapproximation or by grafting.

A permanent injury of the brachial plexus, particularly a penetrating injury, fortunately remains uncommon. In the urban environment, the most common brachial plexus injury is due to stretching. These types occur most frequently as a result of birth injuries (e.g., Erb's palsy) or motor vehicle accidents, particularly those involving motorcycles. The patient prone to dislocating the shoulder joint not uncommonly develops a stretch palsy of the plexus (in most cases, transient). Because the stretch injury for the most part improves without surgical intervention, the patient is referred for aggressive rehabilitation and physical therapy. Surgical intervention is reserved for the patient who does not show improvement within 4 to 6 months or has had a sharp penetrating injury, which merits a high index of suspicion for nerve laceration. (▶Fig. 32.11).

In the acute penetrating injury of the brachial plexus, it can sometimes be difficult to determine the location and the nature of the lesion. Often, however, a good history uncovers the source of the injury. In the case of a penetrating injury with a sharp instrument that results in neural loss, a good physical examination will often detect the part of the plexus that has been injured. When the history is clear and the anatomy well worked out, early surgical intervention for the injury due to sharp

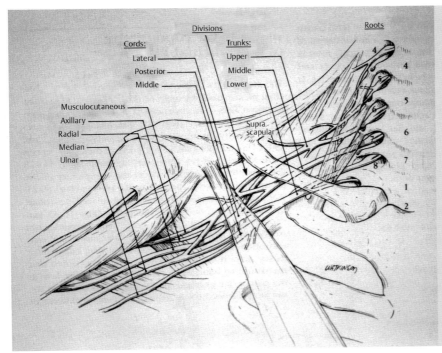

Fig. 32.10 The surgical anatomy of the brachial plexus detailing the relationship of the roots, trunks, divisions, and cords to the scalene muscle and clavicle. (Reproduced with permission from Mackinnon SE, Dellon AL. Classification of Nerve Injuries as the Basis for Treatment Surgery of the Peripheral Nerve. New York, NY: Thieme Medical Publishers, 1988:Figure 16.1.[32])

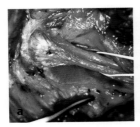
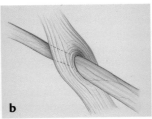
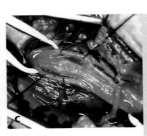

Fig. 32.11 (a) A case of a man shot through the lower neck region with the bullet glancing off the upper trunk of the brachial plexus. At surgery done 3 months later, a tight cicatrix of scar was found encasing the upper trunk; this was opened and removed with the patient having nearly 40% return of function after 6 months of physical therapy. (b) A schematic showing the scar around the upper trunk acting like a napkin ring around the nerve complex. (c) After an internal neurolysis of the trunk.

penetration is indicated. It is helpful to base surgical planning on an electrophysiologic work-up with magnetic resonance imaging (MRI). The work-up should be obtained in the first 24 to 48 hours to determine the level and extent of the injury. The findings of the physical examination and electrophysiologic and radiographic work-up usually make localizing the level of the injury straightforward.[25] Once the level of the lesion has been worked out, the surgeon is in a position to advise the patient as to the need for surgery and the prognosis.

The indications for early intervention in a missile-type penetrating plexus injury are not matters of general consensus. Among the few indications that most authors agree on are injuries that result in a vascular anomaly such as a pseudoaneurysm with resultant compression of the plexus. There is the occasional rare patient with an acute severe pain problem who may need an urgent neurolysis. In a patient with an acute pain syndrome, operation may be indicated for removal of a foreign fragment embedded in the plexus. A review of the war literature gives conflicting indications as to when to explore

a penetrating missile injury of the plexus. A number of these studies in question were completed before the advent of the microscope. Since then, much has changed technically, and today more precise primary repairs of the plexus are not only feasible but also encouraged.

Lesions high in the plexus, those close to the root outlet area, have the worst prognosis and remain the most difficult to repair. MR studies not uncommonly reveal pseudomeningoceles at the root rupture site. The anatomy of this region is such that there is little laxity to the nerves, and primary repairs are therefore difficult. Placement of a graft can be challenging, and any functioning nerve fascicles can be disrupted by the repair. These factors all make for a poor outcome. Surgical exploration of high lesions is rarely indicated. When repair is indicated, it is the sharply transected nerve that has the best chance for successful repair and recovery of some function. Lesions involving the lower plexus have the worst long-term outcome because of the length of nerve that needs to be regenerated. More distal lesions can have partially gratifying results if dealt with promptly, before the nerve has had time to retract. The best outcomes are seen in injuries that only partially disrupt the fascicles. In such lesions the main body of the nerve remains intact, resulting in little retraction. The injured fascicles can be repaired with interposition grafts. Because of the higher exposure, these injuries occur more commonly in the upper trunks and roots.

High-velocity missile injuries to the plexus can significantly disrupt surrounding tissues. For example, if the injury of the plexus is due to the cavitation shock wave generated by the projectile, the disruption mainly occurs in the surrounding tissues. Only rarely is there direct damage to the plexus from impact.[24,26,27]

In a series of gunshot injuries to the brachial plexus, it was shown that the best outcome was achieved in patients who sustained injuries to the upper trunk and lateral and posterior cords.[28] If the injury occurred in the lower trunk and in most medial cord lesions, the results were poor unless the patient exhibited early regeneration with nerve action potentials at operation. Direct injury to the plexus typically results in a poor outcome. Vascular compression, foreign bodies, and external strictures gave the best outcomes if treated aggressively. A number of other authors have shown similar results in gunshot or missile-type injuries.[26,27,28,29,30,31]

Technique

The tight anatomical constraints of the brachial plexus leave little if any room for mobilization, and the surgeon should therefore always be prepared to harvest nerve grafts for interpositioning in areas where gaps appear. As already noted, any attempt to pull the two ends of a divided nerve together and place them under tension will in all likelihood meet with a dismal outcome. On the other hand, in those rare instances in which the surgeon discovers compression of the plexus by a hematoma or foreign body, its removal will often be followed by return of function.

A number of approaches to the brachial plexus have been developed over the years. The most frequently used, because of the ease and extent of the exposure, appears to be the one developed by MacCarty and his group at the Mayo Clinic.[30] The posterior subscapular approach is rarely, if ever, needed in penetrating injuries, with the possible exception of gunshot wounds involving the lower roots and trunks. The brachial plexus can be fully exposed through an S-shaped incision (it is helpful to incorporate the injury scar) that begins vertically on the neck and is carried down to, and then parallel with, the clavicle over to the axillary crease. The length of the incision is modified to include the area of the plexus the operator wishes to visualize. Electrophysiologic monitoring is always employed in plexus exploration; therefore, normal plexus should be visualized to allow monitoring. To visualize the midportion of the plexus, the clavicle can often be dissected free from surrounding tissue and mobilized sufficiently that it need not be cut. When the surgeon is working in the vicinity of the clavicle, care must be exercised not to damage the underlying vascular bundle, which should always be dissected free. The pectoralis major and minor are dissected at their origins and reflected downward toward the chest. For exposure of the cord and terminal branchings, the dissection

is carried further over the axilla. The cephalic vein, which delineates the deltoid and pectoralis muscles, affords easy identification of a plane in which these muscles can be split to obtain greater exposure. The coracobrachialis is reflected free and moved upward rostrally. For lesions higher in the plexus, that is, those that are close to the roots and trunks, the sternocleidomastoid muscle and omohyoid may need to be divided. To visualize the middle and lower elements of the plexus, the anterior scalene muscle has to be divided. Care must be taken to preserve the phrenic nerve, which courses along the scalenus muscle. This nerve should first be identified and then gently retracted with the scalene muscle; it should never be divided, as the morbidity of a paralyzed diaphragm is rarely acceptable (▶ Fig. 32.11).

Once the plexus has been exposed, the site, level, and extent of injury are determined; this is accomplished with the electrophysiologist's assistance. A completely transected nerve is reconstructed with interfascicular grafts, or an epineural repair is performed if the injured nerve can be mobilized sufficiently. In the case of a partially severed nerve, an electrophysiologic analysis is made of the nerve action potentials to determine the extent of conduction. Normally functioning fascicles are dissected and identified, and the remaining damaged fascicles are repaired with interfascicular grafts. When an exposure has been delayed, as in a gunshot wound, the injured nerves are localized. If the nerve remains in continuity but does not show a nerve action potential, an internal neurolysis is done. Typically, the internal nerve is very fibrotic and often difficult to dissect. If the nerve is totally nonviable, both anatomically and electrically, it is resected and a graft placed. If, on electrophysiologic analysis, portions of the nerve prove to conduct, then the nerve is partially split, the nonviable tissue removed, and grafts placed. The key principle in a plexus repair is to preserve as much functioning nerve tissue as possible and employ grafting only to replace tissue, which shows no potential for recovery. Good electrophysiologic monitoring is key, as no other methods are available to identify the viable nerve elements.

With the repairs completed, the layers are closed in reverse order with reattachment of the divided muscles. The clavicle, if split, can be wired or plated together. It has been my experience that the rigid fixation of the clavicle provided by plating seems to be more comfortable for patients. Meticulous hemostasis is critical in the closure. The arm and shoulder are then splinted for 3 to 4 weeks to allow the nerve repairs to obtain good tensile strength. As already emphasized, postoperative physical therapy and rehabilitation remain critical for good recovery of function. For additional details of the surgical anatomy and exposure of the brachial plexus, the reader is referred to Craig and MacCarty's original paper[30] and papers by Kline and Judice,[32] Mackinnon and Dellon,[13] Davis, Onofrio, and MacCarty,[33] and Stevens, Davis, and MacCarty.[34]

To reduce the frustration and postoperative depression that often occurs in plexus injuries, it is essential that the patient, family, and surgeon all have an equal understanding of the long-term goals and what truly can be expected in the event of recovery. It is always the case that the patients' expectations are overly optimistic and often exaggerated. Patients will expect to experience immediate return of lost function when they awaken from surgery. The necessity of thorough counseling and education for the patient and family in the preoperative period is evident. Counseling and education must be continued throughout the lengthy postoperative recovery period. An understanding of what realistic expectations consist in will go a long way toward reducing depression and anxiety; thus, counseling and education are as much a part of the care of the patient as the surgery itself.

32.6 A Final Comment

A common misconception among surgeons concerns the length of time that it takes for an injured nerve to recovery. Established surgeons and house staff commonly state that the duration of the "normal" recovery period is 1 to 2 years. Studies of patients with injuries incurred during the Vietnam conflict and accounts of extensive experience of a number of peripheral nerve surgeons have shown that this estimate is too short. In a long-term follow-up by Eversmann and his colleagues, 14 indicated that only 40 to 45% of cases showed progressive functional recovery in the first 2 years. Longer follow-up disclosed a much higher percentage of recovery; in one case the elapsed time was 8 years. As a result of these findings, patients should be encouraged to continue physical therapy and rehabilitation for as long as possible. The idea that only a year or two is necessary is false and if encouraged can led to unnecessary unsatisfactory outcomes. Surgeons should carefully consider the appropriate duration of follow-up in nerve injuries and not rule out potential recovery in less than 5 years.

The surgical team often ignores the postoperative care period for the patient with a peripheral nerve injury. The care of the patient does not end with either the surgery or with the patient's discharge from the hospital. Peripheral nerve injuries often entail a great deal of pain, with causalgia not being uncommon. For this reason, all my patients receive at least an initial screening by the Pain Service. The basis for this policy is important: a patient with peripheral nerve injury who has minimal pain will participate actively in physical therapy, which is essential in order to prevent contractures, reduce atrophy, and prevent stiffness and thus have a much greater chance of recovery. As it takes a considerable period of time for a nerve to regenerate, it is important to keep the distal structures in the best shape possible so that once the sprouting axons reestablish connection to the distal nerves, structures ready to be innervated await them.

Finally, it must be noted that the patient with a peripheral nerve injury often has associated anesthesia. The importance of educating the patient to the dangers of such anesthesia cannot be overemphasized. Burns, decubitus ulcers, or abrasion injuries can be debilitating but with proper education can be avoided.

References

[1] Brooks DM. Open wounds of the brachial plexus. J Bone Joint Surg Br. 1949; 31B(1):17–33
[2] Burdach E. Beitrag zur mikroskopischen Anatomie der Nerven. Könisberg: Gebrüder Bornträger; 1837
[3] Goodrich JT, Kliot M. History of peripheral and cranial nerves. In: Tubbs RS, Rizk E, Shoja MM, Loukas M, Barbaro N, Spinner RJ, eds. Nerve and Nerve Injuries. Amsterdam, the Netherlands: Elsevier; 2015:3–22
[4] McGillicuddy JE. Techniques of nerve repair. In: Wilkins RH, Rengachary SS, eds. Neurosurgery. New York, NY: McGraw-Hill; 1985:1871–1881
[5] Millesi H. Reappraisal of nerve repair. Surg Clin North Am. 1981; 61(2):321–340
[6] Sunderland S. Nerves and Nerve Injuries. 2nd ed. Edinburgh, UK: Churchill Livingston; 1978
[7] Sunderland S. A classification of peripheral nerve injuries producing loss of function. Brain. 1951; 74(4):491–516
[8] Kline DG. Management of the neuroma in continuity. In: Wilkins RH, Rengachary SS, eds. Neurosurgery. New York, NY: McGraw-Hill; 1985:1864–1871
[9] Kline DG, Hudson AR. Nerve Injuries. Operative results for major nerve injuries, entrapments, and tumors. Philadelphia, PA: W.B. Saunders; 1995
[10] Sedden H. Common causes of nerve injury: open wounds, traction, skeletal. In: Seddon H, ed. Surgical Disorders of the Peripheral Nerves. Baltimore, MD: Williams and Wilkins; 1972:68–88
[11] Seddon HJ. Three types of nerve injury. Brain. 1946; 66:237–288
[12] Gentili F, Hudson AR. Peripheral nerve injuries: types, causes, grading. In: Wilkins RH, Rengachary SS, eds. Neurosurgery. New York, NY: McGraw-Hill; 1985:1802–1812
[13] Mackinnon SE, Dellon AL. Classification of nerve injuries as the basis for treatment. In: Surgery of the Peripheral Nerve. New York, NY: Thieme Medical Publishers; 1988:35–63
[14] Eversmann WW Jr. Long-term follow up of combat-incurred nerve injuries. In: Burkhalter WE, ed. Orthopedic Surgery in Vietnam. Washington, DC: Government Printing Office; 1992: 114-135
[15] Edshage S. Peripheral nerve suture: a technique for improved intraneural topography. Evaluation of some suture materials. Acta Chir Scand Suppl. 1964; 15:331:, 1 [Suppl]
[16] Sunderland S. Funicular suture and funicular exclusion in the repair of severed nerves. Br J Surg. 1953; 40(164):580–587
[17] Smith JW. Microsurgery of peripheral nerves. Plast Reconstr Surg. 1964; 33:317–329
[18] Millesi H, Meissl G, Berger A. The interfascicular nerve-grafting of the median and ulnar nerves. J Bone Joint Surg Am. 1972; 54(4):727–750
[19] Millesi H, Meissl G, Berger A. Further experience with interfascicular grafting of the median, ulnar, and radial nerves. J Bone Joint Surg Am. 1976; 58(2):209–218
[20] Samii M. Modern aspects of peripheral and cranial nerve surgery. Adv Tech Stand Neurosurg. 1975; 2:33–85
[21] Terzis J, Faibisoff B, Williams B. The nerve gap: suture under tension vs. graft. Plast Reconstr Surg. 1975; 56(2):166–170
[22] Sunderland S. The pros and cons of funicular nerve repair. J Hand Surg Br. 1979; 4(3):201–211
[23] Highet WB, Sanders FK. The effects of stretching nerves after suture. Br J Surg. 1943; 30(120):355–369
[24] Omer GE Jr. Nerve injuries associated with gunshot wounds of the extremities. In: Gelberman RH, ed. Operative Nerve Repair and Reconstruction. Philadelphia, PA: J.B. Lippincott; 1991:655–670
[25] Mackinnon SE, Dellon AL. Brachial plexus injuries. In: Surgery of the Peripheral Nerve. New York, NY: Thieme Medical Publishers; 1988:423–454
[26] Brunelli G, Monini L, Brunelli F. Problems in nerve lesions surgery. Microsurgery. 1985; 6(4):187–198
[27] Nelson KG, Jolly PC, Thomas PA. Brachial plexus injuries associated with missile wounds of the chest. A report of 9 cases from Viet Nam. J Trauma. 1968; 8(2):268–275
[28] Kline DG. Civilian gunshot wounds to the brachial plexus. J Neurosurg. 1989; 70(2):166–174
[29] Campbell JB, Lusskin R. Upper extremity paralysis consequent to brachial plexus injury. Partial alleviation through neurolysis or autograft reconstruction. Surg Clin North Am. 1972; 52(5):1235–1245
[30] Craig WM, MacCarty CS. Injuries to the brachial plexus. In: Walters W, ed. Lewis' Practice of Surgery. Vol. 3. Hagerstown, MD: WF Prior Company; 1948:1–15
[31] Nulson FE, Slade HW. Recovery following injury to the brachial plexus. In: Woodhall B, Beebe GW, eds. Peripheral Nerve Regeneration: A Follow-up Study of 3,656 World War II Injuries. Washington, DC: Government Printing Office; 1957:389–408
[32] Kline DG, Judice DJ. Operative management of selected brachial plexus lesions. J Neurosurg. 1983; 58(5):631–649
[33] Davis DH, Onofrio BM, MacCarty CS. Brachial plexus injuries. Mayo Clin Proc. 1978; 53(12):799–807
[34] Stevens JC, Davis DH, MacCarty CS. A 32-year experience with the surgical treatment of selected brachial plexus lesions with emphasis on its reconstruction. Surg Neurol. 1983; 19(4):334–345

33 Acute Management of Compressive Peripheral Neuropathies

Kashif A. Shaikh, Nicholas M. Barbaro, and Richard B. Rodgers

Abstract

Peripheral nerve trauma is a not uncommon neurosurgical emergency. These injuries often affect young, working-aged individuals and can be highly disabling. Long-term outcomes are highly variable. Appropriate initial assessment and management requires an in-depth knowledge of peripheral nerve anatomy as well as a sound understanding of the pathophysiology of acute nerve injury. In this chapter, we review the pathophysiologic aspects of acute peripheral nerve injury, highlight key initial physical examination findings, and discuss the role of ancillary testing, including electromyography/nerve conduction velocity and various modalities of neuroimaging. The indications for and timing of neurosurgical intervention are reviewed across a variety of clinical settings.

Keywords: acute compressive neuropathy, nerve injury peripheral nerve injury, peripheral nerve trauma, traumatic neuropathy

33.1 Introduction

With an annual incidence approaching 50 per 100,000 cases, peripheral nerve trauma is a not uncommon neurosurgical emergency consult.[1] Appropriate initial assessment and management is vital, as these injuries frequently affect young, working-aged individuals and outcomes can be highly variable, ranging from complete recovery to significant limitations and disability. The acute management of traumatic peripheral nerve injuries requires knowledge of normal peripheral nerve anatomy and physiology as well as the an in-depth understanding of the pathophysiology of acute nerve injury.

33.2 Anatomy and Physiology

Although a detailed discussion of the gross anatomy of the peripheral nervous system and its normal variants is beyond the scope of this chapter, it is essential to understand peripheral nerve microanatomy to better assess and manage these injuries[2] (▶Fig. 33.1).

The basic subunit of a given peripheral nerve is the individual axon. Each axon is surrounded by a background substance consisting of a collagen mesh termed the endoneurium. Axons are bundled together into fascicles, which in turn are surrounded by a background substance termed the perineurium. The perineurium is made up of a large number of organized collagen fibers and contributes to the tensile strength of the nerve. Lastly, the entire peripheral nerve is wrapped in a layer of surrounding connective tissue termed the epineurium, which contains the blood supply to the nerve (▶Fig. 33.2). The number of fascicles in a given peripheral nerve can vary from one (monofascicular) to many (polyfascicular) based on the individual nerve and its function[3] (▶Fig. 33.3).

The basic physiology of peripheral nerve conduction is related to the creation and maintenance of an electrochemical gradient. Selective permeability of ion channels in the cell membrane allows an electrochemical potential difference between the intra- and extracellular spaces. This potential difference is responsible for the initiation and transmission of action potentials in response to a given stimulus.[3,4]

Conduction velocity is based on the intrinsic properties of the given nerve, specifically the cross-sectional diameter and degree of myelination. Large-diameter fibers have lower resistance and therefore conduct faster. Myelin decreases capacitance and increases resistance across the cell membrane, serving to increase conduction velocity and minimizing signal attenuation, allowing for fast conduction from node to node (saltatory conduction). Thus, large-diameter myelinated axons have the fastest conduction velocity.[3,5]

33.3 Pathophysiology of Nerve Injury

There are two components to consider in evaluating acute compressive nerve injury: the direct structural trauma, in the form of stretch and/or compression, and the interruption of vascular supply. The response of a given peripheral nerve to an acute compressive insult is based on both intrinsic and extrinsic factors. Extrinsic factors affecting the extent of nerve injury include mechanism of injury, degree of force applied, duration of force applied, and length of involved nerve. Intrinsic properties of a given nerve affecting severity of clinical injury include fiber type and diameter, elasticity and tolerance of stretch, degree of myelination, and extent of vascular supply.[6,7]

Direct structural injury can be limited to the microstructure of the nerve, affecting the nerve at the level of that axon or fascicle, or in severe cases damage the macrostructure including disruption of the epineurium and discontinuity.

Nerve injuries can also result from vascular compromise. Even mild stretch can cause impairment of venous drainage leading to localized hypoxia and edema causing increased intrafascicular pressure. Increased pressure, in turn, limits arterial flow, further worsening hypoxia. Direct disruption of the extrinsic vascular supply can also occur in the setting of extremity injuries such as crushed limb and/or compartment syndrome.

In general, large heavily myelinated axons are more susceptible to injury than smaller-diameter axons with less myelin. This is partially due to the high sensitivity of Schwann cells to ischemia. Nerve fibers with more fascicles are less susceptible to compressive forces because of the ability to redistribute those forces throughout the epineurium.

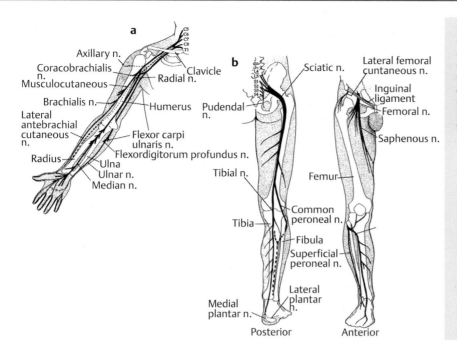

Fig. 33.1 The course of major peripheral nerves in relation to skeletal structures of the **(a)** upper and **(b)** lower extremities. Common sites of injury in the upper extremity include the clavicular region, midhumerus, medial epicondyle, and wrist. Common sites of injury in the lower extremity include the sciatic notch, inguinal ligament, femoral head, popliteal fossa, fibular head, and anterior tibia.

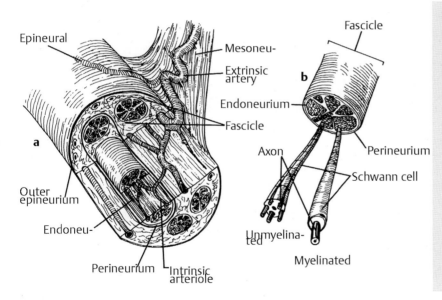

Fig. 33.2 **(a)** Cross-section of a peripheral nerve, with relationships of epi-, peri-, and endoneurium shown. Also shown are the extrinsic and intrinsic vascular supply. **(b)** Cross-section of single fascicle, demonstrating bundles of very thinly myelinated axons and heavily myelinated axons.

33.4 Classification of Peripheral Nerve Injuries

Seddon initially classified peripheral nerve injury on the basis of the structural/functional damage to the nerve.[8,9,10] Class I injuries, termed neuropraxia, involve a temporary interruption of conduction without anatomical axonal disruption. Class II injuries, termed axonotmesis, involve loss of axonal continuity and conduction, with maintenance of the surrouding supportive connective tissues. Class III injuries, termed neurotmesis, involve a complete disruption of the entirety of the nerve. Sunderland later expanded this classification to five degrees of peripheral nerve injury.[8,9] Grade I injuries represent neuropraxic injuries similar to the Seddon classification. Grade II injuries involve damage to the axon with the endoneurium remaining intact. Grade III injuries involve damage to both the axon and the endoneurium. Grade IV injuries involve damage to all the internal nerve structures with only an intact epineurium remaining. Grade V injuries represent complete transection. There is much overlap between the two systems and knowledge of both schemata is important, as the extent of nerve injury has implications for both management and prognosis[8,9,10] (▶ Table 33.1).

Purely neuropraxic injuries recover on the scale of days to weeks as the injured myelin sheath is restored.[11,12] Very mild neuropraxic injuries may even resolve within in a few minutes

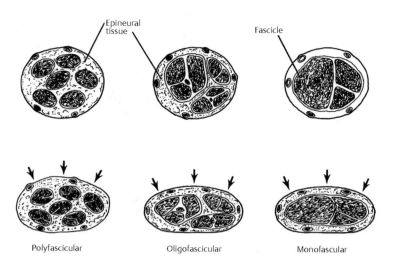

Epineural tissue

Fascicle

Polyfascicular   Oligofascicular   Monofascular

Fig. 33.3 Examples of three different fiber types in the neutral state (top) and under compressive forces as depicted by arrows (bottom). The polyfascicular fiber can distribute compression throughout the epineurial connective tissue and therefore can tolerate greater forces. The monofascicular fiber is affected more severely by compression because of its relative lack of connective tissue. What is less obvious in the figure is the fact that more peripherally located fascicles are more susceptible to compression than those more centrally positioned.

Table 33.1 Classification systems of nerve injuries

Seddon	Sunderland
Neurapraxia: mild injury with reversible loss of function; may be complete or incomplete	First degree: loss of axonal conduction; completely reversible
Axonotmesis: complete interruption of axon with preservation of basement membrane, endo-, peri-, and epineurium; complete injury with distal wallerian degeneration; good potential recovery	Second degree: loss of axon continuity with preservation of endoneurium; good recovery
Neurotmesis: complete anatomical sever, or intact epineurium with internal disruption incompatible with recovery; complete injury; almost always requires surgical repair for any chance of recovery	Third degree: loss of axon and endoneurium, with preservation of perineurium; delayed incomplete recovery
	Fourth degree: Loss of perineurium
	Fifth degree: Loss of epineurium (i.e., transected nerve)

to hours. Axonal injuries, on the other hand, recover over a longer period of time, with the extent and duration of recovery based on the severity of injury and the distance from the site of nerve injury to the innervated muscle with axonal regeneration occurring at approximately 1 mm per day from the axonal stump.[11]

33.5 Evaluation of Compressive Peripheral Nerve Injuries

Evaluation of suspected peripheral nerve injuries begins with ascertaining the history and mechanism of injury. This can provide clues as to the nature and extent of injury. Initial assessment is based on three components: the physical examination, imaging studies, and electrophysiologic testing.[11,12]

33.5.1 Physical Examination

The physical examination is the most important aspect of the initial evaluation. Imaging findings can often be difficult to interpret and nonspecific in the acute setting, and electrophysiologic studies performed early after injury will often appear normal.

A thorough understanding of the basic motor innervation and sensory distributions of a given peripheral nerve and its relationship to adjacent anatomical structures is needed to establish an initial examination and potentially localize site of injury. Documentation of an initial examination is vital. Even in an uncooperative or comatose patient, it is important to establish an initial examination to allow for meaningful comparative serial examinations.

The limb or region being testing should be fully exposed, and ideally, comparison should be made with the unaffected side. Palpation along the known course of a nerve may help reveal site of injury. A Tinel's sign—the presence of easily elicitable neurologic symptoms with light nerve percussion—at a potential site of compression can be suggestive but is not always present.[13] It is also worth noting that a resting pain can radiate leading to false localization.

Detailed description of the muscle innervation of each peripheral nerve is beyond the scope of this chapter. It is important to isolate the muscle and nerve being tested for a precise examination, as patients naturally find compensatory mechanisms to achieve necessary movements.[12]

The sensory examination should include tests of light touch, pain, and vibratory sensation. The examiner must be aware that there is significant overlap in sensory distributions of the peripheral nerves, and this overlap varies by modality. For example, the area of light touch perception of a nerve is larger than the area of sensation of painful stimuli. One must also be aware that the different sensory modalities have varied sensitivity to compressive injury.[12] Disturbances in vibratory sensation occur early and with less severe compression, whereas two-point discrimination is usually the last modality affected before total sensory block. Each peripheral nerve with sensory function has a relatively constant "autologous zone" where sensation will remain impaired even after other sensory nerves have supplied function to the involved skin.

33.5.2 Electrophysiologic Tests

Electrophysiologic testing can be very useful in assessing and following a peripheral nerve injury. These tests can help establish the location and severity of injury, as well as monitor for subclinical improvement when performed serially over time. When performed immediately following injury, the result may be normal.[14] It has generally been considered best to wait at least 2 to 4 weeks following injury to allow for meaningful results; however, recent studies have sought to look closer at the very early subtle findings (prior to the development of fibrillations) to help guide patient counseling and management decisions.[11]

Electromyography (EMG) is a study of electrical activity in the muscle in response to nerve stimulation. It is highest yield if performed after some degree of wallerian degeneration has occurred, as this will then allow signs of denervation to be seen. Fibrillations and positive sharp waves indicate acute denervation. Because motor latencies and potentials differ with severity and time from injury, the EMG can be used to assess both the degree as well as the relative chronicity of injury.[14] As above, it can also be very helpful in following recovery, as serial studies may reveals nascent potentials indicative of axonal regeneration.[11,14]

Nerve conduction velocities (NCVs) test the speed of electrical conduction in a peripheral nerve.[14] This test is performed with surface electrodes to stimulate and record the velocity and amplitude of conduction across a specific region of a nerve as compared with normal standardized values. It is best suited to specifically localize the area or even multiple areas of compression. The study will reveal focal slowing or conduction block across the area of injury, with a decrease in the amplitude of the sensory nerve action potential (SNAP). SNAPs are the most sensitive indicator of nerve compression. The presence of a normal SNAP in a nerve that has lost all motor function indicates that the injury is very proximal, such as in the spinal roots. This occurs because the cell bodies of the sensory nerve fibers are in the dorsal root ganglion, whereas those of the motor axons are in the ventral horn of the spinal cord.

Somatosensory evoked potentials (SSEPs) record the impulses from sensory stimulation to the central nervous system. Although they are designed to assess lesions of sensory pathways of the brain and spinal cord, they can sometimes be helpful in diagnosing a proximal peripheral nerve injury (e.g., root injury).[14,15]

In addition to diagnosis and following recovery, electrophysiologic testing can also be utilized in the operating room during exploration of peripheral nerve injury to assist with localization and also to assess nerve function intraoperatively to guide decision-making during the operation.[14]

33.5.3 Imaging

Initial imaging in the setting of suspected peripheral nerve injury often has already been obtained as part of an assessment of other concominant injuries, such as plain films in the setting of obvious extremity trauma.

In terms of dedicated imaging studies, magnetic resonance imaging (MRI) has largely supplanted computed tomography (CT) as the imaging of choice for suspected nerve and soft-tissue injuries.[16] As technology has advanced, peripheral nerves can now be identified and their courses followed on high-resolution MRI and MR neurography.[11,16,17,18] Signal change within the nerve can sometimes be seen to identify and localize the site of injury.[11,16,17] Extrinsic factors contributing to injury, such as large compartmental hematoma, can also be identified. In addition, MR evaluation of the spine may reveal pseudomeningocele indicative of nerve root avulsion. Studies have evaluated the role of diffusion tensor imaging (DTI) and diffusion tensor tractography (DTT) in evaluating and following nerve regeneration.[11,19,20,21] There is hope that this may ultimately serve as a useful method to detect the very early phases of injury and axonal regeneration, well before EMG changes appear.[11,19,20,21]

Ultrasonography is a potentially useful imaging adjunct and has the advantage of being easily obtainable. An additional benefit is the dynamic quality of ultrasound, allowing assessment of the nerve in the context of its anatomical relationships with movement.[22,23,24,25,26] Work is ongoing to gauge further potential uses of nerve ultrasonography, including intraoperative application.[27] Quality of images obtained and interpretation of the images, however, can be challenging and are highly user dependent.

33.6 Acute Management

In general, the acute management of suspected compression neuropathies is conservative. Urgent or emergent surgical intervention is not commonly performed. There are, however, certain clinical situations that merit early exploration and these will be reviewed.

33.6.1 Fractures/Dislocations

Extremity orthopedic injury is a common cause of acute traumatic peripheral nerve injury. The acute management in these settings is usually dictated by the orthopedic plan for the primary injury. A closed fracture or dislocation with concominant suspected nerve injury should be reduced as soon as possible. As this is often performed in a closed fashion, a decision regarding dedicated nerve exploration can be based on serial physical examinations following reduction. In the case of either open fracture or planned open orthopedic procedure, the involved nerve can be explored at that time if felt to be easily accessible. In general, more harm than good can result from aggressive dissection attempts to find the nerve if not easily accessible from the planned exposure. In terms of prognosis, nerve recovery is better in patients with closed rather than open injuries. This is likely for a variety of reasons, including concomitant vascular injuries, more significant trauma, and higher infection risk associated with open orthopedic fractures.

33.6.2 Compartment Syndrome

A compartment syndrome is defined as increased pressure within a defined space of the body. This can occur within any compartment, including the abdomen and retroperitoneum, but classically the term is used to describe elevated pressure within a fascial compartment in an extremity. This can occur following any trauma to the extremity, including crush injuries, ischemic events, gunshot wounds, and burns.[28]

Symptoms of compartment syndrome typically arise in a delayed fashion, often times several hours following the initial injury, as the acute event incites gradually progressive tissue edema. Clinical suspicion arises in a limb demonstrating any of the "five Ps": pain, paresthesias, paralysis, pallor, pulselessness. A high clinical suspicion is necessary, as a limb demonstrating all five Ps likely has experienced irreversible damage. Diagnosis can be confirmed by measuring compartment pressures. Paresthesias tend to occur when compartment pressures reach 30 mm Hg, with significant edema within the nerve developing between 30 and 50 mm Hg. Compartment pressures greater than 50 mm Hg result in complete conduction block.[28]

Treatment is directed at emergent pressure relief, which usually requires fasciotomies, or several longitudinal incisions in the fascial covering of the compartment. Surgery is usually performed when pressures are greater than 30 mm Hg. Early diagnosis is critical, as pressure relief within 8 hours of symptom onset results in recovery of neurologic function in nearly 80% of patients.

33.6.3 Compressive Hematomas

Hematomas can occur from a variety of traumatic vascular causes, including iatrogenic. Nerve compression can be secondary to an expanding hematoma or as a result of pseudoaneurysm formation following vascular injury.[29,30] As the prevalence of anticoagulation increases, there have been numerous reports of compressive neuropathies related to spontaneous hematoma formation.[31] Nerve injury can result either from direct hematoma compression or from a resultant compartment syndrome secondary to the hematoma.

Urgent surgery in the setting of suspected hematoma compression should be performed in the setting of severe clinical nerve dysfunction or clear worsening of function, as mild to moderate neuropathies often improve with conservative management alone.

33.6.4 Blunt Extrinsic Compression

Blunt extrinsic compression remains the most common cause of peripheral nerve palsy (►Fig. 33.4). There are innumerable potential mechanisms of compression, including iatrogenic operative positioning, blunt trauma over a particularly vulnerable area of nerve course, prolonged or repetitive maintenance of pressure of certain positions, or even tight clothing.[32]

The most classically described compressive peripheral nerve injury is the "Saturday night palsy" or "honeymooner's palsy" in which prolonged pressure over the arm results in radial nerve palsy.[33] The patient in these cases typically reports awakening with a new, often complete, wrist drop.[33]

Another form of compressive neuropathy is termed "crutch palsy," resulting from repetitive and prolonged axillary compression with the use of crutches. This can result in compression neuropathy of the posterior cord of the brachial plexus.[34]

Positioning-related neuropathies in the operating room are not uncommon. Ulnar and peroneal nerves are particularly vulnerable to prolonged compression. Injuries related to tourniquets and even blood pressure cuffs have been reported.[32]

Extrinsic compressive neuropathies are usually best diagnosed with a careful history and physical examination. The initial management of these cases is conservative. Recovery should be followed with EMG and serial examination over the course of weeks.[11,23] The vast majority of these cases will fully recover within 8 weeks.[11,12]

33.7 Surgery

Aside from the above indications for acute exploration, surgery in peripheral nerve compression neuropathies is typically reserved for lack of expected improvement or clinical worsening of neurologic deficit. The optimal timing of surgical intervention is not known, as many of these injuries improve with conservative management. At the same time, however, outcomes of injuries that do not improve with conservative management and ultimately undergo surgical exploration are better the earlier in the course surgery is undertaken. Thus, it is important to try and identify surgical lesions early in the recovery course. Serial EMG has traditionally been used to follow recovery, but it is limited in that significant changes within the nerve must occur before EMG findings are noted.[11] Newer imaging modalities as discussed above such as DTI/DTT will hopefully enable prognostic information to be obtained earlier in the course of injury.[11,19,20,21]

Operative exploration of peripheral nerve injury should involve ample proximal and distal exposure of the involved segment and should include electrophysiologic adjuncts to allow for intraoperative assessment of function throughout the nerve and detection of neuroma-in-continuity. Tourniquets should be avoided, as relative ischemia may worsen injury in the already vulnerable nerve. For a similar reason, excessive manipulation or mobilization of the nerve is generally avoided during neurolysis (►Fig. 33.5). Although beyond the scope of this chapter,

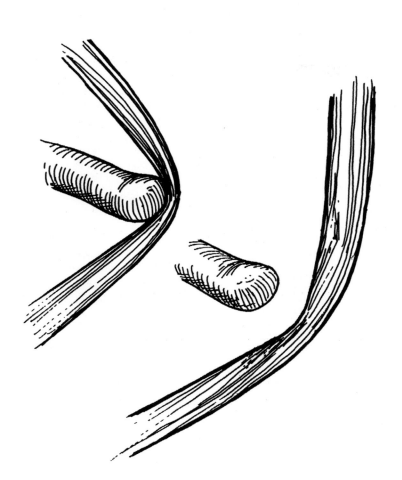

Fig. 33.4 Demonstration that compressive and stretching forces on a peripheral nerve (against skeletal structures, soft tissues, or other masses) can cause permanent changes in the nerve, even after the cause of injury is eliminated.

some traumatic peripheral nerve injuries may not be amenable to direct repair or neurolysis alone and in these situations, nerve transfer procedures can be considered.[35]

33.8 Conclusion

Compressive peripheral nerve injuries are very common. Evaluation requires knowledge of the anatomy, an understanding of the mechanism of injury, and focused physical examination. Imaging studies can be a useful adjunct in certain injury types. Electrophysiologic testing is not as useful in the acute setting but provides invaluable information when performed serially over the course of expected recovery. Advances in imaging are ongoing and may one day allow for the early ascertainment of vital diagnostic and prognostic information.

Although the degree and duration of recovery can be suggested by the severity of the initial injury and is inversely related to the age of the patient, most injuries require an observation period of a few weeks before accurate prognosis can be estimated.

Acute surgical exploration in the acute setting is limited to just a few injury types. Typically, surgical exploration is reserved for lack of expected clinical or electrophysiologic improvement or worsening neurologic deficits. Portions of this chapter, including figures, are adapted with permission from Robertson SC, Traynelis VC. Acute management of compressive peripheral nerve injuries. In: Loftus CM, ed. Neurosurgical Emergencies. Vol. 2. Rolling Meadows, IL: American Association of Neurological Surgeons; 1994:313–326.

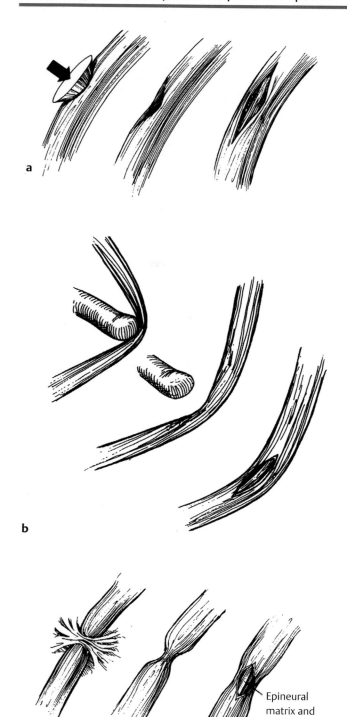

Fig. 33.5 Neurolysis of peripheral nerves with constrictive areas secondary to compression. Three types of compressive injury are shown: **(a)** pure compression, **(b)** compression with stretch, and **(c)** circumferential compression. Neurolysis involves surgical decompression of the involved epineurium, with minimal manipulation of the perineurium or individual fascicles, to restore local function.

References

[1] Kurtzke JF. The current neurologic burden of illness and injury in the United States. Neurology. 1982; 32(11):1207–1214

[2] Omer GE, Jr. Physical diagnosis of peripheral nerve injuries. Orthop Clin North Am. 1981; 12(2):207–228

[3] Kinney. Physiology of the peripheral nerve. In: Youman's Neurological Surgery. Philadelphia, PA: W.B. Saunders; 2003:3809-3818

[4] Menorca RM, Fussell TS, Elfar JC. Nerve physiology: mechanisms of injury and recovery. Hand Clin. 2013; 29(3):317–330

[5] Guyten. Membrane potentials and action potentials. Philadelphia, PA: W.B. Saunders; 1991

[6] Ogata K, Naito M. Blood flow of peripheral nerve effects of dissection, stretching and compression. J Hand Surg [Br]. 1986; 11(1):10–14

[7] Powell HC, Myers RR. Pathology of experimental nerve compression. Lab Invest. 1986; 55(1):91–100

[8] Sunderland S. The anatomy and physiology of nerve injury. Muscle Nerve. 1990; 13(9):771–784

[9] Sunderland S. A classification of peripheral nerve injuries producing loss of function. Brain. 1951; 74(4):491–516

[10] Seddon HJ. A classification of nerve injuries. BMJ. 1942; 2(4260):237–239

[11] Simon NG, Spinner RJ, Kline DG, Kliot M. Advances in the neurological and neurosurgical management of peripheral nerve trauma. J Neurol Neurosurg Psychiatry. 2016; 87(2):198–208

[12] Midha. Peripheral nerve: approach to the patient. In: Youman's Neurological Surgery. Philadelphia, PA: W.B. Saunders; 2003:3819-3830

[13] Tinel J. "Tingling" signs with peripheral nerve injuries. 1915. J Hand Surg [Br]. 2005; 30(1):87–89

[14] Yuen ERL, Slimp J. Electrodiagnostic evaluation of peripheral nerves. In: Youman's Neurological Surgery. Philadelphia, PA: W.B. Saunders; 2003:3851-3872

[15] Kline DG, Hackett ER, May PR. Evaluation of nerve injuries by evoked potentials and electromyography. J Neurosurg. 1969; 31(2):128–136

[16] Spratt JD, Stanley AJ, Grainger AJ, Hide IG, Campbell RS. The role of diagnostic radiology in compressive and entrapment neuropathies. Eur Radiol. 2002; 12(9):2352–2364

[17] West GA, Haynor DR, Goodkin R, et al. Magnetic resonance imaging signal changes in denervated muscles after peripheral nerve injury. Neurosurgery. 1994; 35(6):1077–1085, discussion 1085–1086

[18] Du R, Auguste KI, Chin CT, Engstrom JW, Weinstein PR. Magnetic resonance neurography for the evaluation of peripheral nerve, brachial plexus, and nerve root disorders. J Neurosurg. 2010; 112(2):362–371

[19] Simon NG, Kliot M. Diffusion weighted MRI and tractography for evaluating peripheral nerve degeneration and regeneration. Neural Regen Res. 2014; 9(24):2122–2124

[20] Simon NG, Narvid J, Cage T, et al. Visualizing axon regeneration after peripheral nerve injury with magnetic resonance tractography. Neurology. 2014; 83(15):1382–1384

[21] Simon NG, Cage T, Narvid J, Noss R, Chin C, Kliot M. High-resolution ultrasonography and diffusion tensor tractography map normal nerve fascicles in relation to schwannoma tissue prior to resection. J Neurosurg. 2014; 120(5):1113–1117

[22] Erra C, Granata G, Liotta G, et al. Ultrasound diagnosis of bony nerve entrapment: case series and literature review. Muscle Nerve. 2013; 48(3):445–450

[23] Padua L, Di Pasquale A, Liotta G, et al. Ultrasound as a useful tool in the diagnosis and management of traumatic nerve lesions. Clin Neurophysiol. 2013; 124(6):1237–1243

[24] Padua L, Hobson-Webb LD. Ultrasound as the first choice for peripheral nerve imaging? Neurology. 2013; 80(18):1626–1627

[25] Tagliafico A, Perez MM, Padua L, Klauser A, Zicca A, Martinoli C. Increased reflectivity and loss in bulk of the pronator quadratus muscle does not always indicate anterior interosseous neuropathy on ultrasound. Eur J Radiol. 2013; 82(3):526–529

[26] Zhu J, Padua L, Hobson-Webb LD. Ultrasound as the first choice for peripheral nerve imaging? Neurology. 2013; 81(18):1644

[27] Koenig RW, Schmidt TE, Heinen CP, et al. Intraoperative high-resolution ultrasound: a new technique in the management of peripheral nerve disorders. J Neurosurg. 2011; 114(2):514–521

[28] Gelberman RH, Szabo RM, Williamson RV, Hargens AR, Yaru NC, Minteer-Convery MA. Tissue pressure threshold for peripheral nerve viability. Clin Orthop Relat Res. 1983(178):285–291

[29] Stevens KJ, Banuls M. Sciatic nerve palsy caused by haematoma from iliac bone graft donor site. Eur Spine J. 1994; 3(5):291–293

[30] Pai VS. Traumatic aneurysm of the inferior lateral geniculate artery after total knee replacement. J Arthroplasty. 1999; 14(5):633–634

[31] Hoyt TE, Tiwari R, Kusske JA. Compressive neuropathy as a complication of anticoagulant therapy. Neurosurgery. 1983; 12(3):268–271

[32] Winfree CJ, Kline DG. Intraoperative positioning nerve injuries. Surg Neurol. 2005; 63(1):5–18, –discussion 18

[33] Han BR, Cho YJ, Yang JS, Kang SH, Choi HJ. Clinical features of wrist drop caused by compressive radial neuropathy and its anatomical considerations. J Korean Neurosurg Soc. 2014; 55(3):148–151

[34] Raikin S, Froimson MI. Bilateral brachial plexus compressive neuropathy (crutch palsy). J Orthop Trauma. 1997; 11(2):136–138

[35] Midha R. Emerging techniques for nerve repair: nerve transfers and nerve guidance tubes. Clin Neurosurg. 2006; 53:185–190

34 Spinal Cord Injury and Spinal Cord Injury Without Radiographic Abnormality in Children

Jamal McClendon Jr. and P. David Adelson

Abstract

Although uncommon in children, particularly in comparison with traumatic brain injury, spinal cord injury (SCI) in children presents unique challenges in presentation, clinical and radiologic diagnosis, management, and ultimately rehabilitation for more severe injuries. It is necessary to highlight that despite a high relative incidence, a SCI can present significant morbidity and contribute to mortality, especially if unrecognized because of the unique aspects of pediatric trauma and radiologic presentation. As bony involvement in spine trauma is less common in children compared with adults, this can often lead to an unrecognized SCI that could potentially result in inadvertent worsening. This highlights the need to ensure a meticulous clinical examination and adequate imaging, optimally magnetic resonance imaging (MRI) to assess soft-tissue injury, particularly in children who are nonverbal owing to age and extent and severity of other injuries. Children with a SCI must be managed aggressively to prevent or limit the deterioration from secondary injury. As in all trauma, it is important to maintain rigid immobilization, spinal alignment, and stability, along with cardiopulmonary support and metabolic stabilization, until adequate evaluation is obtained, to ensure identification of any other underlying injuries. This is important throughout the acute care course to optimize outcomes, although very limited in scope because of the lack of any other efficacious methods at present. In the SCI literature, there remains controversy as to the optimal management both for adults and children, especially since children have not been included in large-scale clinical trials. Because SCI in children remains uncommon, it has been difficult to develop pediatric-specific clinical studies for management.

Keywords: imaging, management, mechanism, neuroradiology, pediatric, SCIWORA, spinal cord injury, trauma

34.1 Introduction

Traumatic injury is a major contributor to the cost of health care within the United States and remains the leading cause of death and disability in children.[1] Outcomes have significantly improved with the development of tertiary care trauma centers and protocols that have provided aggressive and targeted treatment for the multisystem involvement following a traumatic injury. Although blunt head trauma is more prevalent in pediatric population, spinal cord injury (SCI) remains a pervasive challenge in children because of neurologic dysfunction but also for the required chronic care. Injury to the cord may occur anywhere along its axis and may lead to permanent neurologic conditions, complications involving multiple organ systems, and lifelong rehabilitative and restorative care.

SCI occurs with a worldwide annual incidence of 15 to 40 cases per million people.[2,3] In the United States, acute SCI affects 12,000 people annually, with a mortality rate of approximately 4,000 before reaching the hospital and another 1,000 in the

hospital.[3] A 2004 study reflected that SCI costs the United States health care system an estimated $40.5 billion annually.[4]

Blunt injury involving the cervical spine is rare in the pediatric population, accounting for 1 to 2% of all pediatric trauma admissions.[5,6,7,8,9,10,11,12,13] Reported characteristics of cervical spine injury in children are strongly age related and vary significantly between infants, young children, and adolescents.[5] Also, pediatric cervical spine injury is more common than thoracic spine injury.

Spinal cord injury without radiographic abnormality (SCIWORA) is described as a SCI without obvious fracture or abnormal alignment seen on plain films or computed tomography (CT). Although more common in children than in adults, the mechanism of injury may be characterized by minimal trauma. It is less commonly diagnosed because of the improvement in imaging, particularly now in the era of advanced magnetic resonance (MR) imaging. The plethora of sequences now available can identify subtle soft-tissue injuries and metabolic disturbances. This form of SCI most requires supportive care, but not lifelong therapy. Diagnosis is based on clinical symptoms, neurologic signs, the complete examination, and radiographic imaging. In this chapter, we will explore the realm of pediatric SCI and discuss SCIWORA. We will also discuss etiology, pathophysiology, mechanism of injury, radiographic findings, and management of SCI. Furthermore, we will explore potential areas of treatment and potential future interventions for SCI.

34.2 Spinal Cord Injury

SCI can result in severe neurologic deficit, deterioration of quality of life, and functional burden to society. Injury to the spinal cord may occur at any region, although patients may have cord-only injuries with no vertebral column involvement or vertebral column and cord injuries. Birth injuries to the spinal cord is also believed to contribute to a significant proportion of SCI in children.[14,15,16] Injuries to the spinal cord must be differentiated from plexus injuries or peripheral nerve pathology. With severe birth trauma, children may suffer injuries at multiple regions of the cord and may involve the peripheral nervous system.[17,18,19,20,21,22,23] Birth injuries account for 4 to 16% of SCI.[14,15] There have been some that have attributed upper cervical or cervicothoracic junction injury resulting in SCI to perinatal mortality.

34.3 Incidence and Prevalence

Based on the 2009 registries involving the Kids' Inpatient Database (KID) and the National Trauma Data Bank (NTDB), the estimated incidence of hospital admission for spinal injury in the United States was 170 per 1 million in the population under 21 years of age.[24] Furthermore, the incidence of SCI was 24 per 1 million. For the KID analyzed from 2000 to 2012, the prevalence for traumatic posterior cervical spine injury was 2.07%, and the mortality rate was 4.87%.[25] For children less than 3 years of age, prevalence for SCI was 0.38%, and those with SCIWORA was 0.19%.[5] Prevalence statistics have relied heavily on large, multi-institutional databases such as the National Pediatric Trauma Registry, the NTDB, and the KID. These data sets have provided meaningful information; however, they are limited to selection bias, convenience sampling, and not fully inclusive of a variety of population/health systems.[25] Cervical spine injury in children increased with age, with approximately 80% of the total cases occurring in adolescents and young adults.[25] The prevalence of SCIWORA decreases in age, with approximately 17% in toddlers and 5.04% in young adults.[25]

SCI has a male predominance. Of those with multisystem trauma and a SCI, there is a higher morbidity and mortality with varying degrees of neurologic deficits. Mortality more commonly occurs in patients with a complete injury.[14,26,27] Mortality following SCI is often secondary to concurrent closed head injury or multisystem trauma and cerebral injury. Although SCI is often thought of as a disease of young adults, with median age at the time of injury at 28.7 years,[28] as the U.S. population ages, there has been an increase in the median age to 38 years at the time of injury.[28]

34.4 Mechanism of Injury

The NTDB reported that for patients less than 3 years of age, motor vehicle collisions were the most common injury mechanism, followed by falls for cervical spine injury.[5] However, cervical spine injuries are only observed in 3.2% of all motor vehicle collisions.[5] Accidents were the most common cause of cervical spine injury, most prevalent in the young adult age group.[25] A meta-analysis evaluated SCIWORA in 433 pediatric patients under 18 years of age reported that the most prevalent mechanism of injury for SCI was sports-related injuries (39.8%), fall (24.2%), and motor vehicle collisions (23.2%).[29]

SCI can occur in various modalities of delivery during the perinatal period. Typically, a mechanical injury or a focal ischemic injury constitutes the majority of cases. Severe traction of the trunk during breech extraction or a difficult forceps delivery both may cause brachial plexus and/or cervical SCI.[30,31,32] Also, 20 to 25% of children born with a SCI were reportedly to have had an uneventful delivery.[18] Persistent hyperextension in utero has been described as a potential etiology for SCI, causing some to believe in early cesarean sections for these children to reduce prevalence in the perinatal period.[33]

Pediatric SCI caused by a motor vehicle collision with a child involved as a passenger, pedestrian, or bicyclist account for 25 to 66% of the reported SCI. Falls are also a common cause of SCI, accounting for 10 to 40%.[14,15,26,27,34,35,36] Sporting and recreational activities account for 4 to 20% of SCI.[26] The peak period for SCI in children is during the summer months, with another peak period around the winter holidays.[27]

34.5 Extent of Injury

Hadley et al described four radiographic patterns for SCI in children: (1) fracture involving the vertebral body or posterior elements only (~ 40%); (2) fracture with subluxation (33%); (3) subluxation without fracture (10%); and (4) SCIWORA (10%).[34] Younger children frequently developed subluxations without

fracture or SCIWORA, although older children were more likely to have a fracture or fracture with subluxation.[34] The location of SCI injury varies depending on age at the time of injury. In the birth to 8 years of age range, the cervical spine is the most commonly injured site, with the upper cervical occurring more frequently in infants and toddlers, whereas in prepubescent and adolescent, the lower cervical spine is more commonly injured. Furthermore, several studies have suggested that very young children suffer craniocervical injury more frequently, and middle-age and older children increase the prevalence of cervicothoracic and distal cord injuries.[15,34,37]

The proportion of complete versus incomplete injuries often depends on the level of injury; however, severity of injury does vary within the literature, as does the most prevalent spinal region to be injured.[14,26,38,39,40,41,42,43] Furthermore, more than one level may be injured in up to 16% of cases.[34] Unfortunately, complete injury is more common in young children.[17,36] This may be a reflection of age at injury and increased protection with skeletal maturity and musculoskeletal development. Pseudosubluxation up to 4 mm can be seen high in the cervical spine and is a normal variant in some children.[44] The relative immaturity of the upper cervical uncovertebral joints makes them susceptible to potential shearing/slippage.[36] These factors individually and in combination make children more likely to develop translational types of injuries of the cervical spine and spinal cord without fracture.

The mortality associated with blunt cervical spine injuries is high, 10.83 to 27%.[5,6,7,25] The mortality rate tended to be higher among younger patients, especially with toddlers.[25] These injuries are often associated with other organ systems, specifically traumatic brain injury (22.1%). Intuitively, patients with American Spinal Injury Association (ASIA) grade A were more likely to have a worse outcome than those of ASIA D on initial presentation.[29]

34.6 Pathobiology

The pathobiology of acute SCI involves a primary mechanical injury resulting in the initial tissue damage in the acute period, followed by the secondary injury that results in further damage over the first few days or weeks. The primary injury involves an array of complex biomechanical forces that cause direct tissue damage to the spinal cord such as a contusion or laceration and/or shear stress loaded on axons or blood vessels, disrupting the normal connectivity and architecture of the spinal cord.[45] The primary insult initiates a postlesional signaling cascade of downstream secondary mechanisms that contribute to the secondary injury.[45] For example, petechial hemorrhage in the gray matter, edema in the white matter, and thrombosis in the microvasculature from the primary injury lead to vasospasm and then ischemia of neuronal tissues.[46] This ischemia leads to further neuronal membrane dysfunction, abnormal continuous activation of neuronal voltage-dependent sodium channels (increasing intracellular sodium), and ultimately cell death.[46] This results in the pathogenesis and resultant tissue damage as part of the secondary injury.

The response to cord injury may also have a significant immune component.[47,48] Disruption of the blood spinal barrier provides opportunity for immune cells (i.e., lymphocytes and macrophages) and microglia to cross. This may reflect a process of secondary injury by apoptosis and necrosis.[47,48] As a result, frequently there is cavitation of the spinal cord in the area of injury.

Hemorrhage and inflammation, marked by the infiltration of polymorphonuclear leukocytes (PMNs), can be seen in the acute period, hours after injury. The early PMN infiltration is followed by a persistent macrophage population in the region of injury up to 2 months after the trauma. In animal studies, demyelination of axon fibers can be localized initially and then becomes widespread in the chronically injured often the integrity of these demyelinated axons is preserved.[49] More severe traumatic cord injury can lead to total disruption of the central gray matter in conjunction with an inflammatory reaction that occurs diffusely in the white matter tracts, resulting in central necrosis and cystic cavitation of the central cord.[50] Depending on the injury location, patients may manifest changes in sensory and/or motor function, and possibly autonomic dysfunction arising from disruption of fiber tracts.[51]

Postmortem studies in children who suffered significant spinal trauma showed spinal, epidural, and subdural hematomas with associated head injuries in 22% of cases, which may have contributed to mortality.[14] Other injuries seen postmortem include cord contusions, cord infarction, laceration, transection, dural disruption, and vertebral artery injury.[21] Spinal cord transection or anatomical discontinuity between proximal and distal segments of the spinal cord frequently is associated with mortality.[52]

The cellular and molecular events that occur in response to SCI have been studied in several animal models. Blunt injury trauma models in animals produce a histologic picture that resembles the typical pathology of SCI in humans. Injury to the cord causes membrane disruption and vascular injury leading to hemorrhage. Spinal neurons typically are subject to necrosis or excitotoxic damage but also apoptosis within 24 hours after SCI.[4] Oligodendrocytes undergo apoptosis in two distinct phases: an early acute phase lasting for 24 to 48 hours after injury and a later subacute phase that can last for several weeks.[4,53,54]

Animal models demonstrated that with blunt cord trauma, damage is limited to various portions of the central gray area, with sparing of the surrounding white matter tracts. A spared rim of axons typically remains at the periphery of the injury. This concussive or compressive force applied to the spinal cord creates immediate cell death of a large portion of neuronal bodies residing in the central gray matter. The surviving axons traversing the surrounding white matter are at risk for secondary injury.[55] The secondary injury cascade influences the functional outcome. These cascade of events include an inflammatory response via the arachidonic acid cascade, the release of excitatory amino acids (glutamate and aspartate), and the lipid peroxidation of cell membranes by various species of oxygen free radicals.[26,56,57,58] Changes in local blood flow as a result of tissue edema and various vasoactive inflammatory mediators may lead to further ischemic injury to the cord.[46] The initiation of apoptosis in neurons and glia is seen even days and weeks following SCI.[59] The comprehensive understanding of this pathophysiology portends to future therapies directed to counteract or eliminate the secondary injury cascade.

The formation of a glial scar can impede axon regeneration.[4] Astrocytes respond with hypertrophy after injury and with increased production of intermediate filaments such as glial fibrillary acidic protein (GFAP).[60] However, reactive astrocytes function to limit the infiltration of inflammatory cells through the blood–brain barrier and facilitate the repair.[4,61,62,63,64] The migration of more mediators forms a glial scar preventing axon regeneration by physically blocking regeneration and accumulating molecules inhibiting axon outgrowth.[65,66]

34.7 Location of Injury

As noted above, whereas upper cervical spine injury (C1–C4) becomes less prevalent with age, lower cervical spine injury (C5–C7) becomes more frequent with age.[25]

34.8 Biomechanics for Regional Prevalence

There have been a variety of proposed mechanisms for SCI at specific regions at particular ages at injury. These different mechanisms are a reflection of the intrinsic differences in the connective tissue, muscular development, and skeletal maturity depending on the age of the individual. Various age groups may develop a unique pathologic entity despite the same mechanism of injury. In the infant, the head is large relative to the neck, and the support for the calvarium takes several months until the muscles and soft tissue develop. Forces of acceleration and deceleration, particularly in a restraint scenario, can create significant momentum at the fulcrum of a weak neck, putting the cervical spine at risk for injury.[27,67,68,69] Additionally, underdeveloped paraspinal and neck musculature, incompletely ossified vertebral column, ligamentous laxity, and disproportionally large heads may play a role in SCI and SCIWORA in young children.[25] Ligamentous laxity is an important factor in the profile of the pediatric spine and may contribute to the increased susceptibility to horizontal shearing from elasticity.[70,71]

In older children, hyperflexion, rotation, traction, hyperextension, vertical load, flexion rotation, and shearing are all mechanistic ways that result in SCI. The force and vector applied to the head and neck may result in the various observed pathologic conditions. For example, diving accidents/trauma cause SCI from a hyperflexion and axial load compression; whiplash and nonaccidental trauma result from a combination of hyperflexion and hyperextension.[36,72]

The histopathologic changes seen after SCI in the human appear to be similar to that described in animal models with the exception of the spinal column injuries and "solid cord lesion" patterns of injury.[49,50,55,73] In a postmortem examination of 12 children with SCI, the histopathology demonstrated a split in the cartilaginous end plate of the vertebral bodies without fracture.[70] The splitting of the cartilaginous end plate was often within the growth zone of a child's vertebral body.[43] Ligamentous injury is more commonly seen than traumatic disk herniation or multiple fractures. Since the immature spine progressively ossifies throughout childhood, young children may be more susceptible to avulsions and epiphyseal separations rather than fractures.[70]

Histologic examination for contusion-type injuries reveals extensive demyelination with relative preservation of the axon fibers, especially small fibers in the dorsal columns.[52] Hematomyelic cavitation, though, may develop, with disruption of the gray matter and relative preservation of the white matter tracts. Spinal cord necrosis, secondary to hyperextension, and cord transection most often occur in the mid- to lower cervical cord or upper thoracic region following birth. There may also be vascular injuries (i.e., dissection) associated with the injury. Cord rupture can occur following birth trauma through application of longitudinal traction.[36,52] When there is disruption of the white matter tracts located at the central portion of the lateral columns with preservation of local gray matter, it may manifest as a central cord syndrome.[20]

34.9 Imaging Findings

The majority of patients with SCI will have some level of radiographic abnormalities. By definition, patients with SCIWORA will have a neurologic deficit without imaging pathology; however, most patients will have some finding. Plain films in the region of interest are extremely important, and a significant amount of information can be obtained from them. The extent of many of these injuries can be further elucidated with multiplanar imaging (i.e., CT, CT myelography, and/or MR imaging). CT helps to identify bony pathology and alignment. CT myelography and MR imaging aid in visualization of compressive cord pathology, alignment, and screening level of injury. MR imaging is the primary method of choice for visualization of soft tissue or nonbony injury, but it is fairly standard to obtain an amalgam of imaging in order to define the extent and severity of the injury.

Betz et al showed that MR imaging was more sensitive in detecting subacute and chronic injuries of the spinal cord than CT.[74] It is useful in the acute and early subacute time to identify ligamentous injury, particularly with high intensity signal abnormalities seen on T2 imaging and short-tau inversion recovery (STIR) imaging. T2 signal within the spinal cord may represent cord edema after injury. MR imaging aids in diagnosis of posttraumatic syrinx, spinal cord hemorrhage, or signal change within the cord. Newer technologies including MR perfusion, diffusion-weighted MR imaging, MR spectroscopy, and MR tractography may provide additional understanding of the structural makeup of the uninjured and injured spinal cord.

Plain films remain essential to the initial work-up following trauma to the child and directs either further diagnostic studies or initiation of treatment. A complete set of plain films of the cervical spine include an anteroposterior (AP), a lateral, and an open-mouth odontoid view. Imaging is considered adequate if there is visualization of the vertebral body of T1. In instances where T1 is not well visualized because of body habitus, the inclusion of a "swimmers" view can be added. AP and lateral films of the thoracic and lumbar spine are obtained in order to assess injuries to the remainder of the spine. Many institutions bypass plain films and obtain CT scans in lieu of increased radiation.

Flexion–extension plain films of the spine assist in determining the stability of a region, and oblique films are useful to denote listhesis or foraminal stenosis. Flexion–extension films are contraindicated in patients with neck pain, and if there is instability seen on the AP or lateral view. Patients with neurologic deficits, fracture seen on plain films, or soft-tissue injury should not receive initial flexion–extension plain films. A cooperative patient who does not have a distracting injury may receive flexion–extension films as long as they can relate pain, paresthesias, or

changes in neurologic function with full range of motion. If inadequate films are obtained because of limited range of motion secondary to spasm or neurologic change during the exercise, rigid immobilization for several weeks followed by repeat examination may facilitate the determination of stability. Advanced imaging in the region of interest in the setting of a neurologic deficit may aid in identifying further injury not seen on plain films.[75]

CT of the spine may provide additional detail not seen on plain films or if T1 is unable to be visualized on the lateral or swimmer's view. One-millimeter-thin cut and three-dimensional reconstructions can define bony pathology with greater extent. Reformatted views in the coronal and sagittal planes provide additional views to observe the region of interest. One limitation is that CT may not identify abnormalities parallel to the axial imagine plane.

CT myelography through administration of intrathecal radiopaque material provides assessment of the integrity of the thecal sac and its contents. There is a risk of neurologic worsening if there is severe stenosis proximal to contrast administration. With this measurable morbidity, it is not the first-line imaging modality following SCI. CT myelography should be considered as an evaluative modality in patients in which MR imaging is contraindicated.

MR imaging has become the advanced imaging modality of choice of the spinal cord following injury, including early evaluation of injured patients, because it identifies pathologic and physiologic changes to the cord and soft tissues. Traumatic disk herniations, cord hemorrhage, cord injury, epidural and subdural hematomas, and ligamentous injury can be identified on MR imaging. Patients with SCI receive MR imaging for evaluation. This information provides detail to the extent of the injury without the invasive nature of myelography. Intravenous contrast for MR imaging is used in the chronic setting to denote blood or scar tissue. Although CT is a better imaging modality for the bone, MR imaging can render important understanding of the relationship between vertebrae and the spinal column with potential cord pathology. MR imaging has been useful to follow longitudinal changes in spinal cord pathology, including contusions, syringohydromyelia, and signal change.

Diagnostic angiography or noninvasive vascular imaging represents second-line modalities when suspected vertebral artery injury may have occurred. There have been reported cases of mortality as a result of vertebral artery injury resulting in quadriplegia, mimicking cord injury.[35,43]

Most often, the clearance of the cervical spine requires negative radiography with no indication of clinical injury to the spine or spinal cord. In adult patients without tenderness along the posterior midline aspect of their spine, no neurologic deficit, a normal level of consciousness without evidence inebriation, no neck pain, full range of motion, and no distracting injuries, the cervical spine can be cleared without radiographic examination.[76] Similarly, these criteria have also been applied to the clearance of pediatric cervical spine injuries.

34.10 SCIWORA

First described by Pang and Wilberger, SCIWORA was initially defined as a syndrome of traumatic myelopathy without vertebral column disruption as visualized on plain films, CT with or without myelography, or flexion–extension plain films.[36] This excludes penetrating trauma and electrical shock. The frequency of its diagnosis depends on clinical awareness and the extent of the radiographic investigation. Again, the prevalence of SCIWORA in children is as high as 20% of SCI. As improved imaging capabilities and increased use of MR continue to advance, there will likely be a smaller prevalence of this conidition.[39,77] The majority, two thirds, of these injuries occur in young children, 8 to 10 years of age, less commonly in adolescents, and rare in adults.[34,35,36,39,78]

SCIWORA may be a challenging pathology to diagnose because of the lack of radiographic abnormalities. The physical examination and clinical findings render the diagnosis without the imaging pathology. The prevalence of SCIWORA in children, compared with adults, is likely related to the physiology of the pediatric spine. Biomechanically, it is more flexible, allowing for increased motion without pathology. The inherent elasticity and hypermobility of the pediatric spine may allow for a transient subluxation at the time of the injury with elastic recoil returning the spine to a relatively normal alignment at the time of presentation.[36,79,80] It has also been suggested that hyperextension in young children may cause a bulge in a cervical disk causing compression of the ventral spinal cord. After the age of 8, many of the unique pediatric anatomical features have matured to an adult orientation, correlating with the reduced prevalence of SCIWORA in older children.

The neurologic findings immediately following SCIWORA may be variable, and signs may manifest in a delayed fashion.[36] There have been reports of delayed, rapid deterioration to complete neurologic dysfunction that may be irreversible. There may be very subtle changes seen on T2 and STIR sequences in patients with SCIWORA.

34.11 Early Resuscitation after SCI

Once a primary SCI has occurred, the goals of management in the acute period are to prevent further insults that would worsen the secondary mechanism and ultimately the secondary injury. Prevention of hypoxemia and hypotension are critical to long-term outcome, but they frequently occur especially with multisystem trauma. Some patients, depending on location of the injury, may require intubation and mechanical ventilation to support a respiratory insufficient state. Once stabilized and ventilatory support is self-sufficient, the child can be extubated; however, there are occasions when tracheostomies will need to be placed for mechanical ventilator weaning or long-term ventilatory assistance at upper cervical SCI or injury that is complicated with pulmonary compromise. Although neurologic complications caused by intubation are rare, and manual inline traction for rigid cervical immobilization is ideal, fiberoptic intubation is preferred to maintain cervical spine alignment.[81,82] For patients needing an emergent airway to provide oxygenation and ventilation, emergent cricothyroidotomy may be necessary for immediate securing of an airway.

Hypotension and hypovolemia are two frequently encountered posttrauma issues associated with SCI. Injury involving the cervical cord and cervicothoracic junction may result in a functional sympathectomy with a loss of motor and sympathetic vasomotor tone. Frequently called "spinal shock," there can be loss of cardiovascular support, systemic vasodilation, and increased venous capacity. Furthermore, loss of sympathetic tone can result in bradyarrhythmia.

For conditions of posttraumatic or hypovolemic shock, the initial management begins with large-bore, peripheral intravenous administration of volume through fluid resuscitation. Central venous catheters provide central venous pressure measures to demonstrate volume status. Additionally, they can be used to float pulmonary artery catheters to obtain pulmonary artery wedge pressure, cardiac output, and vascular resistance, although these methods are less frequently used presently for resuscitation for trauma. Still, maximal information can guide the use of vasoactive medications in the setting of continued shock despite fluid resuscitation.

In children, since they most often have normal functioning cardiovascular and renal systems, fluid status can also be estimated on the basis of urine output. SCI can lead to genitourinary pathology (i.e., retention or incontinence). Urinary catheters or intermittent catheterization on a schedule can assess urine output and prevent distention of the bladder. Although nasogastric tubes are contraindicated in patients with craniofacial or skull base injuries because of potential direct injury, they may be considered to provide trophic feeding or emptying gastric contents.[83] Patients with gastrointestinal ulceration or treatment with high-dose steroids should be treated prophylactically with intravenous H_2 blockers or proton pump inhibitors to diminish gastric secretion. The prevalence of venous thromboembolism in children is low; however, the literature on this population is sparse. Pneumatic compression devices and stockings are utilized to decrease prevalence of venous thromboembolism when heparins are contraindicated. Treatment with chemoprophylaxis is recommended; however, the time for commencement is left at the discretion of the treating physician.

34.12 Neurologic Evaluation

A detailed and complete neurologic evaluation remains the cornerstone for delineating the level of injury, defining the spinal cord syndrome, and obtaining a baseline assessment for all patients with a suspected SCI. Continued assessment is used to follow clinical examination over time. A formal assessment must include motor function of each of the major muscle groups and assessment of rectal function, including sphincter constriction, tone, and bulbocavernous reflex. Diaphragmatic functioning may be assessed on chest plain films or by pulmonary evaluation of tidal volume or vital capacity. Sensory function is tested for all modalities, including temperature, proprioception, and pinprick. Reflexes are also an important component of this assessment.

The ASIA developed a classification scheme to evaluate the motor and sensory function for all spinal levels from C1 through the lowest sacral cord (S4–S5). The ASIA classification scheme for SCI expanded on the original Frankel scale and uses A through E, with A defining complete injury to E where motor and sensory function are preserved. This classification of SCI has led to greater clarity and uniformity in describing injury patterns.[84] The expert panel classified incomplete SCI into five types: a central cord syndrome is associated with a greater loss of upper limb function compared with the lower limbs; Brown–Sequard syndrome results from a hemitransection of the spinal cord; anterior cord syndrome occurs when the injury affects the anterior spinal tracts, including the vestibulospinal tract; and conus medullaris and cauda equina syndromes occur with damage to the conus or spinal roots of the cord.[84] A "complete" injury was defined as no motor or sensory function as well as no anal or perineal sensation or motor representing the lowest sacral cord (S4–S5).

34.13 Associated Cranial Injury

All patients who have had a concurrent blunt head trauma or traumatic brain injury should be maintained in spine precautions until they are "cleared" clinically and/or radiographically.[38] Clearance of the cervical spine with the six criteria has been described above; for reliable patients, plain films including dynamic studies may be necessary for clearance, presuming that adequate films are obtained and patient is without neck pain or neurologic injury.

34.14 Initial Management of Pediatric Spinal Cord Injury

The management of SCI in a child does not differ significantly from that in an adult. The goal of management is to minimize the secondary injury and optimize the milieu for recovery in attempt to prevent further loss of neurologic function. This is done with insuring good oxygenation and blood perfusion to prevent hypotension and hypoxemia and the secondary effects on the spinal cord. Clinical guidelines exist to decompress a compressed spinal cord, maintenance of physiologic stability, and cardiopulmonary and metabolic support.

The initial management consists of rigid immobilization, cardiopulmonary monitoring, and continued assessment of neuraxis. Resuscitation efforts are simultaneously performed, including maintenance of adequate oxygenation and ventilation, and circulatory support. A secondary survey should be performed after the primary survey to ensure no additional concurrent injuries. Secondary insults from systemic injuries may affect the viability of the injured spinal cord, such as hypoperfusion, hypoxemia, or hypothermia. These parameters may cause neurologic deficit and should be considered in any management protocol.

34.15 Treatment for Acute Spinal Cord Injury

Various clinical trials involving methylprednisolone and GM-1 ganglioside have been performed evaluating pharmacologic therapies for the treatment of SCI in adults; however, there is limited information regarding the effectiveness in this population, let alone children. These include the use of methylprednisolone in the Bracken et al National Acute Spinal Cord Injury Study (NASCIS) trials I (low- and high-dose methylprednisolone),[85] II (30 mg/kg bolus followed by 5.4 mg/kg/h for 23 hours of methylprednisolone within 12 hours of injury),[86,87] and III (24-hour infusion versus a 48-hour infusion of maintenance methylprednisolone 5.4 mg/kg/hr)[88] and the GM-1 ganglioside

study.[89,90] These studies were limited and variable on whether they actually improved functional outcome improvement in SCI. The mechanism of action of methylprednisolone in the setting of SCI remains unclear. Theories include stabilization of the cell membrane, maintenance of the blood–brain barrier potentially reducing vasogenic edema, enhancement of spinal cord blood flow, inhibit free radicals, and limit the inflammatory response after injury.[91,92,93,94,95,96,97,98,99] GM-1 ganglioside is a naturally occurring salt in cell membranes especially abundant in the central nervous system. Its proposed mechanism(s) of action in the treatment of acute SCI include antiexcitotoxicity effects, apoptosis prevention, potentiation of neuritic sprouting, and effects on nerve growth factors.

A prospective, multicenter study has shown that early decompression within first 24 hours is associated with better neurologic outcomes than later surgery for compressive pathology.[100] There have been off-label attempts at management of acute SCI, including lumbar drain placement to decrease intradural pressure and optimize blood flow to the spinal cord, high-dose dexamethasone, and artic sun cooling.

The optimal mean arterial pressure for spinal cord perfusion after trauma remains unclear.[101] The 2013 American Association of Neurological Surgeons and Congress of Neurological Surgeons (AANS/CNS) guidelines for cervical SCI treatment recommended mean arterial pressure of acute SCI patients between 85 and 90 mm Hg.[101,102,103] Future understanding of vasopressor management protocols for patients with SCI will be important not only for optimizing spinal cord perfusion and patient outcomes but also for minimizing potential complications related to the vasoactive medication.[101]

Werndle et al performed a prospective trial examining intraspinal pressure and spinal cord perfusion pressure through monitoring.[104] The intraspinal pressure waveform resembled the respective intracranial pressure waveform. The morphology of the intraspinal pressure pulse waveform reflected intracranial pressure waveform shape and was composed of the three peaks (percussion, tidal, and dicrotic waves), and the behavior of P2 changed with increased intraspinal pressure.[105] This has the potential to be used for monitoring pressure after SCI.

SCI results in a deleterious accumulation of intracellular sodium through voltage-gated sodium channels within axons, and dysfunction of membrane-bound Na^+,K^+-ATPase pump with a reduction in sodium efflux.[45,106,107] This drives the influx of intracellular calcium, ultimately leading to structural and functional injury.[45,108] Pharmaceuticals inhibiting these mechanisms may portend to improved outcomes.

In addition to promising areas of research, alternative treatment modalities are on the horizon to aid in recovery of function. Neuroprosthetics represent engineering and biomedical innovation that may increase functional independence for patients with chronic SCI. This new frontier will continue to increase in importance as it continues to develop.

34.16 Treatment of SCIWORA

Surgical intervention requiring a stabilization procedure is not performed without structural pathology or demonstrated instability. The treatment of this form of SCI focuses on secondary prevention. The physician can do very little to ameliorate the primary injury and focuses on the recovery and secondary injury prevention with resuscitation and maintenance of systemic parameters. It is uncommon to have a diagnosis of SCIWORA with instability; widened facets or listhesis may be seen on plain films or CT. SCIWORA is treated with rigid immobilization and optimization of local milieu. Rigid immobilization up to 3 months followed by assessment for late instability is recommended to limit motion and secondary injury.[36]

Prevention of the primary injury is the most fruitful way to prevent a SCI; however, preservation of function and viable neurologic tissue from secondary insult can possibly improve outcomes.

34.17 Complications

SCI patients often require significant resources depending on the magnitude of injury. The child is susceptible not only in the acute period to posttraumatic complications but also to long-term problems that require ongoing rehabilitation and supportive care. Pulmonary complications (i.e., pneumonia), gastrointestinal complications (i.e., ulcers), musculoskeletal complications (pressure sores), peripheral vascular complications (venous thromboembolism), and genitourinary complications (urinary tract infection) cause significant morbidity in this population. Patients may require 24-hour care and may require intensive physical therapy and rehabilitative services to maintain function.

Chronic complications following SCI include chronic pulmonary dysfunction that may persist years after injury. Patients with upper cervical injuries may require lifelong ventilator dependence. Common delayed or chronic complications of the gastrointestinal tract include ulceration, which is most often neurogenic in origin, and constipation. SCI patients are often placed on a bowel regimen for prevention and depending on level of injury may require rectal stimulation. Furthermore, genitourinary pathology ranges from sexual dysfunction to urinary retention requiring catheterization to prevent infection, incontinence/retention, or failure.[42]

SCI patients are susceptible to delayed neurologic deterioration. In the acute phase, deterioration is often from compromised blood flow to the spinal cord.[36] In the chronic phase, a posttraumatic syrinx may result.[34] Musculoskeletal pain and spasticity are also significant problems that interfere with activities of daily living and can contribute to significant morbidity. Medically intractable spasticity (i.e., failure of oral baclofen) may require delivery of intrathecal baclofen and/or intramuscular botulinum toxin.

Chronic neuropathic pain is a potential pathologic complication after SCI. Estimates of post SCI pain (of any type) range from between 13 and 94%.[109,110,111] In one study, one third of patients will develop at-level and one third of patient will develop below-level neuropathic pain 12 months after injury.[112] The at-level pain was more prevalent in the early months after SCI and was more likely to resolve with time than below-level.[112] The chronic neuropathic pain must be differentiated from musculoskeletal pain occurring in 50 to 70% of those reporting chronic pain, although not as severe or functionally limiting.[109,113]

Pain is rated third behind decreased ambulation/mobility and decreased sexual function as the most difficult SCI complication.[28,109] Treatment of neuropathic pain can occur with pharmaceutical agents or potentially neuromodulation strategies.

34.18 Outcome

Long-term outcome in children is determined by the severity of the initial injury.[14] Physical therapy and rehabilitation services should be started early to assist the patient to become independent and functional for their activities of daily living and then ultimately within society. Early mobilization is paramount. The majority of patients with complete SCI will have no improvement. It is the hope that with continued development of neuronal sprouting, axonal regeneration, and remyelination, improved clinical results will result in vivo. Those children who present neurologically intact without acute neurologic sequelae occasionally suffer a delayed deterioration.

34.19 New Therapies for Acute Spinal Cord Injury

Recently, there have been a number of therapies that were investigated in clinical trials, bringing hope to patients with SCI.[45,114] Riluzole is a sodium channel–blocking agent used to treat amyotrophic lateral sclerosis and has been trialed as treatment for acute SCI.[115] It is U.S. Food and Drug Administration approved to be used in amyotrophic lateral sclerosis (ALS) to improve survival by modulating excitatory neurotransmission and providing neuroprotective mechanisms.[115] Preclinical studies with SCI have demonstrated functional recovery by preventing the aberrant release of sodium and glutamate imbalance.[116,117] The mechanism of influx of sodium ions as a cause for secondary injury is the rationale for use of sodium channel–blocking agent to reduce injury.[45]

The Riluzole in Acute Spinal Cord Injury Study (RISCIS) is a randomized, double-blind, placebo-controlled parallel multicenter trial commencing after satisfactory phase I results.[45,118] Stem cell treatment is a potential option for SCI, and a variety of different stem cell types have been evaluated in animal and human models. It is likely that no single therapy will solve the challenges presented in SCI. The goal for stem cells is to prevent apoptosis or replace injured cells, particularly oligodendrocytes, which could facilitate remyelination of spared axons and inhibition of a glial scar. Furthermore, strategies that reduce extent of glial scar or diminish its inhibitory effects could be used to support axon regeneration. Also, strategies modulating the immune repose and blocking effect of inhibitory molecules have been investigated.

Therapeutic strategies involving transplantation of stem cells after SCI focuses on the replacement of injured neurons and oligodendrocytes (facilitate myelination), support survival of cells at the lesion site, and optimizing the milieu within the injured cord to facilitate axonal regeneration.[4] Limited evidence has been obtained of clinically significant benefits on stem cell therapies, although none have been approved for SCI. The current data suggest that stem cell transplantation is safe but of limited or no therapeutic efficacy.[4]

The goal of future therapy in acute SCI involves the development of new compounds that inhibit secondary injury. There exists a short period of time in the acute period where prompt administration of therapeutic substance(s) may exert some positive effect on outcome. Reducing acute inflammation and optimizing the local milieu for axonal sprouting and trophic factor response are important targets. For chronic SCI, the focus of therapeutic strategies depends on the promotion of neural connections.

34.20 Conclusion

SCI continues to have a major impact on the health care system. From patient morbidity and mortality to the delivery of care and the need for lifelong financial support, there continues to be major implications for patients, families, and society. The long-standing need for care is paramount. SCI results in a multitude of changes affecting several different cell types, leading to a complex pathologic picture. No single treatment modality will probably achieve regeneration of injured cord.

Patients with a SCI must be managed aggressively to prevent or limit the deterioration from secondary injury. Rigid immobilization, cardiopulmonary support, and metabolic stabilization are paramount in this process to optimize outcomes, although very limited in scope because of the lack of any other efficacious methods at present. Radiographs and advanced imaging aid in the diagnosis. Methylprednisolone is no longer the standard of care; however, there are a number of novel treatments that may have functional impact. Each passing year allows for a richer understanding of the pathophysiology of SCI that provides opportunities for therapeutic interventions. Research is critical to our knowledge regarding the disease, and clinical trials provide the basis for treatment and improved patient functional outcome.

References

[1] McCarthy A, Curtis K, Holland AJ. Paediatric trauma systems and their impact on the health outcomes of severely injured children: an integrative review. Injury. 2016; 47(3):574–585

[2] Tator CH. Update on the pathophysiology and pathology of acute spinal cord injury. Brain Pathol. 1995; 5(4):407–413

[3] Ackery A, Tator C, Krassioukov A. A global perspective on spinal cord injury epidemiology. J Neurotrauma. 2004; 21(10):1355–1370

[4] Sahni V, Kessler JA. Stem cell therapies for spinal cord injury. Nat Rev Neurol. 2010; 6(7):363–372

[5] Polk-Williams A, Carr BG, Blinman TA, Masiakos PT, Wiebe DJ, Nance ML. Cervical spine injury in young children: a National Trauma Data Bank review. J Pediatr Surg. 2008; 43(9):1718–1721

[6] Platzer P, Jaindl M, Thalhammer G, et al. Cervical spine injuries in pediatric patients. J Trauma. 2007; 62(2):389–396, discussion 394–396

[7] Brown RL, Brunn MA, Garcia VF. Cervical spine injuries in children: a review of 103 patients treated consecutively at a level 1 pediatric trauma center. J Pediatr Surg. 2001; 36(8):1107–1114

[8] Carreon LY, Glassman SD, Campbell MJ. Pediatric spine fractures: a review of 137 hospital admissions. J Spinal Disord Tech. 2004; 17(6):477–482

[9] Cirak B, Ziegfeld S, Knight VM, Chang D, Avellino AM, Paidas CN. Spinal injuries in children. J Pediatr Surg. 2004; 39(4):607–612

[10] Givens TG, Polley KA, Smith GF, Hardin WD, Jr. Pediatric cervical spine injury: a three-year experience. J Trauma. 1996; 41(2):310–314

[11] Kokoska ER, Keller MS, Rallo MC, Weber TR. Characteristics of pediatric cervical spine injuries. J Pediatr Surg. 2001; 36(1):100–105

[12] Mohseni S, Talving P, Branco BC, et al. Effect of age on cervical spine injury in pediatric population: a National Trauma Data Bank review. J Pediatr Surg. 2011; 46(9):1771–1776

[13] Vitale MG, Goss JM, Matsumoto H, Roye DP, Jr. Epidemiology of pediatric spinal cord injury in the United States: years 1997 and 2000. J Pediatr Orthop. 2006; 26(6):745–749

[14] Osenbach RK, Menezes AH. Pediatric spinal cord and vertebral column injury. Neurosurgery. 1992; 30(3):385–390

[15] Ruge JR, Sinson GP, McLone DG, Cerullo LJ. Pediatric spinal injury: the very young. J Neurosurg. 1988; 68(1):25–30

[16] Gordon N, Marsden B. Spinal cord injury at birth. Neuropadiatrie. 1970; 2(1):112–118

[17] Burke DC. Traumatic spinal paralysis in children. Paraplegia. 1974; 11(4):268–276

[18] Shulman ST, Madden JD, Esterly JR, Shanklin DR. Transection of spinal cord. A rare obstetrical complication of cephalic delivery. Arch Dis Child. 1971; 46(247):291–294

[19] Towbin A. Spinal injury related to the syndrome of sudden death ("crib-death") in infants. Am J Clin Pathol. 1968; 49(4):562–567

[20] Sladky JT, Rorke LB. Perinatal hypoxic/ischemic spinal cord injury. Pediatr Pathol. 1986; 6(1):87–101

[21] Towbin A. Spinal cord and brain stem injury at birth. Arch Pathol. 1964; 77:620–632

[22] Allen JP. Birth injury to the spinal cord. Northwest Med. 1970; 69(5):323–326

[23] LeBlanc HJ, Nadell J. Spinal cord injuries in children. Surg Neurol. 1974; 2(6):411–414

[24] Piatt JH, Jr. Pediatric spinal injury in the US: epidemiology and disparities. J Neurosurg Pediatr. 2015; 16(4):463–471

[25] Shin JI, Lee NJ, Cho SK. Pediatric cervical spine and spinal cord injury: a national database study. Spine. 2016; 41(4):283–292

[26] Anderson JM, Schutt AH. Spinal injury in children: a review of 156 cases seen from 1950 through 1978. Mayo Clin Proc. 1980; 55(8):499–504

[27] Hill SA, Miller CA, Kosnik EJ, Hunt WE. Pediatric neck injuries. A clinical study. J Neurosurg. 1984; 60(4):700–706

[28] Watson JC, Sandroni P. Central neuropathic pain syndromes. Mayo Clin Proc. 2016; 91(3):372–385

[29] Carroll T, Smith CD, Liu X, et al. Spinal cord injuries without radiologic abnormality in children: a systematic review. Spinal Cord. 2015; 53(12):842–848

[30] Byers RK. Spinal-cord injuries during birth. Dev Med Child Neurol. 1975; 17(1):103–110

[31] Stern WE, Rand RW. Birth injuries to the spinal cord: a report of 2 cases and review of the literature. Am J Obstet Gynecol. 1959; 78:498–512

[32] Norman MC, Wedderburn LC. Fetal spinal cord injury with cephalic delivery. Obstet Gynecol. 1973; 42(3):355–358

[33] Abroms IF, Bresnan MJ, Zuckerman JE, Fischer EG, Strand R. Cervical cord injuries secondary to hyperextension of the head in breech presentations. Obstet Gynecol. 1973; 41(3):369–378

[34] Hadley MN, Zabramski JM, Browner CM, Rekate H, Sonntag VK. Pediatric spinal trauma. Review of 122 cases of spinal cord and vertebral column injuries. J Neurosurg. 1988; 68(1):18–24

[35] McPhee IB. Spinal fractures and dislocations in children and adolescents. Spine. 1981; 6(6):533–537

[36] Pang D, Wilberger JE, Jr. Spinal cord injury without radiographic abnormalities in children. J Neurosurg. 1982; 57(1):114–129

[37] Osenbach RK, Menezes AH. Spinal cord injury without radiographic abnormality in children. Pediatr Neurosci. 1989; 15(4):168–174, discussion 175

[38] Kewalramani LS, Tori JA. Spinal cord trauma in children. Neurologic patterns, radiologic features, and pathomechanics of injury. Spine. 1980; 5(1):11–18

[39] Kewalramani LS, Kraus JF, Sterling HM. Acute spinal-cord lesions in a pediatric population: epidemiological and clinical features. Paraplegia. 1980; 18(3):206–219

[40] Hubbard DD. Injuries of the spine in children and adolescents. Clin Orthop Relat Res. 1974(100):56–65

[41] Stauffer ES, Mazur JM. Cervical spine injuries in children. Pediatr Ann. 1982; 11(6):502–508, 510–511

[42] Melzak J. Paraplegia among children. Lancet. 1969; 2(7610):45–48

[43] Hachen HJ. Spinal cord injury in children and adolescents: diagnostic pitfalls and therapeutic considerations in the acute stage [proceedings]. Paraplegia. 1977; 15(1):55–64

[44] Gaufin LM, Goodman SJ. Cervical spine injuries in infants. Problems in management. J Neurosurg. 1975; 42(2):179–184

[45] Fehlings MG, Nakashima H, Nagoshi N, Chow DS, Grossman RG, Kopjar B. Rationale, design and critical end points for the Riluzole in Acute Spinal Cord Injury Study (RISCIS): a randomized, double-blinded, placebo-controlled parallel multi-center trial. Spinal Cord. 2016; 54(1):8–15

[46] Tator CH, Fehlings MG. Review of the secondary injury theory of acute spinal cord trauma with emphasis on vascular mechanisms. J Neurosurg. 1991; 75(1):15–26

[47] Blight AR. Macrophages and inflammatory damage in spinal cord injury. J Neurotrauma. 1992; 9(Suppl 1):S83–S91

[48] Popovich PG, Wei P, Stokes BT. Cellular inflammatory response after spinal cord injury in Sprague-Dawley and Lewis rats. J Comp Neurol. 1997; 377(3):443–464

[49] Wakefield CL, Eidelberg E. Electron microscopic observations of the delayed effects of spinal cord compression. Exp Neurol. 1975; 48(3 Pt 1):637–646

[50] Janssen L, Hansebout RR. Pathogenesis of spinal cord injury and newer treatments. A review. Spine. 1989; 14(1):23–32

[51] Schwab ME. Repairing the injured spinal cord. Science. 2002; 295(5557):1029–1031

[52] Bunge RP, Puckett WR, Becerra JL, Marcillo A, Quencer RM. Observations on the pathology of human spinal cord injury. A review and classification of 22 new cases with details from a case of chronic cord compression with extensive focal demyelination. Adv Neurol. 1993; 59:75–89

[53] Liu XZ, Xu XM, Hu R, et al. Neuronal and glial apoptosis after traumatic spinal cord injury. J Neurosci. 1997; 17(14):5395–5406

[54] Emery E, Aldana P, Bunge MB, et al. Apoptosis after traumatic human spinal cord injury. J Neurosurg. 1998; 89(6):911–920

[55] Ducker TB, Lucas JT, Wallace CA. Recovery from spinal cord injury. Clin Neurosurg. 1983; 30:495–513

[56] Schwab ME, Bartholdi D. Degeneration and regeneration of axons in the lesioned spinal cord. Physiol Rev. 1996; 76(2):319–370

[57] Hall ED, Yonkers PA, Andrus PK, Cox JW, Anderson DK. Biochemistry and pharmacology of lipid antioxidants in acute brain and spinal cord injury. J Neurotrauma. 1992; 9(Suppl 2):S425–S442

[58] Wrathall JR, Teng YD, Choiniere D. Amelioration of functional deficits from spinal cord trauma with systemically administered NBQX, an antagonist of non-N-methyl-D-aspartate receptors. Exp Neurol. 1996; 137(1):119–126

[59] Choi JU, Hoffman HJ, Hendrick EB, Humphreys RP, Keith WS. Traumatic infarction of the spinal cord in children. J Neurosurg. 1986; 65(5):608–610

[60] Fawcett JW, Asher RA. The glial scar and central nervous system repair. Brain Res Bull. 1999; 49(6):377–391

[61] Faulkner JR, Herrmann JE, Woo MJ, Tansey KE, Doan NB, Sofroniew MV. Reactive astrocytes protect tissue and preserve function after spinal cord injury. J Neurosci. 2004; 24(9):2143–2155

[62] Herrmann JE, Imura T, Song B, et al. STAT3 is a critical regulator of astrogliosis and scar formation after spinal cord injury. J Neurosci. 2008; 28(28):7231–7243

[63] Okada S, Nakamura M, Katoh H, et al. Conditional ablation of Stat3 or Socs3 discloses a dual role for reactive astrocytes after spinal cord injury. Nat Med. 2006; 12(7):829–834

[64] Sahni V, Mukhopadhyay A, Tysseling V, et al. BMPR1a and BMPR1b signaling exert opposing effects on gliosis after spinal cord injury. J Neurosci. 2010; 30(5):1839–1855

[65] Busch SA, Silver J. The role of extracellular matrix in CNS regeneration. Curr Opin Neurobiol. 2007; 17(1):120–127

[66] Zuo J, Neubauer D, Dyess K, Ferguson TA, Muir D. Degradation of chondroitin sulfate proteoglycan enhances the neurite-promoting potential of spinal cord tissue. Exp Neurol. 1998; 154(2):654–662

[67] Cattell HS, Filtzer DL. Pseudosubluxation and other normal variations in the cervical spine in children. A study of one hundred and sixty children. J Bone Joint Surg Am. 1965; 47(7):1295–1309

[68] Pennecot GF, Gouraud D, Hardy JR, Pouliquen JC. Roentgenographical study of the stability of the cervical spine in children. J Pediatr Orthop. 1984; 4(3):346–352

[69] Bailey DK. The normal cervical spine in infants and children. Radiology. 1952; 59(5):712–719

[70] Aufdermaur M. Spinal injuries in juveniles. Necropsy findings in twelve cases. J Bone Joint Surg Br. 1974; 56B(3):513–519

[71] Baker DH, Berdon WE. Special trauma problems in children. Radiol Clin North Am. 1966; 4(2):289–305

[72] Caffey J. The whiplash shaken infant syndrome: manual shaking by the extremities with whiplash-induced intracranial and intraocular bleedings, linked with residual permanent brain damage and mental retardation. Pediatrics. 1974; 54(4):396–403

[73] Behrmann DL, Bresnahan JC, Beattie MS, Shah BR. Spinal cord injury produced by consistent mechanical displacement of the cord in rats: behavioral and histologic analysis. J Neurotrauma. 1992; 9(3):197–217

[74] Betz RR, Gelman AJ, DeFilipp GJ, Mesgarzadeh M, Clancy M, Steel HH. Magnetic resonance imaging (MRI) in the evaluation of spinal cord injured children and adolescents. Paraplegia. 1987; 25(2):92–99

[75] Bates D, Ruggieri P. Imaging modalities for evaluation of the spine. Radiol Clin North Am. 1991; 29(4):675–690

[76] Hoffman JR, Mower WR, Wolfson AB, Todd KH, Zucker MI; National Emergency X-Radiography Utilization Study Group. Validity of a set of clinical criteria to rule out injury to the cervical spine in patients with blunt trauma. N Engl J Med. 2000; 343(2):94–99

[77] Dickman CA, Rekate HL, Sonntag VK, Zabramski JM. Pediatric spinal trauma: vertebral column and spinal cord injuries in children. Pediatr Neurosci. 1989; 15(5):237–255, discussion 56

[78] Walsh JW, Stevens DB, Young AB. Traumatic paraplegia in children without contiguous spinal fracture or dislocation. Neurosurgery. 1983; 12(4):439–445

[79] Glasauer FE, Cares HL. Biomechanical features of traumatic paraplegia in infancy. J Trauma. 1973; 13(2):166–170

[80] Papavasiliou V. Traumatic subluxation of the cervical spine during childhood. Orthop Clin North Am. 1978; 9(4):945–954

[81] Meschino A, Devitt JH, Koch JP, Szalai JP, Schwartz ML. The safety of awake tracheal intubation in cervical spine injury. Can J Anaesth. 1992; 39(2):114–117

[82] Mulder DS, Wallace DH, Woolhouse FM. The use of the fiberoptic bronchoscope to facilitate endotracheal intubation following head and neck trauma. J Trauma. 1975; 15(8):638–640

[83] Chiles BW, III, Cooper PR. Acute spinal injury. N Engl J Med. 1996; 334(8):514–520

[84] Hadley MN, Walters BC, Grabb PA, et al. Guidelines for the management of acute cervical spine and spinal cord injuries. Clin Neurosurg. 2002; 49:407–498

[85] Bracken MB, Shepard MJ, Collins WF, et al. A randomized, controlled trial of methylprednisolone or naloxone in the treatment of acute spinal-cord injury. Results of the Second National Acute Spinal Cord Injury Study. N Engl J Med. 1990; 322(20):1405–1411

[86] Bracken MB, Shepard MJ, Collins WF, Jr, et al. Methylprednisolone or naloxone treatment after acute spinal cord injury: 1-year follow-up data. Results of the second National Acute Spinal Cord Injury Study. J Neurosurg. 1992; 76(1):23–31

[87] Bracken MB, Holford TR. Effects of timing of methylprednisolone or naloxone administration on recovery of segmental and long-tract neurological function in NASCIS 2. J Neurosurg. 1993; 79(4):500–507

[88] Bracken MB, Shepard MJ, Holford TR, et al. Administration of methylprednisolone for 24 or 48 hours or tirilazad mesylate for 48 hours in the treatment of acute spinal cord injury. Results of the Third National Acute Spinal Cord Injury Randomized Controlled Trial. National Acute Spinal Cord Injury Study. JAMA. 1997; 277(20):1597–1604

[89] Bracken MB. Steroids for acute spinal cord injury. Cochrane Database Syst Rev. 2012; 1):CD001046

[90] Geisler FH, Coleman WP, Grieco G, Poonian D; Sygen Study Group. The Sygen multicenter acute spinal cord injury study. Spine. 2001; 26(24, Suppl):S87–S98

[91] Means ED, Anderson DK, Waters TR, Kalaf L. Effect of methylprednisolone in compression trauma to the feline spinal cord. J Neurosurg. 1981; 55(2):200–208

[92] Hall ED. The neuroprotective pharmacology of methylprednisolone. J Neurosurg. 1992; 76(1):13–22

[93] Hall ED, Wolf DL, Braughler JM. Effects of a single large dose of methylprednisolone sodium succinate on experimental posttraumatic spinal cord ischemia. Dose-response and time-action analysis. J Neurosurg. 1984; 61(1):124–130

[94] Young W, Flamm ES. Effect of high-dose corticosteroid therapy on blood flow, evoked potentials, and extracellular calcium in experimental spinal injury. J Neurosurg. 1982; 57(5):667–673

[95] Faden AI, Jacobs TP, Holaday JW. Opiate antagonist improves neurologic recovery after spinal injury. Science. 1981; 211(4481):493–494

[96] Tempel GE, Martin HF, III. The beneficial effects of a thromboxane receptor antagonist on spinal cord perfusion following experimental cord injury. J Neurol Sci. 1992; 109(2):162–167

[97] Sharma HS, Olsson Y, Cervós-Navarro J. Early perifocal cell changes and edema in traumatic injury of the spinal cord are reduced by indomethacin, an inhibitor of prostaglandin synthesis. Experimental study in the rat. Acta Neuropathol. 1993; 85(2):145–153

[98] Winkler T, Sharma HS, Stålberg E, Olsson Y. Indomethacin, an inhibitor of prostaglandin synthesis attenuates alteration in spinal cord evoked potentials and edema formation after trauma to the

spinal cord: an experimental study in the rat. Neuroscience. 1993; 52(4):1057–1067

[99] Guth L, Zhang Z, Roberts E. Key role for pregnenolone in combination therapy that promotes recovery after spinal cord injury. Proc Natl Acad Sci U S A. 1994; 91(25):12308–12312

[100] Fehlings MG, Vaccaro A, Wilson JR, et al. Early versus delayed decompression for traumatic cervical spinal cord injury: results of the Surgical Timing in Acute Spinal Cord Injury Study (STASCIS). PLoS One. 2012; 7(2):e32037

[101] Readdy WJ, Whetstone WD, Ferguson AR, et al. Complications and outcomes of vasopressor usage in acute traumatic central cord syndrome. J Neurosurg Spine. 2015;1–7

[102] Aarabi B, Hadley MN, Dhall SS, et al. Management of acute traumatic central cord syndrome (ATCCS). Neurosurgery. 2013; 72(Suppl 2):195–204

[103] Ryken TC, Hurlbert RJ, Hadley MN, et al. The acute cardiopulmonary management of patients with cervical spinal cord injuries. Neurosurgery. 2013; 72(Suppl 2):84–92

[104] Werndle MC, Saadoun S, Phang I, et al. Monitoring of spinal cord perfusion pressure in acute spinal cord injury: initial findings of the injured spinal cord pressure evaluation study*. Crit Care Med. 2014; 42(3):646–655

[105] Varsos GV, Werndle MC, Czosnyka ZH, et al. Intraspinal pressure and spinal cord perfusion pressure after spinal cord injury: an observational study. J Neurosurg Spine. 2015; 23(6):763–771

[106] Agrawal SK, Fehlings MG. Mechanisms of secondary injury to spinal cord axons in vitro: role of Na+, Na(+)-K(+)-ATPase, the Na(+)-H+ exchanger, and the Na(+)-Ca2+ exchanger. J Neurosci. 1996; 16(2):545–552

[107] Tietze KJ, Putcha L. Factors affecting drug bioavailability in space. J Clin Pharmacol. 1994; 34(6):671–676

[108] Stys PK. General mechanisms of axonal damage and its prevention. J Neurol Sci. 2005; 233(1–2):3–13

[109] Siddall PJ, McClelland JM, Rutkowski SB, Cousins MJ. A longitudinal study of the prevalence and characteristics of pain in the first 5 years following spinal cord injury. Pain. 2003; 103(3):249–257

[110] Berić A, Dimitrijević MR, Lindblom U. Central dysesthesia syndrome in spinal cord injury patients. Pain. 1988; 34(2):109–116

[111] Davis L, Martin J. Studies upon spinal cord injuries; the nature and treatment of pain. J Neurosurg. 1947; 4(6):483–491

[112] Finnerup NB, Norrbrink C, Trok K, et al. Phenotypes and predictors of pain following traumatic spinal cord injury: a prospective study. J Pain. 2014; 15(1):40–48

[113] Rintala DH, Loubser PG, Castro J, Hart KA, Fuhrer MJ. Chronic pain in a community-based sample of men with spinal cord injury: prevalence, severity, and relationship with impairment, disability, handicap, and subjective well-being. Arch Phys Med Rehabil. 1998; 79(6):604–614

[114] Baptiste DC, Fehlings MG. Pharmacological approaches to repair the injured spinal cord. J Neurotrauma. 2006; 23(3–4):318–334

[115] Miller RG, Mitchell JD, Moore DH. Riluzole for amyotrophic lateral sclerosis (ALS)/motor neuron disease (MND). Cochrane Database Syst Rev. 2012(3):CD001447

[116] Schwartz G, Fehlings MG. Evaluation of the neuroprotective effects of sodium channel blockers after spinal cord injury: improved behavioral and neuroanatomical recovery with riluzole. J Neurosurg. 2001; 94(2, Suppl):245–256

[117] Wu Y, Satkunendrarajah K, Teng Y, Chow DS, Buttigieg J, Fehlings MG. Delayed post-injury administration of riluzole is neuroprotective in a preclinical rodent model of cervical spinal cord injury. J Neurotrauma. 2013; 30(6):441–452

[118] Grossman RG, Fehlings MG, Frankowski RF, et al. A prospective, multicenter, phase I matched-comparison group trial of safety, pharmacokinetics, and preliminary efficacy of riluzole in patients with traumatic spinal cord injury. J Neurotrauma. 2014; 31(3):239–255

35 Acute Shunt Malfunction

Ahmed J. Awad, Rajiv R. Iyer, and George I. Jallo

Abstract

The risk for shunt infections has decreased owing to the introduction of smaller devices and the advances in sterile techniques while performing shunt surgeries. However, having a foreign body implanted into the human body still carries the risk for potential infection. Any patient with a shunt who presents to the emergency room or office with new neurologic symptoms should be evaluated for a possible shunt malfunction. In an acute setting, when a patient with a shunt presents with a potential neurologic complaint, the diagnosis should be shunt malfunction until proven otherwise. Imaging studies are often essential for the diagnosis of shunt malfunction. There are three main causes of acute shunt malfunction: obstruction of the proximal/ventricular catheter; obstruction distal to the proximal catheter, including the valve and distal catheter; and disconnection, breakage, or migration of any component of the shunt system. Each of these etiologies requires a unique management algorithm.

Keywords: CSF, drainage, obstruction, shunt series, shunt revision, tap, ventricle, ventriculostomy

35.1 Introduction

The risk for shunt infections has decreased over the past few decades owing to the introduction of smaller devices and the advances in sterile techniques while performing shunt surgeries. However, having a foreign body implanted into the human body still carries the risk for potential infection. Shunt malfunction is very common in the practice of pediatric neurosurgery, as shunt malfunction signs and symptoms are the most common presentation of shunt infection. Clinical trials have demonstrated that the failure rate of implanted shunts may be as high as 40% within the first year, with mechanical malfunctions constituting more than half of all failures.[1,2,3,4] Despite the frequency of shunt malfunctions, misdiagnosis or mismanagement of acute shunt malfunction still occurs and can result in irreparable neurologic damage or even death. Thus, understanding the presentation of acute shunt malfunction and the management options that are available remains vitally important to the neurosurgeon. This chapter addresses the presentation, diagnosis, and management of acute shunt malfunction, excluding infectious causes and failures due to overdrainage, which are addressed in other chapters. We will specifically discuss the management protocols for acute shunt malfunctions at our institution.

35.2 Clinical Presentation and Diagnosis

The possible clinical presentations of acute shunt malfunction are innumerable. Any patient with a shunt who presents to the emergency room or office with new neurologic symptoms should be evaluated for a possible shunt malfunction. In an acute setting, when a patient with a shunt presents with a potential neurologic complaint, the diagnosis should be shunt malfunction until proven otherwise.

In the emergency room, each patient with a suspected shunt malfunction undergoes a thorough history and neurologic examination and is immediately scheduled for a reduced radiation dose noncontrast head computed tomography (CT) scan or fast/limited magnetic resonance imaging (MRI) study and a shunt series (a series of radiographs that follow the course of the shunt from the head to its distal location). A neurosurgical consult is often obtained while the child undergoes these studies. Important aspects to elucidate on history are reason for shunting, date of first shunt placement, number of revisions and reasons for revision, date of last revision and presenting signs or symptoms at that time, shunt type and setting and whether these were recently changed, and others.

Common complaints related to shunt malfunction include nausea, vomiting, seizures, visual changes, malaise, and altered level of consciousness and depend upon factors such as age of the patient, severity of shunt malfunction, and etiology of hydrocephalus. Family members are particularly sensitive to symptoms of shunt malfunction. Statements such as "this is what happens when his/her shunt malfunctions" or "this same thing happened before his/her last shunt revision" are often highly prognostic.

The physical examination includes vital signs, which may demonstrate bradycardia or abnormalities in blood pressure and respiratory rate in severe cases. Other aspects of the physical examination include palpation of the shunt along its entire course. Fluid collections around the valve or ventricular insertion site often herald a shunt obstruction, as do abdominal ascites. Occasionally, disconnections can also be palpated on physical examination. Fontanelles, if present, can be palpated to estimate intracranial pressure (ICP).

During the neurologic examination, a funduscopic examination can be attempted to assess for papilledema. Cranial nerve examination can sometimes detect abnormalities such as abducens nerve paresis or upgaze palsy seen with hydrocephalus and increased ICP. Other neurologic signs, such as ataxia, may also be indicators of shunt malfunction.

Although some pediatric neurosurgeons do not believe that shunt pumping is useful in assessing shunt function,[5] we believe that in certain cases, pumping the shunt can indicate shunt malfunction, particularly if the patient is well known to the practitioner. We advocate, however, performing shunt pumping only after an imaging study has demonstrated the presence of hydrocephalus and volume of cerebrospinal fluid (CSF) surrounding the proximal catheter, as the potential for obstructing a functional shunt with shunt pumping is theoretically higher in a patient with very small ventricles or a malpositioned ventricular catheter. Furthermore, the results obtained from shunt pumping should never be used to definitively rule out a possible shunt malfunction.

35.3 Radiographic Studies

Imaging studies are often essential for the diagnosis of shunt malfunction. As mentioned previously, most patients who present to the emergency room undergo both an X-ray shunt series and an intracranial imaging study (CT or MRI).

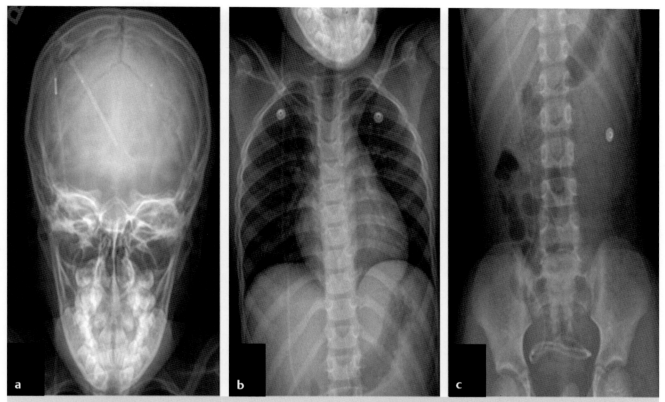

Fig. 35.1 (a–c) Example shunt series. Multiple plain radiographs (shunt series) demonstrating continuous course of a ventriculoperitoneal shunt tubing from head to abdomen.

Plain radiographs can be obtained easily and efficiently. A plain radiograph shunt series allows for the determination of the type of shunt system in place, including the valve, valve setting, and general location of the catheters (▶ Fig. 35.1). A shunt series may also demonstrate disconnections, breaks, or kinks in the shunt system, which may lead directly to shunt malfunction. Comparison with prior films can also be of critical importance, for example, a fixed-position, coiled peritoneal catheter could serve as an etiology of shunt malfunction.

Most patients with a suspected shunt malfunction will also undergo a head CT or rapid MRI to determine the shape and size of the ventricular system. In the majority of cases, even in cases of frank ventriculomegaly, brain imaging should be compared with prior scans with knowledge of the clinical history at each time point of previous imaging. Prior to the advent of electronically stored radiographic information, we asked all families to hold on to copies of old head CT scans and other imaging studies and to bring these copies with them to any emergency room or clinic visit. Comparison with prior scans aids in the interpretation of current imaging in the setting of suspected shunt malfunction. An increase in the caliber of the ventricular system from a baseline examination obtained when the patient was asymptomatic, in addition to a clinical suspicion of shunt malfunction, warrants shunt exploration in the majority of cases.

Additional imaging findings that may require attention include overdrainage signs such as subdural hygromas or slit ventricles, as well as a malpositioned proximal catheter. Occasionally, shunt malfunction occurs despite the presence of small ventricles. In some patients, ventricular compliance is low enough such that increased ICP and shunt obstruction occur without ventriculomegaly nor changes in ventricular size.

Radionuclide studies can be performed to identify the presence of a shunt obstruction but are rarely indicated in the acute setting. In certain cases, when distal malfunction is suspected, abdominal CT or ultrasonography may demonstrate an abdominal pseudocyst, ascites, visceral perforation, or malposition of the distal catheter. Ultrasound may be used in infants with a patent fontanelle and also to determine the presence of abdominal collections such as pseudocysts.

35.4 Shunt Tap

A shunt tap procedure can be performed quickly at the bedside with minimal complications.[6] Shunt taps can be both diagnostic and therapeutic. For most shunt taps, we use a 23- or 25-gauge butterfly needle attached to a 25-cm length of tubing. The area over the shunt reservoir is prepped with Betadine (Purdue Pharma L.P., Stamford, CT) or a similar antiseptic solution, and the shunt bulb is entered at a steep angle under sterile conditions. With the needle in place, the tubing is extended upward to act as a manometer to estimate the ICP based upon the flow of CSF into the tubing. If CSF overflows out the distal end of the tubing, then the ICP is estimated to be greater than 25 cm H_2O, suggesting increased ICP. The end of the butterfly tubing can then be placed below the level of the shunt valve to assess for proximal flow. Sood et al have shown that assessing the "drip interval" with this method is very effective for diagnosis of proximal shunt malfunction.[7]

If there is no immediate return of fluid, then a 3-mL syringe can be connected to the tubing and an attempt can be made at aspirating CSF from the valve using the smaller syringe. Inability to aspirate CSF is often a sign of proximal malfunction. Distal malfunction can sometimes be diagnosed by manually occluding the inlet portion of the valve and allowing the fluid column in the tubing to flow distally. Slow or absent distal flow can be an indicator of distal malfunction. CSF obtained from the shunt tap is always sent to the laboratory for cell count, Gram stain, culture, glucose, and protein.

35.5 Causes of Acute Malfunction

There are three main causes of acute shunt malfunction: (1) obstruction of the proximal/ventricular catheter; (2) obstruction distal to the proximal catheter, including the valve and distal catheter; and (3) disconnection, breakage, or migration of any component of the shunt system. Each of these etiologies requires a unique management algorithm.

35.5.1 Proximal Obstruction

Obstruction of the proximal catheter is the most common cause of acute shunt malfunction. Debris from the ventricles or the choroid plexus can often occlude the perforations of the proximal catheter, resulting in obstruction of CSF drainage. Proximal obstruction can sometimes be diagnosed solely by clinical examination when a fluid collection is palpated over the cranial burr hole. Most often, however, diagnosis requires analysis of imaging studies (▶ Fig. 35.2) and results from a shunt tap. Occasionally, the diagnosis is not made until intraoperative interrogation of the shunt system is performed.

The treatment of acute shunt malfunction due to proximal catheter obstruction is replacement of the ventricular catheter in the operating room. The procedure is scheduled as a level I emergency; thus, the patient should be taken expeditiously to the operating room. Both proximal and distal sites are prepped, and the cranial incision is opened. The valve is disconnected from the ventricular catheter, and proximal obstruction is confirmed by the lack of CSF flow from the ventricular catheter. The ventricular catheter is then carefully removed and replaced.

Removal of the proximal catheter can be difficult in cases of delayed shunt malfunction owing to the presence of adhesions and gliosis around the catheter. Gentle traction combined with cauterization of surface scar tissue is often sufficient to release the catheter. In some cases, a stylet may be placed down the proximal catheter and low intermittent monopolar cautery is applied to free the catheter.

Cannulation of the ventricle can also prove to be difficult in some cases. For most cases of proximal shunt obstruction, where catheter position is appropriate, we prefer to "soft-pass" a new catheter down the original shunt tract. While an assistant removes the proximal catheter, the surgeon places a new catheter, with the stylet pulled back a few centimeters, through the hole in the cortex to the appropriate depth or until CSF emanates from the new catheter. In cases where new proximal catheter positioning is sought, the original burr hole should be enlarged and surface scar tissue should be removed before placing the new ventricular catheter. Additionally, the trajectory of the existing proximal catheter can be used as a guide for the new trajectory. After CSF flow is confirmed from the new proximal catheter and before reattaching the proximal catheter to the valve, the patency of the valve and distal catheter should be assessed with a blunt needle and manometer filled with saline.

Postoperatively, patients are observed overnight and often sent home the following day. Postoperative imaging can be performed to confirm placement of the ventricular catheter and resolution of ventriculomegaly. In most cases, however, resolution of clinical symptoms and signs is a reliable indicator of reconstituted shunt function.

35.5.2 Distal Obstruction

Distal obstruction can occur at the level of the shunt valve or distal catheter. Debris can clog the valve, causing it to malfunction. Similarly the distal catheter can become occluded by debris, contents of the abdominal cavity, or even a blood clot in the case of atrial catheters.

Less commonly, kinking of the distal catheter at its connection to the valve or entry site in the abdomen or chest can be the cause of distal obstruction and shunt malfunction. These kinks are usually identifiable on a shunt series. In certain cases, abdominal CT is utilized to confirm distal malfunction due to poor CSF absorption or malpositioning of the catheter.

Distal obstruction is most often diagnosed by the presence of increased ventricular caliber on an imaging study and the presence of good proximal CSF flow with a shunt tap. Since CSF can be readily and relatively easily accessed with a shunt tap, the management of patients with a distal obstruction can proceed in a less urgent fashion than with proximal shunt obstruction. Following a large-volume shunt tap to normalize ICP, patients can be monitored closely while studies are performed and preparations are made for definitive operative intervention.

Replacement of the distal catheter or valve in the operating room is the treatment for distal shunt obstruction. In some cases, because of multiple prior abdominal resulting in scarring, or poor CSF absorption, plans should be made preoperatively for insertion of the distal catheter into an alternative location. In cases where numerous revisions have previously been performed, we often ask our colleagues from general surgery or thoracic surgery to assist us with placement of the distal catheter into an alternative site, such as the internal jugular vein, subclavian vein, or pleural space.

Prior to closure, the proximal catheter should always be interrogated because a concomitant partial proximal obstruction may exist concurrently with a distal obstruction. In uncomplicated revisions, patients are monitored for 24 hours and then sent home. Postoperative imaging is advisable but is not requisite.

35.5.3 Disconnection, Fracture, and Migration

Disconnection, fracture, and migration of the proximal or distal shunt catheters can sometimes be detected on physical examination but are most often diagnosed upon careful inspection of plain radiographs (▶ Fig. 35.3). Disconnections can

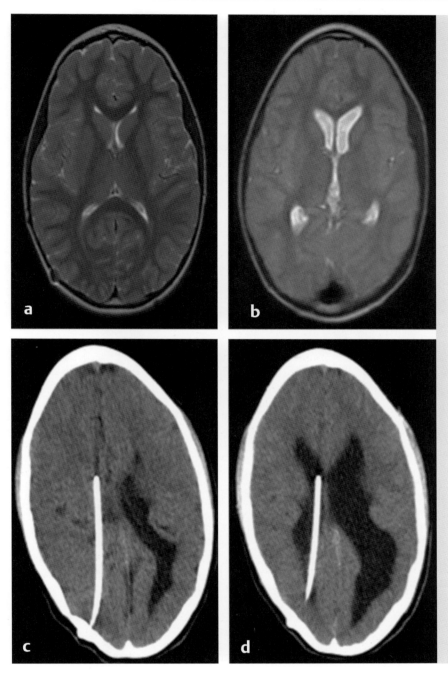

Fig. 35.2 (a, b) Ventriculomegaly associated with shunt malfunction. T2-weighted magnetic resonance images demonstrating baseline ventricular caliber **(a)** and ventricular caliber during shunt malfunction **(b)**, aiding in the diagnosis of shunt malfunction. **(c, d)** Computed tomography (CT) images demonstrating baseline ventricular caliber **(c)** and ventricular caliber during shunt malfunction **(d)**, aiding in the diagnosis of shunt malfunction.

occur at either the proximal catheter–valve connection or the distal catheter–valve connection. These may result from poorly assembled connections between the valve and catheters, or as the child grows, from excessive tension on one of the components of the shunt system. Intraoperative repair of disconnections should specifically address both of these issues.

Fracture of the shunt catheter or valve can result acutely from local trauma or more often as a late complication of repeated biomechanical stress along with calcification and aging of the shunt components. Fractures often occur at sites where the shunt is in close contact with bony surfaces

such as the clavicle or rib cage. The treatment of a fractured shunt catheter or valve is removal of the fractured pieces and replacement.

Migration of either the proximal and the distal catheter can occur. Migration of the proximal catheter often results in shunt obstruction by occlusion of the inlet ports with brain tissue. Distal migrations are more common and have been described in a variety of locations, particularly with ventriculoperitoneal shunts.[8,9,10,11,12,13] Treatment of catheter migration requires replacement and, if possible, retrieval of the migrated fragment.

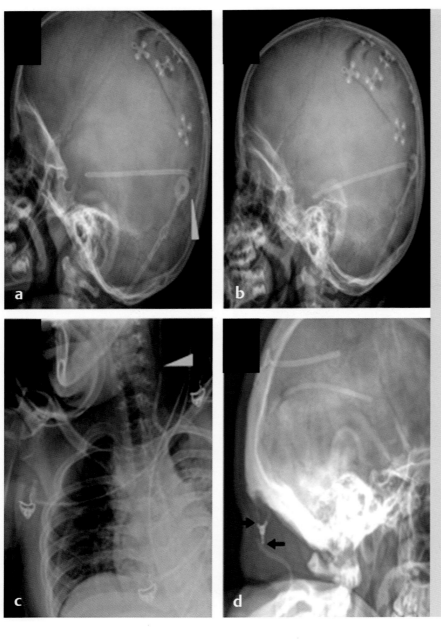

Fig. 35.3 (a, b) Shunt disconnection and fracture. Plain skull radiographs demonstrating disconnection of the proximal catheter from the shunt reservoir (arrowhead) **(a)** and reconnection following surgical revision **(b)**. **(c)** Plain chest radiograph demonstrating ventriculoperitoneal shunt fracture (arrowhead) as it courses along the neck. **(d)** Lateral skull radiograph demonstrating multiple sites of shunt disconnection (arrows) at a Y-connection point in a patient with multiple ventricular catheters.

35.6 Management of the Unstable Patient

It is not uncommon to encounter patients with an acute shunt malfunction who present with acute distress and who demonstrate vital sign instability or overt herniation. These situations call for immediate action, often before any imaging studies can be obtained. Standard protocols for management of the airway, breathing, and circulation (ABC) should be performed while urgent action is taken to address management of ICP by removal of CSF.

An emergent shunt tap should be performed if it is found that the shunt does not pump properly. If CSF can be withdrawn from the reservoir, then enough CSF should be slowly removed until the ICPs are normalized and vital signs have stabilized. If CSF cannot be removed and the patient's situation is dire, a small-gauge spinal needle can be carefully placed, percutaneously, through the shunt burr hole and along, or through, the proximal shunt catheter directly into the ventricle. Again, CSF should be removed slowly until ICPs and vital signs have normalized.

CSF can also be accessed by placement of an emergent intraventricular catheter at the bedside using standard techniques. In infants, alternatively, an emergent fontanelle tap can be performed. This, however, is rarely necessary in a patient with patent sutures because of the increased compliance of the calvarium.

Following stabilization, the patient should be scheduled immediately for the operating room for shunt revision surgery. If the patient is sufficiently stabilized by appropriate measures, one may elect to proceed with imaging studies prior to the procedure, to identify the site of malfunction.

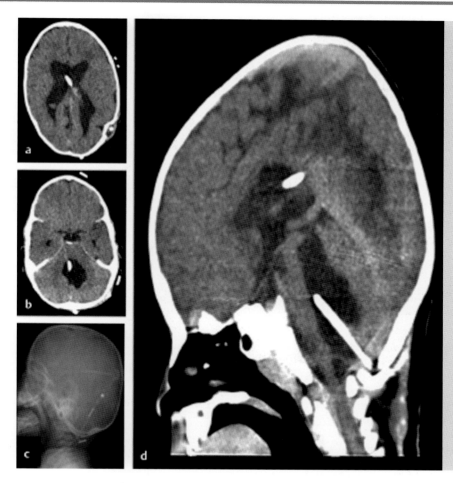

Fig. 35.4 (a–c) Complex hydrocephalus. Axial noncontrast computed tomography CT image **(a, b)** and lateral skull radiograph **(c)** demonstrating lateral and fourth ventricular catheters coursing independently as two shunt systems. **(d)** Sagittal head CT image demonstrating multiple proximal catheters needed to treat a patient with complex hydrocephalus.

35.7 Special Situations

35.7.1 External Ventricular Drainage

In certain cases, where continuous monitoring of ICP is necessary, the shunt system can be removed and replaced with either an intraventricular catheter or externalized shunt system. This is commonly done for infected shunt systems that require removal and rarely necessary for mechanical malfunctions. However, in complex cases of shunt malfunction, it is sometimes advisable to proceed with external ventricular drainage and continuous ICP monitoring before deciding upon a definitive shunt revision.

35.7.2 Endoscopic Third Ventriculostomy

Endoscopic third ventriculostomy (ETV) can be performed for cases where there is a history of obstructive hydrocephalus, particularly due to aqueductal stenosis, and multiple shunt malfunctions with revisions. ETV can often be combined with removal of the entire shunt system and with or without placement of an externalized intraventricular catheter for postoperative ICP monitoring. Recent studies have demonstrated high ETV success rates in patients presenting with shunt failure due to an obstructive hydrocephalus. Several studied demonstrated similar success rates in patients undergoing primary ETV and

ETV as treatment for shunt failure.[14,15,16] ETV was particularly efficacious (64–80%) for patients presenting with an infected shunt.[14,15,16] The use of ETV in an emergent setting, however, should only be performed at centers with significant experience with this technique.

35.7.3 Multiple Shunt Systems

The presence of multiple shunt systems for compartmentalized hydrocephalus adds to the complexity of the management of acute shunt malfunction (▶Fig. 35.4). Scenarios involving the investigation of multiple shunt systems, whether independent or T-connected, require special attention to ventricular asymmetry on imaging studies and can sometimes require shunt taps for each system. Replacement or revision of more than one system may be necessary and requires special attention to positioning in the operating room in order to replace multiple shunt parts in a single sitting.

35.7.4 Slit Ventricle Syndrome

Patients with *slit ventricle syndrome* have symptoms of elevated ICP with small or "slitlike" ventricles on imaging studies (▶Fig. 35.5). The exact etiology of slit ventricle syndrome is debatable and may be related to intermittent proximal catheter obstruction due to surrounding ventricular collapse, or shunt

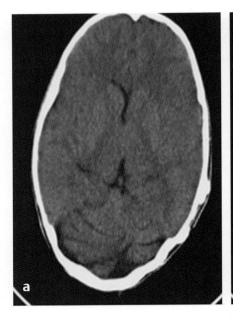
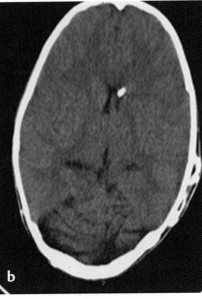

Fig. 35.5 (a, b) Slit ventricle syndrome. Axial noncontrast head computed tomography images demonstrating slitlike ventricles in a patient with shunted hydrocephalus presenting with symptoms of shunt malfunction.

obstruction with increased ICP in the setting of a noncompliant ventricular system. In the latter cases, significant increases in ICP may occur without significant change in ventricular size. The diagnosis of shunt malfunction in the presence of slit ventricles can be challenging with standard techniques such as shunt tapping because of difficulty with result interpretation and often requires intraoperative exploration of the shunt system to confirm.

Several treatment options have been proposed for slit ventricle syndrome, including subtemporal decompression, lumboperitoneal shunting, and even shunt removal. Recent clinical studies, though, have demonstrated high success rates in slit ventricle syndrome with use of a programmable valves. Kamiryo et al first reported successful use of a programmable valve system to normalize ICP in a patient with slit ventricle syndrome.[17] Kamikawa et al subsequently demonstrated high rates of success in 20 patients with a history of multiple shunt revisions, including two cases where the shunt system was altogether eliminated.[18]

References

[1] Hanlo PW, Cinalli G, Vandertop WP, et al. Treatment of hydrocephalus determined by the European Orbis Sigma Valve II survey: a multicenter prospective 5-year shunt survival study in children and adults in whom a flow-regulating shunt was used. J Neurosurg. 2003; 99(1):52–57

[2] Kestle J, Drake J, Milner R, et al. Long-term follow-up data from the Shunt Design Trial. Pediatr Neurosurg. 2000; 33(5):230–236

[3] Kestle JR, Walker ML; Strata Investigators. A multicenter prospective cohort study of the Strata valve for the management of hydrocephalus in pediatric patients. J Neurosurg. 2005; 102(2, Suppl):141–145

[4] Pollack IF, Albright AL, Adelson PD; Hakim-Medos Investigator Group. A randomized, controlled study of a programmable shunt valve versus a conventional valve for patients with hydrocephalus. Neurosurgery. 1999; 45(6):1399–1408, discussion 1408–1411

[5] Piatt JH, Jr. Physical examination of patients with cerebrospinal fluid shunts: is there useful information in pumping the shunt? Pediatrics. 1992; 89(3):470–473

[6] McComb JG. Acute shunt malfunction. Neurosurg Emerg. 1994; 2:327–334

[7] Sood S, Kim S, Ham SD, Canady AI, Greninger N. Useful components of the shunt tap test for evaluation of shunt malfunction. Childs Nerv Syst. 1993; 9(3):157–161, discussion 162

[8] Adeolu AA, Komolafe EO, Abiodun AA, Adetiloye VA. Symptomatic pleural effusion without intrathoracic migration of ventriculoperitoneal shunt catheter. Childs Nerv Syst. 2006; 22(2):186–188

[9] Akcora B, Serarslan Y, Sangun O. Bowel perforation and transanal protrusion of a ventriculoperitoneal shunt catheter. Pediatr Neurosurg. 2006; 42(2):129–131

[10] Kim MS, Oh CW, Hur JW, Lee JW, Lee HK. Migration of the distal catheter of a ventriculoperitoneal shunt into the heart: case report. Surg Neurol. 2005; 63(2):185–187

[11] Park CK, Wang KC, Seo JK, Cho BK. Transoral protrusion of a peritoneal catheter: a case report and literature review. Childs Nerv Syst. 2000; 16(3):184–189

[12] Taub E, Lavyne MH. Thoracic complications of ventriculoperitoneal shunts: case report and review of the literature. Neurosurgery. 1994; 34(1):181–183, discussion 183–184

[13] Yuksel KZ, Senoglu M, Yuksel M, Ozkan KU. Hydrocele of the canal of Nuck as a result of a rare ventriculoperitoneal shunt complication. Pediatr Neurosurg. 2006; 42(3):193–196

[14] O'Brien DF, Javadpour M, Collins DR, Spennato P, Mallucci CL. Endoscopic third ventriculostomy: an outcome analysis of primary cases and procedures performed after ventriculoperitoneal shunt malfunction. J Neurosurg. 2005; 103(5, Suppl):393–400

[15] Bilginer B, Oguz KK, Akalan N. Endoscopic third ventriculostomy for malfunction in previously shunted infants. Childs Nerv Syst. 2009; 25(6):683–688

[16] Marton E, Feletti A, Basaldella L, Longatti P. Endoscopic third ventriculostomy in previously shunted children: a retrospective study. Childs Nerv Syst. 2010; 26(7):937–943

[17] Kamiryo T, Fujii Y, Kusaka M, Kashiwagi S, Ito H. Intracranial pressure monitoring using a programmable pressure valve and a telemetric intracranial pressure sensor in a case of slit ventricle syndrome after multiple shunt revisions. Childs Nerv Syst. 1991; 7(4):233–234

[18] Kamikawa S, Kuwamura K, Fujita A, Ohta K, Eguchi T, Tamaki N. [The management of slit-like ventricle with the Medos programmable Hakim valve and the ventriculofiberscope] [in Japanese]. No Shinkei Geka. 1998; 26(4):349–356

36 The Perinatal Management of a Child Born with a Myelomeningocele

Kimberly A. Foster and Frederick A. Boop

Abstract

Myelomeningocele (MMC) is the most severe central nervous system (CNS) congenital malformation compatible with life. No definitive studies demonstrate emergent operative repair of the MMC improves outcome; however, evidence does support emergent measures to optimize the patient's condition at the time of repair, with surgical repair on an urgent basis. This includes covering the defect with a sterile dressing, the initiation of broad-spectrum intravenous antibiotics, and rapid transport to a facility accustomed to caring for pediatric neurosurgical patients. Preoperative ultrasound assessment of the head, spine, kidneys, and, when indicated, the heart will alert the surgeon to associated abnormalities that may require additional attention. Many children with MMC require treatment of hydrocephalus, most commonly with ventriculoperitoneal shunting. Other conditions, such as tethered cord, Chiari malformation–related sequelae, and urologic and orthopedic abnormalities, may require treatment throughout the life of a patient with MMC.

Keywords: Chiari malformation, fetal surgery, hydrocephalus, myelomeningocele, neural tube defect, spina bifida, tethered cord, ventriculoperitoneal shunt

36.1 Introduction

Myelomeningocele (MMC) represents the most severe central nervous system (CNS) congenital malformation compatible with life. Although most neurosurgeons would agree that the operative repair of a leaking MMC is better classified as "urgent" rather than "emergent," CNS infection remains one of the leading causes of morbidity and mortality in the perinatal period in infants born with neural tube defects (NTDs). It is therefore germane that the treatment of the child born with a NTD is included in a textbook of neurosurgical emergencies. Delay of care may lead to CNS infection[1]; evidence suggests that infants who survive meningitis, ventriculitis, and possible sepsis may have long-term developmental and cognitive dysfunction.[2] Measures taken immediately following delivery can effectively reduce the risk of a perinatal infection and complication. Furthermore, evidence suggests that prenatal diagnosis, intrauterine management, and the mode of delivery may impact the long-term prognosis of the MMC child.

NTDs are the most common congenital abnormalities of the CNS, and MMC is the most common NTD. In the United States, the incidence of MMC is between 0.3 and 1.4 per 1,000 live births and has remained relatively stable since the introduction of folic acid supplementation.[3] Incidence varies depending on race and demographics, more commonly occurring in Caucasians compared with African Americans. Overall rates have declined because of improved nutrition, mandatory folate fortification, and elective termination. The risk of recurrence is 1 to 2% for parents having a previously affected child,[4] and a female with MMC has a 3% risk of having a child with MMC.[5]

MMC, and other open NTDs, are mainly caused by a failure of primary neurulation. To date, the cause of MMC remains unknown and may be the net result of multiple aberrant embryologic events.[4,6,7] Epidemiologic and laboratory studies have cited a variety of causes for MMC, and although MMC is most often an isolated malformation, the causes are multifactorial. Genetic transmission can be autosomal dominant, autosomal recessive, or X-linked recessive, but with a low concordance between monozygotic twins, MMC is most likely polygenic.[8]

Although many cellular pathways and embryologic events have been implicated, folate (vitamin B_6) appears critical to the pathogenesis of MMC. Double-blind randomized and nonrandomized studies have shown a 70% reduction in the recurrence rates for mothers of spina bifida children given folate supplements as compared with similar mothers given a placebo.[9] Subsequent studies have demonstrated a 60% reduction in first-time dysraphic births in mothers receiving similar supplements.[10] The United States Public Health Service recommends that all women of childbearing age who are capable of becoming pregnant consume 0.4 to 1.0 mg of folic acid per day.[9] Given that many pregnancies in the United States are unplanned, it would only be through general dietary supplementation that a reduction in the incidence of MMC through this mechanism could be accomplished. Teratogens, such as certain anticonvulsants (valproic acid) have been associated with higher incidence of MMC, possibly through their effect on folate metabolism.[11]

Debate has surrounded the treatment of MMC. Some neurosurgeons have attempted to look for elements within the disorder that might influence outcome as a means of determining which children should be treated aggressively and which children should be allowed to die.[12,13] The most notable such study was that of Lorber, published in 1971,[14] in which he categorized patients into two groups, with paralysis at or above L2, marked hydrocephalus, kyphosis, and other congenital anomalies or birth injuries being used as criteria for nonsurgical management. His results demonstrated that of those with adverse criteria, half died. Forty percent had a normal intelligence quotient (IQ). Of those who had no adverse criteria, one fourth died, half had severe sequelae, and 14% were mentally deficient. He surmised that treatment should be offered only to those patients who could "look forward to life without grave handicaps." The Groningen Protocol, developed in the Netherlands in 2004 to administer active euthanasia to select infants thought to have a "hopeless prognosis," included children with hydrocephalus and MMC.[15] McLone demonstrated that earlier selection criteria are unable to predict which patients will have favorable outcomes and, therefore, should not be used.[16] In his study, in which 89 children had aggressive care, including repair of the MMC within the first 24 hours of life, the surgical mortality was 2% and the overall mortality at a minimum of 3.5 years of follow-up was 14%. In this population, 80% required shunting, 73% had a normal or above-average IQ, 54% were able to ambulate, and 87% achieved social urinary continence; moreover, parents of children with MMC rarely regret a decision to treat their child with MMC. In North America as of 2017, most infants with MMC are treated. This chapter offers specific guidelines as to the perinatal management of these children based upon our current state of knowledge.

36.2 Prenatal Diagnosis

The wider utilization of prenatal ultrasonography and screening of high-risk pregnancies has resulted in the earlier diagnosis of spinal dysraphism.[17] Maternal serum α-fetoprotein (AFP) analysis, performed at 16 to 18 weeks of gestation with a 75% sensitivity for the detection of open NTDs, is often the first step in diagnosis.[18] Prenatal ultrasound carries a sensitivity of nearly 100%, with visualization of the placode and bony anomalies or indirect cranial signs associated with MMC.[18] Amniocentesis for amniotic AFP, acetylcholinesterase, and chromosomal analysis are also highly sensitive.[19] After diagnosis, decisions regarding the future management of the pregnancy should involve consultation and discussion with pediatricians, neurosurgeons, and geneticists. Options include fetal surgery evaluation, early intervention postnatally, no intervention, and termination of the pregnancy, as discussed below.

Progressive hydrocephalus is uncommon in the fetus and appears to be more likely to occur the higher the spinal level of the defect; however, if there is increasing ventriculomegaly, early intervention may take the form of cesarean section of the preterm infant once the lungs have reached maturity. Should fetal distress occur prior to lung maturation, cesarean delivery may still be warranted following appropriate consideration of the complex ethical issues. The once actively debated issue of in utero diversion of cerebrospinal fluid (CSF) via ventriculoamniotic shunt has not shown benefit and therefore has been abandoned.[20]

For children who have reached term, the best mode of delivery remains unclear. In a nonrandomized study, it was demonstrated that the mode of delivery does not affect intellectual outcome in these infants.[21] Another prospective nonrandomized study conducted by Luthy et al confirmed this, but it also demonstrated that children with a NTD who were exposed to the forces of labor were 2.2 times more likely to have a severe paralysis than were those delivered by cesarean section before the onset of labor.[22] This suggested that the stress of labor and delivery may be harmful to the exposed spinal neural elements and has been the rationale behind recommending elective cesarean section for mothers of infants in whom the lesion is recognized antenatally. Studies have not been conducted examining the possible relationship between mode of delivery and perinatal CNS infections in children with a MMC born to mothers infected with group B streptococcus; however, a relationship is plausible and may exist, lending further credence to elective cesarean section for the delivery of children with MMC. Conversely, there have also been multiple nonrandomized studies that have shown no clear benefit of cesarean section,[23,24,25,26,27] except in cases of breech position or severe hydrocephalus. Nonetheless, the optimal mode of delivery for mother and patient remains unclear and should be considered on a case-by-case basis.

36.3 Postnatal Diagnosis and Evaluation

If the diagnosis of MMC has not been made prenatally, it generally becomes obvious upon inspection of the newborn. Three important questions then need to be addressed. First, does the fluid space communicate with the environment? Although in the authors' experience the majority of these lesions leak CSF, it can sometimes be difficult to establish this on initial examination. Careful inspection of the child while crying or gentle pressure on the anterior fontanelle may reveal CSF leaking from the lesion. Palpation of the lesion itself or probing with an instrument is neither helpful nor recommended. A sterile gauze placed over the lesion during the remainder of the examination may become moist with serum or CSF, but frank wetness establishes the diagnosis of an "open" lesion. Closed lesions can be treatable electively, as the risk of meningitis and/or ventriculitis associated with CSF leakage does not exist.

Second, what is the neurologic status of the child? This is critical to establish once the child is born, whether or not the MMC was discovered in utero. Determining the exact level of sensorimotor dysfunction can be difficult, but the prognosis for sensorimotor function is generally predicted by anatomical level, with the exception of cervicothoracic MMC. Stimulation, either by sound or by touch, may elicit reflex movements that give the parents a false sense of optimism. In fact, simple observation is often the best estimate of the child's functional level. The orthopedic deformities, which result from the unopposed actions of certain muscle groups, may be of localizing value. Lesions above T12 will cause flaccid hips, legs, and feet. Lesions below L1–L2 will cause fixed flexion deformity of the hips due to functional iliopsoas unopposed by the gluteal musculature. Lesions below L3–L4 will result in genu recurvatum, and lesions below L4–L5 may cause degrees of talipes equinovarus or pes cavus. All patients with spinal dysraphism are presumed to have some degree of neurogenic bladder dysfunction. In the presence of a dyssynergic bladder, the practice of trying to expel urine by suprapubic pressure (Credé's maneuver) may cause ureteral reflux and is to be discouraged.[28]

Third, does the child have associated congenital anomalies, neurologic or otherwise? Ten percent of children with spina bifida will have a chromosomal abnormality, and 15% will harbor other anomalies outside of the nervous system.[22,29] A thorough examination of the cardiovascular, gastrointestinal, pulmonary, and genitorurinary systems is mandatory before consideration can be given to surgical intervention. Within the nervous system itself, greater than 80% of children with MMC have hydrocephalus,[30,31] and 70 to 90% require a shunt,[30,32] although the need for shunting in some children has recently been debated. An associated Chiari II hindbrain abnormality occurs in 90% of children, but these rarely require operative intervention. Tandem abnormalities of the spinal cord such as diastematomyelia, syringomyelia, dermoid tumors, lipomas, or spinal arachnoid cysts are not uncommon.

When the head is large, the scalp veins dilated, and the fontanelle full, the diagnosis of hydrocephalus is easily made; however, hydrocephalus may exist in the absence of clinical signs, being recognized only by the sonographic presence of ventricular enlargement. In some instances, it may not develop until several days following MMC closure, and so it remains important to follow the child closely, with routine ultrasound evaluation at short intervals to evaluate for hydrocephalus. Similarly, the clinical manifestations of the Chiari II hindbrain malformation may be subtle and not apparent for months to years following birth. Whether stridor, poor feeding, lower cranial nerve palsies, or apneic spells are due to direct compression of the brainstem (by the cerebellar tonsils) or are secondary to intrinsic malformation of the medulla may be difficult to discern. It is absolutely critical to first rule out unrecognized hydrocephalus or a shunt malfunction when children manifest Chiari II–like symptoms, as pressure from above may be the cause. Which symptoms will respond to decompressive suboccipital surgery remains a matter of contention. In general, brainstem dysfunction is a poor prognostic sign, and of the 15 to 30% of children who die within the first 5 years of life, most will die from complications of the hindbrain malformation.[32,33,34]

36.4 Neuroimaging

The favored imaging modality for fetal imaging because of its sensitivity in detecting tissue–water interfaces, and its low radiation exposure to the fetus, the fetal ultrasound serves as an excellent tool in the early detection of NTDs.[20] Signs of MMC seen on ultrasound prompt a more detailed examination of the fetus. Biochemical markers, fetal chromosomal studies, and magnetic resonance imaging (MRI) are all appropriate tools in the antenatal diagnosis of MMC and may be useful in the diagnosis of other developmental abnormalities.

When considering preoperative investigations of the newborn child with open NTD, one should keep in mind the principles of minimal handling and patient comfort. Laborious, time-consuming, costly, and invasive tests are unnecessary in the immediate management of the infant with open NTD; however, a plain chest–abdomen–pelvis X-ray is simple to perform and often taken to verify the placement of an umbilical vein or artery catheter and can incorporate the spinal column at the level of the lesion to demonstrate the presence and severity of an associated spinal deformity. We perform important ultrasound examinations before closure; a head ultrasound serves as an excellent baseline examination of the ventricles and may provide information relating to the posterior fossa malformations. An ultrasound of the spine in these neonates may demonstrate the presence of syringomyelia, diastematomyelia, or a dermoid tumor and can accurately determine the level of the conus medullaris (▶ Fig. 36.1).[35,36] On a dedicated renal ultrasound, the kidneys and bladder can be visualized, revealing the number and position of the kidneys and the presence of concomitant urologic abnormalities, including hydronephrosis and/or an overdistended bladder. Transcranial Doppler flow studies of the major branches of the circle of Willis may also reflect abnormal cerebral perfusion in the face of progressive hydrocephalus because resistance to blood flow in these vessels increases in the face of increasing intracranial pressure.[37] MRI of the complete neuraxis can be performed, but the child does not need this preoperatively, as it rarely, if ever, changes immediate management.

36.5 Counseling and Timing of Surgery

The neurosurgeon is an integral member of the antenatal counseling team. The neurosurgeon offers an intimate relationship with the condition, including a detailed knowledge of the structural abnormality, experience regarding related conditions, and information on long-term quality of life issues and the treatment of patients at various stages of life. Other members of the team should include a genetic counselor, a neonatologist or pediatrician, and an obstetrician. A team composed of these members will be able to provide detailed information in an impartial manner to the family regarding the nature of the condition, obstetric management, postnatal care, quality-of-life issues and can address concerns regarding elective termination. It is estimated that as many as 50% of pregnancies affected by NTDs and nearly one quarter of those affected by spina bifida are terminated electively.[38,39]

It is important to emphasize to all caretakers that the burden of care begins with closure of the MMC and that care is a lifelong commitment. Treatment comes at a substantial financial and time cost to both the family and the health care system. In fact, costs have been estimated to exceed $340,000 per lifetime per patient and an annual cost of nearly $500 million to the health care system.[9] These children require lifelong multidisciplinary support, sometimes in an institutionalized environment. Time spent with the family in these early stages may cultivate understanding and acceptance of this chronic condition. This, in turn, will create less strain on the family, better acceptance of the child, fewer institutionalized children, and, ultimately, less burden on the health care system. It has been demonstrated that parental satisfaction and their likelihood of taking responsibility for the child are directly related to the quality of information given initially and their degree of involvement in the decision-making process.[40] A survey by McLone revealed that parents do not fully understand the nature of their child's affliction until as long as 6 months after the child's birth.[16] In this regard, they ultimately must rely upon the advice of their physicians.

The prognosis of children with spina bifida varies dramatically with the level of the lesion and the presence of associated anomalies, but several general statistics can be presented to parents. Current data suggest that more than 90% of newborn infants with MMC will survive beyond infancy,[41] and rare deaths in infancy are caused by the Chiari malformation or shunt failure. Overall long-term mortality is between 30 and 60%.[32,33] Three out of four will have normal IQ,[32,42] and 60% of those with normal IQ have some learning disability.[43] Over 80% of adults are independent in activities of daily living (ADLs), and although one third will attend college, only one third are gainfully employed.[44] Although ambulation status correlates with sensorimotor level, nearly 90% of children (given a high percentage of low lumbosacral level) are ambulatory.[45] By adolescence, half of the children with MMC will be wheelchair dependent. Fortunately, nearly 90% will achieve social urinary continence with the use of drugs and intermittent catheterizations (CIC).[32,46,47] Half of all patients have complete bowel continence, and most have control a majority of the time.[32] Genital sensation is reported in over two thirds of males.

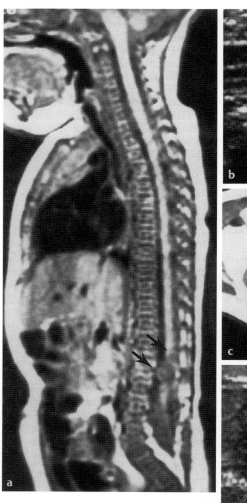

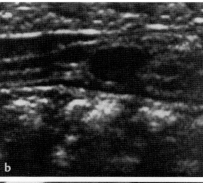

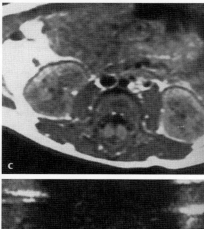

Fig. 36.1 (a) Sagittal T1-weighted magnetic resonance imaging (MRI) of a neonate demonstrates a tethered spinal cord with cystic intramedullary lesions of the distal spinal cord. (b) Ultrasound of the lumbar spine in the same infant confirms the presence of a tethered spinal cord and demonstrates the cystic abnormalities within the conus medullaris. (c) Axial T1-weighted MRI of the spine in another infant demonstrates a diastematomyelia. (d) Axial ultrasound of the spine through the same region confirms the presence of a diastematomyelia.

Rates of ventricular shunting are debated and variable, many reports claiming 80 to 90% requiring a shunt, whereas other studies showing 60 to 70%. This rate may be different and, in fact, lower depending on the geographic location of the child.[48] Recently, some neurosurgeons have attempted endoscopic third ventriculostomy (ETV) for hydrocephalus related to MMC, although results are still early and there may be some degree of permissive ventriculomegaly at some institutions. Long-term results are necessary to understand the role of ETV in this disease process.[49,50] Nonetheless, in shunted children, shunt failure rates are up to 40, 60, and 85% at 1, 5, and 10 years post shunting, respectively.[51] Shunt infection rates are variable, particularly upon the geographic location of the child.[52,53,54]

Some children may require multiple operations in their first 10 years of life, for myriad orthopedic, neurosurgical, or urologic complications. Up to 30% of children require a tethered cord surgery, noted by the progression of symptoms (although MRI can be obtained, children with MMC will nearly always appear tethered on imaging), and perhaps up to 5% develop syringomyelia.[51] Physicians should emphasize to caretakers

that although surgery on the spine and the brain will not restore function, it may prevent further deterioration. To this point, the early introduction of the team approach is helpful and reassures the parents that their child can live a productive and rewarding life; multidisciplinary spina bifida clinics, attended by neurosurgery, orthopedics, physical medicine and rehabilitation, urology, and social work, are now a mainstay at many institutions.

In the immediate postnatal period, the physician may rarely encounter the situation in which caretakers choose to withhold treatment; this presents a medical, ethical, moral, and legal dilemma. Some series have documented that all untreated children will die within 12 months,[55] whereas evidence from the developing world shows that this not to be the case, and although the rate is unknown, the authors have witnessed children survive to scar over their MMC and live into adolescence and adulthood. Moreover, infants do not die immediately and those who will pass may have a slow, lingering death that is trying for the patient, caretakers, and health care team. Recognizing that withholding treatment is a difficult dilemma, the American Academy of Pediatrics has suggested that the decision to withhold or withdraw life-sustaining treatment should be made only after thorough review from consultants with medical, legal, ethical, and social expertise.[56]

Considering the aforementioned complex issues, it is perhaps surprising that surgical management of the MMC patient has remained largely unchanged since the closure of MMC became widespread in the mid-1970s. Since that time, researchers and physicians have come to learn much more about the disease and the accompanying sequelae of spina bifida patients. For instance, the in utero exposure of the neural tissue to the amniotic fluid may perhaps damage the tissue and alter its development.[57,58] By minimizing spinal cord exposure to the uterine environment, one might be able to alleviate some of the morbidity associated with the disease.

In 1997, the first open intrauterine MMC repairs (IUMRs) were performed at Vanderbilt University Medical Center and Children's Hospital of Philadelphia, and intrauterine repair has been conducted at some institutions for over 15 years.[59,60,61] Subsequently, a randomized, controlled, multicenter trial, known as the Management of Myelomeningocele Study (MOMS), has been completed.[62] The results of this study have shown a reduction in the rate of Chiari malformation, reduced need for ventricular shunting for hydrocephalus, and decreased incidence of secondary injury to the lower spinal cord (damage at the placode itself). The utility of intrauterine surgery is limited by many factors, including high cost, maternal and fetal risk, potential for complications in future pregnancies, and the need for early recognition of the MMC. The American College of Obstetricians and Gynecologists recommends fetal surgery be offered and conducted at highly experienced centers only, with a specialized multidisciplinary team including trained obstetricians, anesthesiologists, neurosurgeons, and an experienced intensive care unit.[63]

Although results of IUMR seem promising in select patients, currently the standard of care in the child with an open NTD includes delivery via cesarean section followed by closure of the defect at some point after delivery. Although the exact timing of surgical closure is somewhat controversial, it has become clear that the surgical treatment of the child with an open NTD should be considered urgent, not emergent.[16,55,64] Current standard of care is to operate within 72 hours of birth, without a risk of complication.[65] A retrospective comparison of IQ in relation to history of ventriculitis suggests that CNS infections may be the major cause of mental retardation in children with MMC; however, conditions can be optimized such that the risk of CNS infection is minimized.[66,67] Time also permits caretakers to receive appropriate counseling and become involved in the decision-making process.

Importantly, the decision as to the timing of surgery requires a consideration for the situation. For example, a child with a low lesion, no hydrocephalus or associated abnormalities, and well-informed caretakers, who has been delivered in a tertiary referral institution with on-site neurosurgical facilities, should have surgery as soon as possible (often the subsequent day). Conversely, a child with a high lesion, associated hydrocephalus, cardiovascular anomalies, poorly informed caretakers, born to a single, adolescent mother recovering from a cesarean section in a peripheral hospital may benefit from a slight delay in surgery as medical and social issues are addressed.[68]

36.6 Immediate Treatment

Following the birth and stabilization of the neonate with an open NTD, the child should be placed in the prone position in an infant warmer with the head of the bed level. Positioning the child on, or direct pressure over, the unrepaired MMC should be avoided. The closed spinal defect, on the other hand, need not be treated with special care unless the covering tissues are thin and fragile. In such a case, the defect should be covered with a sterile dressing to prevent accidental injury and as a reminder to nursing staff and caretakers of the repair.

In the case of a leaking MMC, the defect should be covered with a sterile saline-soaked gauze. If the defect is large, the infant may lose significant amounts of body heat and fluid, even in the presence of an infant warmer; this can be obviated by covering the defect and lower torso with a plastic drape. For a leaking MMC, the early institution of broad-spectrum intravenous antibiotics has been demonstrated to significantly reduce the likelihood of a perinatal ventriculitis, the major contributor to perinatal mortality in these infants. Should it occur, ventriculitis is likely to be caused by *Escherichia coli*, group B streptococcus, or *Staphylococcus* species.[67] The antibiotics chosen should have good CSF penetration and coverage of these organisms, based on patterns of resistance within one's hospital. Studies have not shown a significant advantage of one antibiotic over another, and at our institution the neonatologists will decide, taking many factors into consideration.

If the child is at a community hospital, the aforementioned steps should be conducted and the child should be transported to the nearest facility dedicated to the treatment of the pediatric neurosurgical patient. Prior to surgery, the infant should have a thorough physical examination by a neonatologist and neurosurgeon, with attention to associated congenital anomalies such as renal or cardiac defects.

Historically, the presence of urine was mandatory preoperatively to verify that the infant had functional kidneys, although this should not be an absolute criterion in the modern era. Currently the authors' preoperative spina bifida protocol includes an ultrasound of the head, spine, kidneys, and bladder. If cyanosis or a cardiac murmur is recognized, an echocardiogram is included. The presence of a secondary spinal lesion or a significant intracranial process as evidenced by screening ultrasound may dictate further anatomical definition by computed tomography (CT) or MRI. A preoperative complete blood count should be seen prior to surgery, both to verify that the hematocrit is sufficient and to observe the white blood cell count (WBC). In neonates, a low WBC may be the harbinger of impending sepsis, as may hypothermia, and may temper the timing of surgery or the decision to place a ventricular shunt concomitant with the MMC repair.

36.7 Operative Technique

Following administration of general endotracheal anesthesia, the infant is placed on the operating table in the prone position with bolsters under the chest and the iliac spines. As noted above, intravenous antibiotics with broad CNS coverage should have been initiated and are continued for the purpose of surgery. If a simultaneous shunt is to be placed, a modified lateral

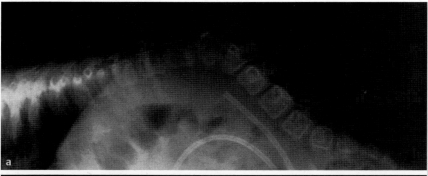

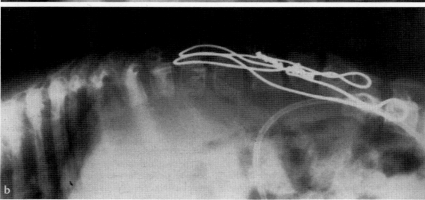

Fig. 36.2 (a) A lateral thoracolumbar X-ray demonstrates a congenital kyphosis in a child born with spina bifida. (b) The kyphosis is corrected by incising through the disk spaces and anterior longitudinal ligament, leaving the posterior longitudinal ligament intact. Following reduction of the deformity, wires placed laterally around the pedicles serve to maintain the reduction. Blood loss for the case was less than 50 mL. The vertebral end plates remain intact, allowing for normal spinal growth.

decubitus position will allow access to the peritoneal cavity and to the MMC at a single setting,[69] although some surgeons may prefer to completely reposition and redrape the child for purposes of shunting after the MMC is repaired. If the child has fixed contractures of the hips, the bolsters should be built up so that the contracted joints are supported. If there is accompanying ventriculomegaly, the table should be placed in slight Trendelenburg position throughout the procedure to prevent excessive drainage of CSF. A warming device should be placed on the bed underneath the infant to assist in maintaining body temperature throughout the case. Intravenous and irrigating fluids should be euthermic. In the preparation of the patient's skin, one should avoid scrubbing the neural placode and should avoid prepping with sclerosing agents such as alcohol or alcohol-containing soaps. Gentle irrigation with an iodine solution (Betadine solution; Purdue Pharma L.P., Stamford, CT) or antibiotic solution with bacitracin will suffice. Draping should be generous in the event that rotational flaps or relaxing incisions are necessary. With the maintenance of meticulous hemostasis, it is rarely necessary to transfuse a child for this surgery. For a detailed description of the operative procedure, the reader is referred to the superb article by McLone.[70]

Once the neural placode has been dissected free of its surrounding tissues, it should be carefully inspected for abnormalities. If a thickened filum terminale is identified, it should be sectioned. Chadduck and Reding reported a congenital dermoid within the filum terminale associated with a MMC, recognized at the time of sectioning.[71] Next, the reconstitution of the pial edges of the neural placode into a "sausage" or "taco" shape is recommended. This will not restore neural function but will simplify the repair of a tethered spinal cord later in life should the patient become symptomatic from retethering in the future.

The dural cuff is developed and closed, and attempts should be made to also bring together a fascial layer of closure over the neural tube. Dural substitute or grafting is rarely necessary and does not appear to reduce the rate of subsequent tethering. It may increase CSF leak or infection rates; the authors do not recommend use of grafting. If the facets are widely splayed and prominent, they may require resection or fracturing to achieve this layer of closure without jeopardizing skin closure. Up to 10% of infants will have a significant kyphotic deformity of the spine at the level of the MMC, complicating the skin closure. Techniques of vertebrectomy and kyphectomy have been described to assist in closure.[72,73] These are almost always associated with significant blood loss and the need for transfusions. A technique preferred by the authors, performed in conjunction with a pediatric orthopedic spine colleague (R. E. McCarthy, personal communication), involves freeing the paraspinous muscles from their abnormal position lateral to the vertebra to expose the anterior spine. Incisions are then made through the disk spaces and anterior longitudinal ligament (ALL) at the involved levels, leaving the posterior longitudinal ligament intact. This dissection is through a relatively avascular plane and is advantageous in that it leaves the end plates intact, allowing for normal growth of the vertebral segments. Once the disks and ALL are incised, the kyphosis can be manually reduced. A posterior tension band is then created to maintain the reduction by placing heavy sutures or wire around the pedicles above and below the kyphus (▶Fig. 36.2). The paraspinous muscles are then closed over the defect dorsally, allowing the muscle to function as spine extensors, as they were intended, rather than as flexors.

In closing the skin, most defects can be closed primarily if the available skin and subcutaneous tissues are undermined far

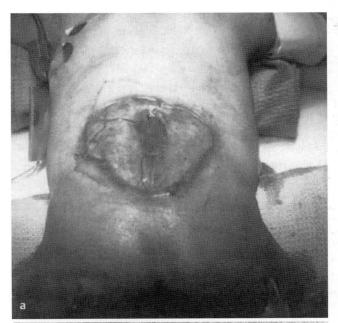

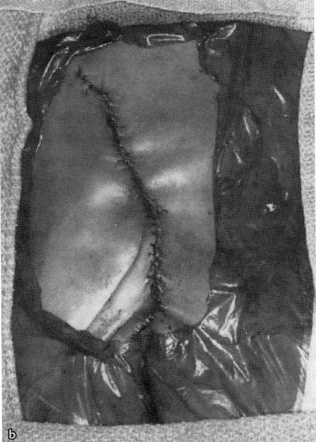

Fig. 36.3 (a) A newborn with a large thoracic myelomeningocele is positioned on the operating table on bolsters with the head in slight Trendelenburg. (b) The same infant with primary closure of the skin following repair of the defect. Note that by undermining the skin and subcutaneous tissues far laterally, this lesion did not require rotational flaps or relaxing incisions.

enough laterally (▶Fig. 36.3). Often redundant skin will need to be trimmed, and the closure can be performed in a vertical, horizontal, or Z-plasty manner.[74] There is rarely the need for rotational flaps or relaxing incisions. In rare instances, a particularly challenging defect may be encountered and the assistance of a plastic surgeon is worthwhile. At our institution, the neurosurgeon makes a decision to consult plastic surgery based on preoperative evaluation of the defect.

In the past, it was considered standard practice to delay shunting of the lateral ventricles (a procedure that a large majority of these infants will require) for several days until it has been established that the child has not developed ventriculitis. In children with hydrocephalus evident at birth or shortly thereafter, such a practice of delayed shunting may necessitate daily ventricular taps and can jeopardize the lumbar wound closure from antecedent CSF pressure. This delay in shunting also demands that the patient and caretakers endure a second intubation and anesthetic in the perinatal period. Several studies have shown no significant difference in the shunt infection rate in infants shunted at the time of MMC repair compared with those undergoing a delayed procedure.[69,75,76,77] A CSF-diverting procedure performed at the time of repair has the advantage of decreasing the risk of hydrocephalus on brain development and decreasing the potential for CSF leakage, fistula formation, or infection; therefore, it is recommended that ventricular shunting be performed at the same operative setting unless there is doubt about the necessity of shunting. Children born with a small or normal head circumference at birth and with small ventricles on ultrasound should be watched for the development of hydrocephalus. Also, evidence of infection should delay closure until 48 to 72 hours of intravenous antibiotics can be administered and should also delay placement of any implants for the treatment of hydrocephalus, with proof of resolved meningitis/ventriculitis before permanent shunting. The use of external ventricular drainage--to reduce the risk of infection, leak after closure, and/or as a bridge to shunting--has met with mixed results.[78,79]

Despite early closure, up to 18% of patients experience wound complications, including dehiscence, pseudomeningocele formation, CSF leak, and infection. These complications have negative effects on outcome and significantly increase the length of hospital stay for these patients.[80] Attempts have been made to determine factors that can reduce the number of wound complications; however, most studies have focused on variations of surgical technique in closure.[81] Miller et al showed that simultaneous MMC closure and placement of a ventriculoperitoneal shunt significantly reduced wound complications and spinal fluid leakage.[82] Specifically, they noted that 17% of patients who had a shunt placed in a delayed fashion had a CSF leak at the site of their MMC closure, whereas none of the patients who had simultaneous closure and shunting developed this problem. In addition, there was no significant increase in shunt-related complications between simultaneous and sequential closure and shunting patients, as total shunt complication (e.g., shunt malfunction and CSF infection) rates were 24% and 29%, respectively. One caveat was that there was a higher percentage of patients with shunt malfunction in the simultaneous group (19%)

than the sequential group (8%), although this did not reach statistical significance.

These recommendations are for children receiving care in an institution similar to the authors'—a large tertiary center in the developed world. Children cared for in resource-poor centers or countries certainly have unique considerations, and the medical, social, and cultural climate for physician, caretaker, and patient must be carefully considered. For instance, Albright and Okechi published a series of over 30 Kenyan children with lumbosacral MMC with pre- and postoperative motor function documentation, finding that distal cordectomy (in which the placode is truncated and not included in repair) may serve to decrease the rate of future tethering without subjecting children to a significant loss in motor function.[83] In sharp contrast, the use of intraoperative neurophysiologic monitoring is advocated at many centers in the United States, for preservation of every possible nerve fiber.[84] This may not be practical in all settings, and the technique by which MMC is repaired continues to evolve, depending upon the setting in which neurosurgical care is being delivered.

36.8 Postoperative Care

Postoperatively, these children are observed overnight in the neonatal intensive care unit (NICU). In the postoperative period, they are seen by neonatology, urology, orthopedics, rehabilitation, social services, and other members of the multidisciplinary spina bifida team. If a local spina bifida support group exists, it may be useful to introduce the parents to representatives of this group.

The infant is nursed in the prone position to avoid pressure necrosis of the tenuous skin over the spine. Should necrosis of the wound edges occur, it should not be débrided but instead covered with a dry dressing. In time, the wound edges will reepithelialize and the eschar will fall off. In the event the wound leaks CSF, consideration of a shunt should be given immediately. If the wound leaks in the presence of a preexisting shunt, it is likely that the shunt has malfunctioned and may require revision.

If the infant has difficulty with bladder distention, a clean intermittent bladder catheterization (CIC) schedule should be instituted. This can be easily taught to most parents prior to discharge. The family should also be instructed in the care of the neurogenic bowel and skin. Finally, every effort should be made to return the infant to his/her mother as soon as possible. These infants are generally separated from the mother at the time of birth, and it is often several days before the mother is reunited with her child. The practice of "rooming-in," available in many NICUs, should be encouraged.

36.9 Conclusion

Over the last few decades, the incidence of MMC is on the decline in the developed world. This is no doubt due in large part to increasing folate supplementation but also to some degree related to improvements in access to prenatal care, education of parents and physicians, technological advances such as the availability of prenatal ultrasound and maternal serum AFP measurements, and prevalence of elective pregnancy termination.

There are no definitive studies to demonstrate *emergent* operative repair of the MMC improves outcome. Evidence does suggest, however, that *emergent* measures to optimize the patient's condition at the time of repair, with surgical repair on an *urgent* basis, are indicated. This includes covering the defect with a sterile dressing, the initiation of broad-spectrum intravenous antibiotics, and rapid transport to a facility accustomed to caring for pediatric neurosurgical patients. Preoperative ultrasound assessment of the head, spine, kidneys, and, when indicated, the heart, will alert the surgeon to associated abnormalities that may require additional attention. Studies indicate that there are no good "selection criteria" upon which to base a decision not to treat these children. Currently, pediatric neurosurgical centers now aggressively treat nearly all children born with a MMC. Only the rare child with severe, multiorgan disease sequelae, coupled with strong desires of a well-informed family, should prompt consideration of nontreatment. In such instances, the neurosurgeon should take advantage of available legal, social, and ethical services.

Although the general approach to surgical repair has remain largely unchanged, advances in the treatment of hydrocephalus and intrauterine repair techniques continue to change the face of the care of the child with MMC. Undoubtedly, studies from both the developed and developing world, taking into consideration many facets of MMC pathophysiology and management, will shape the future care and approach to children with spina bifida.

References

[1] Rodrigues AB, Krebs VL, Matushita H, de Carvalho WB. Short-term prognostic factors in myelomeningocele patients. Childs Nerv Syst. 2016; 32(4):675–680

[2] Pinto FC, Matushita H, Furlan AL, et al. Surgical treatment of myelomeningocele carried out at 'time zero' immediately after birth. Pediatr Neurosurg. 2009; 45(2):114–118

[3] Boulet SL, Yang Q, Mai C, et al; National Birth Defects Prevention Network. Trends in the postfortification prevalence of spina bifida and anencephaly in the United States. Birth Defects Res A Clin Mol Teratol. 2008; 82(7):527–532

[4] Campbell LR, Dayton DH, Sohal GS. Neural tube defects: a review of human and animal studies on the etiology of neural tube defects. Teratology. 1986; 34(2):171–187

[5] Shurtleff DB, Lemire RJ. Epidemiology, etiologic factors, and prenatal diagnosis of open spinal dysraphism. Neurosurg Clin N Am. 1995; 6(2):183–193

[6] Copp AJ, Brook FA, Estibeiro JP, Shum AS, Cockroft DL. The embryonic development of mammalian neural tube defects. Prog Neurobiol. 1990; 35(5):363–403

[7] Dias MS, Walker ML. The embryogenesis of complex dysraphic malformations: a disorder of gastrulation? Pediatr Neurosurg. 1992; 18(5–6):229–253

[8] Myrianthopoulos NC, Melnick M. Studies in neural tube defects. I. Epidemiologic and etiologic aspects. Am J Med Genet. 1987; 26(4):783–796

[9] Control USDoHaHSCfD. Recommendations for the use of folic acid to reduce the number of cases of spina bifida and other neural tube defects. MMWR Recomm Rep. 1992; 41(RR-14):1–7

[10] Werler MM, Shapiro S, Mitchell AA. Periconceptional folic acid exposure and risk of occurrent neural tube defects. JAMA. 1993; 269(10):1257–1261

[11] Steegers-Theunissen RP. Folate metabolism and neural tube defects: a review. Eur J Obstet Gynecol Reprod Biol. 1995; 61(1):39–48

[12] Foltz EL, Kronmal R, Shurtleff DB. Chapter 10. To treat or not to treat: a neurosurgeon's perspective of myelomeningocele. Clin Neurosurg. 1973; 20:147–163

[13] Freeman JM. Chapter 9. To treat or not to treat: ethical dilemmas of the infant with a myelomeningocele. Clin Neurosurg. 1973; 20:134–146

[14] Lorber J. Results of treatment of myelomeningocele. An analysis of 524 unselected cases, with special reference to possible selection for treatment. Dev Med Child Neurol. 1971; 13(3):279–303

[15] Eduard Verhagen AA. Neonatal euthanasia: lessons from the Groningen Protocol. Semin Fetal Neonatal Med. 2014; 19(5):296–299

[16] McLone DG. Treatment of myelomeningocele: arguments against selection. Clin Neurosurg. 1986; 33:359–370

[17] Hogge WA, Dungan JS, Brooks MP, et al. Diagnosis and management of prenatally detected myelomeningocele: a preliminary report. Am J Obstet Gynecol. 1990; 163(3):1061–1064, discussion 1064–1065

[18] Cuckle HS. Screening for neural tube defects. Ciba Found Symp. 1994; 181:253–266, discussion 266–269

[19] Wilson RD. Prenatal evaluation for fetal surgery. Curr Opin Obstet Gynecol. 2002; 14(2):187–193

[20] Hansen AR, Madsen JR. Antenatal neurosurgical counseling: approach to the unborn patient. Pediatr Clin North Am. 2004; 51(2):491–505

[21] Bensen JT, Dillard RG, Burton BK. Open spina bifida: does cesarean section delivery improve prognosis? Obstet Gynecol. 1988; 71(4):532–534

[22] Luthy DA, Wardinsky T, Shurtleff DB, et al. Cesarean section before the onset of labor and subsequent motor function in infants with meningomyelocele diagnosed antenatally. N Engl J Med. 1991; 324(10):662–666

[23] Cochrane D, Aronyk K, Sawatzky B, Wilson D, Steinbok P. The effects of labor and delivery on spinal cord function and ambulation in patients with meningomyelocele. Childs Nerv Syst. 1991; 7(6):312–315

[24] Cuppen I, Eggink AJ, Lotgering FK, Rotteveel JJ, Mullaart RA, Roeleveld N. Influence of birth mode on early neurological outcome in infants with myelomeningocele. Eur J Obstet Gynecol Reprod Biol. 2011; 156(1):18–22

[25] Hadi HA, Loy RA, Long EM, Jr, Martin SA, Devoe LD. Outcome of fetal meningomyelocele after vaginal delivery. J Reprod Med. 1987; 32(8):597–600

[26] Lewis D, Tolosa JE, Kaufmann M, Goodman M, Farrell C, Berghella V. Elective cesarean delivery and long-term motor function or ambulation status in infants with meningomyelocele. Obstet Gynecol. 2004; 103(3):469–473

[27] Merrill DC, Goodwin P, Burson JM, Sato Y, Williamson R, Weiner CP. The optimal route of delivery for fetal meningomyelocele. Am J Obstet Gynecol. 1998; 179(1):235–240

[28] Bauer SB, Colodny AH, Retik AB. The management of vesicoureteral reflux in children with myelodysplasia. J Urol. 1982; 128(1):102–105

[29] Nyberg DA, Mack LA, Hirsch J, Pagon RO, Shepard TH. Fetal hydrocephalus: sonographic detection and clinical significance of associated anomalies. Radiology. 1987; 163(1):187–191

[30] Rintoul NE, Sutton LN, Hubbard AM, et al. A new look at myelomeningoceles: functional level, vertebral level, shunting, and the implications for fetal intervention. Pediatrics. 2002; 109(3):409–413

[31] Swank M, Dias L. Myelomeningocele: a review of the orthopaedic aspects of 206 patients treated from birth with no selection criteria. Dev Med Child Neurol. 1992; 34(12):1047–1052

[32] Bowman RM, McLone DG, Grant JA, Tomita T, Ito JA. Spina bifida outcome: a 25-year prospective. Pediatr Neurosurg. 2001; 34(3):114–120

[33] Oakeshott P, Hunt GM, Poulton A, Reid F. Expectation of life and unexpected death in open spina bifida: a 40-year complete, non-selective, longitudinal cohort study. Dev Med Child Neurol. 2010; 52(8):749–753

[34] Steinbok P, Irvine B, Cochrane DD, Irwin BJ. Long-term outcome and complications of children born with meningomyelocele. Childs Nerv Syst. 1992; 8(2):92–96

[35] Glasier CM, Chadduck WM, Burrows PE. Diagnosis of diastematomyelia with high-resolution spinal ultrasound. Childs Nerv Syst. 1986; 2(5):255–257

[36] Glasier CM, Chadduck WM, Leithiser RE, Jr, Williamson SL, Seibert JJ. Screening spinal ultrasound in newborns with neural tube defects. J Ultrasound Med. 1990; 9(6):339–343

[37] Chadduck WM, Seibert JJ, Adametz J, Glasier CM, Crabtree M, Stansell CA. Cranial Doppler ultrasonography correlates with criteria for ventriculoperitoneal shunting. Surg Neurol. 1989; 31(2):122–128

[38] Forrester MB, Merz RD. Prenatal diagnosis and elective termination of neural tube defects in Hawaii, 1986–1997. Fetal Diagn Ther. 2000; 15(3):146–151

[39] Roberts HE, Moore CA, Cragan JD, Fernhoff PM, Khoury MJ. Impact of prenatal diagnosis on the birth prevalence of neural tube defects, Atlanta, 1990–1991. Pediatrics. 1995; 96(5 Pt 1):880–883

[40] Charney EB. Parental attitudes toward management of newborns with myelomeningocele. Dev Med Child Neurol. 1990; 32(1):14–19

[41] McLone DG. Continuing concepts in the management of spina bifida. Pediatr Neurosurg. 1992; 18(5–6):254–256

[42] Oakeshott P, Hunt GM. Long-term outcome in open spina bifida. Br J Gen Pract. 2003; 53(493):632–636

[43] Fletcher JM, Francis DJ, Thompson NM, Davidson KC, Miner ME. Verbal and nonverbal skill discrepancies in hydrocephalic children. J Clin Exp Neuropsychol. 1992; 14(4):593–609

[44] McLone D, Naidich TP. Myelomeningocele: outcome and late complications. In: McLaurin, Schut I, Venes JL, Epstein F, eds. Pediatric Neurosurgery. Vol. 68. Philadelphia, PA: W.B. Saunders; 1989:80-82

[45] Findley TW, Agre JC, Habeck RV, Schmalz R, Birkebak RR, McNally MC. Ambulation in the adolescent with myelomeningocele. I: early childhood predictors. Arch Phys Med Rehabil. 1987; 68(8):518–522

[46] Samuelsson L, Skoog M. Ambulation in patients with myelomeningocele: a multivariate statistical analysis. J Pediatr Orthop. 1988; 8(5):569–575

[47] Spindel MR, Bauer SB, Dyro FM, et al. The changing neurourologic lesion in myelodysplasia. JAMA. 1987; 258(12):1630–1633

[48] Kumar R, Singh SN. Spinal dysraphism: trends in northern India. Pediatr Neurosurg. 2003; 38(3):133–145

[49] Perez da Rosa S, Millward CP, Chiappa V, Martinez de Leon M, Ibáñez Botella G, Ros López B. Endoscopic third ventriculostomy in children with myelomeningocele: a case series. Pediatr Neurosurg. 2015; 50(3):113–118

[50] Stone SS, Warf BC. Combined endoscopic third ventriculostomy and choroid plexus cauterization as primary treatment for infant hydrocephalus: a prospective North American series. J Neurosurg Pediatr. 2014; 14(5):439–446

[51] Dias MS, McLone DG Myelomeningocele. In: Albright AL, Pollack IF, Adelson PD, eds. Principles and Practice of Pediatric Neurosurgery. New York, NY: Thieme; 2014: 338–366

[52] Gamache FW, Jr. Treatment of hydrocephalus in patients with meningomyelocele or encephalocele: a recent series. Childs Nerv Syst. 1995; 11(8):487–488

[53] Ochieng' N, Okechi H, Ferson S, Albright AL. Bacteria causing ventriculoperitoneal shunt infections in a Kenyan population. J Neurosurg Pediatr. 2015; 15(2):150–155

[54] Tuli S, Drake J, Lamberti-Pasculli M. Long-term outcome of hydrocephalus management in myelomeningoceles. Childs Nerv Syst. 2003; 19(5–6):286–291

[55] Sutton LN, Charney EB, Bruce DA, Schut L. Myelomeningocele—the question of selection. Clin Neurosurg. 1986; 33:371–381

[56] Noetzel MJ. Myelomeningocele: current concepts of management. Clin Perinatol. 1989; 16(2):311–329

[57] Drewek MJ, Bruner JP, Whetsell WO, Tulipan N. Quantitative analysis of the toxicity of human amniotic fluid to cultured rat spinal cord. Pediatr Neurosurg. 1997; 27(4):190–193

[58] Heffez DS, Aryanpur J, Hutchins GM, Freeman JM. The paralysis associated with myelomeningocele: clinical and experimental data implicating a preventable spinal cord injury. Neurosurgery. 1990; 26(6):987–992

[59] Adzick NS, Sutton LN, Crombleholme TM, Flake AW. Successful fetal surgery for spina bifida. Lancet. 1998; 352(9141):1675–1676

[60] Tulipan N. Intrauterine myelomeningocele repair. Clin Perinatol. 2003; 30(3):521–530

[61] Walsh DS, Adzick NS, Sutton LN, Johnson MP. The rationale for in utero repair of myelomeningocele. Fetal Diagn Ther. 2001; 16(5):312–322

[62] Adzick NS, Thom EA, Spong CY, et al; MOMS Investigators. A randomized trial of prenatal versus postnatal repair of myelomeningocele. N Engl J Med. 2011; 364(11):993–1004

[63] American College of Obstetricians and Gynecologists. ACOG Committee opinion no. 550: maternal-fetal surgery for myelomeningocele. Obstet Gynecol. 2013; 121(1):218–219

[64] John W, Sharrard W, Zachary RB, Lorber J, Bruce AM. A controlled trial of immediate and delayed closure of spina bifida cystica. Arch Dis Child. 1963; 38(197):18–22

[65] Charney EB, Weller SC, Sutton LN, Bruce DA, Schut LB. Management of the newborn with myelomeningocele: time for a decision-making process. Pediatrics. 1985; 75(1):58–64

[66] Brau RH, Rodríguez R, Ramírez MV, González R, Martínez V. Experience in the management of myelomeningocele in Puerto Rico. J Neurosurg. 1990; 72(5):726–731

[67] Charney EB, Melchionni JB, Antonucci DL. Ventriculitis in newborns with myelomeningocele. Am J Dis Child. 1991; 145(3):287–290

[68] Okorie NM, MacKinnon AE, Lonton AP, Dickson JA. Late back closure in myelomeningoceles—better results for the more severely affected? Z Kinderchir. 1987; 42(Suppl 1):41–42

[69] Chadduck WM, Reding DL. Experience with simultaneous ventriculo-peritoneal shunt placement and myelomeningocele repair. J Pediatr Surg. 1988; 23(10):913–916

[70] McLone D. Repair of the myelomeningocele. In: Rengachery SS, WIlkins RH, eds. Neurosurgical Operative Atlas. Vol. 3. Philadelphia, PA: Williams and Wilkins; 1993:41–48

[71] Chadduck WM, Roloson GJ. Dermoid in the filum terminale of a newborn with myelomeningocele. Pediatr Neurosurg. 1993; 19(2):81–83

[72] Hwang SW, Thomas JG, Blumberg TJ, et al. Kyphectomy in patients with myelomeningocele treated with pedicle screw-only constructs: case reports and review. J Neurosurg Pediatr. 2011; 8(1):63–70

[73] Samagh SP, Cheng I, Elzik M, Kondrashov DG, Rinsky LA. Kyphectomy in the treatment of patients with myelomeningocele. Spine J. 2011; 11(3):e5–e11

[74] Cruz NI, Ariyan S, Duncan CC, Cuono CB. Repair of lumbosacral myelomeningoceles with double Z-rhomboid flaps. Technical note. J Neurosurg. 1983; 59(4):714–717

[75] Bell WO, Arbit E, Fraser RA. One-stage meningomyelocele closure and ventriculoperitoneal shunt placement. Surg Neurol. 1987; 27(3):233–236

[76] Epstein NE, Rosenthal AD, Zito J, Osipoff M. Shunt placement and myelomeningocele repair: simultaneous vs sequential shunting. Review of 12 cases. Childs Nerv Syst. 1985; 1(3):145–147

[77] Hubballah MY, Hoffman HJ. Early repair of myelomeningocele and simultaneous insertion of ventriculoperitoneal shunt: technique and results. Neurosurgery. 1987; 20(1):21–23

[78] Demir N, Peker E, Gülşen İ, Ağengin K, Tuncer O. Factors affecting infection development after meningomyelocele repair in newborns and the efficacy of antibiotic prophylaxis. Childs Nerv Syst. 2015; 31(8):1355–1359

[79] Talamonti G, D'Aliberti G, Collice M. Myelomeningocele: long-term neurosurgical treatment and follow-up in 202 patients. J Neurosurg. 2007; 107(5, Suppl):368–386

[80] Kshettry VR. Letter to the editor: validity of the results of a perioperative protocol to reduce shunt infections. Acta Neurochir (Wien). 2014; 156(4):789

[81] Emsen IM. Closure of large myelomeningocele defects using the O-S flap technique. J Craniofac Surg. 2015; 26(7):2167–2170

[82] Miller PD, Pollack IF, Pang D, Albright AL. Comparison of simultaneous versus delayed ventriculoperitoneal shunt insertion in children undergoing myelomeningocele repair. J Child Neurol. 1996; 11(5):370–372

[83] Albright AL, Okechi H. Distal cordectomies as treatment for lumbosacral myelomeningoceles. J Neurosurg Pediatr. 2014; 13(2):192–195

[84] Jackson EM, Schwartz DM, Sestokas AK, et al. Intraoperative neurophysiological monitoring in patients undergoing tethered cord surgery after fetal myelomeningocele repair. J Neurosurg Pediatr. 2014; 13(4):355–361

37 Recognition and Management of Intrathecal Baclofen and Narcotic Withdrawal Syndromes

Douglas E. Anderson and Drew A. Spencer

Abstract

Neurosurgeons are commonly called upon to evaluate and treat chronic pain and spasticity caused by a wide spectrum of frequently encountered pathologies. Implantable intrathecal baclofen and narcotic delivery systems can significantly improve symptoms and functional status in carefully selected patients with pain or spasticity. Pump and catheter placement and subsequent management require an experienced, multidisciplinary team. Medication withdrawal syndromes related to system complications and failure are rare and usually preventable but can be life-threatening when they occur. In this chapter, we review briefly the basic neuropharmacology of baclofen and morphine when given intrathecally, common etiologies associated with intrathecal pump and delivery failure, and the prompt recognition and management of these syndromes.

Keywords: baclofen, chronic pain, intrathecal pump, morphine, spasticity, withdrawal

37.1 Introduction

Spasticity and chronic pain are familiar conditions to the neurosurgeon, as they arise from a variety of frequently encountered conditions, including spinal cord injury, multiple sclerosis, cerebral palsy, degenerative spinal disease, and many others. The advent of implantable pumps for the administration of intrathecal (IT) baclofen and narcotic medications has proven to be an important therapeutic addition for patients suffering from these conditions. There are three drugs on the market approved by the Federal Drug Administration (FDA) for IT therapy for pain and spasticity: baclofen, morphine, and ziconotide. Ziconotide, a non-narcotic medicine approved for IT use in the treatment of chronic pain, although associated with potential side effects, has no associated withdrawal syndromes.

Patients who suffer from conditions with attendant intractable spasticity despite maximal doses of oral baclofen commonly experience marked improvement in functional status and clinically graded spasticity after both bolus and continuous dosing.[1,2] Patients with an implanted IT narcotic pump experience consistent improvement in chronic nociceptive, neuropathic, or mixed pain control over those managed with other regimens.[3,4] Still, patient selection is critical and complex. Patients with noncancerous chronic pain being considered for IT pump placement should undergo evaluation for psychiatric comorbidities such as depression, anxiety, addiction, suicidal ideation, or personality disorder. These patients have been shown to have a much less robust response to IT therapy.[5] Experienced and vigilant multidisciplinary teams must manage patients with IT pumps, as rare complications are possible that can precipitate acute medication withdrawal syndromes. Early recognition and treatment of withdrawal syndromes is imperative.

The most widely used IT pump system is the Medtronic SynchroMed II pump. The pump itself houses a drug reservoir, battery, pump apparatus, and the programmable components capable of coordinating dosage. A small-caliber catheter connects to the pump, is tunneled subcutaneously, anchored at the fascial or interspinous ligamentous entry point, and enters the lumbar IT space ending in the upper lumbar or lower thoracic levels. Newer pump models are magnetic resonance imaging (MRI) compatible, such that MR images can be collected when clinically indicated.[6,7,8] Programming data are stored permanently in the pump's internal memory, which allows trained clinicians to interrogate and obtain information about pump status or alter the rate timing of drug delivery as clinically indicated. Pumps eventually require replacement at the end of their battery life, but current technology, including rechargeable battery technology, extends this interval to an average of almost 7 years.

37.2 Pharmacology and Indications

37.2.1 Pharmacology of Baclofen

Baclofen is an antispasmodic agent that causes central nervous system (CNS) depression and skeletal muscle relaxation via γ-aminobutyric acid type B (GABA$_B$) receptor activation at spinal cord sites. It is thought that GABA$_B$ receptor agonism blocks the release of excitatory neurotransmitters at the synapse, thereby directly inhibiting muscle contraction and the initiation of spasticity. An IT bolus of baclofen produces measurable antispasmodic effect in 30 to 60 minutes, with a peak spasmolytic effect seen at approximately 4 hours after dosing. Drug effect can last 4 to 8 hours, depending on the patient's symptoms, and the dose and speed of drug administration. Usually a test dose is 25 to 50 µg. After the start of continuous IT infusion, antispasmodic action is seen in 6 to 8 hours. Maximum efficacy is observed within 24 to 48 hours. The half-life of IT baclofen is 2 to 5 hours.[9] Tolerance occurs in approximately 22% of patients, requiring dose adjustments during the first 18 months of therapy.[10] Most patients achieve an effective basal dose, with rare instances requiring drug holidays or other adjunct strategies.[11,12]

37.2.2 Pharmacology of Morphine

Morphine is a natural opiate that acts primarily on the mu (µ)-opioid receptor located throughout the peripheral and central nervous systems, including terminal afferent axons located in the substantia gelatinosa of the spinal cord. Morphine binds to receptors on the primary afferent neurons (presynaptic) and cells within the dorsal horn of the spinal cord (postsynaptic) to inhibit the release of neurotransmitters such as substance P and calcitonin gene–related peptide and finally hyperpolarize postsynaptic neurons. Activation of µ-opioid receptors results in analgesia and sedation, with a high incidence of tolerance and dependence. Tolerance is a well-documented

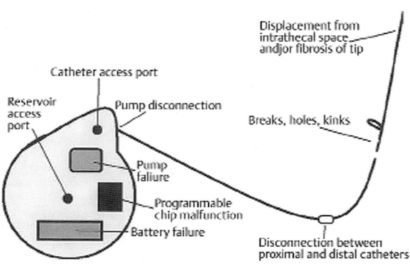

Fig. 37.1 Possible etiologies of pump failure.

obstacle to effective therapy in all opiate or opioid medications, requiring frequent dose titration or cycling of medications. The half-life of IT morphine is relatively short, 1.5 hours.[13]

37.2.3 Indications for Intrathecal Pumps

Implantable pumps are indicated for patients with intractable pain or spasticity who have had a positive response to oral medication but require larger doses, have intolerable side effects from oral medicines, or inadequate pain relief. Continuous IT administration of analgesic medications was initially utilized in cases of terminal malignancy but is now an option for patients with chronic pain of multiple etiologies. IT administration offers potential benefits, including decreased medication dose, fewer systemic side effects, and continuous steady-state administration, and avoids the pitfalls of oral therapy in carefully selected patients.[5] However, the potential side effects of IT opioids are substantial and include sedation, sweating, delayed gastric emptying, urinary retention, pruritus, nausea and vomiting, and respiratory depression. The possibility of respiratory depression has put a damper on IT morphine use. In the face of long life expectancies in patients with pain of nonmalignant origin, the frequency of these side effects and occurrence of tolerance have caused many clinicians to carefully reconsider this therapeutic option in this patient population.

37.3 Complications Leading to Baclofen and Morphine Withdrawal

IT drug delivery using an implantable pump and IT catheter is associated with a variety of complications that can cause acute pharmacologic withdrawal and life-threatening clinical syndromes (▶Fig. 37.1).

37.3.1 Catheter-Related Complications

Catheter-related complications remain the most common mechanical cause of baclofen or morphine pump failure that may lead to withdrawal.[14] These complications occur at varying rates, typically between 20 and 25%, but have been reported to occur in up to 75% of patients.[14,15,16,17] Catheters are susceptible to kinking, breakage or shearing, disconnection from the pump, and retraction out of the IT space despite the standard use of a soft-tissue anchor.[18] Plain anteroposterior (AP) and lateral radiographs can reveal the cause of some catheter-related failures. However, it is sometimes necessary to perform contrast-enhanced evaluations with fluoroscopy or computed tomography (CT) to further isolate the source of the problem.

37.3.2 Infectious Complications

Infection is typically the second-most reported complication and is a risk to all implanted components, with both pump and catheter infections adversely affecting IT pumps. This occurs in a small percentage of cases; however, some articles document a perioperative infection incidence of approximately 10%.[19,20] Most infections are localized with a small risk of meningitis, but if suspected, immediate standard intravenous antibiotic administration followed by obtaining cerebrospinal fluid (CSF) for culture and sensitivity studies is essential.[3] In rare cases, patients can present with fulminant sepsis.[21] Infection almost invariably requires pump removal and delayed reimplantation after complete resolution of the infection. Because infection is associated with pump removal, it is essential to begin drug replacement to prevent withdrawal.

37.3.3 Other Complications

Errors in pump programming are a rare but potentially devastating cause of withdrawal or toxicity. Rarely, frequent use of MRI can affect pump function as well, interfering with the memory/programming components, which can have downstream effects on other internal hardware.[6] Battery fatigue or failure is typically recognized by the pump system warning signals and is a predictable phenomenon that is almost always treated on an elective basis. The internal motor that delivers medication is a reported source of failure with patterns varying from complete and instant failure to intermittent symptom recurrence.[21] In patients receiving radiation treatment (28–36 Gy), the pump's programming components may be damaged or the battery may be depleted.[22] Others have found doses up to 45 Gy to be safe in patients with IT pumps, but they still recommend that pumps be carefully monitored both during and after treatment.[6] Breakdown or corrosion of the pump housing and/or components is extremely rare, as the materials used are chosen specifically for their inert properties when implanted, but has been noted in the literature.[14,21,23]

37.4 Recognition and Treatment of Clinical Withdrawal Syndromes

37.4.1 Baclofen

Side effects associated with IT baclofen therapy include light-headedness, drowsiness, confusion, muscle weakness, and ataxia. Treatment protocols for overdose include standard life support measures, the use of the parasympathomimetic, reversible cholinesterase inhibitor, physostigmine 2 mg intravenously, and CSF drainage via lumbar drain.[24]

Acute withdrawal symptoms include sudden increase in spasticity, pruritus, fever leading to hyperthermia, or epileptic seizures. Withdrawal is seldom life-threatening. High doses of benzodiazepines can be used to ameliorate withdrawal, while diagnosis of IT pump system failure is pursued. Some report that oral baclofen may not be adequate or tolerated in acute withdrawal such that administration of baclofen via lumbar puncture is indicated. Fulminant clinical scenarios with high fever, altered mental status, and rigidity profound enough to cause rhabdomyolysis are rare but have also been reported.[14,17] Clearly, in the case of life-threatening syndromes, one follows the standard concepts of maintaining airway, ventilation, and circulatory support. One group described cardiac arrest after severe withdrawal in a patient who fortunately recovered after a prolonged hospitalization.[25] Definitive treatment of withdrawal due to pump complications consists of restoration of a functioning IT delivery system. To determine the site of IT drug delivery failure, one can follow a systematic checklist[26]:

1. Interrogate the pump and check programming and filling status of the pump with the system telemetry to rule out programming errors and or empty pump reservoir.
2. Perform AP and lateral X-rays looking for disconnections, kinks, and dislodgment of the catheter.
3. If the X-rays are nondiagnostic, it is possible to check pump rotor function using real-time fluoroscopy after programming a 90-degree pump rotor rotation and visual radiographic observation.
4. If the pump is functional, one can attempt side port aspiration of 2 to 3 mL of CSF (necessary to remove baclofen from the catheter and the possibility of baclofen overdose during subsequent tests). If successful, one can then program an IT baclofen bolus through the pump–catheter system as a therapeutic trial.
5. Fluoroscopy with iodinated contrast injection of 3 mL of through the accessory port is indicated to analyze catheter continuity, connectedness, and IT position (again, 2–3 mL of CSF should be aspirated to avoid IT baclofen bolus). Disconnection of the catheter from the pump, leaks or perforations, as well as catheter tip dislodgments or migration can sometimes be visualized after contrast injection. Contrast-enhanced CT imaging of the entire pump and catheter system can reveal several potential abnormalities with more accuracy than plain films or fluoroscope.

With resolution or replacement of malfunctioning components of the IT system, almost all patients can be returned to their previous state of both symptom control and steady-state medication level.[21]

37.4.2 Morphine

Side effects of morphine therapy include urinary retention, constipation, pruritus, respiratory depression, nausea, hypotension, vomiting, and reduced libido. Treatment of IT morphine overdose includes standard life supporting measures, continuous intravenous naloxone infusion, lumbar catheter drainage of CSF, and control of hypertension and status epilepticus.[27]

Signs of withdrawal include severe pain, agitation, gastrointestinal distress, hyperthermia, palpitations, and in some cases pulmonary edema.[5,9,11] Opiates can be parenterally administered, with rapid reversal of the withdrawal process. Gradual weaning of IT morphine requires 3 to 6 weeks of gradual titration.

37.5 Conclusion

IT drug therapy for the treatment of chronic spasticity and pain is a safe and useful therapeutic intervention that has the potential to improve the quality of life significantly for complex patient populations. Under the guidance of an experienced, multidisciplinary team, appropriately selected patients can see a dramatic improvement in their functional status. Patients with implanted IT pumps frequently report improved symptoms and outcomes over those treated with long-term oral therapy and experience relatively few serious complications.[3,4,5,11] Management of this patient population requires intimate knowledge of the pump system and placement technique, careful coordination of follow-up care and pump maintenance, and swift diagnosis and treatment when drug withdrawal syndromes or other complications arise.

References

[1] McCormick ZL, Chu SK, Binler D, et al. Intrathecal versus oral baclofen: a matched cohort study of spasticity, pain, sleep, fatigue, and quality of life. PM R. 2016; 8(6):553–562

[2] Morota N, Ihara S, Ogiwara H. Neurosurgical management of childhood spasticity: functional posterior rhizotomy and intrathecal baclofen infusion therapy. Neurol Med Chir (Tokyo). 2015; 55(8):624–639

[3] Brogan SE, Winter NB. Patient-controlled intrathecal analgesia for the management of breakthrough cancer pain: a retrospective review and commentary. Pain Med. 2011; 12(12):1758–1768

[4] Smith TJ, Coyne PJ. Implantable drug delivery systems (IDDS) after failure of comprehensive medical management (CMM) can palliate symptoms in the most refractory cancer pain patients. J Palliat Med. 2005; 8(4):736–742

[5] Czernicki M, Sinovich G, Mihaylov I, et al. Intrathecal drug delivery for chronic pain management-scope, limitations and future. J Clin Monit Comput. 2015; 29(2):241–249

[6] Kosturakis A, Gebhardt R. SynchroMed II intrathecal pump memory errors due to repeated magnetic resonance imaging. Pain Physician. 2012; 15(6):475–477

[7] De Andres J, Villanueva V, Palmisani S, et al. The safety of magnetic resonance imaging in patients with programmable implanted intrathecal drug delivery systems: a 3-year prospective study. Anesth Analg. 2011; 112(5):1124–1129

[8] Diehn FE, Wood CP, Watson RE, Jr, Mauck WD, Burke MM, Hunt CH. Clinical safety of magnetic resonance imaging in patients with implanted SynchroMed EL infusion pumps. Neuroradiology. 2011; 53(2):117–122

[9] Gracies JM, Nance P, Elovic E, McGuire J, Simpson DM. Traditional pharmacological treatments for spasticity. Part II: general and regional treatments. Muscle Nerve Suppl. 1997; 6:S92–S120

[10] Brown J, Klapow J, Doleys D, Lowery D, Tutak U. Disease-specific and generic health outcomes: a model for the evaluation of long-term intrathecal opioid therapy in noncancer low back pain patients. Clin J Pain. 1999; 15(2):122–131

[11] Ver Donck A, Vranken JH, Puylaert M, Hayek S, Mekhail N, Van Zundert J. Intrathecal drug administration in chronic pain syndromes. Pain Pract. 2014; 14(5):461–476

[12] Kroin JS, Bianchi GD, Penn RD. Intrathecal baclofen down-regulates GABAB receptors in the rat substantia gelatinosa. J Neurosurg. 1993; 79(4):544–549

[13] Sjöström S, Tamsen A, Persson MP, Hartvig P. Pharmacokinetics of intrathecal morphine and meperidine in humans. Anesthesiology. 1987; 67(6):889–895

[14] Stetkarova I, Brabec K, Vasko P, Mencl L. Intrathecal baclofen in spinal spasticity: frequency and severity of withdrawal syndrome. Pain Physician. 2015; 18(4):E633–E641

[15] Borrini L, Bensmail D, Thiebaut JB, Hugeron C, Rech C, Jourdan C. Occurrence of adverse events in long-term intrathecal baclofen infusion: a 1-year follow-up study of 158 adults. Arch Phys Med Rehabil. 2014; 95(6):1032–1038

[16] Follett KA, Burchiel K, Deer T, et al. Prevention of intrathecal drug delivery catheter-related complications. Neuromodulation. 2003; 6(1):32–41

[17] Watve SV, Sivan M, Raza WA, Jamil FF. Management of acute overdose or withdrawal state in intrathecal baclofen therapy. Spinal Cord. 2012; 50(2):107–111

[18] Awaad Y, Rizk T, Siddiqui I, Roosen N, McIntosh K, Waines GM. Complications of intrathecal baclofen pump: prevention and cure. ISRN Neurol. 2012; 2012:575168

[19] Michael FM, Mohapatra AN, Venkitasamy L, Chandrasekar K, Seldon T, Venkatachalam S. Contusive spinal cord injury up regulates mu-opioid receptor (mor) gene expression in the brain and down regulates its expression in the spinal cord: possible implications in spinal cord injury research. Neurol Res. 2015; 37(9):788–796

[20] Malheiro L, Gomes A, Barbosa P, Santos L, Sarmento A. Infectious complications of intrathecal drug administration systems for spasticity and chronic pain: 145 patients from a tertiary care center. Neuromodulation. 2015; 18(5):421–427

[21] Riordan J, Murphy P. Intrathecal pump: an abrupt intermittent pump failure. neuromodulation. 2015; 18(5):433–435

[22] Wu H, Wang D. Radiation-induced alarm and failure of an implanted programmable intrathecal pump. Clin J Pain. 2007; 23(9):826–828

[23] Medtronic. Targeted Drug Delivery Systems. http://professional.medtronic.com/ppr/intrathecal-drug-delivery-systems/index.htm#tabs-3. Published 2014. Accessed January 20, 2016

[24] Müller-Schwefe G, Penn RD. Physostigmine in the treatment of intrathecal baclofen overdose. Report of three cases. J Neurosurg. 1989; 71(2):273–275

[25] Cardoso AL, Quintaneiro C, Seabra H, Teixeira C. Cardiac arrest due to baclofen withdrawal syndrome. BMJ Case Rep. 2014; 2014

[26] Dahlgren R, Francel P. Recognition and management of intrathecal baclofen withdrawal syndrome. In: Loftus CM, ed. Neurosurgical Emergencies. 2nd ed. New York, NY: Thieme; 2007:358–362

[27] Sauter K, Kaufman HH, Bloomfield SM, Cline S, Banks D. Treatment of high-dose intrathecal morphine overdose. Case report. J Neurosurg. 1994; 81(1):143–146

Index

Note: Page numbers set **bold** or *italic* indicate headings or figures, respectively.